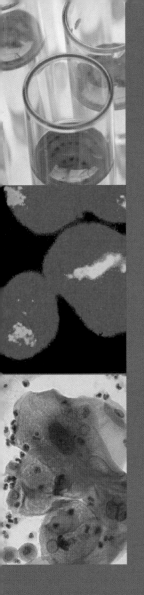

THE SCIENCE OF
LABORATORY
DIAGNOSIS

Second Edition

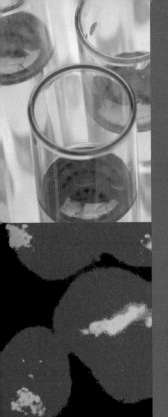

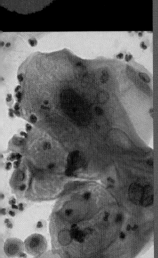

THE SCIENCE OF
LABORATORY
DIAGNOSIS

Second Edition

Edited by

David Burnett

Micropathology Ltd.
University of Warwick Science Park,
Sir William Lyon's Road,
Coventry CV4 7EZ, UK

John Crocker

Department of Cellular Pathology,
Birmingham Heartlands Hospital,
Bordesley Green East, Birmingham, UK

John Wiley & Sons, Ltd

Other Wiley Editorial Offices

John Wiley & Sons Inc., 111 River Street, Hoboken, NJ 07030, USA

Jossey-Bass, 989 Market Street, San Francisco, CA 94103-1741, USA

Wiley-VCH Verlag GmbH, Boschstr. 12, D-69469 Weinheim, Germany

John Wiley & Sons Australia Ltd, 33 Park Road, Milton, Queensland 4064, Australia

John Wiley & Sons (Asia) Pte Ltd, 2 Clementi Loop #02-01, Jin Xing Distripark, Singapore 129809

John Wiley & Sons Canada Ltd, 22 Worcester Road, Etobicoke, Ontario, Canada M9W 1L1

Wiley also publishes its books in a variety of electronic formats. Some content that appears in print may not
be available in electronic books.

British Library Cataloguing in Publication Data

A catalogue record for this book is available from the British Library

ISBN 0 470 85912 1

Typeset in 10/12 pt Times by Thomson Press, New Delhi, India
Printed and bound in Spain by Grafos SpA, Barcelona
This book is printed on acid-free paper responsibly manufactured from sustainable forestry
in which at least two trees are planted for each one used for paper production.

With love to our families

"Faith" is a fine invention
When Gentlemen can *see*–
But *Microscopes* are prudent
In an Emergency

Emily Dickinson

Contents

Preface to the first edition

It has been the experience of ourselves and our colleagues for some years that people at all levels come to work in our laboratories but have no experience of such environments. We have felt that there was a need for the text, across all disciplines of pathology, which would explain the 'whys and wherefores' of laboratory medicine. We emphasize that this text is not intended to be a 'recipe book'; its purpose is, however, very much to explain the basic principles of laboratory techniques and the interpretation of results obtained from them. We have tried to ensure that this book is of use to as diverse a range of readers as possible. This should include undergraduate and postgraduate students, trainee pathologists, surgeons and physicians, as well as laboratory scientific staff. The contents are multidisciplinary and there is overlap between some chapters and sections. This is deliberate as it reflects the true state of modern pathology. We feel that it is important that pathologists in each sub-specialty should be more aware of activity in their colleagues' laboratories. This book intends to represent standard methods and fairly recent advances within them. It is again stressed that compartmentalization of pathology and laboratory medicine is artificial although often convenient. However, it is our hope that workers in one speciality will be stimulated by reading other sections. For example, histopathologists working in the field of lymphoma need to understand large area of haematology and microbiology. The former, of course, impinges on the management of lymphoma patients, as does microbiology when opportunist infections occur after chemotherapy. Furthermore, clinical chemists need to relate their findings in relation to haematology and so on.

Another feature of this book is that there is, in some areas, overlap between chapters and sections; this is wholly intentional and again reflects the present state of laboratory medicine. Also, the applications, contexts and interpretation of shared methods will inevitably differ depending upon the discipline. The reader will notice that particularly in sections covering subjects such as electron microscopy and molecular techniques where methodologies are shared extensively between different disciplines. Indeed, failure to engage in cross-field communication will have an evitable deleterious effect on advances in routine and research methodologies. To our knowledge this book is unique and we hope it will give insight to many people training and trained in laboratory medicine concerning not only their own field but also those of others. Most chapters include a list of principal articles although in some cases this has been deemed unnecessary; furthermore, the occasional chapter has an extended reading list which may reflect its complexity or wide-ranging content. We should, of course, like to express our gratitude to all of our section editors and chapter authors. Naturally, we are indebted to our Publisher, John Harrison and his staff. Our thanks are also extended to Mrs Ruth Fry, Mrs Vivien Garland and Mrs Valerie Griffiths for secretarial help and answering endless telephone calls.

John Crocker
David Burnett

John Crocker (1952–2004)

John Crocker demonstrated, from an early stage in his relatively short life, a keen intellect and a deep interest in science and much besides. He was awarded an exhibition to King's College, Cambridge at the age of only sixteen. There he read Medicine. His first publication, the first of over 250, was in his third year at Cambridge, the result of his undergraduate pathology project. It was at Cambridge that John met his life-long partner and wife, Kate. After qualifying, John decided to train as a pathologist. His first post was at the East Birmingham Hospital (now the Birmingham Heartlands Hospital), to which he returned as a consultant after seven years in the Department of Pathology at the University of Birmingham, during which he obtained his M.D. It was here that he developed his research interest into lymphomas.

John enjoyed working at the Department of Histopathology at the Heartlands Hospital, particularly because of the rapport with his supportive colleagues. Despite contributing hugely to the usual diagnostic, teaching and administrative duties of the department, John managed to maintain a very active research career, collaborating with other pathologists and scientist, particularly those at the Universities of Warwick, Birmingham and Wolverhampton; the latter two awarding him personal chairs. With Jane Starczynski and colleagues he developed diagnostic techniques unique in the Region. His contributions to pathology were recognised by the unusual honour of admission, in 1995, as an honorary member of The Royal College of Physicians. With genuine interests including astronomy, music, modern literature, marine biology, computers, art, photography, chemistry and geology, it is clear that John was something of a polymath. His eclectic nature was brought to bear on his work and his belief that pathologists of all disciplines have much to learn from each other and indeed, from other scientific disciplines, was the philosophy behind the book you hold in your hands. Regrettably, John died before this second edition went to press. All his family, friends and colleagues will remember him not only as an extremely bright and enthusiastic scientist, but also a jovial, kindly man with a deep sense of compassion. I should like to dedicate this second edition to his memory.

David Burnett. March 2005

Preface to the second edition

It has been 6 years since the first edition of this book and we now have a new publisher, John Wiley & Sons, who agreed that it was timely to update this volume.

Authors are always keen to have the opportunity to improve what they have written and this is reflected here. It has also been an opportunity to bring certain areas up-to-date because of rapid developments in those fields, although, inevitably, there are some chapters that have changed little. Some chapters now have different or additional authors. The reasons for this are several. In some cases, authors have recruited new collaborators and some authors have retired since publication of the first edition. Tragically, one original author, Graeme Bird, has died. Nevertheless, the essence of the book remains the same, although the style has inevitably changed to suit the current publishers, whom we would like to thank for all their support, especially Dr Joan Marsh. We would also like to thank Ruth Fry for her secretarial assistance.

John Crocker
David Burnett

Contributors list

Derek C Allen *Histopathology Laboratory, Belfast City Hospital, Belfast BT9 7AD, UK*

Hazel Appleton *Health Protection Agency, Specialist and Reference Microbiology Division, 61 Colindale Avenue, London NW9 5HT, UK*

Dugald R Baird *Formerly Department of Microbiology, Lanarkshire Acute Hospitals NHS Trust, Hairmyres Hospital, Eaglesham Road, East Kilbride G75 8RG, UK*

Diana M Barnes *Hedley Atkins/Cancer Research UK Breast Pathology Laboratory, Guy's Hospital, St. Thomas Street, London SE1 9RT, UK*

Supratik Basu *Pathology Laboratory, Warwick Hospital, Lakin Road, Warwick CV34 5BJ, UK*

Paul C Boreland *Microbiology Department, Ulster Hospital, Dundonald, Beifast BT16 1RH*

Brian Boullier *Illuminate Communications, The Beacons, Leeds Road, Lightcliffe, Halifax HX3 8NU, UK*

Eric Y Bridson *Formerly Oxoid Ltd, 3 Bellever Hill, Camberley, Surrey BU15 2HB, UK*

David Burnett *Micropathology Ltd. University of Warwick Science Park, Sir William Lyon's Road, Coventry CV4 7EZ, UK*

Joan Butler *Honorary Lecturer, Guy's, King's and St. Thomas's School of Medicine, London*

Catherine Caveen *Department of Haematology, Warwick Hospital, Lakin Road, Warwick CV34 5BJ, UK*

G S Challand *Department of Clinical Biochemistry, Royal Berkshire Hospital, Reading, Berkshire RG1 5AN, UK*

Susan M Chambers *Department of Clinical Biochemistry, Kings College Hospital, Denmark Hill, London SE5 9RS, UK*

Ian Chant *Department of Haematology, Warwick Hospital, Lakin Road, Warwick CV34 5BJ, UK*

John Crocker *Department of Cellular Pathology, Birmingham Heartlands Hospital, Bordesley Green East, Birmingham B9 5SS, UK*

Roger P Eglin *National Transfusion Microbiology Laboratories National Blood Service, Colindale Ave Colindale, London NW95BG*

Mohammad S Enayat *Molecular Haemostasis Laboratory, Birmingham Children's Hospital NHS Trust, Ladywood, Birmingham B16 8ET, UK*

Brian Eyden *Department of Histopathology, Christie Hospital NHS Trust, Manchester M20 4BX, UK*

Stephen Finn *Department of Histopathology, Trinity College Dublin, Dublin, Ireland*

Richard Flavin *Department of Histopathology, Trinity College, Dublin, Dublin, Ireland*

Cheryl E Gillett *Hedley Atkins/Cancer Research UK Breast Pathology Laboratory, Guy's Hospital, St. Thomas Street, London SE1 9RT, UK*

Robert WA Girdwood *formerly Scottish Parasite Diagnostic Laboratory, Stobhill Hospital, Balornack Road, Glasgow, G21 3UW*

Ian M Gould *Department of Medical Microbiology, Medical School, Foresterhill, Aberdeen AB9 2ZB, UK*

Trevor Gray *Histopathology Department, Queen's Medical Centre, University Hospital NHS Trust, Nottingham NG7 2UH, UK*

Peter W Hamilton *Department of Pathology, The Queens University of Belfast, Grosvenor Road, Belfast BT12 6BL, UK*

Neil Hand *Histopathology Department, Queen's Medical Centre, University Hospital NHS Trust, Nottingham NG7 2UH, UK*

Mark Hathaway *National Blood Service, Vincent Drive, Selly Oak, Birmingham B15 2SG, UK*

Andrew J Hay *Department of Microbiology, Raigmore Hospital, Old Perth Road, Inverness IV2 6DJ, UK*

Ivor Hickey *School of Biology and Biochemistry, Medical Biology Centre, Queen's University Belfast, 97 Lisburn Road, Belfast BT9 7BL, UK*

Alan D Hirst *Department of Biochemistry, Bradford Royal Infirmary, Duckworth Lane, Bradford BD9 6RJ, UK*

Richard E Holliman *Department of Medical Microbiology, St. George's Hospital and Medical School, Blackshaw Road, London SW17 0QT, UK*

Darrel Ho-Yen *Department of Microbiology, Raigmore Hospital, Old Perth Road, Inverness IV2 6DJ, UK*

A P Huissoon *Regional Immunology Department, Birmingham Heartlands Hospital, Bordesley Green East, Birmingham B9 5SS, UK*

Mervyn Humphries *Northern Ireland Regional Genetics Centre, Leukaemia Cytogenetics Laboratory, Floor A, Belfast City Hospital, Tower Block, Lisburn Road, Belfast BT9 7AB, UK*

William L Irving *Department of Virology, University of Nottingham, Nottingham, UK*

Nick Jackson *Department of Haemotology, University Hospitals Coventry and Warwickshire NHS Trust, Clifford Bridge Road, Coventry, UK*

Julie D Johnson *Department of Medical Microbiology, St. George's Hospital and Medical School, Blackshaw Road, London SW17 0QT, UK*

Alex W L Joss *Microbiology Department, Raigmore Hospital NHS Trust, Perth Road, Inverness IV2 3UJ, UK*

Paul E Klapper *Department of Virology, Health Protection Agency, Leeds Laboratory, Bridle Path, York Road, Leeds LS15 7TR, UK*

Goura Kudesia *Department of Virology, Northern General Hospital NHS Trust, Herries Road, Sheffield S5 7BQ, UK*

William J Marshall *Consultant Clinical Biochemist, The London clinic, 20 Devonshire Place, London W79 6BW*

Cara M Martin *Department of Histopathology, Trinity College Dublin, Dublin, Ireland*

Graham Martin *Haemotology Department, GloucesterHospitals NHS Trust, Great Western Road, Gloucester GL1 3NN*

Siraj A Misbah *Department of Immunology, Churchill Hospital, Old Road, Headington, Oxford OX3 7LJ, UK*

Jonathan North *Department of Immunology, City Hospital, Dudley Road, Birmingham B18 7QH, UK*

Marie M Ogilvie *Division of Medical Microbiology, College of Medicine and Veterinary Medicine, University of Edinburgh, Edinburgh, UK*

John O'Leary *Department of Pathology, The Coombe Women's Hospital, Dublin, Ireland; and Department of Histopathology, Trinity College Dublin, Dublin, Ireland*

Esther O'Regan *Department of Histopathology, Trinity College Dublin, Dublin, Ireland*

Jacqueline C Osipiw *Department of Clinical Biochemistry, Royal Berkshire Hospital, Reading, Berkshire RG1 5AN, UK*

Alan Pawley *Virology Laboratory, Queen's Medical Centre Trust, Nottingham, UK*

Steven J Picton *Affymetrix UK Ltd, Wooburn Green, High Wycombe HP10 0HH, UK*

Paul Revell *Department of Haematology, Staffordshire General Hospital, Weston Road, Stafford ST16 3SA, UK*

Bernard F Rocks *Department of Clinical Pathology, Royal Sussex County Hospital, Brighton, Sussex BN2 5BE, UK*

Peter E Rose *Department of Haematology, Pathology Laboratory, Warwick Hospital, Lakin Road, Warwick CV34 5BJ, UK*

Jessica Schroeder *Department of Clinical Biochemistry, Royal Berkshire Hospital, Reading, RG1 5AN*

Anne Sermon *Department of Haematology, Nottingham City Hospital, Hucknall Road, Nottingham NG5 1PB, UK*

Orla Sheils *Department of Histopathology, Trinity College Dublin, Dublin, Ireland*

Jon Sherlock *Applied Biosystems, Applera, UK*

Roy A Sherwood *Department of Clinical Biochemistry, King's College School of Medicine and Dentistry, Bessemer Road, London SE5 9PJ, UK*

Barrie Sims *Department of Histopathology, Staffordshire General Hospital, Weston Road, Stafford ST16 3SA, UK*

Paul J Smith *Department of Cellular Pathology, Birmingham Heartlands Hospital, Bordesley Green East, Birmingham B9 5SS, UK*

Paul Smyth *Department of Histopathology, Trinity College Dublin, Dublin, Ireland*

Jane Starczynski *Department of Cellular Pathology, Birmingham Heartlands Hospital, Bordesley Green East, Birmingham B9 5SS, UK*

Andrew Taylor *Trace Element Laboratory, School of Biological Sciences, University of Surrey, Guildford, Surrey GU2 5XH, and Clinical Laboratory, Royal Surrey County Hospital, Guildford, Surrey GU2 5XX, UK*

Steven Walton *Department of Haematology, Warwick Hospital, Lakin Road, Warwick CV34 5BJ, UK*

Adrian T Warfield *Department of Histopathology, Birmingham Heartlands Hospital, Bordesley Green East, Birmingham B9 5SS, UK*

Janine L Warfield *Birmingham Heartlands Hospital, Bordesley Green East, Birmingham B9 5SS, UK*

David W Warnock *Division of Bacterial and Mycotic Diseases, National Center for Infectious Diseases, Centers for Disease Control and Prevention, Atlanta, GA 30333, USA*

Frank Wells *Biochemistry Department, Warwick Hospital, Lakin Road, Warwick, CV34 5BJ*

Keith Whaley *Department of Immunology, Leicester Royal Infirmary, Leicester LE1 5WW, UK*

SECTION 1

HISTOPATHOLOGY

1

Specimen handling and preparation for routine diagnostic histopathology

PJ Smith and JL Warfield

Introduction

Diagnostic histopathology is a specialty that, even nowadays, has remained a particularly labour-intensive faculty benefiting over the years from only a modest development in time-saving, automated technology. Tissue-processing and section-staining machines, an integral part of any routine histology laboratory, have become increasingly more sophisticated in terms of their application and their contribution to the Health and Safety-conscious environment in which we work. The manual inscription of tissue processing cassettes and microscope slides is fast becoming antiquated since the introduction of stand-alone and computer-linked transcription systems. Automatic coverslipping is also commonplace in many laboratories, minimizing personal exposure to organic solvents and allowing staff, otherwise involved in section mounting, to concentrate their efforts in the remaining manual areas of the department.

The modern routine histopathology laboratory, although having benefited from a degree of automation and continually evolving enhancements to its standard equipment, remains an area that is sensitive to increases in workload activity. Spare capacity relates directly to processing capability and the number of staff available to perform the associated tasks required to produce stained histopathological sections for subsequent microscopical examination and diagnosis by a pathologist. Many modern laboratories have experienced significant increases in workload activity over the past few years, as a result of waiting list initiatives and mergers, without a directly proportional rise in staffing levels. It is inevitable that these laboratories, like our own, have had to streamline their methodologies and repertoires in order to exist in today's high-throughput working environment and still continue to provide an efficient and effective quality service.

It is the intention of this chapter to provide a simple insight into tissue preparation in the modern histopathology laboratory, with the emphasis on efficiency, effectiveness and quality of service. It is not our intention to explain in any particular depth of philosophy, chemistry or minor details of the processes involved in tissue preparation, but to give an overall picture of these processes. This should enable the reader to put the techniques into perspective and act as an aid to the standardization of routine histopathology in the diagnostic laboratory.

The preparation of tissue samples for diagnosis will be described under the following headings:

1. Specimen management systems.

2. Specimen receipt and handling.

3. Fixation and decalcification.

4. Tissue processing and embedding.

5. Microtomy.

6. Special techniques.

The Science of Laboratory Diagnosis, Second Edition   Edited by David Burnett and John Crocker

Specimen management systems

Most modern histopathology laboratories have their own departmental information technology system for the storage and retrieval of patient demographic and specimen data. The manual or computerized patient registration system should be situated within the booking-in area of the laboratory. This accommodation should be separate from the 'cut-up' room and, ideally, housed in an office environment, either self-contained or integrated into the clerical area of the laboratory.

Computer-based information systems

One of the fundamental functions of a computer-based specimen management system is to facilitate the allocation of unique hospital and laboratory patient/specimen-specific identifiers—the patient hospital registration number and the laboratory number. The hospital registration number should be present on the histology request form and the accompanying specimen. The laboratory number is usually allocated automatically by the software, but may be manually entered. The laboratory number remains with the specimen throughout the histological process and is transferred to the request form, specimen pot(s), tissue cassette(s), microscope slide(s) and the final diagnostic report belonging to the patient.

The pathologists, laboratory manager, secretaries and laboratory areas require terminals to facilitate the input and coding of diagnostic reports, patient/specimen enquiries, work list generation, input of additional technical procedures, specimen/request tracking (audit trail), tissue/condition specific list generation and the collection of data for workload activity, weighted activity and costing.

Manual data entry

Manual data entry, using a surgical day book, and the manual labelling of tissue cassettes and microscope slides has more drawbacks than a computerized laboratory system. Manual systems rely on neat, clear handwriting and the accurate allocation of progressive laboratory numbers by an individual. Transcription errors may occur during the transfer of the laboratory number to tissue cassettes and microscope slides if the handwriting in the day book, or on the request form, is of a poor standard. Poor or illegible marking of tissue cassettes may result in the mismatching of tissue blocks with request forms and slides, resulting, as a worst case scenario, in a patient being misdiagnosed if similar tissues are involved or in the wasting of precious laboratory time while the situation is resolved. It is essential in all laboratories, regardless of whether a manual or computerized system is the order of the day, that stringent control measures are in place to ensure the integrity of the final diagnostic report.

Manual systems require provision of a cross-reference file for report retrieval, a diagnostic index and ample storage facilities for the filing of reports and request forms.

The quality of information processed by the service department is only as good as the quality of information on the request form and/or the information provided by the hospital patient administration or order communications systems in the case of computer networking.

On completion of manual or computerized data entry, the request forms are matched with their respective specimen pot(s) and the pots themselves marked indelibly with the laboratory number. Some laboratories may allocate the laboratory number, prior to booking in, using pre-printed rolls of self-adhesive sequential numbers.

Automatic cassette markers and slide writers

Cassette markers and slide writers are commercially available and can be utilized by all laboratories. Manual data entry laboratories would rely on manual input into these machines, as would those laboratories with less common generic computer systems. Laboratories with more sophisticated systems can interface specifically with these machines, so that cassette marking and slide writing become totally automatic procedures linked to, for example, data entry and work list generation, respectively. The advent of these machines has enabled clear, concise labelling of cassettes and slides and has reduced transcription error to a minimum (Figure 1.1).

Specimen receipt and handling

The trimming or cut-up room

A purpose-designed room, the 'cut-up' or 'trimming' room, should be available for the receipt and handling of all tissue specimens requiring histopathological diagnosis. This room should be totally separate from other laboratory accommodation, well illuminated, well ventilated and provide areas for specimen unbagging and matching and specimen dissection. The storage of formalin-fixed ('wet') tissues, following dissection, may

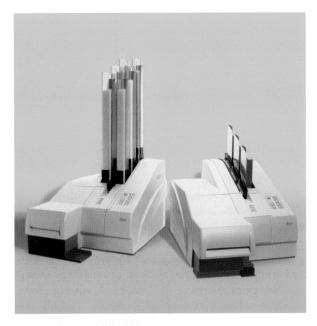

Figure 1.1 Leica IP C and IP S cassette and slide writers

(tweezers) for the handling of biopsies and tissue slices. Personal protective equipment (PPE) should include gowns or theatre pyjamas, aprons, surgical and cut-resistant gloves, goggles, visors, surgical masks and respirators (used in conjunction with specimen discard).

The 'cut-up' room may, where space is available, house the tissue-processing machines. Processors can be of the totally enclosed variety, and Health and Safety approved, or of the 'open' variety, which should be enclosed in a ventilated cabinet in order to contain solvent fumes.

Fixation and decalcification

When tissues are removed from the body they undergo a series of degenerative changes known as *autolysis* and *putrefaction*. Autolysis is the breakdown of cells and tissue components by the body's own enzymes and putrefaction is the degenerative change brought about in tissue as a consequence of bacterial action.

also be a function of the 'cut-up' room. Custom-built, ventilated specimen stores are commercially available and can be incorporated into larger 'cut-up' rooms or be conveniently housed in a separate, enclosed area used specifically for specimen storage.

The containment of formaldehyde is of prime concern in this area and is legislated for under the Health and Safety Act, 1974, in conjunction with the Containment of Substances Hazardous to Health (COSHH) Regulations. Formaldehyde is the most commonly used of all fixatives in the modern histology laboratory and will be discussed later. Hitherto, the specimen 'cut-up' area should be provided with an extraction facility in the form of a dissection bench fitted with an extraction system that pulls fumes away from the user. The bench should include an integral sink, with hot and cold running water, for washing specimens and cleansing the area after disinfection with the appropriate chemical agent. The dissection area of the bench should slope towards the sink to facilitate the drainage of formalin away from the fixed specimens and should include a polypropylene, or cut-resistant, dissection board for the examination and trimming of the fixed biopsies and whole organs.

A standard cut-up kit should include a stainless steel ruler, scalpel and PM40 handle and blades, steel-handled knives, a brain knife, scissors, bowel scissors, probes, a magnifying illuminator, bowel clamps, and forceps

The aims of fixation

Fixation should arrest autolysis and putrefaction and preserve the cells and tissue components in as 'lifelike' a state as possible. The fixative should not cause excessive shrinkage, swelling or hardening of the tissue and should stabilize the tissue against the rigours of processing. Finally, the fixative should complement and enhance subsequent histological staining, immunohistochemical and molecular biology procedures. This is broadly the remit of an 'ideal' fixative. However, in reality fixation is a compromise of these various requirements.

Types of fixative

Simple fixatives are single-chemical solutions, e.g. methanol, ethanol, glacial acetic acid and formaldehyde, which have no additives and which, used on their own, may produce some of the artefacts mentioned previously. *Compound fixatives* are mixtures of simple fixatives which have been formulated to offset and minimize fixation artefacts, e.g. Carnoy's fluid (ethanol–chloroform–acetic acid), which is recommended for the fixation of nucleic acids.

Simple and compound fixatives react with proteins in two ways. *Coagulants*, as suggested by their name, coagulate tissue protein, e.g. ethanol. *Non-coagulant fixatives*, e.g. formaldehyde, form cross-links with tissue protein.

Duration of fixation

Adequate fixation is essential for all subsequent histological techniques. A delay in a tissue being placed in a fixative, or inadequate infiltration of the fixative prior to processing, may affect the morphological interpretation, histochemical or immunohistochemical analysis. The length of fixation depends on the density of the tissue and the speed of penetration of the fixative. Softer, less dense tissues are penetrated more quickly than dense fibrous tissues and bone. The penetration rate of fixatives varies from one to another, e.g. glutaraldehde and Carnoy's fluid are more rapid in their action than formaldehyde. To facilitate thorough fixation, it is commonplace in histology laboratories to describe and then slice large dense specimens. Alternatively, the fixative can be injected into a whole organ and heated using a microwave oven or incubator.

Formaldehyde as the routine fixative of choice

The most widely utilized fixative in routine histopathology departments is 10% formalin (4% formaldehyde) and its derivatives. Formaldehyde is soluble in water to a maximum of 40% by weight (100% formalin) and is commercially available as a 40% solution to which 10–14% methanol has been added as a stabilizer. 10 parts of 100% formalin is normally diluted with 90 parts water, physiological saline or phosphate buffer to obtain the 10% working solution. Non-buffered formalin becomes acidic on standing, due to the formation of formic acid. Formic acid reacts with blood, in blood-rich tissues such as spleen, to produce a black pigment called acid formalin haematin. This usually occurs after prolonged fixation and the use of buffered formalin solutions will alleviate this fixation artefact.

Formalin has a pungent odour, is a strong eye, skin and mucous membrane irritant and, in some workers, may cause contact dermatitis. Personnel involved with formalin usage should undergo annual respiratory sensitizer screening. Maximum recommended exposure limits are one part per million and exposure levels should be monitored on a regular basis. Formalin solutions should be carefully handled in well-ventilated rooms/fume hoods and protective clothing such as gloves, laboratory coats, goggles and respirators should be worn.

Formalin reacts to form cross-links between proteins. Soluble proteins are fixed to structural proteins, giving strength to the tissue and enabling subsequent processing. Formalin does not fix carbohydrates but it does fix glycogen when it is held to a fixed protein. It is a good fixative for complex lipids.

Heat and agitation speeds up the process of fixation. The recommended time for fixation of tissues in formalin is 24–48 hours, the optimum time being 7–10 days. Modern enclosed tissue processing machines allow for the heating of reagents (40–45°C) during processing and, thus, the process of fixation can be expedited. Tissues received in the laboratory should be completely submerged in 5–10 times their volume of fixative.

No fixative is ideal but 10% formalin has the advantages of preserving a wide range of tissues. Formalin is tolerant and adequate histochemistry can be subsequently performed. Tissue may be stored for long periods without harmful effects on the nucleus, cytoplasm or overall morphology of the tissue. It is not the fixative of choice for immunohistochemistry or molecular biology, but many of the problems may be overcome with appropriate pre-treatments of the tissue.

Other commonly used fixatives

- *Gluteraldehyde* is often the fixative of choice for tissue requiring electron microscopy, as it gives good preservation of the ultrastructure of the cell. It is a respiratory sensitizer and is strongly linked to industrial asthma. Appropriate safety measures should be observed when handling glutaraldehyde. Its use as a disinfectant has, in the main, been outlawed in hospitals.

- *Osmium tetroxide* is used as a secondary fixative in electron microscopy, usually after primary fixation in glutaraldehyde. It fixes lipids and also preserves the fine structure of the cell. Osmium tetroxide is toxic and appropriate safety precautions should be taken when handling it.

- *Potassium dichromate* may be used to identify adrenal medullary tumours, both macroscopically and microscopically. It reacts with adrenal medullary catecholamines, producing a black or brown precipitate which is water-insoluble. It is not suitable as a general fixative as it penetrates tissue slowly and causes shrinkage.

- *Alcohol* penetrates tissue rapidly and may be used in conjunction with other fixatives to increase the speed of fixation. *Absolute ethanol* preserves glycogen but it causes distortion of nuclear detail and shrinkage of cytoplasm. Carnoy's fixative is a good fixative for nucleic acids but causes shrinkage of the tissue and lysis of red blood cells. It consists of absolute ethanol, chloroform and glacial acetic acid.

- *Various additives* in fixatives may be used. For example, tannic acid, phenol or heavy metal solutions may be added to formalin to increase the rate of penetration, improve preservation or enhance subsequent staining procedures.

- *Vapour fixation* using volatile fixatives enables retention of soluble substances *in situ*, by converting them into insoluble products before they come into contact with solvents. This method is often used in conjunction with freeze drying. Suitable fixatives for this technique include formaldehyde, osmium tetroxide and alcohol.

- *Microwave ovens* can be used in fixation, either to preserve the tissue with the action of the heat itself or to speed up the process of fixation, as described earlier.

Decalcification

Bone or tissues containing calcified material require decalcification prior to processing to enable standard microtomy (in tissues where quantification of calcium is required, undecalcified bone sectioning may be carried out). Various decalcifying fluids can be used, including acids, e.g. nitric acid, chelating agents, e.g. ethylene diamino-tetraacetic acid (EDTA), a combination of both, or commercially produced solutions. Heat applied to decalcifying solutions, using a microwave oven or incubator, may be used to speed up the decalcification process. Prolonged time in a decalcifying fluid, especially acidic solutions, may damage the morphology of the tissue and adversely affect the quality of subsequent techniques. The end-point of decalcification can be found by either chemical testing of the solution, X-ray of the tissue or, more commonly, manual assessment.

Tissue processing and embedding

Fixed, stabilized, tissue will subsequently undergo microtomy involving the preparation of 1–6 μm thick tissue sections for examination microscopically. To facilitate this process, the tissue must be supported internally and externally. Although freezing protocols

are available for both fixed and unfixed tissue samples, these methods are normally utilized for the demonstration of fixation-labile components or for rapid diagnostic techniques. For general histopathological diagnosis, tissues are commonly subjected to a series of reagents, culminating in their infiltration, and subsequent envelopment by a rigid support medium. The most widely used fixatives are variations of 10% aqueous formalin and, as such, it is the aim of tissue processing to substitute the aqueous fixative within the specimen by non-water-miscible paraffin wax. To achieve this, the specimen is subjected to the following stages:

1. Dehydration—alcohol replaces the aqueous fixative within the tissue.

2. Clearing—an ante-medium, such as xylene, replaces the alcohol.

3. Infiltration—paraffin wax replaces the clearing agent and infiltrates the tissue.

4. Embedding—infiltrated tissue is encapsulated by paraffin wax to provide a rigid support for microtomy.

To ensure good tissue processing it is essential that tissue slices are no more than 2–3 mm thick for rapid/urgent processing schedules and 3–5 mm thick for routine overnight and weekend schedules. Poor processing will occur if tissue is crammed into the processing cassette, by prohibiting the reagents to circulate adequately. Tiny biopsies may be placed into commercially available biopsy bags or mesh biopsy cassettes which, in turn, are placed inside the processing cassette (Figure 1.2a, b).

Factors affecting tissue processing

Temperature

At low temperatures processing reagents are more viscous and hence their tissue diffusion rates are slower. An elevated processing temperature increases the kinetic energy of reagent molecules, decreases reagent viscosity and increases the rate of diffusion of reagent into the tissue. Gentle heating of the dehydration and clearing reagents, in the range 37–45°C, will substantially reduce processing times but may increase tissue shrinkage due to the effect of heat on collagen.

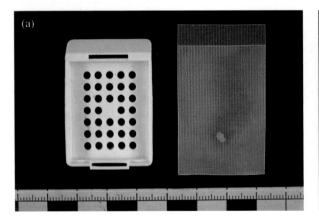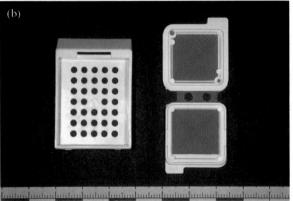

Figure 1.2   (a) Tissue processing cassette and biopsy bag. (b) Cell safe biopsy container

High temperatures at the infiltration stage may cause undue tissue shrinkage and hardening. This can be resolved by employing temperatures of 2–3°C above the melting point of the infiltration media to minimize these effects. However, blood and muscle may still become brittle during infiltration and the combined effect of the fixation regime, the dehydrating agent and tissue type must also be considered.

Vacuum and pressure

Modern enclosed tissue processing machines incorporate a switchable vacuum and pressure cycle. In practice, the application of pressure during dehydration and clearing has little effect on diffusion of reagents, although it may have an increased effect at the infiltration stage. However, the application of a vacuum enhances dehydration, clearing and infiltration.

Agitation

The maximum surface area of tissue should be available for fluid/reagent exchange and circulation during processing. This is not achieved in situations where tissue cassettes lie at the bottom of a container, are static in the reagent or are packed tightly into the processing basket. Maximum surface area for fluid exchange is impaired and circulation of reagent around the tissue is impeded, resulting in stagnation, i.e. the reagent surrounding the tissue remains at a lower concentration and a much longer time is required for satisfactory processing.

To achieve consistent processing results, the tissue cassettes should be loosely packed, suspended and agitated in the reagent to prevent stagnation and allow circulation of the medium. Agitation can be facilitated by magnetic stirrers and rotors for manual processing, whereas modern processing machines utilize either rotational, up-and-down, side-to-side and/or tidal flow motion.

Dehydration, clearing, infiltration and embedding

Dehydration

The majority of tissue fixatives are made up in aqueous solution and the function of the dehydrating agent is to remove free and bound water molecules from the tissue specimen. The most commonly employed dehydrating agent, for routine paraffin processing, is 99.85% ethanol which, due to its expense, is purchased by laboratories in the form of the less expensive 99% industrial methylated spirit (IMS) containing 2% methanol. Certain lipids and water-soluble proteins are removed from the tissue during this stage.

Tissues are processed through a rising concentration gradient of ethanol to 99% IMS (absolute ethanol). The fixation regime employed and the tissue type will dictate the strength of the first IMS bath. Routine histological processing schedules employ 70% IMS as the first step in tissue dehydration. Delicate tissues may need to be processed slowly from 50% IMS, whereas tissues that have been fixed in an alcoholic reagent such as Carnoy's fixative may be immersed directly into several changes of 99% IMS.

Dehydration time is dependent on the size and type of tissue specimen. In general, tissue blocks of 1 mm thickness require 30 minutes in each graded alcohol and tissue blocks of 5 mm thickness require up to 90 minutes in each graded alcohol.

Clearing

The clearing agent is a reagent that is miscible with paraffin wax and acts as a link between the dehydrating agent (non-miscible) and the paraffin wax itself. The most commonly used clearing agents for routine tissue processing are hydrocarbons such as xylene, toluene, chloroform and petroleum solvents. These reagents are all controlled substances under the COSHH regulations, are flammable, cause skin degreasing and have varying degrees of toxicity. Toluene is a possible carcinogen, chloroform has a narcotic effect and xylene, although not proved to be a carcinogen, may cause headaches as a side-effect to inhalation of the vapour where adequate extraction facilities are not provided (usually in cover-slipping and manual staining areas).

For the reasons stated previously, xylene is probably the most widely used clearing agent. It is compatible with all the major enclosed tissue processors and is relatively cheap. Xylene should be purchased as the benzene- (carcinogenic) and sulphur-free reagent. Prolonged exposure to xylene may cause excessive tissue hardening and tissue processing schedules should be formulated to minimize this effect. Tissues of 1–2 mm thickness require two or three changes of xylene over 0.5–1 hours and specimen blocks of 3–5 mm thickness require three changes over a 2–4 hour period for normal processing. The heat and vacuum facilities on modern tissue processing machines will substantially reduce these times.

Infiltration

Paraffin wax is the infiltration and embedding medium of choice for routine histopathology. It is a mixture of polycrystalline straight-chain hydrocarbons, produced from the distillation and cracking of crude mineral oil. Paraffin wax is categorized by its melting point, which, in turn, reflects the admix of molecular weights of its constituent hydrocarbons. Melting points, although not wholly accurate, are in the range 39–68°C and, as a general rule, the higher the melting point the harder the wax. Softer tissues benefit from infiltration by lower melting point waxes and harder tissues from infiltration by those with a higher melting point. However, routine histopathological processing is partly a compromise, due to the variation in size and hardness of the tissue samples

to be processed and the preferred clearing agent. To this end, paraffin wax of melting point 56–58°C is normally employed. Infiltration times are illustrated below in Table 1.1. Infiltration times are greatly reduced by the application of a vacuum. This is essential for specimens of lung, where the vacuum forces out trapped air molecules from the tissue.

Additives have been included in some paraffin waxes to improve their crystalline consistency by reducing their hardness and brittleness and, hence, improve their cutting (microtomy) characteristics. These substances include, among others, thermoplastic resins, plastic polymers and dimethyl sulphoxide (DMSO), which aids infiltration and allows thin sectioning.

Embedding

Paraffin wax for tissue embedding should be clean, filtered and held at 2–4°C above its melting point. On completion of processing the tissue basket is transferred to a heated reservoir or free-standing bath of paraffin wax. Tissues are removed from their cassettes, one at a time only, with heated forceps and placed face down in a prefilled mould of molten paraffin wax. The mould is placed on a refrigerated surface or ice tray to facilitate the clamping of the tissue to its base. A variety of moulds are available and include: stainless steel moulds of graded capacities which receive the processing/embedding cassette, the latter acting as the tissue support platform; Leuckhart's L pieces; ice trays; metal boats; and peel-away plastic moulds. Moulds are left on the cold plate until the wax solidifies or, where a form of refrigeration is not available, can be immersed in cold water once a thick enough crust has formed on the surface of the wax. Commercial embedding centres, which combine a heated mould store, a molten wax reservoir/dispenser and a cold plate, are readily available (Figure 1.3). Once the wax has solidified, the tissue blocks may be gently removed from their moulds and prepared for microtomy.

It is a general rule, for appropriate orientation of tissue specimens, that the surface of the tissue facing downward in the cassette should be placed face down in the mould. Orientation is extremely important for effective diagnosis. A skin biopsy should be embedded at right angles to its surface to give the correct plane for sectioning. Cylindrical/tubular tissue, such as Fallopian tube or vas deferens, should be embedded on end in order that transverse sections may be cut through their walls and lumena. Dyes or special inks can be utilized to mark resection planes and allow for correct tissue orientation.

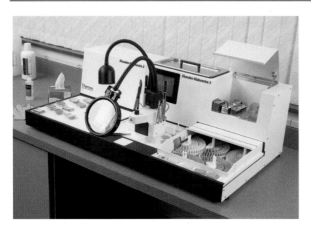

Figure 1.3   Shandon Histocentre 3 tissue embedding centre

Automatic tissue processors

Carousel-type 'open' tissue processors (Figure 1.4a) have mostly been replaced by 'enclosed' (Figure 1.4b), Health and Safety-compliant processing machines with larger cassette capacities. Open processors release reagent vapours into the atmosphere as the tissue basket moves between stations and, therefore, should be contained within a well-ventilated area/extraction facility. Agitation is effected by a rotational or dunking motion and vacuum is available on the final wax infiltration baths. Tissues are processed through the solvents at room temperature.

Enclosed processors are stand-alone/modular units which fully contain reagent fumes during tissue processing by means of water/vapour traps and charcoal adsorption filters. Reagents are pumped into and out of a processing chamber/retort. Agitation is provided in the form of tidal flow of reagents in and out of the retort or by a side-to-side rotational motion. Ingress of reagents can be enhanced by alternating, programmable vacuum and pressure cycles, of which vacuum is the most effective, and the dehydrating and clearing steps can be substantially reduced by the ability to heat the reagents (25–45°C). Microprocessor technology enables multiple processing schedules to be stored and retrieved and, on some machines, allows for simultaneous use of add-on units running a variety of schedules under the control of a command module.

'Routine overnight' and 'rapid' tissue processing schedules

Table 1.1 shows a comparison of 'routine overnight' and 'rapid' schedules for open and enclosed automatic

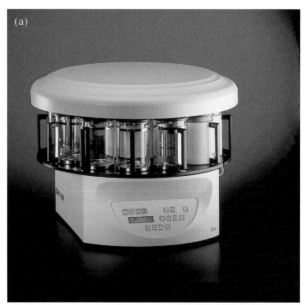

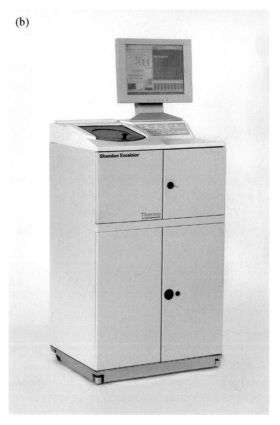

Figure 1.4   (a) Leica TP1020 tissue processor. (b) Shandon Excelsior enclosed tissue processor

tissue processing. The replenishment of processing reagents and infiltration media is dependent on the volume of reagent used per step and the quantities of tissue cassettes being processed. Appropriate safety

Table 1.1 'Routine overnight' and 'rapid' schedules for tissue processing

Reagent	Open tissue processor			Enclosed tissue processor		
	Routine overnight (minutes)	Rapid (minutes)	Vacuum	Routine overnight (minutes)	Rapid (minutes)	Vacuum
10% Formol saline	60	30	No	30*	15	Yes
70% Alcohol	60	0	No	30*	0	Yes
95% Alcohol	60	0	No	30*	15	Yes
100% Alcohol	60	15	No	30*	15	Yes
100% Alcohol	60	15	No	30*	15	Yes
100% Alcohol	60	30	No	60*	15	Yes
100% Alcohol	60	30	No	60*	15	Yes
Xylene	30	15	No	30*	10	Yes
Xylene	60	15	No	30*	15	Yes
Xylene	60	30	No	30*	15	Yes
Paraffin wax	60	30	No	30*	15	Yes
Paraffin wax	60	30	Yes	60*	30	Yes
Paraffin wax	90	30	Yes	60*	30	Yes

*Processing temperature of 45°C.

precautions should be taken and the use of personal protective equipment is essential when decanting these solutions.

Microwave processing

The utilization of microwave technology for the rapid processing of tissue has been with us for a number of years now. It is particularly useful in conjunction with one-stop clinics, where an expeditious diagnostic biopsy report is required before the patient is discharged. Urgent biopsies and same-day biopsy reporting turn-around times also benefit from this technology and, importantly, the quality of the final preparation is not compromised.

Microtomy

Microtomy is the production of thin sections, 1–5 microns (µm) in thickness, from paraffin wax-embedded tissue blocks. This process utilizes a microtome in conjunction with a microtome knife or disposable microtome blade and blade holder. Microtomes are of the 'rotary' or 'base sledge' variety and are commercially available from a large number of laboratory equipment suppliers. The microtome knife has largely been superseded, in routine histopathology departments, by the disposable microtome blade. Microtome knives need to be specially sharpened, either manually (a highly skilled

procedure) or by machine, which can be extremely time-consuming in an age where workload activity demands the streamlining of histopathology services.

Microtomes

The *rotary microtome* (Figure 1.5) is a general-purpose machine for the production of semi-thin tissue sections

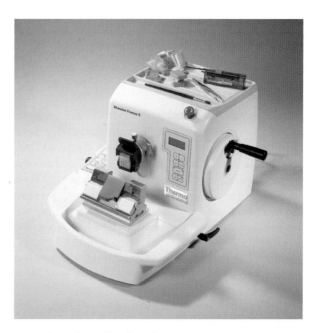

Figure 1.5 Shandon Finesse E rotary microtome

for light microscopy. The manual rotation of the laterally mounted wheel causes the advance mechanism to move the block holder towards the rigidly mounted knife at a pre-set thickness of cut (section thickness). The block moves up and down against the knife in a vertical plane with the production of flat sections on the downward stroke, usually 3–5 µm thick for routine histological purposes. The speed of the block against the knife is controlled by the rate at which the hand wheel is rotated. Heavy duty, motorized, rotary microtomes are also available for use in conjunction with the production of semi-thin (0.5–1 µm) resin-embedded sections for light microscopy, where the constant speed of the block against the knife can be controlled automatically. The section thickness range of these microtomes is usually 0.5–60 µm.

The *sledge microtome*, although best suited for the sectioning of hard tissues and some softer resins, is equally suitable for the sectioning and ribboning of soft tissues and biopsies. The heavy construction of these machines means that they do not succumb easily to vibration and the knife clamp can be angled away from the direction of cut, which aids in sectioning hard tissues. The block holder is mounted on two parallel runners and the block holder advanced by either a manual specimen advance on the handle itself or by a lever mounted on the side of the block carrier, which moves against a static stanchion. The block is passes forwards and backwards against the knife, using a push-and-pull motion. Sections are cut at 3–5 µm for routine histology.

Microtome knives

Conventional steel microtome knives have, in the main, been replaced by disposable blades for routine histopathology.

Steel knives are manufactured from a high-grade carbon or tool-quality steel that should be free from impurities and rust-resistant. Knives are tempered (hardened) from the tip inwards and the degree of hardness measured using the Vickers scale (usually 400–900 on the scale). The degree of hardness can vary between manufacturers and between individual knives from the same manufacturer. A hardness of 700 is desirable, 400 being soft and 900 being considered brittle, for routine use. Steel knives come in a variety of profiles, dependent on their intended use (Figure 1.6):

- *Profile A* is biconcave and was employed for sectioning celloidin embedded tissues. It is rarely used in routine histopathology.

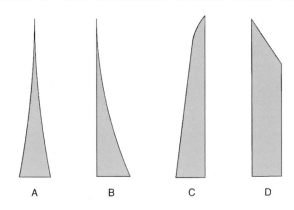

Figure 1.6 Microtome knife profiles

- *Profile B* is plano-concave and can be used to section wax-embedded soft tissues, celloidin-embedded tissues and botanical specimens. Profiles A and B produce the sharpest edges.

- *Profile C* is wedge-shaped and is the most commonly utilized steel knife for routine histopathology. It is a more rigid knife than profiles A and B and is used for paraffin wax sectioning of all tissues, as well as being employed in cryostats for sectioning frozen material (see below). This profile cannot be ground as sharp as profiles A and B.

- *Profile D* is tool-edge or plane-shaped and is used for sectioning hard materials, such as resins and extremely hard paraffin wax tissue blocks. This knife produces the least sharp edge when ground.

The sharpening and honing of the above knives, by the various manual and automated methods available, is suggested as further reading.

Disposable blades are modified, thickened razor blades produced from high-quality stainless steel and give reproducible, compression-free, good quality sections. The thin blade is held rigidly in its own special holder to minimize vibration during microtomy. The blades may be coated with platinum or chromium for a longer cutting life. These blades appear to be the first choice, nowadays, for routine histopathology.

Other knives include *tungsten carbide* for resin work and production of undecalcified bone sections; *glass*, *diamond* and *sapphire knives* for use with araldite- and epoxy resin-embedded material for electron microscopy or for small, narrow blocks of acrylic- or polyester resin-embedded tissues for light microscopy.

Paraffin wax sectioning

A freshly honed microtome knife or new disposable blade with a sharp, blemish-free edge is essential for quality sectioning. All operations concerning the placement or removal of the block into and out of the block holder should be carried out with the safety of the user in mind. Blades are extremely dangerous and should be treated with respect. The hand wheel of rotary microtomes should be clamped and the block carrier on sledge microtomes should be positioned, and clamped where available, at the end of the microtome furthest from the blade during these procedures.

Some laboratories employ a 'rough-cutting' microtome to trim down the tissue block until a representative cross-sectional area of the tissue is obtained. Sections are removed at 10–15 µm intervals, until the full face of the tissue is available, followed by several sections at 4–5 µm to ensure a smooth block surface (avoids rough cutting artefact). The block holder of the rough cutter is set in the same plane as the rest of the laboratory microtomes. Rough cutting and sectioning may be performed on the same microtome or even the same blade. Section cutting should be performed on a separate area of the blade or knife to that which was used for rough cutting purposes.

Blocks for diagnostic sectioning are pre-cooled on an ice tray or chiller plate prior to cutting. Chilling causes compression of the block and offers a more rigid block face to the knife for ease of sectioning. Section thickness is commonly set at 3–5 µm. As the knife edge passes through the block face, the tissue sections move up (sledge microtome) or down (rotary microtome) the knife face. As the block hits the knife edge, the friction produced causes a 'melting front' in the wax and, thus, subsequent sections adhere to each other, creating a ribbon. This ribbon of sections is supported, removed from the knife edge and floated on to a 48–50°C waterbath with cutting forceps. The sections are teased apart at their points of adhesion and attached to glass microscope slides by part submersion of the slide in the water. Excess water is drained from the slide, which is left to dry face up on a 60°C hotplate, not in direct contact, until all traces of water have disappeared. The slide is then placed in contact with the hotplate for 5–10 minutes to facilitate adhesion of the paraffin wax section to the glass. Sections are now ready for staining by haematoxylin and eosin (H&E) or a whole host of other tinctorial and immunocytochemical methods that the histologist has at his/her disposal. Section mounting, as mentioned earlier, may be automated.

Macroblock (large block) sectioning

Sub-specialization/team reporting in conjunction with minimum data set production is the suggested approach for histological diagnosis. The sampling, processing and sectioning of whole cross-sections of a tumour is now a widely adopted histological technique which proffers more accurate information on tumour orientation and distances from resection margins. The method has a wide application, but is particularly useful in breast, prostate and bowel pathology.

The processing of macroblocks requires megacassettes, large slides and separate archiving facilities. Processing times are increased and sections are cut on modified sledge or rotary microtomes. Staining is facilitated mainly by hand.

Special techniques

Frozen sectioning of fresh tissues

The majority of routine histopathology laboratories include amongst their repertoires a diagnostic frozen section service for suspected tumour patients. A diagnosis can be telephoned to the surgeon within 10–20 minutes of receipt of the tissue sample and, hence, aid the clinical management of the patient. The *cryostat* (Figure 1.7), a rotary or rocking microtome housed

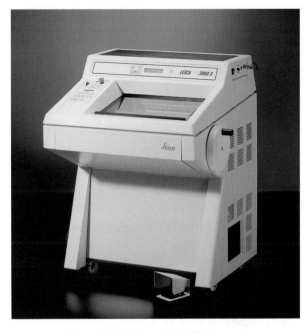

Figure 1.7   Leica CM3050S Cryostat

within a refrigerated chamber, is utilized for this procedure. The temperature of the specimen and specimen holder, knife and chamber can normally be set independently, or a single temperature may be pre-selected for the whole. Fresh tissue for rapid diagnosis is received from the operating theatre, frozen on to the specimen holder using carbon dioxide, liquid nitrogen or a commercial freezing spray, and transferred to the cryostat for sectioning. If conditions are optimal for the tissue being sectioned, then it is possible to cut sections as thin as 1 µm. Fresh tissues should be dissected and frozen in the confines of a microbiological safety cabinet. Most modern cryostats incorporate a 4 hour formalin decontamination cycle for the disinfection of the chamber after sectioning unsuspected infectious cases (some tuberculous lesions can closely mimic tumour macroscopically).

The *freezing microtome* (Figure 1.8) may be utilized for the semi-thin sectioning of fresh tissues, where there

surface of the tissue as the specimen holder is advanced by a preset thickness. The tissue is frozen *in situ* by means of an attached carbon dioxide cylinder or a circulating coolant. Consistent thin sections are difficult to obtain.

Undecalcified bone sectioning

This requires the production of 4–5 µm sections of undecalcified bone embedded in an acrylic or polyester resin. Although a base sledge microtome may be used for this purpose, it is more common to employ a *heavy-duty motorized microtome* (Figure 1.9). D profile (tool

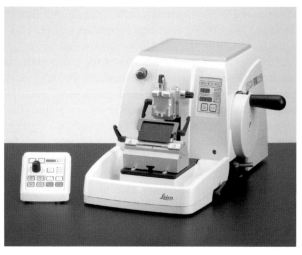

Figure 1.9 Leica RM2255 motorized heavy duty rotary microtome

edge), tungsten, glass or diamond knives are commonly used for the sectioning of this tissue.

Electron microscopy

Electron microscopy requires the production of ultra-thin resin-embedded sections using an *ultramicrotome*. Hard epoxy or araldite resins are usually employed and section thickness is measured in nanometres (nm). Sectioning is facilitated by the use of glass or diamond knives and section thickness monitored by observing the interference colour produced by the section in contact with water, i.e. gold (90–120 nm), silver (60–90 nm) and grey (<60 nm). Sections are picked up and stained on

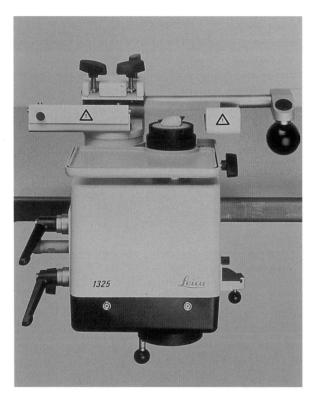

Figure 1.8 Leica 1325 freezing microtome

is a requirement to demonstrate substances that are normally removed during routine processing (e.g. lipids). This type of microtome has a static specimen holder, with the knife itself being manually drawn across the

special copper and/or rhodium grids. The stains employ heavy metal salts, such as lead citrate and uranyl acetate, which impregnate certain tissue structures. These heavy metals deflect an electron beam, produced by the electron microscope. This produces shades of black and grey areas within the tissue section, where ultra-structural elements have been impregnated by the heavy metals. The electron microscope incorporates a camera system that can photograph areas of interest within the section, the final result being the electron micrograph. This is an extremely simplistic overview of electron microscopy.

Further reading

Bancroft JD, Gamble M. *Theory and Practice of Histological Techniques*, 5th edn. 2002: Churchill Livingstone, Edinburgh.

Acknowledgements

Photographs by courtesy of Thermo Electron Anatomical Pathology, Leica UK Ltd, and Dr AT Warfield, Histopathology, University Hospital Birmingham, UK.

2

General stains

Barrie Sims

Why stain?

Thin tissue sections, when examined under the micro-scope, show very little differentiation between the composite structures. Staining the tissues with contrasting coloured dyes allows the structures to be visualized under the light microscope. Additionally, the demonstration of various cell products, cell inclusions or micro-organisms requires the use of specialized staining procedures.

The majority of diagnostic routine histopathology is performed on paraffin wax-embedded tissues. Exceptional to this is the use of frozen sections. These are necessary either for urgent diagnosis or to demonstrate substances that are lost, destroyed or inhibited by the process of fixation and embedding.

Following microtomy, the paraffin wax section is still infiltrated with wax. Wax present in the sections obscures the tissue structure and is largely impermeable to stains. The majority of staining methods are water- or alcohol-based, therefore the removal of the wax is necessary. Once sections have dried onto the slide, the sections are treated with xylene to remove the wax. Rinsing the sections in graded alcohols removes the xylene and allows the sections to hydrate in water. This process is often referred to in methodology by a variety of terms, e.g. 'de-wax sections'; 'sections to water'; 'hydrate sections'.

Basic staining mechanisms

In diagnostic histopathology, staining methods may be grouped into four main processes (vital staining, i.e.

where dye is applied to living tissues, is rarely used, if at all).

Elective solubility

This is the mechanism by which stains that are dissolved in a solvent are more soluble in the tissue component than they are in the solvent. This mechanism is primarily used in the demonstration of fat in frozen sections. The dyes used are usually of the Sudan type (Sudan III, Sudan IV).

Metallic impregnation

The deposition of metallic silver onto tissue elements may be used to demonstrate a wide variety of structures and substances.

Cells that have the ability to reduce an ammoniacal silver solution, without the need for an external reducing agent, are termed 'argentaffin'. Melanin and the Kultschitzky cells of the gastrointestinal tract are typical examples.

Cells or structures that require the use of an external reducing agent are termed 'argyrophil'. Metallic impregnation is used widely in the demonstration of reticular fibres, basement membranes, fungi, cellular inclusions and nerve cells and their processes.

Histochemical reactions

These are methods in which there is a clear understanding of the mechanisms involved in the reaction.

The Science of Laboratory Diagnosis, Second Edition   Edited by David Burnett and John Crocker
© 2005 John Wiley & Sons, Ltd

The final reaction may utilize a dye or may in itself produce a coloured reaction. For example, Schiff reagent, used in the demonstration of aldehydes, uses the dye basic fuchsin in the reaction, which colours the aldehyde sites magenta; whereas in Perls' reaction for ferric iron deposits (Figure 2.1), the interaction between potassium ferrocyanide (a constituent of Perls' solution) and the ferric iron in the tissues produces the pigment Prussian blue at the site of ferric iron.

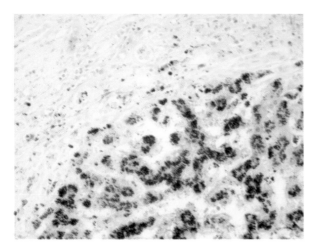

Figure 2.1 Perls' reaction for ferric iron. The deposits of ferric iron are stained blue

Many enzymes may be demonstrated by the incubation of sections (frozen or wax) in substrates containing a substance upon which the enzyme reacts, producing a primary reaction product (PRP). A second reagent then couples with the PRP to produce a coloured deposit at the site of activity. Control sections that are known to contain (positive) or not contain (negative) the substance are used to determine the specificity of the reaction. Substances known to inhibit the reaction may also be used to improve the specificity of the reaction.

Staining with dyes

The majority of staining procedures in routine diagnostic pathology will fall into this group. In many cases the understanding behind the mechanism of staining is not clearly defined and the results will often depend upon the skill and knowledge of the histotechnologist.

Classification

Dyes may be classified as natural or synthetic. Natural dyes include haematoxylin, whilst synthetic dyes will include the greater majority of dyes used in histotechnique (e.g. eosin, methylene blue and basic fuchsin). Dyes may also be classified as acidic, basic or neutral.

Acidic and basic dyes

Simplistically, acidic dyes (anionic) are attracted to tissue elements with basic properties such as the cytoplasm of cells. Basic dyes (cationic) will be attracted to structures of an acidic nature such as the DNA in the cell nucleus. By using a combination of acid and basic dyes of a contrasting colour, the nucleus and cytoplasm can be differentiated. This forms the basis of the stain haematoxylin and eosin (H&E), a method used in most diagnostic histopathology laboratories to demonstrate general structure.

Neutral dyes

Neutral dyes are produced by the combination of solutions of acid and basic dyes. The resulting product stains both acidic and basic structures from a single solution. Romanowsky stains used, for example, in demonstrating cells in bone marrow, are a combination of methylene blue and eosin.

Metachromasia

Dyes that combine with certain tissue elements producing a colour that is different from the original dye are termed 'metachromatic'. Metachromatic staining methods may be used for the demonstration of connective tissue mucins, mast cell granules, amyloid and cartilage. Generally metachromasia is lost during dehydration of sections prior to the application of a coverglass. Using an aqueous mounting medium will usually prevent this. There are a number of variations to metachromatic methods that retain the metachromasia during dehydration.

Fluorescence

The majority of staining methods are visualized using visible light. Dyes that have the ability to absorb ultraviolet light and then transmit that light into the visible spectrum are termed 'fluorescent'. Fluorescent dyes may be used to demonstrate *Mycobacterium tuberculosis* amyloid (and tissue antigens when applied to immunocytochemical techniques). Fluorescent microscopes are required to view the preparations and a darkened room is necessary for optimum clarity. Fluorescent staining is often short-lived and photography is used to provide a permanent record.

Direct dyes

Dyes that have the ability to combine with tissue structures from simple aqueous or alcoholic solutions are termed 'direct' dyes. Eosin and many other aniline dyes exhibit this property.

Indirect dyes

Dyes that have no direct affinity for the tissue structures and require the use of an intermediary substance to allow staining are termed 'indirect' dyes. The intermediary substance is referred to as a 'mordant' (similar to a catalyst). The dye combines with the mordant, which combines with the tissue element, producing a dye–mordant–tissue complex. Haematoxylin, without the use of a mordant, is a weak tissue stain. The addition to the haematoxylin solution of metals such as aluminium potassium sulphate or ferric chloride can create powerful, versatile stains.

Haematoxylin staining

Haematoxylin solutions need to be oxidized (sometimes referred to as 'ripened') before they are used to stain tissues. Oxidation can either be performed chemically by the addition of oxidizing agents such as sodium iodate, or naturally using sunlight (which can take several months). The process of oxidation converts haematoxylin into haematein. Preparations of haematoxylin usually are only partly oxidized, further oxidation continuing with time. The use of part oxidation increases the shelf-life of the solution.

   Depending upon the mordant used, haematoxylin can demonstrate a number of different structures.

Alum haematoxylins

These are produced by the addition of aluminium potassium sulphate or aluminium ammonium sulphate to the haematoxylin solution. Alum haematoxylins are used to stain cell nuclei blue. There are various formulations available such as Harris's, Ehrlich's, Mayer's,

Delafield's, Cole's and Gill's. Alum haematoxylins need to be 'blued' (see later) for the nuclei to stain blue.

Iron haematoxylins

Produced by the addition of ferric chloride or ferric ammonium sulphate to the haematoxylin solution. The resultant solution produces a dense black stain, which may be used to demonstrate cell nuclei, elastin, muscle striations and myelin. The resultant stain is more resistant to acid extraction than alum haematoxylins and is used where acidic counterstains are used, such as the van Gieson method for connective tissues. The structure demonstrated would depend upon the reagent used to differentiate (removal of excess dye from the background of the section until only the structure required is demonstrated). Acid differentiators will remove sufficient dye to demonstrate cell nuclei. By re-applying the mordant solution to the section, there is a progressive removal of the haematoxylin from the section. This will allow myelin, elastin and muscle striations to be demonstrated. Alum haematoxylins can be converted to iron haematoxylins by treatment of the section with an iron solution prior to the haematoxylin. The celestine blue-haemalum sequence is such an example.

Lead haematoxylin

Haematoxylin solutions containing lead will demonstrate endocrine cells.

Phosphotungstic acid haematoxylin

This will demonstrate muscle striations, fibrin, nuclei, myelin, cilia, neuroglial cells and amoebae. Tungstophosphoric acid is used as the mordant and haematein or haematoxylin as the dye. The use of haematein removes the need for oxidation.

Commercial preparations

Many haematoxylin solutions are now commercially available. This avoids the need for time-consuming preparation in the laboratory and the handling of toxic substances. New formulae have removed the use of harmful or toxic substances (e.g. mercury) from the preparation, making the solutions more environmentally friendly.

Regressive and progressive staining

Regressive

A regressive stain will usually be applied to the section for a period of time that will initially stain all the tissue structures. Selectively removing the excess stain reveals the elements to be demonstrated. The removal of the excess stain is called 'differentiation'. The use of solvents (alcohol), dilute acid and acid/alcohol solutions or the mordanting solution may achieve this.

Progressive

A progressive stain will increasingly stain tissue elements, depending upon the time in the staining solution. Progressive stains do not overstain the tissues and the staining period is stopped after a given period of time. Mayer's haemalum is a progressive nuclear stain that is often used as a nuclear counterstain in other techniques, e.g. periodic acid–Schiff (PAS) method.

Common staining methods

Routine staining methods may be grouped into nine categories (see Table 2.1).

Table 2.1   Categories of routine staining methods

General structure
Connective tissue fibres
Carbohydrates and mucosubstances
Pigments
Micro-organisms
Extracellular substances (fibrin, amyloid)
Lipids
Cytoplasmic granules
Neurological

General structure

The haematoxylin and eosin method (commonly referred to as H&E) is one of the most widely used of the general structure stains used in diagnostic histopathology (see Figure 2.2). The procedure broadly

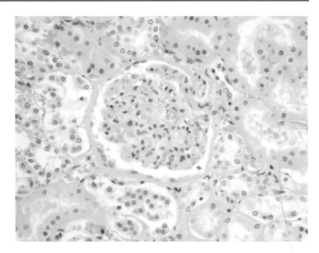

Figure 2.2   Haematoxylin and eosin-stained section of kidney showing a centrally placed glomerulus. Nuclei are stained blue (the differing intensities dependant upon the amount of nuclear chromatin present) and the general structure pink. Red blood cells are salmon pink

Table 2.2   Protocol for H&E staining

1. De-wax the sections with xylene, treat with graded alcohols and wash in water
2. Stain the nuclei with an alum haematoxylin (e.g. Harris's, Gill's, etc.)
3. Rinse in water to remove the excess stain
4. Remove excess dye from the tissues (differentiate) until only nuclei are demonstrated (a mixture of 0.5–1.0% hydrochloric acid in 70% alcohol is frequently used).
5. Wash the sections until nuclei are blue. The term 'blueing' is used to describe the process whereby cell nuclei, stained with an alum haematoxylin, are washed either in water or a weak alkali until the nuclei change from red to blue. The reaction is analogous to the changes in colour shown by litmus
6. Stain the cell cytoplasm with eosin (there a number of formulations that may be used to suit local conditions and pH of the water)
7. Following a brief wash in water (or directly to alcohol) the sections are returned to xylene and a coverglass applied

follows the regime shown in Table 2.2. The process of washing and dehydration following eosin staining will remove eosin from the section. Careful control of this process allows the various structures (muscle, collagen and red blood cells) to be selectively demonstrated in different intensities of pink to red.

Simple staining solutions

A 0.5–1% aqueous solution of methylene blue (for example) will stain all tissue structures blue. Selective removal of the dye using washing and alcohols will demonstrate tissue elements in differing intensities of blue.

Romanowsky stain

This is neutral dye (see above) which when applied to paraffin wax sections can produce a similar staining reaction to that of H&E.

Connective tissue fibres and muscle

Collagen and muscle

van Gieson van Gieson and its variants are the most commonly used stains for collagen and muscle. The staining solution is a mixture of picric acid and acid fuchsin. Because of the acidic nature of the van Gieson solution, an iron haematoxylin is used for nuclear staining. Muscle and red blood cells are stained yellow whilst collagen is stained red; nuclei are black.

Trichromes Will demonstrate collagen and muscle differentially (Figure 2.3). Muscle staining is red, whilst collagen may be blue or green, depending upon the staining regime used. Mercury-based fixatiion usually

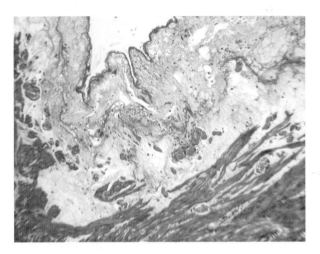

Figure 2.3 Demonstration of connective tissues is using a trichrome method. Muscle fibres are stained red, collagen blue, nuclei black and red blood cells bright red

produces superior results to those of formaldehyde. The stain requires skill to perform. The theory behind trichrome staining is varied and complex and beyond the reaches of this chapter.

Phosphotungstic acid haematoxylin (PTAH) Often used in the demonstration of muscle tissues, PTAH will stain muscle striations and myofibrils blue. Collagen is stained red.

Reticular fibres

Silver impregnation Reticular fibres are primarily demonstrated using silver impregnation methods (Figure 2.4). There are a wide variety of silver methods

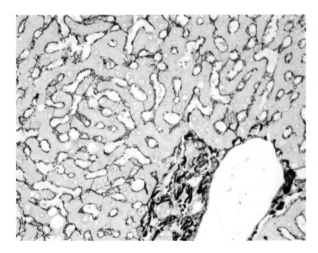

Figure 2.4 Silver impregnation of reticular fibres in a section of liver. A fine black network of fibres outlines the cells. The coarser staining (bottom right) is collagen

available; however, the methodology is similar (see Table 2.3). Counterstaining of the nuclei is optional. Reticular fibres are blackened and other structures are rendered in shades of brown (unless toned). Nuclei may be impregnated. The preparation of the ammoniacal silver solution requires skill and must be done fresh. The periodic acid–Schiff (PAS) reaction will also demonstrate reticular fibres.

Basement membranes The demonstration of glomerular basement membranes is required during the diagnosis of glomerular disease. The sections are oxidized with periodic acid and impregnated with a methenamine silver solution. The reaction is progressive

Table 2.3 Protocol for silver impregnation staining

1. *De-wax* sections and rinse in distilled water
2. *Oxidize* with potassium permanganate
3. *Bleach* with oxalic acid
4. *Sensitize* with iron alum
5. *Impregnate* with an ammoniacal silver nitrate solution
6. *Reduce* with formaldehyde
7. *Fix* with sodium thiosulphate
8. *Tone* (optional) with chloroauric acid (gold chloride)
9. *Wash*, dehydrate with alcohol, treat with xylene and coverglass

and halted at the desired point of impregnation. Sections cut at 1–2 μm are required to enable fine basement membrane structures to be visualized. The PAS reaction may also be used to demonstrate basement membranes.

Elastin   A number of dyes may be used to demonstrate elastin tissue. These may vary from haematoxylin (Verhoeff's method); rescorcin fuchsin (Weigert's, Miller's); aldehyde fuchsin and orcein. Verhoeff's method, although popular, has difficulty in demonstrating both coarse and fine fibres in the same section. The Miller's variant of Weigert's elastin stain produces consistently good, reliable results. This method consistently scores higher than other methods in quality assurance studies [United Kingdom National Quality External Quality Assurance Service for Cellular Pathology Technique (UKNEQAS-CPT); *website: www.ukneqas-cpt.co.uk*]. Orcein has proved popular for demonstrating elastin in skin. van Gieson's connective tissue stain is often used to counterstain the elastin stain.

Carbohydrates and mucosubstances

Periodic acid–Schiff reaction (PAS)

The PAS reaction is used throughout pathology to demonstrate a wide range of substances. Periodic acid breaks the carbon bonds of adjacent 1:2 glycol groups by oxidation revealing aldehydes. The aldehydes will cause the colourless Schiff reagent to re-colour and stain sites of activity a deep magenta colour. Because many substances contain 1:2 glycol groups, the stain is not very selective. To improve the selectivity of the reaction for some substances, it is necessary to extract or block that substance in a duplicate section using enzymes or chemicals.

Glycogen

The PAS reaction is frequently used for the demonstration of glycogen. To demonstrate the sites of glycogen deposition, it is necessary to pre-treat a duplicate section with diastase. The diastase will extract the glycogen and, when both sections are stained, the digested section will show an absence of PAS staining at the sites of glycogen.

Methenamine silver can be used in a similar way, demonstrating glycogen as a black product. Best's carmine is another popular method for glycogen.

Mucosubstances

Mucosubstances are commonly found as mixtures of various types and include mucins. Mucins are found in many tissue sites (e.g. glandular tissue and connective tissue). The demonstration of the various mucins will depend upon their particular characteristics. Neutral mucins may be stained by the PAS reaction (Fig. 2.5),

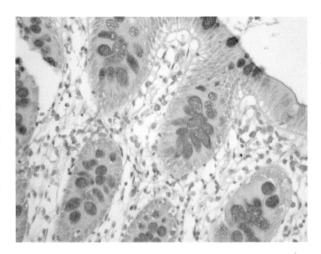

Figure 2.5 Demonstration of mucin staining using a combination of the periodic acid–Schiff (PAS) method and Alcian blue. Neutral mucins are stained magenta, acid mucins blue and mixtures deep purple blue

whilst acid mucins may be demonstrated with alcian blue.

Alcian blue, prepared at different pH's, will differentiate between general acid mucins and sulphated mucins. Alcian blue prepared with differing concentrations of magnesium chloride will demonstrate mucosubstances such as hyaluronic acid, chondroitin sulphate, keratin sulphate and heparin.

Connective tissue mucins may also be demonstrated with metachromatic dyes such as toluidine blue, whilst Southgate's mucicarmine will demonstrate carboxylated or weakly acidic mucins.

Blocking techniques to prevent staining of particular chemical groups (e.g. carboxyl) are used to improve specificity by the absence of staining in the treated sections.

Demonstration of pigments

Pigments may be found in normal and pathological material and may be formed naturally or as an artefact of tissue fixation or staining.

Artefacts

These usually occur during fixation and may be created by acid solutions of formaldehyde reacting with blood (formalin pigment). They may be avoided by the use of neutrally buffered formalin solutions. Mercury-based fixatives (e.g. Zenker) will leave a deposit of mercury salts within tissues. Both of these pigments are easily removed before staining commences. Table 2.4 lists some common pigments and the methods used to demonstrate them.

Microorganisms

Microorganisms that can be demonstrated histologically include bacteria, viral inclusions, fungi and spirochaetes. Simple stains such as methylene blue will often provide a quick and easy means of identifying the presence of organisms within a section. However, methylene blue will provide information regarding only their morphology.

Bacteria

Bacteria are divided into Gram-positive or Gram-negative, according to their staining reaction with Gram's crystal violet stain. Gram-positive bacteria retain the stain following differentiation in either acetone or alcohol, whilst Gram-negative bacteria are decolorized. Following staining with the crystal violet stain, where iodine is used as a mordant or 'trapping agent', precipitating the dye within the cytoplasm of Gram-positive bacteria, a red counterstain is used to demonstrate Gram-negative bacteria. The technique requires skill, as it is possible to over-differentiate the crystal violet, rendering Gram-positive bacteria red.

Acid alcohol-fast bacilli

These organisms are commonly demonstrated using the Ziehl–Neelsen (ZN) method. Basic fuchsin and phenol are mixed to produce 'strong carbol fuchsin'. Following staining (with or without the use of heat) the section is differentiated with a solution of acid alcohol until the section is decolourized. A counterstain (blue or green) will demonstrate other organisms and general structure.

A fluorescent method (auramine-rhodanine) may also be used. Viewed under a fluorescent microscope the organism fluoresces yellow/green. This method is more sensitive than the standard ZN as isolated organisms are identified more easily. It is usually necessary to follow up the method with a standard ZN once the location of the organisms has been identified.

Viral inclusions

There are no specific staining methods for viral inclusions, as many of the methods will stain other structures. Phloxine tartrazine has been used to demonstrate viral

Table 2.4 Demonstration of some common pigments

Pigment	Demonstration method
Haemosiderin	Perls' Prussian blue
Bile pigment	Gmelin
Melanin	Masson Fontana
Lipofuschins	Schmorl's ferric ferrocyanide
	PAS
	Masson Fontana
	Sudan black
	Long Ziehl–Neelson
Amine precursor uptake and decarboxylation (APUD) cell granules in neuroendocrine cells	Lead haematoxylin
	Masson Fontana
	Diazo
	Grimelius
	Bodian
Chromaffin cells	Chromaffin reaction
	Giemsa
Copper	Rubeanic acid
	Rhodanine
Asbestos	Perl's Prussian blue
	Birefringence

inclusion bodies and orcein is regularly used for the demonstration of hepatitis B. The demonstration of viral inclusions has largely been replaced by immunocytochemical methods.

Fungi

Fungi may be quite apparent in H&E-stained sections but can be more selectively stained by PAS, Grocott's methenamine silver (Fig. 2.6), Southgate's mucicarmine

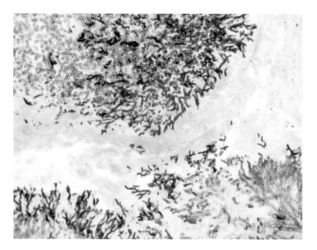

Figure 2.6 Silver impregnation of fungal hyphae. Grocott's method

(for *Cryptococcus*), Gram's stain, Ziehl–Neelsen and Giemsa.

Spirochaetes

Spirochaetes are probably the most difficult organisms to demonstrate in tissue sections. The classical method of Levaditi was performed on tissue blocks that were impregnated with silver. Subsequent embedding and sectioning revealed the spirochaetes as being black.

There are a number of silver methods described for demonstrating spirochaetes in tissue sections. All of these methods require a substantial degree of skill to perform successfully. Some of these methods have been adapted to demonstrate *Helicobacter.*

Extracellular substances (fibrin and amyloid)

Fibrin

Fibrin stains strongly with eosin and is moderately PAS-positive. Fibrin threads stain strongly with phospho-

tungstic acid haematoxylin. 'Fibrinoid' is a term applied to a hyaline substance found to give similar staining reactions to those of fibrin.

Lendrum's martius scarlet blue method demonstrates red blood cells as yellow, younger fibrin and fibrinoid as red, collagen and older fibrin as blue. The method requires skilful differentiation. The original method recommended mercury-based fixation; however, acceptable results can be achieved with non-mercury, formaldehyde solutions.

Amyloid

Amyloid stains pink in H&E sections, is moderately PAS-positive and stains yellow-to-brown on van Gieson staining. Amyloid is most routinely demonstrated using Congo red. There are a number of formulations staining amyloid pink to red. Under polarized light, Congo red-stained amyloid is dichroic, producing yellow-to-green birefringence.

Methyl violet or toluidine blue stain amyloid metachromatically (purplish red to violet).

Thioflavine T is a fluorescent dye exhibiting bright yellow fluorescence. This method is not specific but is highly sensitive.

Lipids

Lipids may be found in both normal and pathological tissues.

Simple lipids are normally lost during paraffin wax processing and frozen sections are required to demonstrate their presence. Simple lipids are demonstrated using fat-soluble dyes (e.g. Sudan dyes). The principle of the staining relies on the fact that the dye is more soluble in the fat than the solvent it is made up in (elective solubility).

Compound lipids, in which other products are present (e.g. phospholipids), may resist processing and be demonstrable by a number of methods in paraffin sections. Myelin (phospholipid) can be demonstrated with Luxol fast blue or haematoxylin-based stains.

Cytoplasmic granules

Mast cell granules

Mast cell granules are metachromatic and can be demonstrated using toluidine blue, thionin or azure A. The granules exhibit purple-to-red metachromasia with nuclei and other structures stained blue. Other connective tissues and some epithelial mucins may also be demonstrated. Alcian blue may also be used to demonstrate the granules. Chloroacetate esterase is recommended by Bancroft as the method of choice.

Paneth cell granules

Paneth cell granules are acidophilic and seen easily in well-differentiated H&E-stained sections. The phloxine tartrazine method of Lendrum stains the granules red against a yellow background.

Pancreatic cell granules

Tinctorial staining of the islet cells of the pancreas has largely been replaced with more specific immunocytochemical methods. Some traditional methods include chrome alum haematoxylin and aldehyde fuchsin for B cells, Grimelius for A cells, and the Hellerström and Hellman method for D cells.

Pituitary cell granules

Immunocytochemical methods have again largely replaced traditional staining methods. PAS–orange G was a popular method, best performed upon dichromate-based fixatives (Helly's fluid). PAS would stain pituitary basophils magenta, the orange G the acidophils orange, and the chromophobes were unstained. Trichromes have also been used to demonstrate the cell types.

Eosinophils

Eosinophils are acidophil and clearly demonstrated in well-differentiated H&Es. Chromotrope and Romanowsky stains have also been employed.

Neurological tissues

In routine diagnostic histopathology, the demonstration of neurological elements by conventional staining methods is largely confined to those of nerve cells, their processes and myelin. Immunocytochemical methods have largely replaced some of the more capricious silver impregnation techniques (Table 2.5).

Table 2.5 Some common neurological stains

Structure	Method
Neurones and processes	Silver impregnation
Nissl substance	Cresyl fast violet
Myelin	Luxol fast blue
	Solochrome cyanin
	PTAH
	Iron haematoxylin

Conclusions

Conventional staining methods still have an important role to play in diagnosis of tissue pathology. Diagnostic laboratories now use a combination of tinctorial staining and immunocytochemical staining to provide the necessary information for histopathologists to arrive at an informed diagnostic opinion. The morphological appearance of tissue stained with H&E provided the precursor for subsequent investigations.

Although immunocytochemistry has superseded a number of historical staining methods there are still a large number of investigations that rely solely on conventional staining with dyes.

Further reading

This chapter is intended to provide a very basic introduction to staining. For more in-depth information the following books are suggested:

Bancroft JD, Gamble M. *Theory and Practice of Histological Techniques*, 5th edn. 2002: Churchill-Livingstone, Edinburgh.

Culling CFA, Allison RT, Barr WT . *Cellular Pathology Technique*, 4th edn. 1885: Butterworths, London.

Advanced reading

Horobin RW, Kiernan JA (eds.) *Conn's Biological Stains. A Handbook of Dyes, Stains and Fluorochromes for Use in Biology and Medicine*, 10th edn. 2002: Bios Scientific, Oxford, UK.

Acknowledgements

I would like to express my thanks to Dr Stephen Harris, Consultant Histopathologist, Staffordshire General Hospital, for his help during the preparation of the manuscript, and to Jim Elsam, HTEQA Services, for providing the digital images.

3

Enzyme histochemistry

Trevor Gray and **Neil Hand**

Introduction

Enzymes are large tertiary proteins that act as catalysts for most biological reactions and are vital in cellular metabolism while maintaining homeostasis in man. There are over 700 known enzymes, each catalysing a specific reaction by acting on specific molecules (substrates). The resulting reaction product may act as a new substrate for a different enzyme, as illustrated by the Krebs's cycle. After each metabolic reaction, the enzyme in each case is left unaltered for further interactions.

Biochemists routinely study enzyme levels in solutions derived from bodily fluids, tissue cultures and resected tissue for diagnostic and research investigations. This gives valuable evidence in detecting and monitoring disease processes and assessing drug-induced physiological changes. The results obtained by biochemical analyses are, however, related to a heterogeneous population of cells found in tissues and do not give specific cellular values. A more accurate assessment of intracellular enzyme location and biological activity can be undertaken using enzyme histochemistry. This relies on applying an enzyme detection system to tissue sections or smears. This technique produces a final coloured reaction product that is localized to the cells with an intensity proportional to the enzyme activity. Unlike biochemical methods, this intensity is difficult to measure, but the qualitative microscopic appearances as seen by an experienced pathologist are more relevant in the histological detection and assessment of several disease processes.

The main problem with enzyme histochemistry is the retention of enzyme function during tissue preparation and histochemical staining. Numerous histological methods have been developed for specific enzymes and, although these methods are not difficult, the non-standard tissue handling procedures required have resulted in these techniques being usually performed in specialized laboratories.

Other non-enzyme histochemical methods for enzyme detection on standard paraffin sections include immunohistochemistry and mRNA *in situ* hybridization. These methods can identify the presence or production of cellular enzymes but neither can show the biological activity of the enzyme.

Structure and classification

Structure

Enzymes are high molecular weight globular proteins that may be found free within the cytoplasm (*lysoenzymes*), or bound to cellular membranes (*desmoenzymes*). Non-proteinous components (*prosthetic groups*) may be attached to the enzyme, which may help form an active quaternary structure. The functional property of the enzyme depends on maintaining the shape and charge of its 'active site' at the site of enzyme/substrate interaction.

Various co-factors are necessary for most enzyme reactions. Activators such as ions of calcium, magnesium, manganese, sodium, potassium and others help with electron transfer during the enzymatic reaction. Co-enzymes are molecules that combine with a non-active 'apoenzyme', producing a sterically active site by

The Science of Laboratory Diagnosis, Second Edition   Edited by David Burnett and John Crocker
© 2005 John Wiley & Sons, Ltd

altering the apoenzyme's quaternary structure. The co-enzyme can also combine with the substrate and may play an active part in the metabolic reaction. Most of the B vitamins are co-enzymes.

Classification

There are several ways of classifying enzymes, the most accurate being the enzyme code number, based on the systematic name of the enzyme. This contains the name of the specific substrate reacted upon, followed by a word with the suffix 'ase', specifying the type of reaction involved. In diagnostic enzyme histochemistry, a shorter trivial name is more commonly used due to the small number of enzymes investigated.

Six major enzyme groups are classified according to their effect on the substrate; oxidoreductases, transferases, hydrolases, lyases, isomerases and ligases. Probably the most important groups to the diagnostic enzyme histochemist are oxidoreductases (previously known as oxidases and dehydrogenases) and hydrolases. These are often called 'oxidative' and 'hydrolytic' enzymes, respectively.

Preservation and preparation

Enzyme preservation

The cumulative effects of the processing stages required in the production of a conventional paraffin-embedded tissue block, such as fixation, dehydration and embedding in paraffin wax, are not conducive to preserving functional enzymes. These procedures usually result in complete loss of enzyme activity, although chloroacetate esterase and peroxidase are sufficiently resistant to damage by paraffin processing. Consequently, the demonstrations of most enzymes are usually performed on frozen sections, but other preparations such as smears may also be employed.

It is important to remember that various enzymes react differently to external influences, but most enzymes are rapidly lost if fresh tissue is left at room temperature. Many oxidative enzymes, which are diagnostically important when investigating muscle disease, are located in mitochondria. When fresh tissue is deprived of oxygen, the mitochondrial membranes are quickly damaged and reduction in enzyme activity occurs. It is therefore important to quickly freeze the tissue, which is usually fresh, as most oxidative enzymes cannot withstand conventional fixation. Hydrolytic

enzymes are contained in lysosomes but are damaged by freezing and subsequent thawing of blocks or sections with a release of enzymes. Diffusion of hydrolytic enzymes can be minimized and localization improved if the tissue is treated with a fixative before cryotomy, although some loss of enzyme activity will occur. In practice, enzyme histochemical staining is often carried out on unfixed cryostat sections, especially in clinical circumstances where a delay in diagnosis is undesirable, or different enzymes are required to be demonstrated in the same sample. However, localization of some enzymes may be improved by briefly fixing the tissue section after cryotomy.

If fixation is employed, the fixative should be at 4°C and used for the shortest time possible. Formol calcium is often recommended for tissue blocks, as this helps maintain cell membrane integrity, although buffered formalin or formal saline is satisfactory in most cases. Cryotomy and enzyme activity may be further improved by washing the fixed tissue in a sucrose buffer solution before freezing. For optimal results, it is important to keep these solutions close to the physiological pH of the tissue. A variety of fixatives in addition to formol calcium have been used on smears and cryostat sections, including acetone, formalin vapour and formalin–alcohol mixtures. The choice of fixative depends on the particular enzyme investigated, and is a compromise between enzyme activity and morphological appearance. Even after short fixation times, most oxidative enzymes are rendered inactive but, as previously mentioned, fixation may be used after demonstrating these enzymes to help preserve cellular morphology and the localization of the final reaction product.

Tissue preparation

Several different methods are available for the examination of enzymes, but in this chapter only frozen sections, smears and paraffin sections will be considered. As previously outlined, the enzymes required to be demonstrated will mainly decide the type of preparation employed.

Frozen sections

The most common specimen preparation in enzyme histochemistry is the use of frozen sections, usually cut with a cryostat. Tissue is required to be rapidly snap-frozen as slow freezing will cause ice crystal artefacts: faster freezing produces smaller ice crystals. Muscle biopsies account for most diagnostic enzyme histochemistry samples, yet are very prone to ice crystal artefact. The optimal method for freezing muscle is to use isopentane that has been frozen with liquid nitrogen and allowed to partly thaw. The solid fraction acts as a thermal buffer, keeping the temperature of the liquid fraction stable ($-150°C$) during freezing of the tissue. The tissue (fixed or unfixed) is orientated on a cork disc in OCT gel and immersed in the thawing isopentane until the gel and specimen freezes. The cork is similarly attached to the block holder using OCT compound and then placed inside the cryostat ready for sectioning at $-23°C$. Liquid nitrogen alone should not be used, as it has a low rate of thermal conductivity, producing a gaseous thermal barrier around the tissue, which in turn induces cellular damage by allowing large ice crystals to form.

Smears

Smears may be prepared by various methods from blood, bone marrow and tissue cell suspensions. Imprint smears of tissue, e.g. lymph nodes, are also useful where fresh tissue is cut and the new surface touched gently against a clean glass slide. Most smears are air-dried and lightly fixed (depending on the enzymes required) for a few seconds, usually with cold acetone, before cytochemical staining of the cells.

Paraffin wax sections

Most enzymes will not withstand the effects of standard paraffin wax processing and therefore this mode of preparation is not often useful. Peroxidase and chloroacetate esterase are, however, sufficiently hardy to survive routine paraffin wax embedding and may be easily shown. Some other enzymes may be partly preserved using a specialized schedule with waxes of a low melting point, but this is seldom used.

Histochemical techniques

These histological methods are unique in that the enzymes are never stained; only the reaction products are demonstrated. For meaningful results, careful optimization of the enzyme reaction and colouring of the reaction product is essential.

The process involves cleavage of a substrate by the tissue-bound enzyme to form a primary reaction product (PRP). This PRP can then react with a chemical known as a capture agent to form a final reaction product (FRP), which should be insoluble and at the site of the enzyme. Numerous factors influence the reactions and all must be carefully controlled. The pH of the incubating solutions is critical for most enzyme reactions and is maintained using suitable buffers. Varying the temperature can alter the enzyme reaction rate, with some methods requiring incubation at $37°C$, while others are performed at room temperature. The sub-optimal room temperature allows more time for completion of FRP formation with the PRP and capture agent, thus improving localization of the FRP to the enzyme site by decreasing the enzyme reaction rate. Substrates and capture agents should be chosen to prevent interactions and both should be readily diffusible across cell membranes. Both substrate and capture agent should be used at a concentration that would prevent local depletion during rapid enzyme activity, but not at a concentration that would inhibit the enzyme reaction. The selection of a capture agent is dependent upon the enzyme method used and the type of tissue in which the enzyme is found. For example, when using the metal precipitation method on muscle, the calcium salt is preferred to the lead salt, as the latter can bind non-specifically with the muscle. Often there is also a choice of substrates, but many naturally occurring substrates, although cheap, may be non-specific or produce PRPs that are not totally insoluble. Specially synthesized substrates usually produce superior results.

It is important to include positive control tissue during histochemical staining so that the quality of the reagents and the accuracy of the protocol employed can be assessed. Omission of the substrate from the incubating medium or the inclusion of specific inhibitors will act as a negative control.

Enzyme reaction methods

In histopathology most enzymes are demonstrated using either (a) simultaneous coupling or (b) post-incubation coupling.

Simultaneous coupling

Simultaneous coupling only requires one solution containing both the substrate and a capturing agent, with the required co-factors. The tissue-bound enzyme reacts with the substrate in solution to produce a PRP. The PRP may be either insoluble or soluble, as the capture agent (also in solution) binds with the PRP instantaneously to form a FRP. This insoluble FRP is bound to the enzyme site and may be coloured or colourless, although the latter would require an additional colouring step for visualization.

Post-incubation coupling

Occasionally it is not possible to have the substrate and capturing agent in one solution, as the conditions required for PRP production may be different from that required for FRP production. Sometimes the capturing agent may also interfere with or inhibit the enzyme function. In post-incubation coupling methods, the initial solution only contains the substrate and any cofactors required. The PRP produced must be insoluble, as false negatives or gross diffusion of the FRP will occur. A secondary solution that contains the capture agent is then applied to produce the FRP as above. In practice it is difficult to find suitable substrates for post-incubation coupling methods, with a result that it is rarely used.

Demonstration methods

The coloured FRPs are normally produced by one of the following methods:

1. Metal precipitation.

2. Azo-dye.

3. Tetrazolium salt.

4. Indigogenic method.

Other methods include:

5. The oxidation of 3,3-diaminobenzidine (DAB) by cytochrome oxidase or the peroxidases to form a brown pigment.

6. The metabolism of glycogen by phosphorylase to produce a polysaccharide that is coloured blue/black with iodine.

Metal precipitation methods

Metal precipitation methods are routinely used to identify phosphatases, e.g. acid phosphatase, alkaline phosphatase and adenosine triphosphatase (ATPase; Figure 3.1).

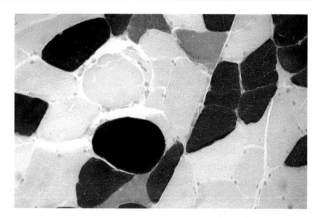

Figure 3.1 Frozen sections showing differential staining of muscle fibres for ATPase following incubation at pH 4.2 with a metal precipitation technique

They rely on the release of phosphate ions from the substrate, which then react with lead or calcium salts in solution (capture agent) to form the insoluble FRP of lead or calcium phosphate.

Lead phosphate is colourless but is blackened with ammonium sulphide solution to form lead sulphide. Calcium phosphate is insoluble at alkaline pH and needs to be converted to cobalt phosphate with cobalt chloride solution, before treating with ammonium sulphide to form black cobalt sulphide. Both these methods are liable to fade with time, but may be recoloured with ammonium sulphide.

The acetyl cholinesterase method using the substrate acetyl thiocholine can be regarded as a metal precipitate method that produces a PRP of thiocholine, which reacts with copper sulphate and potassium ferricyanide, respectively, to form brown copper ferrocyanide.

Azo-dye methods

The azo-dye methods are used to identify acid and alkaline phosphatases, non-specific esterase and chloroacetate esterase. The different substrates contain a naphthol group that can be cleaved by one of the above enzymes. Various diazonium salts or freshly hexazotized pararosaniline are used that react with the naphthol group to form a coloured insoluble azo dye. Typically, the diazonium salts used include Fast Red TR, Fast Blue RR, Fast Blue B and Fast Garnet GBC, which have to be aqueously mounted. The azo dye formed from the hexazotized pararosaniline is the method of choice, as it can be mounted in a synthetic resin, which improves optical localization at light microscopy. Diazonium salts may be used with either simultaneous or post-incubation coupling methods.

Tetrazolium salt methods

Tetrazolium salts are colourless, water-soluble salts that accept enzymatically-released hydrogen from the substrate to form highly coloured water-insoluble micro-crystalline deposits known as formazans. Many oxidative enzymes, such as succinic dehydrogenase, are demonstrated using tetrazolium salts such as methyl-thiazolyldiphenyl tetrazolium (MTT; Figure 3.2) and nitro blue tetrazolium (NBT). As with diazonium

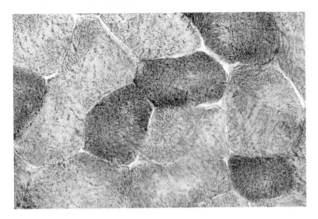

Figure 3.2 Frozen section of muscle stained for NADH diaphorase using the tetrazolium salt MTT

salts, several factors influence their selection, but NBT is often used in preference to MTT, as it can be mounted in a synthetic resin.

Indigogenic method

The various substrates contain an indoxyl group, which is released as a PRP, which in turn is oxidized by the capture agent potassium ferricyanide to form a turquoise FRP (Figure 3.3). The incubation solution also includes potassium ferrocyanide, which prevents over-oxidation of the FRP.

Diagnostic applications of enzyme histochemistry

Enzyme histochemistry may be used for a variety of diagnostic applications such as:

1. Skeletal muscle fibre typing.

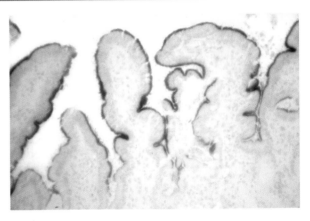

Figure 3.3 Frozen section of jejunum showing lactase activity on the microvilli, stained turquoise using the indigogenic method

2. Nerves and ganglia in suspected Hirschsprung's disease.

3. Gastrointestinal tissue to assess malabsorption.

4. Demonstration of lymphoid and myeloid cells.

5. Identification of early liver degeneration.

The first two applications are the most common, but are unusually confined to specialized diagnostic centres.

Skeletal muscle

The use of enzyme histochemistry in the diagnosis of neuromuscular diseases and congenital myopathies has become firmly established, with many histopathological appearances only recognized and described after the introduction of enzyme histochemistry.

Traditional tinctorial staining of striated muscle is sufficient to show inflammatory responses and variation in fibre size, but is unable to differentiate between the various muscle fibre types. This is important, as many disease processes are confined to, or show alteration of, specific muscle fibre types. This can be in the form of atrophy or hypertrophy, and in certain diseases alteration of the internal cellular structure. The application of enzyme histochemical methods on transversely cut skeletal muscle enables several different fibre types to be distinguished, which, in conjunction with examining their distribution and size, can assist in diagnosis.

Striated muscle fibres may be broadly divided into Type 1 and Type 2, depending on the level of ATPase activity shown at pH 9.4. If ATPase staining is applied after pre-incubating in a buffer at pH 4.2 or 4.6, further differentiation of Type 2 fibres into subtypes 2A, 2B and 2C may be achieved (Figure 3.1). Another important enzyme to demonstrate is phosphorylase, which in McArdle's disease is deficient in striated muscle cells but still present in smooth muscle cells of blood vessels, and hence serves as a useful inherent control. NADH diaphorase (reduced nicotinamide adenine dinucleotide) is used to study the internal structure of muscle cells, as it demonstrates mitochondria and the sarcoplasmic reticulum network (Figure 3.2). When this is compared with the myofibrillar distribution shown by ATPase, various pathological conditions may become apparent. Abnormal enzyme distribution patterns are often described in terms of their appearances that are specific to a particular disease entity, such as 'target fibres', 'ring fibres', and 'central cores'. Cytochrome oxidase, succinic dehydrogenase, and lactate dehydrogenase are more specific for mitochondria and may prove helpful in identifying mitochondrial myopathies. A summary of the differential enzyme staining of skeletal muscle is shown in Table 3.1.

Table 3.1 Diagnostic enzyme histochemistry

Tissue	Enzyme	Method	Substrate	pH	Colour	Demonstrates
Striated muscle	Myofibrillar ATPase	Metal precipitation (calcium chloride)	Adenosine triphosphate (ATP)	9.4	Black/brown	Type 1 fibres—pale Type 2a & 2b & 2c fibres—dark
		Metal precipitation (calcium chloride) pre-incubation @ pH 4.6				Type 1—dark Type 2b & 2c fibres—intermediate Type 2a fibres—pale
		Metal precipitation (calcium chloride) pre-incubation @ pH 4.2				Type 1 fibres—dark Type 2c fibres—intermediate Type 2a & 2b fibres—pale
	NADH Diaphorase	Tetrazolium salt (MTT)	NADH	7.0	Black	Mitochondria (Type 1 fibres—darker) Sarcoplasmic reticulum
	Succinic dehydrogenase	Tetrazolium salt (MTT)	Sodium succinate	7.0	Black	Mitochondria (Type 1 fibres—darker) for
	Cytochrome oxidase	Oxidation of DAB	Cytochrome c	7.4	Brown	mitochondrial abnormalities
	Myophosphorylase	Metabolism of glycogen (iodine)	Glucose-1 phosphate	5.9	Purple/black	Negative staining muscle fibres in McArdle's disease
	Myoadenylate deaminase	Tetrazolium salt (NBT)	Adenosine-5 monophosphate (AMP)	6.1	Blue	Absent in some metabolic disorders
	Aldolase		Disodium fructose 1,6 diphosphate	8.6		
	Phosphofructo-kinase		Fructose-6 phosphate	7.0		
Nerves	Acetyl cholinesterase	Potassium ferri-cyanide–copper sulphate reaction (metal precipitation)	Acetyl thiocholine iodide	6.0	Red/brown	Nerve fibres and cells In rectum, colon (Hirschsprung's) and muscle diseases
Jejunum	Lactase	Indigogenic method (potassium ferricyanide)	5-Bromo-4-chloro-3-indoxyl-β, D fucoside	6.0	Turquoise	Reduced or negative with malabsorption
	Sucrase	Azo dye (pararosaniline)	6-Bromo-2-naphthyl-α, D glucoside	6.0	Red	

Recently, immunohistochemical methods have been developed for reliable muscle fibre typing on paraffin-processed tissue. While this may have important diagnostic potential for such processed tissue, it does not allow identification of the other diagnostically important enzymes or the ability to show their metabolic activity.

Nerves and ganglia

In normal colon and rectum, ganglion cells and associated nerves are present that are responsible for colonic motility. In Hirschsprung's disease in children, there is an absence of ganglia from between the circular and longitudinal smooth muscle junction (myenteric plexus) and in the submucosa. There is also a marked increase in the number and thickening of non-argyrophilic nerve fibres in the submucosa and the lamina propria. The ganglion cells can be readily identified on an H&E section but nerve fibres are much more difficult. Both ganglion cells and nerve fibres contain cholinesterase, which may be demonstrated using the quick acetyl cholinesterase method. Identification of Hirschsprung's is normally required to confirm the initial diagnosis and later during corrective surgery, when the resection boundaries have to be identified before removal of the abnormal bowel. As this is performed during surgery using small rectal suction biopsies, speed is important. Cryostat H&E-stained sections are usually sufficient to detect the absence or presence of large ganglion cells, but any superficial biopsies that are not discarded as the acetyl cholinesterase method is used to show the abnormal nerve fibres in the lamina propria (Figure 3.4).

The same method can be used to demonstrate motor end plate abnormalities in striated muscle biopsies.

Gastrointestinal tissue

To achieve a definitive diagnosis on gastrointestinal biopsies where malabsorption is suspected, morphological information alone is insufficient. Various enzymes on the brush border of villi are useful, but the disaccharidases, lactase, trehalase and sucrase are particularly important. These enzymes reflect changes to enterocyte injury; lactase (Figure 3.3) is the most sensitive, whereas sucrase is the most resistant and therefore histochemical staining for these two diasaccharidases is helpful. These methods can also be use to detect primary lactase or sucrase deficiencies, although clinically the biochemical

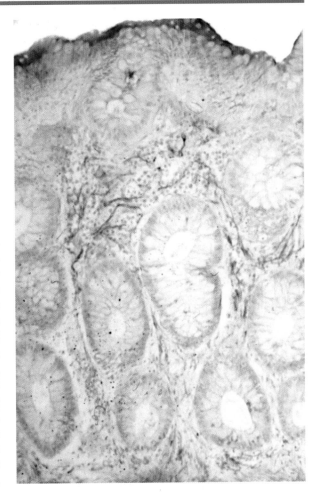

Figure 3.4 Frozen section of rectal tissue with Hirschsprung's disease, stained for acetyl cholinesterase demonstrating the thickened nerve fibres

assay of these disaccharides is usually more important than histochemical identification.

Acid phosphatase found in the lysosomes of enterocytes and in macrophages in the lamina propria may also be a useful enzyme to demonstrate when considering malabsorption. To assess and monitor malabsorption properly, jejunum is required to be orientated so that the villi are sectioned longitudinally.

Lymphoid and myeloid cells

Several enzymes, including non-specific esterase, acid phosphatase and chloroacetate esterase, are used for the cytochemical identification and evaluation of cells in smear preparations, as shown in Table 3.2. In addition to enzyme activity, specific cells may be differentiated by their staining pattern, i.e. focal or diffuse.

Table 3.2 Enzyme histochemical staining for white blood cells

Enzyme	Method	Substrate	pH	Colour	Comments
Chloroacetate Esterase	Azo dye (pararosaniline)	Naphthol AS-D chloroacetate	6.3	Red	Mast cells stain first followed by eosinophils and neutrophils
Acid phosphatase	Azo dye (pararosaniline)	Naphthol AS-BI phosphate	5.0	Red	Monocytes stain diffusely T cells have a single small spot
Alkaline phosphatase	Azo dye (Fast Red TR)		8.0	Red	Neutrophils
Non-specific esterase	Azo Dye (pararosaniline)	α-Naphthyl acetate	7.6	Red	Monocytes

Immunohistochemistry is now the method of choice for identifying these cells in histopathology, but some haematology departments still use the enzyme histochemical methods. Chloroacetate esterase, which as previously mentioned survives paraffin embedding, can distinguish lymphoid and myeloid cells, as the former is not demonstrated. Mast cells are also easily recognized by their strong staining, morphology and granularity using this enzyme histochemical method (Figure 3.5).

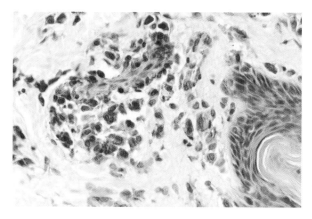

Figure 3.5 Paraffin section of skin showing mast cells in the dermis stained red for chloroacetate esterase using naphthol AS-D chloroacetate and hexazonium pararosaniline

Liver degeneration

The absence of enzyme activity in frozen sections of liver may be useful in identifying early hepatocyte damage and cirrhotic changes. Where there is marked cirrhotic change, a control sample is important as there may be not be any normal hepatocytes present to act as an internal control. Redistribution of enzyme activity, such as acid phosphatase located in the nucleus, is also an early sign of cell damage and eventual necrosis, due to lysosomal degeneration.

Conclusion

Enzyme histochemistry still plays a vital role in histopathology, especially in the detection and diagnosis of muscle disease, even though new immunohistochemical methods are now available. In immunocytochemistry and molecular biology, enzyme histochemical techniques are routinely used in the detection systems. The formazan method for succinic dehydrogenase has been successfully used on fresh macro heart slices to identify infarction on post mortem tissue. Forensic scientists have also used enzyme histochemical methods to help determine the date and time when a wound was induced. In research, a much wider range of enzymes are studied, using diverse techniques such as electron microscopy and flow cytometry, in addition to light microscopy.

References

Bancroft JD. Enzyme histochemistry and its diagnostic applications. In *Theory and Practice of Histological Techniques*, 5th edn, Bancroft JD, Gamble M (eds). 2002: Churchill Livingstone, London, 593–620.

Bancroft JD, Hand NM. *Enzyme Histochemistry*. RMS Microscopy Handbook No. 14. 1987: Oxford University Press, Oxford.

Behan WMH, Cossar DW, Madden HA, McKay IC. Validation of a simple, rapid, and economical technique for distinguishing type 1 and 2 fibres in fixed and frozen skeletal muscle. *J Clin Pathol* 2002; **55**: 375–380.

Dawson IMP. Fixation: what should the pathologist do? *Histochem J* 1972; **4**: 381–385.

Filipe MI, Lake BD. *Histochem in Pathology*, 2nd edn. 1990: Churchill Livingstone, Edinburgh.

Hayhoe FGJ, Quaglino D. *Haematological Cytochemistry*, 2nd edn. 1988: Churchill Livingstone, Edinburgh.

4

Immunohistochemistry

Jane Starczynski and **John Crocker**

Introduction

In terms of normal function and of disease states, study of the simple morphology of sections or cells is generally sufficient for analysis. As described in Chapters 3 and 5, ancillary techniques, such as histochemistry, enzyme histochemistry and electron microscopy, may be most helpful in understanding further the nature and functional state of a cell or tissue type. However, in the 1970s it became apparent that more detailed assessment of the products of cell function was both necessary and possible. In histopathology, the advent of immunohistochemistry (IHC) was exciting and opened large new vistas in the investigation of biopsy and surgical excision specimens. The principle which underlies all IHC is that of demonstrating antigen by means of its binding to an antibody which, in turn, is linked to a label that can be visualized histologically (Figure 4.1). Thus, the site of the antigen in question is highlighted. IHC methods can conveniently be classified into three main groups, viz. direct, indirect and complex, and range from those visualized using UV-activated fluorescence to those that are chromogenic. In addition, particulate material, such as heavy metal, may be used at both the light and electron microscope levels.

Direct methods

In these, antibody directed against a certain molecule or part of a molecule (epitope) is bound to a section. The antibody has a 'reporter agent' bound to it and is thus visualized directly. The method is relatively insensitive in that there is no 'amplification' of the antigenic signal involved. The direct technique has largely been abandoned in routine IHC; however, it is still the method of choice for flow cytometry (see Chapter 8).

Indirect methods

The indirect methods involve the use of layers of antibody to demonstrate the antigen concerned. This is illustrated classically by the build-up of layers of antibodies directed against antigens of differing species specificity, giving an 'inverted cone' of molecules, thus amplifying the original signal greatly. Thus, for example, rabbit anti-human antigen as the first step is further reacted with, say, a labelled swine anti-rabbit antibody. This gives greater sensitivity than direct methods but has largely been superseded by more complex methods.

Multi-stage methods

Multi-stage methods involve building layers of antibodies and labels to amplify the signal at the site of antibody binding. Examples of these include the enzyme bridge methods, peroxidase–antiperoxidase (PAP) and alkaline phosphatase–anti-alkaline phosphatase (APAAP) techniques, and avidin/streptavidin–biotin-based systems. In all of these reactions the signal sensitivity is much greater than in direct and indirect techniques, the 'inverted cone' of amplification being much greater with multilayering of molecules.

The Science of Laboratory Diagnosis, Second Edition Edited by David Burnett and John Crocker
© 2005 John Wiley & Sons, Ltd

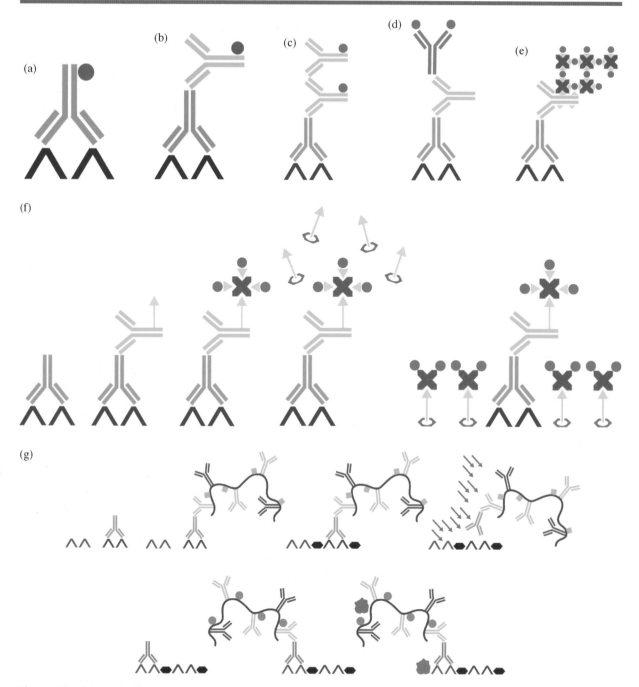

Figure 4.1 Schematic diagram to show some of the more commonly used IHC sequences. (a) Direct method: labelled primary antibody reacts with tissue antigen. (b) Two-step indirect method: enzyme-labelled secondary antibody reacts with primary antibody bound to tissue antigen. (c) Three-step indirect method: enzyme-labelled tertiary antibody reacts with enzyme-labelled secondary antibody. (d) The APAAP complex reacts with secondary antibody. Primary antibody and the antibody of the immune complex must be raised in the same species. (e) In the ABC method, the avidin– or streptavidin–biotin–enzyme complex reacts with the biotinylated secondary antibody. (f) In the catalysed signal amplification (CSA) sequence, the primary antibody is followed by a biotinylated secondary antibody, then (strept)avidin complex, then the amplification reagent and, finally, the (strept)avidin–enzyme complex. (g) Dual staining for two epitopes, using CSA methodology. The first antibody is applied, followed by the first 'spine' molecule, then an appropriate chromogen. Then a blocking agent is applied. The second primary antibody is then used, with a second 'spine' molecule and a second chromogen. (h) Key to (a)–(f). Reproduced by permission of DAKO Cytomation Ltd

(h)

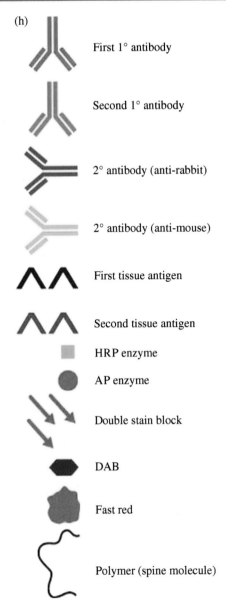

First 1° antibody

Second 1° antibody

2° antibody (anti-rabbit)

2° antibody (anti-mouse)

First tissue antigen

Second tissue antigen

HRP enzyme

AP enzyme

Double stain block

DAB

Fast red

Polymer (spine molecule)

Figure 4.1 (*Continued*)

'Reporter and linkage molecules'

In order to visualize the antigen, albeit indirectly, it is necessary to produce a visual signal to localize the binding site in the cells or tissues. Accordingly, a range of 'reporter' systems has been developed over the years. These are described, more-or-less chronologically, below.

Fluorescent molecules

The original reporter was the fluorescent dye, fluorescein, tagged to the appropriate antibody. The antigen could then be visualized by fluorescence microscopy (see Chapter 6). A limitation of using fluorescent reporter molecules is their photoinstability, the signal gradually fading on exposure to daylight. It should be noted that the antigenic rather than fluorescent properties of fluorescein are now being used to good effect in non-biotin-based detection systems for IHC. There are now multiple fluorophores with different excitation and emission frequencies that can be used to allow simultaneous labelling of multiple antigens within the same tissue.

Immunofluorescence has relatively limited use in the diagnostic laboratory today but is still seen in the assessment of renal (Figure 4.2) and skin biopsies,

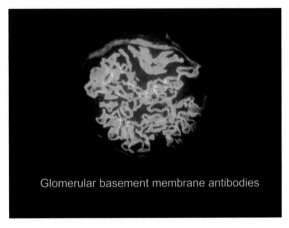

Glomerular basement membrane antibodies

Figure 4.2 A photomicrograph of a glomerulus from a renal biopsy. The patient had IgA glomerulopathy and delicate immunostaining can be seen in this frozen section, reacted for IgA (fluorescent green). Reproduced by courtesy of Dr. Aarnoud Huissoon

perhaps because the material lends itself to the demonstration of linear or membranous antigen. It is still used extensively for antigen localization in research and, with the ability simultaneously to localize multiple antigens within the same tissue/cell, provides useful information on cellular and protein interactions.

Peroxidase

Horseradish peroxidase (HRP) is an extraordinarily well-suited molecule for the investigation of human disease. First, it is not of mammalian origin, being derived, of course, from a plant! This means that the chances of antigenic cross-reaction are lessened; however, it must be noted that enzymatic activity of HRP is similar to that in mammals and this can cause problems when the enzyme is demonstrated in tissues or cells (see below). Second, it can be demonstrated readily through its reaction with a variety of substrates producing a coloured reaction product that can be visualized microscopically, e.g. 3,3′-diaminobenzidine (DAB) in the presence of hydrogen peroxide. Finally, it is a molecule that can be used at the ultrastructural level. HRP labelling has been used in direct, indirect and multi-stage techniques. For some years, the mainstay of histopathology laboratories was the peroxidase–antiperoxidase (PAP) method. However, this has probably been overtaken generally by the more 'amplifying' avidin–biotin (ABC) technique.

A problem with the use of HRP lies in the presence of peroxidatic activity endogenous to human and other tissues, which will lead to a positive reaction, e.g. neutrophil polymorphs have endogenous peroxidase activity. Fortunately, this activity can largely be 'blocked' by pre-treatment of the section with blocking reagents, notably hydrogen peroxide or hydrochloric acid in methanol and sodium azide. Even when this is done, certain cells, notably neutrophil polymorphs and mast cells, which are very rich in peroxidase, may still give false positive results.

Alkaline phosphatase

Alkaline phosphatase (AP) is another enzyme that has found widespread use in IHC, especially in cell preparations. This latter is largely because of the high sensitivity of the resulting alkaline phosphatase-anti-alkaline phosphatase (APAAP) interaction. AP can give vivid colour reaction products with certain substrates, but in general these suffer from the problem that, unlike say the DAB reaction product, they are soluble. This means that sections must be mounted in aqueous media; these previously remained liquid and created problems with long-term storage, but permanent mountants are now available. Again, there may be problems with endogenous tissue alkaline phosphatase, but this may be blocked with agents such as levamisole.

Gold–silver

Antibodies can be bound to fine, uniform aggregates of the element gold and this will in turn react with silver

from argentous compounds, by virtue of differing electropositivity. This gives a very sensitive reaction sequence which found extensive use at the light microscope level some 10 years ago, when it was used in studies as a labelling method for low-expression epitopes, such as those on cell surfaces. It must be stated, however, that the method never found widespread diagnostic application and generally remained as a research tool. Furthermore, it has largely been replaced by the avidin–biotin complex (ABC) series of methods. However, a major use of immunogold technique lies in the field of immuno-electron microscopy, where metallic particles can be seen to localize on antigenic sites; indeed, it is possible to demonstrate more than one antigen in the same preparation by using antibodies linked to gold particles of different sizes.

Avidin–biotin

The avidin–biotin methods rely on the high-affinity binding between avidin (or streptavidin) and biotin. This exquisitely high affinity is central to their application as an intermediate stage in amplification, high-sensitivity methods such as ABC (Figure 4.3). The

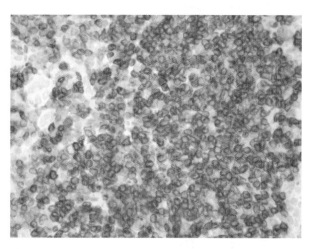

Figure 4.3 A photomicrograph of a follicular lymphoma, immunostained for the bcl-2 oncoprotein, using ABC methodology

secondary antibodies are biotinylated, with the tertiary avidin layer conjugated to a reporter molecule such as HRP or AP. The ABC method has found widespread use in both diagnostic and research laboratories and is probably the standard at present. One potential problem with ABC-based systems is that both avidin and biotin can be found within some normal tissue. It is important to consider this when working with these tissues and the use of avidin/biotin blocks can be used to counter this problem.

Tyramine signal amplification (TSA)

TSA is a very sensitive method that results in striking signal amplification, up to 10^3 times greater than other methods. In this system, HRP acts as a catalyst in the deposition of tyramide, bound to either a fluorochrome or biotin in both direct and indirect reactions. This is of great value when the target antigen is expressed at low levels and may be below the threshold for detection using standard IHC methods.

Non-biotin systems

It has previously been noted that there can be problems with endogenous enzyme activity and endogenous molecules within normal tissue. More recent methods have been developed using labels that are not usually found in normal tissue. Fluorescein has found favour recently as a coupling reagent, not by virtue of its fluorescence but as an antigen: this molecule has the obvious advantage in that it clearly does not have a human analogue!

A novel approach to signal amplification has been the introduction of polymer-based systems. These allow multiple enzyme (HRP/AP) labels to be attached to the secondary antibody via a polymer backbone. This type of system is a two-step procedure and thus saves time over conventional avidin/biotin systems, whilst the multiple enzyme labels maintain the sensitivity.

Non-specific antibody binding

Readers should note that primary antibodies may bind non-specifically to tissue sections, largely by means of their Fc fractions. The problem is much more likely to occur with polyclonal than with monoclonal reagents. This can generally overcome by means of 'blocking' with the appropriate non-immune serum.

'Antigen-retrieval' methods

Enzyme pre-treatment

In the late 1970s it was found that immunostaining could often be enhanced by pre-treatment of sections with certain proteolytic enzymes, such as pronase or trypsin. The precise basis for such processes is uncertain, but it is assumed that certain antigenic groups are 'unmasked' biochemically by removal of obscuring side-chains, enabling access of the primary antibody. The enzymes are highly lytic and 'titration' prior to regular use is essential to avoid tissue disruption.

Microwave pre-treatment

In the 1990s it became apparent that certain epitopes could conveniently be 'unmasked' by the use of controlled microwave irradiation of tissue sections in aqueous media. As with enzyme pre-treatment, the mechanism behind the success of microwaves is far from clear; nonetheless, this technique has found very wide application in the last few years. Like enzyme methods, microwave treatment not only in some cases improves visualization of certain antigens but may also enable detection when *none* was possible before. As with enzyme treatment, 'titration' of microwave timing is necessary.

Another recent development has been the use of pressure-cooking of sections to improve immunostaining. This is presumably rather more hazardous than the careful use of microwave ovens! Pressure cooking can also be performed in microwave ovens; autoclaving, steaming and simple boiling have also been used in some centres.

With retrieval methodology, it is essential to use precoated microscope slides to avoid loss of tissue from the slide surface. Positively charged slides are available commercially; alternatives include coating the slides with poly-L-lysine, APES or Vectabond.

Controls

It is most important to set up certain essential controls before testing any new antibody and, ideally, at least some of these constraints should be applied on a day-to-day diagnostic basis. *Positive controls* involve the inclusion of sections known to have elements reactive with the antibody in question. This is the most important and regularly used control in everyday diagnostic IHC. It is useful sometimes to prepare a composite paraffin wax-embedded tissue block containing an assortment of small pieces of known positive controls and mounted on the same slide as the test section. This enables the pathologist to see both positively- and negatively-stained structures at the same time.

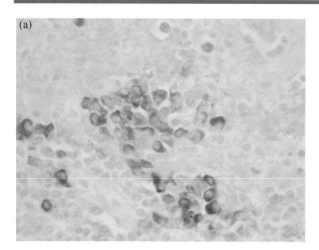
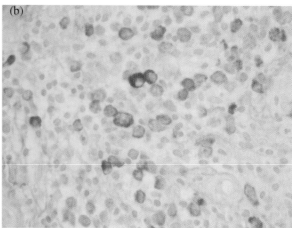

Figure 4.4 Sections double-stained to show brown (DAB, Menarini) cytoplamic reactivity for κ Ig light chain and steel-grey (Vector SG) cytoplasmic activity for λ light chain. In (a), plasma cells in a 'reactive' tonsil show a mixture of cells, some containing one chain and some the other. In (b), all of the plasma cells (in a skin biopsy) contain the κ-chain and are, therefore, clonal

When a new antibody is being evaluated prior to diagnostic or research use, a range of more rigorous controls are required. These would include: 'blocking' with the pure antigen/epitope (i.e. pre-adsorbing the antibody with its target antigen); omission of the primary antibody (or replacement with an isotype-matched control) or further antibodies in the sequence and application of the chromogenic reaction alone. Such controls check for the specificity of primary antibody binding and on the need for its presence in a positive reaction result.

Dual-labelling methods

It is often important to be able to demonstrate more than one antigen or epitope in a particular cell or tissue. An example lies in the demonstration of κ (kappa) and λ (lambda) light chains to determine clonality in a lymphocytoid lesion (Figure 4.4). The question asked is, of course, 'Is it a section of benign or malignant lymphoid tissue?'. The exhibition of monoclonality in/on cells from a section must in everyday terms indicate malignancy and the ability to demonstrate or fail to demonstrate this will influence patient management. To demonstrate more than one antigen/epitope, chromogenic substrates of different colours are used and the preparation assessed accordingly. IHC can also be combined with other techniques, such as the 'AgNOR'

method (see Chapter 8), conventional histochemistry and *in situ* hybridization.

Polyclonal versus monoclonal antibodies

The early work on IHC was performed using polyclonal antisera, raised in mammals against antigenic preparations. These antisera were polytypic and thus tended to give staining patterns which were often not 'clean' on sections, with binding of different constituent antibodies to rather variable microscopic sites. The method of 'affinity purification', where the polyclonal antibody was run through a column containing the target antigen, bound to matrix, improved the specificity of the reagents. With the advent of monoclonal antibodies, far 'cleaner' and more specific localization of epitopes, and thus better delineation of cell and tissue species, became possible.

A major early problem, however, was that unlike many polyclonal antibodies, most monoclonal antibodies could not successfully be applied to routine, archival paraffin wax-embedded sections. Accordingly, most early studies depended upon the availability of frozen section material, with its relatively poor morphological preservation. Nowadays, however, with the advent of higher affinity monoclonal antibodies, many can successfully be applied to paraffin sections, especially following the use of antigen retrieval methods.

Nonetheless, frozen sections may still offer an advantage over paraffin wax sections in that the former can offer better visualization of *surface* antigens.

Applications of immunohistochemistry

It would be far beyond the scope and intent of this book to give a comprehensive account of the myriad applications of IHC in the diagnostic laboratory. Suffice it to say that this technology can be used in diagnosis and as an indicator of prognosis in routine cellular pathology. IHC has enabled us to distinguish between lymphomas and small cell carcinomas, melanomas and seminomas, mesotheliomas and adenocarcinomas, and B and T cell lymphomas. Furthermore, we can identify microorganisms as far-ranging as *Cytomegalovirus* to *Toxoplasma* and, as discussed in Chapter 8, we can assess cell proliferation and apoptotic state. In addition, hormones, hormone receptors, growth factors, adhesion molecules and oncogene products can be demonstrated by IHC, as can ligands for certain molecules. As a caveat, however, it must be stressed that shared epitopes do not necessarily indicate shared lineages. For example, the Reed–Sternberg cells of Hodgkin's disease and adenocarcinoma cells both express CD15, yet it is not suggested that these cell types are of common lineage! An increasingly important field for the application of IHC lies in the field of assessment of prognosis, which can help the clinician to tailor more accurately the most suitable therapy for a particular malignancy. Examples lie in the assessment of growth fraction by means of the antibody Ki67. Also, for example, the expression of the bcl-2 oncoprotein confers a relatively poor prognosis in high-grade lymphomas. Investigation of oestrogen and progesterone receptor and HER2 status are also of great importance in the treatment of breast carcinomas.

Quality control

In today's world of tightening laboratory standards, external quality control as well as routine internal surveillance are highly desirable. Many countries have external quality assessment schemes which, in general, depend on the assessment of staining of selected antigens by the 'target' laboratory. The specimens are a combination of straightforward cases and of sections where more difficulty may be expected (e.g. the staining of surface Ig light chains on antigen-presenting cells).

This should enable laboratories to improve and standardize their technique in the light of peer review.

Automation

Immunohistochemistry came into the arena of automation relatively late (Figure 4.5). This was probably

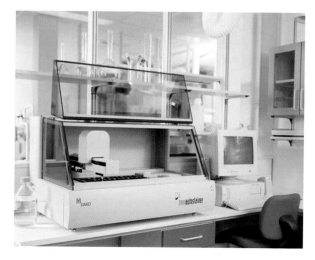

Figure 4.5 An automatic immunostainer, as produced by Dako Cytomation Ltd. Reproduced by permission of DAKO Cytomation Ltd

because initially relatively few antibodies were available that were suitable for routine use. Recently, however, any busy laboratory will have a large panel of reagents being applied to numerous section in any diagnostic 'run' and the call for automation has risen.

The earlier devices were semi-automated and largely served to save time. manipulation and reagent volumes by reducing, for example, the tedium of multiple buffer washes and so forth. Later, more automated machines have come onto the market. These are, of course, much more expensive than their predecessors but are microprocessor-controlled, programmable to the user's requirements and enable the processing, in some instances, of sections simultaneously with others undergoing other types of staining.

Imaging

It is now possible, increasingly, to quantify IHC staining. In the past, this has been most difficult, because of our

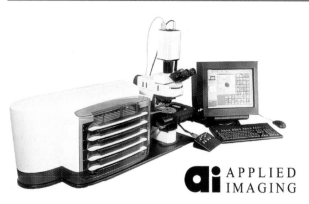

APPLIED
IMAGING

Figure 4.6   Applied Imaging's Ariol SL-50. Reproduced by permission of Applied Imaging

poor understanding of the stoichiometry of IHC reactions, especially at the chromogen-binding level. However, systems are now available, e.g. Applied Imaging's Ariol SL-50 (Figure 4.6), which allows quantification and analysis of IHC (and FISH) slides with high-throughput hardware and image analysis software. This also allows 'virtual networking', enabling multiple pathologists to evaluate panels of slides scanned by the system and to report their findings directly back into hospital systems.

Further reading

Leong AS-Y, Cooper K, Leong FJW-M. *Manual of Diagnostic Antibodies for Immunohistology*. 2003: Greenwich Medical Media, London.

Polak JM, van Noorden S. *Introduction to Immunocytochemistry*. 1997: Bios Scientific, Oxford.

Boenisch T (ed.). *Immunochemical Staining Methods*, 3rd edn 2001: DAKO corporation, California.

Dabbs DJ. *Diagnostic Immunohistochemistry*. 2002: Churchill Livingstone, New York.

5

Electron microscopy in pathology

Brian Eyden

Introduction

Human tissues or fluids containing human cells are sampled mainly for diagnostic purposes, i.e. for the identification of distinct categories of disease that can be recognized and treated by clinicians. A microscopically verified diagnosis is often necessary for optimizing patient management and, in the field of cancer at least, many purely clinical diagnoses are re-assigned by histopathological microscopical investigation.

The light microscopical examination of haematoxylin and eosin (H&E)-stained sections of tissue embedded in paraffin wax is the most important technical procedure for human solid tissue diagnosis. Here, a pathologist assesses cell and matrix appearances, including architecture, in the context of gross findings and clinical data to render a diagnosis. While light microscopy of H&E sections remains the basis of histological diagnosis, newer techniques, such as electron microscopy (EM), immunohistochemistry, AgNOR-staining, flow cytometry, cytogenetics and 'molecular' techniques [gene rearrangement analysis, fluorescence *in situ* hybridization and polymerase chain reaction (PCR) analysis] can now provide additional information to refine our understanding of disease and diagnosis.

Diagnostic electron microscopy has been important since the late 1960s and early 1970s. From the early 1980s, however, immunohistochemistry in particular has become an indispensable technique and has been responsible for a decline in the practice of EM. It is seen as the more convenient and useful technique and has therefore attracted resources that might otherwise have been directed towards EM. However, EM provides a unique kind of information—on morphology at the sub-cellular level—and can thus provide new information on disease, some of which has diagnostic applications. Partly, this is because there remain many conditions where purely morphological characteristics are important in diagnosis (Tables 5.1 and 5.2) but also because of the limitations of immunohistochemistry, a technique of particular importance in tumour diagnosis.

The current literature testifies to the continuing value of EM in both research and the diagnosis of cases of human disease that are problematical by light microscopy (Dar *et al.*, 1992; Hashimoto, 1994; Kandel *et al.*, 1998; Mierau, 1999; Eyden, 1999, 2002; Lloreta-Trull *et al.*, 2000; Tucker, 2000; Al-Sarraj *et al.*, 2001). The lack of an ultrastructural input arguably diminishes the performance of a diagnostic department, since EM can continually confirm or refute the light microscopy-based interpretations of pathologists. It thus raises the confidence with which a given diagnosis is held. It is a saying of some truth that EM makes pathologists *better* pathologists.

The extent to which EM is made use of in a routine diagnostic department is determined by the available expertise (both technical and interpretational) and significantly by the philosophy and background of the departmental head. There are those who have used EM in the past but now no longer rely on it, preferring immunohistochemistry and the newer molecular techniques to solve diagnostic problems—this despite the fact that immunohistochemistry continues to change in terms of technology and there is a question about the specificity of many of the antibodies used. By contrast, others use EM to a greater extent, and these usually

The Science of Laboratory Diagnosis, Second Edition   Edited by David Burnett and John Crocker
© 2005 John Wiley & Sons, Ltd

Table 5.1　Ultrastructural markers of cellular differentiation used in the identification of tumours

Cell type	Ultrastructural features
Squamous epithelium	Desmosomes, tonofibrils, basal lamina
Glandular epithelium	Apical junctional complex, microvilli, mucigen granules
Type 2 pneumocyte	Surfactant bodies (myelinosomes)
Mesothelium	Long, sinuous, smooth microvilli
Neuroendocrine cell	Neuroendocrine ("dense-core") granules
Schwann cell	Slender processes coated with external lamina
Adipocyte	Fat droplets, lamina
Striated muscle cell	Sarcomeres consisting of actin and myosin arrays and Z-disks
Smooth muscle cell	Fine myofilaments with focal densities, external lamina
Myofibroblast	Rough endoplasmic reticulum, myofilaments, fibronexus junctions
Fibroblast	Rough endoplasmic reticulum, collagen secretion granules
Endothelium	Weibel–Palade bodies
Neurone	Neuroendocrine granules, smooth endoplasmic reticulum, microtubules, synaptic junctions
Melanocyte	Melanosomes
Juxtaglomerular cell	Rhomboidal granules
Leydig cell	Crystals, lipid, smooth endoplasmic reticulum, tubular cristae
Granulosa cell	Desmosomes
Langerhans cell	Birbeck granules
Plasma cell	Golgi apparatus, rough endoplasmic reticulum
Macrophage	Lysosomes, filopodial processes
Lymphocyte	'Undifferentiated' cell (no distinctive organelles)

Adapted from Cameron and Toner (1998)

occupy positions in large or specialized institutions where either the large work-load or the referral nature of many of the specimens gives larger numbers of difficult cases.

Quantitating the value of EM is difficult. It has been said that up to 5% of all tumours, for instance, may be problematical enough to merit EM investigation, while 25% of non-neoplastic renal specimens may need EM (Pearson *et al.*, 1994). Whatever the numbers, EM should be applied whenever there is an interpretational difficulty in the H&E section. EM is always worth doing in these circumstances because it is never possible to predict in an individual case what results may emerge, and sometimes one experiences the delight of totally unexpected and new findings. Further, EM and immunohistochemistry (and all the other newer techniques) should be seen as complementary, and it is a widely expressed sentiment that information from, for example, both immunohistochemistry and EM can give a more complete picture of a lesion than either technique on its own. Sometimes the picture is complicated by the use of both techniques—they may conflict—but this can be regarded as a stimulus for further research.

Principles of EM technique and organization

Transmission electron microscopy—resolving power

Nearly all ultrastructural diagnostic work uses transmission electron microscopy (TEM), to demonstrate specific or characteristic cellular and matrix features, which may enhance our understanding and diagnosis of disease (Tables 5.1 and 5.2). In addition to TEM, there are some, although far fewer, applications in what one might call 'specialized' techniques: scanning EM, which is another 'morphological' kind of EM, and other techniques, giving information on elemental content (X-ray microanalysis) or biomolecular composition (immunocytochemistry and ultrastructural histochemistry) (Table 5.3). EM 'versions' of light microscopy procedures have also been developed, such as morphometry for providing quantitative information at the ultrastructural level (e.g. of nuclear irregularity in lymphomas).

In spite of the development of newer 'functional' ultrastructural techniques, EM is still mostly a morphological technique, like H&E histopathology. Like light

Table 5.2 Application of electron microscopy to non-neoplastic conditions

Renal disease	Capillary basement membrane thickness (e.g. thin basement membrane disease)
	Presence and location of immune deposits (e.g. membranous glomerulonephritis [GN)]
	Presence of extracellular fibrils (e.g. amyloid) cellular inclusions (e.g. myelin figures in Fabry's disease) Staging of certain diseases (e.g. membranous GN) foot processes (extensive fusion may be indicative of minimal change GN)
Neuromuscular disorders	Mitochondrial, congenital and metabolic myopathies
Skin disorders	Disorders of keratinization
	Mechanobullous dermatoses
	Hair and nail defects
Connective tissue disorders	Stromal disorders involving alterations of collagen, proteoglycans and elastin amyloidosis
Haematopoietic disorders	Platelet disorders
	Granulocytic anomalies
Inborn errors of metabolism	Accumulation of metabolites
	Potential for prenatal detection
Paediatric liver biopsies	Metabolic liver disease
	Reye's syndrome
Endomyocardial biopsies	Cardiomyopathies, amyloidosis
Respiratory diseases	Ciliary abnormalities
	Identification of lung particulates
Disorders of the central and peripheral nervous system	Dementias, neuropathies, CADISIL[*]
Reproductive medicine	Spermatozoan abnormalities
Infectious agents	Viruses, bacteria, protozoa, fungi

[*]Cerebral autosomal dominant arteriopathy with subcortical infarcts and leucoencephalopathy
Adapted from Cameron and Toner (1998)

Table 5.3 Specialised ultrastructural techniques and procedures

- Scanning electron microscopy
- Immunoelectron microscopy
- Ultrastructural histochemistry
- X-ray microanalysis and electron-diffraction
- Freeze-fracture/freeze-etching
- Ultrastructural *in situ* hybridization
- Ultrastructural morphometry

microscope. Consequently, structural details of the cell and matrix as small as a few nanometres in size can be imaged, which are beyond the ability of light microscopy to detect. Over the years, therefore, cell and matrix structures, which are distinctive or specific for a cell or a disease, have been identified and this accumulated mass of information forms the basis of diagnostic electron microscopy in both tumours and non-neoplastic disease (Tables 5.1 and 5.2).

microscopy, EM uses sections subjected to a form of radiation for observation. The radiation (the electron beam) interacts with the material in the section to produce an image, which can be interpreted to give information on the nature of the specimen. The significance of EM is that it uses an electron beam. Since resolving power is determined by radiation wavelength, in practice the resolving power of an electron microscope is about 100 times greater than that of a light

Image formation

In TEM, electrons in the illuminating ('incident') beam, on contacting the section, produce a number of interactions. Many simply pass through the section virtually unchanged. Others are deflected from their path ('elastically scattered') by areas or points of electron density in the section and filtered off from the post-incident beam by an appropriately positioned aperture (Figure 5.1a). The post-incident beam, therefore, possesses areas lacking electrons in comparison with the incident beam

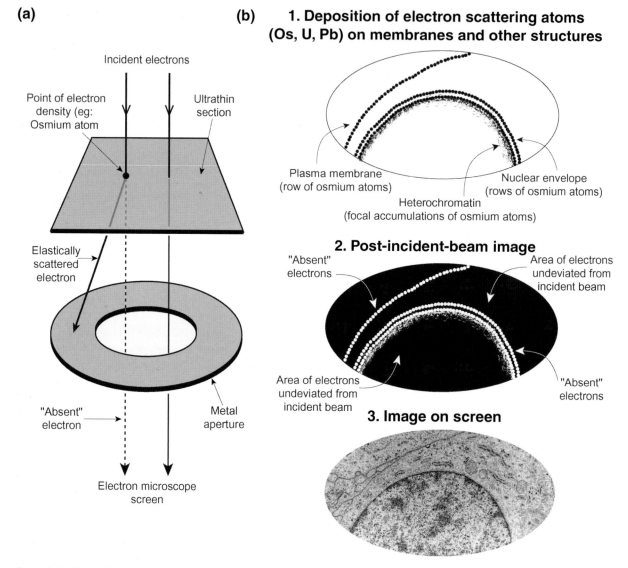

Figure 5.1 Image formation in the transmission electron microscope. Electrons in the incident beam contact the ultrathin section (a). Some pass through undeviated from their incident path (a), while those impacting on a point of density in the section (e.g. a heavy metal atom) are deviated out of the incident path (elastically scattered) and prevented from going onto the viewing screen by a metal aperture (a). The post-incident beam therefore contains information due to the combination of undeviated and elastically scattered electrons (b). Drawing by Paul Chantry

(Figure 5.1b), and this difference forms the basis of the image. Density within a section may be innate, as in a focus of mineralisation, or it can be introduced by chemical treatment of the tissue in the section. Mostly, this is done using osmium tetroxide solution (see Technique below) in which osmium atoms selectively attach to biological materials such as membranes. Consequently, a row of osmium atoms attached to a cell membrane will produce an image reflecting this line of 'absent' electrons in the post-incident beam

(Figure 5.1b), which in turn becomes a line on the electron microscope screen as electrons impact on the fluorescent coating of the viewing screen and are converted to visible light.

Technique

The techniques used to prepare tissue for thin-sectioning TEM have become fairly standardized in recent years. As in light microscopy, tissue needs to be fixed promptly to avoid autolysis and is first fixed in an aldehyde, a predominantly cross-linking protein fixative. It is accepted that glutaraldehyde, of a number of commercially available aldehydes, gives the best compromise of ultrastructural preservation and convenience of use. However, fixation of a biopsy or a resection specimen in glutaraldehyde requires staff and time in attending a surgical theatre or ward. Depending on staffing levels, it may be necessary to retrieve tissue from the main specimen in histological formalin. Provided this is buffered to physiological pH, the specimen is fairly small and the sample for EM is not taken from deep within a large specimen (where autolysis may alter tissue structure), preservation can be very good. The option of sampling from tissue in histological formalin precludes embedding the entire specimen in wax and requires a small representative piece to be held back for the eventuality of a diagnostic problem being encountered at the H&E level of investigation. This may not be feasible in a busy institution.

The specimen fixed in glutaraldehyde or retrieved from formalin needs to be cut up into small pieces ('mm-cubes'), since subsequent processing reagents tend to be slowly penetrating. The small samples available for study constitute one of the major limitations of EM. Following aldehyde fixation, selective contrast is introduced by an osmium tetroxide solution and sometimes also a uranyl acetate solution. These heavy metal atoms selectively attach to cell structures and thereby provide electron-scattering power and contrast. Although the reactions of these reagents with biological constituents are complex, osmium tetroxide is known to be a lipid fixative and one of its main functions is to delineate membranes by depositing osmium atoms on to bimolecular leaflets. Uranyl acetate is a phospholipid fixative and so also enhances membrane delineation, although, in addition, it fixes nucleic acids and thereby gives density to ribosomes and dexyribonucleoprotein ('chromatin') in the nucleus.

Following this *en bloc* staining and fixing, tissue is dehydrated in ethanol or acetone and infiltrated with a liquid epoxy resin, sometimes with a transitional solvent such as propylene oxide, toluene, or the less commonly used but less toxic limonene. The epoxy resin-infiltrated block of tissue is then thermally polymerized to a solid state. The infiltration steps can be carried out manually with tissue in small, capped, glass vials, with reagents replaced by pipette, or by an automated tissue processor. Recently introduced microwave-based instruments can process tissue to a polymerized block in a matter of

hours, comparable with typical immunohistochemistry procedures.

The epoxy resin blocks have the physical properties enabling sections to be cut on an ultramicrotome on hand-made disposable glass or permanent diamond knives. Sections with a thickness of about 80 nm are thin enough for the passage of electrons required for image formation, yet strong enough to withstand the heating effect of exposure to high-energy electrons. Sections are usually picked up on 3 mm diameter copper mesh grids, stained for additional contrast in uranyl acetate and lead citrate solutions (Maunsbach and Afzelius, 1999) and are then ready for examination in the electron microscope.

Handling of tissues before fixation

The processes of sampling and tissue handling prior to fixation can be crucial to obtaining well-selected and well-preserved tissue. This is of the highest importance, since interpretation is greatly facilitated by the quality of structural preservation. In spite of the desirability of using glutaraldehyde or even buffered histological formalin, it is sometimes necessary to retrieve tissue from the wax block. It is routine policy in some busy diagnostic institutions to block everything into wax, and this particularly applies to small specimens, where it is especially appropriate not to sample for EM in order to avoid compromising the light microscopy examination.

The rather brutal regime of hot xylene and wax inevitably damages some ultrastructure but some cell constituents can survive wax—desmosomes, tonofibrils, myofilaments, intermediate filaments, lumina, Birbeck granules, neuroendocrine granules and melanosomes. Certain purely membranous structures, such as smooth endoplasmic reticulum and mitochondria, are often poorly preserved but some plasma membranes can be well preserved or delineated and thus recognizable. A variation on retrieving from wax is the so called 'pop-off' method, in which an H&E section can be processed for electron microscopy and osmicated, dehydrated and infiltrated with resin on the glass slide. The section can then be 'popped off' into a conventional epoxy resin mould for subsequent ultrathin sectioning (see Further Reading). This technique can also be applied to smears, but is technically demanding.

Tissue that has been dried or frozen without cryopreservative agents, or left overnight before fixation, can be expected to be useless for EM (except that certain microorganisms may survive; see Figure 5.7b). However, cryoprotected tissue, which is frozen, then thawed, can give good ultrastructural results. Many other samples can be, or need to be, fixed in glutaraldehyde. The buffy coat from peripheral blood, semen, nasal and bronchial brushings, and the small fragments of tissue than can be seen in a fine-needle aspiration sample in a syringe are, from a procedural point of view, just as easily fixed in glutaraldehyde as formalin. Some specimens do not need to be fixed at all. Hermansky–Pudlak syndrome, a complex condition which includes platelet dysfunction, can be demonstrated simply by drying a platelet preparation on a film-coated grid and examining directly in the electron microscope for the distinctive granules and abnormal granule number (see Figure 5.9d).

Preliminaries to examining ultrathin sections

In solid-tissue histopathology, EM is seldom performed in isolation from other sources of diagnostic information. The pathologist needs to have all appropriate clinical information, must know the detailed histological appearances of the lesion and, in the case of tumours, will usually have immunohistochemical findings to hand when EM is being carried out. The idea of doing EM *before* immunohistochemistry in order to eliminate unnecessary immunostains is potentially useful and arguably logical but seems not to have become popular.

It is usual to precede ultramicrotomy with the cutting of 'semi-thin' sections. These are usually 1–2 µm in thickness, stained with toluidine blue or a similar stain, and examined in the light microscope. They provide confirmation that tissue is present of comparable morphology to that seen in the H&E section, or that cells are present which are expected on the basis of the clinical background where there is no H&E of a solid-tissue counterpart (e.g. in a body fluid specimen). With this procedure, unwanted foci of collagen or necrosis, commonly found in tumours, can be avoided. Finally, semi-thin sections can provide information on the quality of tissue preservation. Pale-staining cells and nuclei often indicate good preservation, whereas sharply delineated nuclei with clear interiors often indicate poor preservation (Eyden, 2002). In the investigation of a tumour, therefore, semi-thin sections from several blocks should be cut, and the most appropriate chosen on the basis of tumour cell content and quality of preservation. In complex lesions, it is desirable to cut ultrathin sections from blocks representing all of the histologically different areas.

Having ensured appropriate selection for ultramicrotomy, the pathologist or scientist examines ultrathin sections for cell structures or matrix constituents regarded as characteristic or specific for certain conditions. The identification of these structures relies on a detailed interpretational knowledge of cell and tissue ultrastructure, as well as a knowledge of the ultrastructural characteristics of specific diseases: this is an expertise which tends to be accumulated over a number of years. Where, in the UK for example, clinical scientists or biomedical scientists examine ultrathin sections under instruction from pathologists, close liaison and communication between these parties is essential. In the work-up of a complex tumour, for example, diagnostic ideas may change in the course of a few days as immunostains continue to become available.

Applications of transmission electron microscopy

Tumours

In tumour diagnosis, successful characterization of a given tumour depends on finding its distinctive cell and/or matrix structures. These are regarded as being the same as those found in the 'normal cellular counterpart'. So, for example, an intestinal carcinoid can be diagnosed by the neuroendocrine granules found in normal enteroendocrine cells (Figure 5.2), mammary carcinoma by the desmosomes, tonofibrils, basal lamina, lumina and mucigen granules (Figures 5.3a and 5.5) as in normal breast epithelium, and malignant melanoma by finding the melanosomes characteristic of normal melanocytes (Figure 5.3b). This is not to say that these tumours arise from these differentiated normal cells; rather, they are thought to originate from more primitively differentiated stem cells. A wide variety of tumours can be identified on the basis of their distinctive or specific ultrastructure (Table 5.1). Examples of specific organelles useful in tumour diagnosis are shown in Figures 5.2–5.5.

There are pitfalls in the ultrastructural diagnosis of tumours. Clearly, many tumours lose expected features as they become less differentiated. A typical examination protocol is carefully to examine one block (one grid of ultrathin sections) for 1 hour. However, tumours with decreasing levels of differentiation may need more extensive searching—several hours and multiple blocks, depending on the pathologist's perception of the clinical need of the diagnostic result. As a further complication, tumours may also express unexpected features, and thus show 'divergent' or 'anomalous' differentiation. The diagnostician must, therefore, have a knowledge of

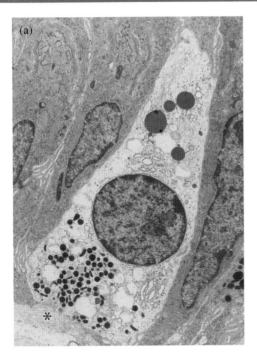
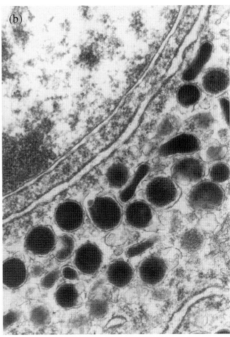

Figure 5.2 (a) Normal enteroendocrine cell from the normal human small intestine. The highly electron-dense inclusions near the basal pole of the cell (*) are neuroendocrine, hormone-containing granules. Note rounded and rod-shaped granules (×8700). (b) Small intestinal carcinoid tumour (metastatic to a mesenteric lymph node). Note the same kind of neuroendocrine granule morphology (×60 700)

these tumour features from personal experience and the literature. Nonetheless, EM is of greatest value in those tumours which, in the H&E section, appear poorly differentiated: these will tend to show weak or negative immunostaining for expected markers, and immunohistochemical confirmation of an H&E diagnosis may therefore be lacking. EM is also extremely important when immunostaining fails to indicate a clearly defined phenotype for reasons of uncertain antibody specificity, uncertainty in whether the staining is weakly positive or negative, or unexpected ('aberrant') staining. For example, variants of malignant melanoma, lymphoma and sarcoma exist which stain positively for the epithelial intermediate filament, cytokeratin, and ultrastructural investigation may be necessary to clarify the differentiation.

It is important to be aware of the presence of non-neoplastic cells in tumour tissue. Micrographs of endothelial cells and pericytes in vessel walls have appeared in the literature misinterpreted as tumour cells. Cells of normal tissues being invaded by tumour, or regenerating normal tissue cells (e.g. striated muscle cells), and inflammatory or reactive cells (e.g. macrophages, lymphocytes, plasma cells, myofibroblasts) must also be dis-

criminated as non-neoplastic. These will tend to be well differentiated, and such cells must be viewed with suspicion, especially if encountered in a poorly differentiated tumour.

Although any tumour showing some interpretational uncertainty by light microscopy merits assessment by EM, the technique has shown particular usefulness in a number of tumour groups—'anaplastic' round-epithelioid cell tumours; small-round-cell tumours; spindle-cell tumours; and the broad category of mesenchymal or soft-tissue lesions, including sarcomas. A number of the latter are fibroblastic and can be expected to show little immunopositivity other than for vimentin, a rather non-specific marker. Electron microscopy can also assist in suggesting the primary site of a metastatic neoplasm, while in central nervous system tumours, the identification of meningeal, Schwannian, neuronal, glial or ependymal features by EM is important for the neuropathologist, since immunohistochemistry has limited value in discriminating between these tumours (Cameron and Toner, 1998; Al-Sarraj *et al.*, 2001).

Finally, the value of EM in simple confirmation of a suspected diagnosis should not be underestimated. Diagnosing a lesion is not a black-and-white issue:

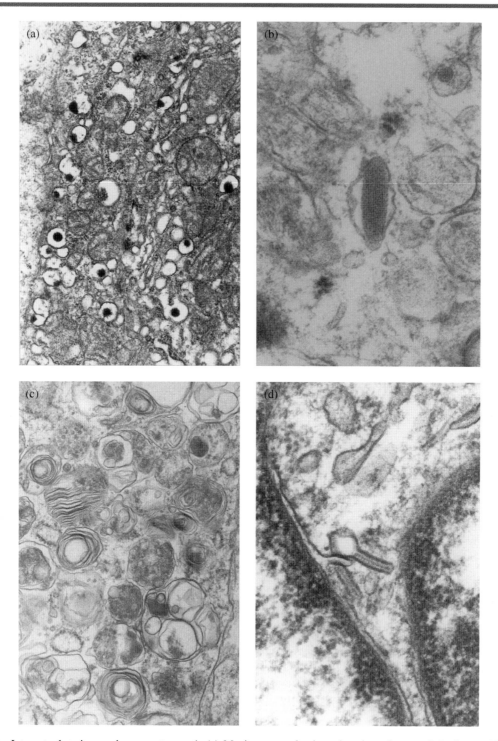

Figure 5.3   Intracytoplasmic membrane systems—1. (a) Mucigen granules in a ductal carcinoma of the breast. They have a dense proteinaceous core in a clear space. In keeping with their exocrine nature, they are often found near lumina, into which they discharge their contents (×24 000). (b) Melanosomes constitute the ultrastructural hallmark for melanocytic differentiation. This melanosome in a spindle-cell malignant melanoma is non-pigmented and is lying free in the cytoplasmic matrix (×98 000). Multiple melanosomes within a secondary lysosome (a compound melanosome) are evidence of uptake of exocytosed melanosomes, and are often found within macrophages or fibroblasts. (c) Lysosomes are markers of macrophages but many tumours ('granular cell tumours') can show abundant secondary lysosomes. This figure shows secondary lysosomes in a gastrointestinal stromal tumour (×36 000). (d) Birbeck granule in a Langerhans cell granulomatosis (×69 000)

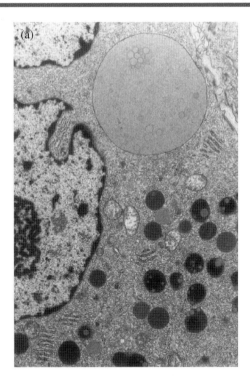
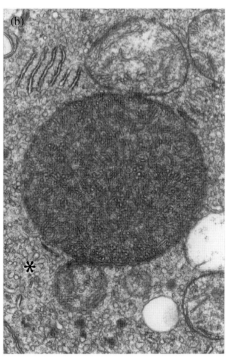

Figure 5.4 Intracytoplasmic membrane systems—2. Black adenoma of the adrenal cortex in a patient with Cushing's syndrome. The steroidogenic phenotype consists of lipid (a), smooth endoplasmic reticulum (* in b) and mitochondria with tubular cristae (see the giant mitochondrion in b), and is mainly found in Leydig cells, hilar cells and adrenocortical tumours. Lipofuscin is also common in these tumours and is responsible for the pigmentation in this tumour. Note also the short stacks of rough endoplasmic reticulum (a, ×10 000; b, ×30 000)

pathologists hold diagnoses with a certain level of confidence, and this can be increased by an ultrastructural input.

Non-neoplastic disease

Currently, EM applied to non-neoplastic disease is perhaps in a more secure position than EM applied to tumours, since in tumour pathology, immunohistochemistry and molecular techniques are encroaching on to formerly secure ultrastructural territory. Whereas in tumour diagnosis the primary objective is often the determination of the tumour's cellular differentiation, in non-neoplastic disease there are many applications where multiple forms of structural change within a single organelle, cell or tissue can be identified (cilia, glomerular epithelium, striated muscle cell, peripheral nerve), which are indicative of different diseases. Hence, EM can have a more critical rôle, and one perhaps less dependent on immunohistochemistry and molecular biology. Figures 5.6–5.9 include examples of diagnostic EM applied to non-neoplastic disease. Similar points

of procedure apply to examining non-neoplastic disease in terms of confirmation of the presence of lesional cells and their quality of preservation from semi-thin sections, just as in tumours. Many non-neoplastic diseases, however, are studied by means of fluids, and here a judgement needs to be made of the cells to be expected in semi-thin sections on the basis of the clinical background.

EM has long had a value in identifying microorganisms. Among the most clinically significant in terms of numerical incidence are viruses, which have traditionally been identified using the quick and precise technique of negative staining (see Chapter 18 for details). Other microscopic organisms can have their diagnosis confirmed or details of their structure revealed by EM: they include bacteria such as spirochaetes (Figure 5.7a), protozoa such as *Cryptosporidium*, microsporidia and *Leishmania* (in AIDS), and fungi such as *Candida* and *Pneumocystis* (Figure 5.7b).

The distinction between diagnosis, on the one hand, and research or technological development, on the other, is sometimes blurred, and EM has a role in such development. It has usefulness, for example, in assessing

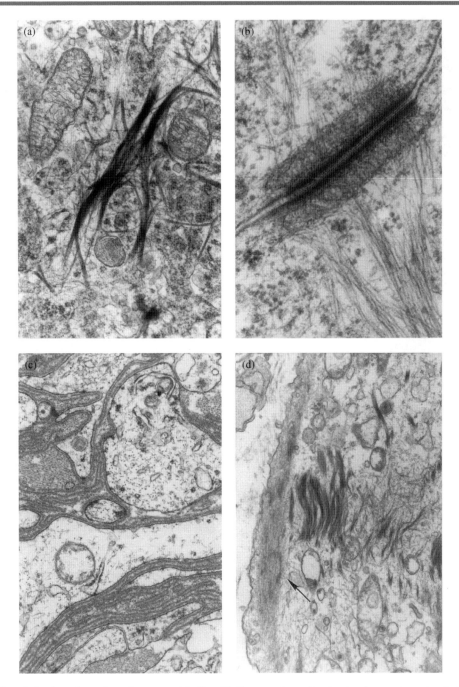

Figure 5.5 Cytoskeletal and surface features. (a) Tonofibrils are the ultrastructural counterpart of the cytokeratin immunostaining that can help to identify epithelial differentiation in tumours. Tonofibrils often contact desmosomes and thereby promote cellular cohesion, a feature typical of carcinomas. Pseudo-angiosarcomatous squamous cell carcinoma (×31 900). (b) The desmosome is the most important intercellular junction for identifying epithelial differentiation. It has submembranous plaques, an 'intermediate line' in the space between apposed plasma membranes, and tonofibrils attaching the plaques to the perinuclear cytoskeleton. Epithelial mesothelioma (×99 000). (c) Lamina is a distinctive coating of cells such as epithelium, endothelium, Schwann and perineurial cells, adipocytes and muscle cells. It is absent from fibroblasts, myofibroblasts, chondroblasts, osteoblasts and neurones, and thus has diagnostic importance. In this benign Schwannoma, multiple layers of lamina surround cell processes (×30 000). (d) Smooth-muscle myofilaments with their distinctive focal densities are important markers of smooth-muscle cell differentiation. They are also seen in myoepithelial cells, pericytes, myofibroblasts and interstitial cells of Cajal, and their tumours. Note the finer myofilaments (arrow) in contrast to the coarser cytokeratin filaments forming tonofibrils in this spindle-cell squamous carcinoma (×20 100)

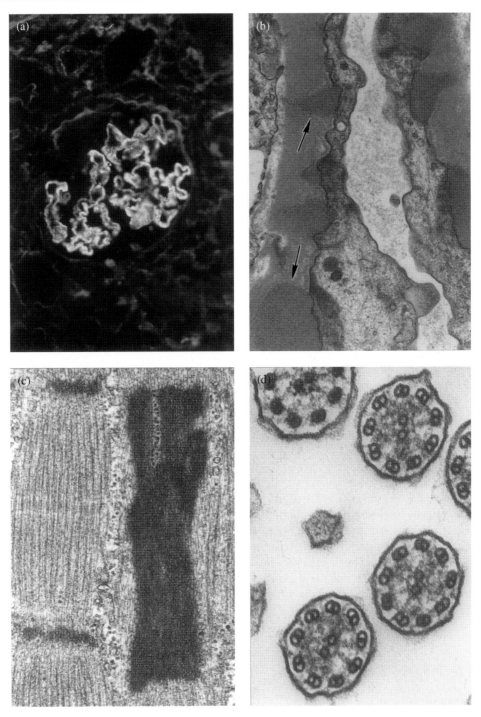

Figure 5.6   Non-neoplastic electron microscopy—tissue pathology. (a,b) Membranous glomerulonephritis. (a) Immune deposits after immunofluorescence light microscopy using a fluorescein-labelled anti-IgG antibody. (b) Corresponding transmission electron micrograph of glutaraldehyde-fixed tissue showing subepithelial immune deposits (arrows) of a discrete organization mirroring the light microscopy. Note thickening of the basement membrane and loss of podocyte foot processes (×25 000). Photographs courtesy of Dr Alan Curry. (c) Nemaline rod myopathy in a 15 year-old girl. Clinical presentation included a delay in motor milestones, walking on toes, frequent falls and leg-aches after exercise. The nemaline rod here is dense, shows cross-striations and is regarded as an abnormality of the Z-disk. Normal Z-disks and sarcomeres are seen here for comparison (×60 000). Photograph courtesy of Dr Liz Curtis. (d) Primary ciliary dyskinesia syndrome. Note absence of dynein arms from peripheral doublets (×160 000). Photograph courtesy of Ann Dewar

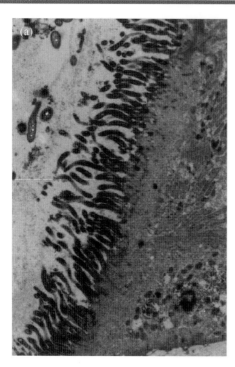 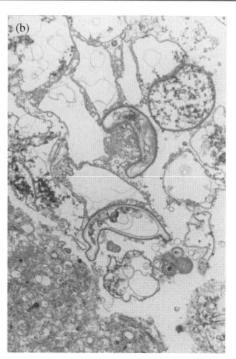

Figure 5.7   Non-neoplastic electron microscopy—infectious organisms. (a) Spirochaetosis in a biopsy from the large intestine (×8 800). (b) *Pneumocystis* from autopsy lung tissue. This tissue had inadvertently been left overnight without fixation. Consequently, although most of the tissue is poorly preserved (as expected), the *Pneumocystis* organisms are still identifiable by their distinctive curved profiles. Here, appearance in an immunocompromised cancer patient suggests an opportunist infection (×7 500)

the quality of structural preservation of oocytes in ovarian cortex surgically removed and cryopreserved *in vitro* in young female cancer patients for the duration of their chemotherapy. Antenatal diagnosis can be achieved from cells harvested from amniotic fluid (Cameron and Toner, 1998), while there is a growing interest in the ultrastructural characterization of stem cells in the emerging field of tissue engineering.

Specialized techniques and procedures

Table 5.3 lists techniques which are designated as 'specialised' in that they are not as widely used in diagnostic laboratories as TEM, and which have fewer truly diagnostic applications. In many instances, the images from these techniques confirm a fairly secure diagnosis based primarily on clinical and histopathological findings, but they often nevertheless add new details, which can enhance the understanding of disease. They are clearly of potential value in research, and it

should be remembered that research findings are sometimes precursors of diagnostic tests. These techniques tend to be found in diagnostic laboratories that may also have research responsibilities, where research has led to expertise in the technique, and personnel trained and experienced in the technique are onhand to exploit the technique in rare diagnostic questions when they arise (see Further Reading).

Scanning electron microscopy (SEM)

SEM gives three-dimensional information, especially on surface features, and very often, therefore, the images are more easily interpretable (Figure 5.8a) than those from TEM, where there is a need to extrapolate an interpretation from thin sections and where also there may be interpretational difficulty due to suboptimal orientation. Tissue is usually fixed in a similar way to that for TEM, but at the end of the dehydration stage, ethanol is replaced with liquid carbon dioxide, most usually under pressure in a *critical point dryer*. At the critical

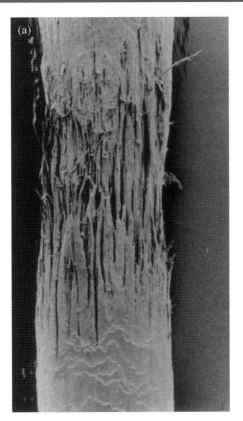 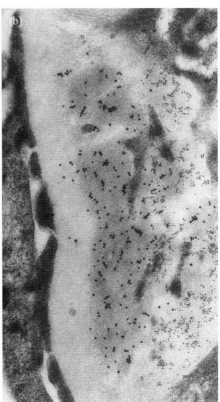

Figure 5.8 Special techniques—1. (a) Scanning electron microscopy. Human hair shaft. The patient was investigated for pili torti, where the hair shaft is twisted and fragile, but SEM analysis indicated trichorrhexis nodosa, with damage presumed to be due to mechanical or chemical trauma ($\times 830$). (b) Immunoelectron microscopy. Double-staining TEM of mesangial region of a glomerulus from a patient with mesangial IgA nephropathy to show double immunolocalization of type IV collagen (10 nm gold) within the mesangial matrix and IgA (20 nm gold) within the electron-dense deposit ($\times 33\,000$). Micrographs courtesy of Dr Jill Moss and Ian Shore

point, liquid and gaseous carbon dioxide form a continuum, which allows drying of the specimen in a way that avoids the distortions of cell and tissue structure which would otherwise arise from conventional drying. The dried specimen is then coated with a thin layer of evaporated metal (gold, palladium, platinum or chromium), which helps to remove the build-up of charge during exposure to the electron beam. The tissue, usually fixed to a metal base (a *stub*), is then ready to be inserted into the scanning electron microscope. In contrast to the incident beam in a TEM, the electron beam in SEM is scanned over the specimen in a raster-type ('TV') fashion. This causes the emission of secondary electrons, which are collected by an electron-detector and converted into an observable image on a cathode ray tube. In addition to surface contour and detail, scanning electron microscopes offer the advantage of lower magnification

(tens or hundreds) compared with those traditionally available for TEM and so can be used for whole pathological specimens.

Diagnostic applications of SEM are limited. They include the examination of human hair (Fig. 5.8a) and the identification of respiratory particulates, particularly asbestos fibres, which can also be studied by X-ray microanalysis for identifying chemical or elemental composition. The findings may have legal significance in connection with industrial exposure (Ingram *et al.*, 1989). The claimed ability to distinguish B and T cells and mesothelioma and adenocarcinoma on the basis of differential cell surface morphology has not been widely exploited in routine practice. Table 5.4 gives some of the many examples of SEM applied to human cells and tissues which have contributed data to understanding disease without leading to true routine diagnostic tests.

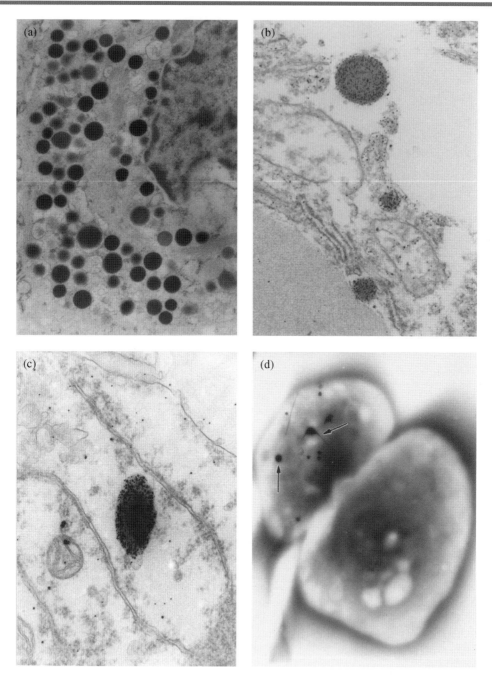

Figure 5.9   Special techniques—2. Ultrastructural histochemistry. (a) Uranaffin procedure for neuroendocrine granules in a mucoid carcinoma of breast (×25 700). (b) EM Grimelius stain to distinguish neuroendocrine granules from lactational secretion granules in an amphicrine carcinoma of breast (×39 600). (c) Warthin–Starry stain modified for EM to demonstrate melanin in a malignant melanoma (×45 000). (d) Whole, unfixed, unstained platelets on a Formvar-coated grid. The patient had acquired Hermansky–Pudlak-like syndrome secondary to a myelodysplastic condition. The granules (arrows) are rich in calcium, which provides inherent electron density. Mean granule count was 3.8 per platelet (normal value, 5.3). Note dense granules in one platelet and absence in the adjacent platelet, and one granule with "tails" (×17 700). Micrograph courtesy of Bart E Wagner

Table 5.4 Applications of SEM to human clinical material

- Asbestos fibres and other respiratory particulates
- Distinguishing B and T cells through cell surface morphology
- Mesothelial and adenocarcinomatous microvilli
- Spermatozoan abnormalities
- Urothelium and urothelial carcinoma
- Endometrial hyperplasia
- Benign prostatic hyperplasia, and intraluminal crystals in prostatic carcinoma
- Renal papillae/ducts of Bellini
- Oesophageal and intestinal surfaces
- *Giardia lamblia* on the duodenal surface
- Spirochaetosis
- *Cryptosporidium*
- Crohn's disease
- Acute appendicitis
- Synovial tissue and cells in rheumatoid arthritis and gout
- Calcium pyrophosphate crystals in cartilage and meniscal tissue
- Mitochondria in oncocytes
- Leukaemic cell (hairy cell) surfaces

Immunoelectron microscopy

Immunoelectron microscopy (ultrastructural immunolabelling, 'immunoEM') provides simultaneously the morphological data of conventional TEM and information on biomolecular composition as in light microscopical immunohistochemistry. ImmunoEM data, like those from SEM, tend to be confirmatory, or add to the scientific understanding of a clinical condition. However, the potential of the technique to confirm a diagnosis, to remove some interpretational uncertainty and to enhance the confidence with which a diagnosis is held, is very great. In practice, however, staffing levels and funding currently available to EM compromise the use of diagnostic immunoEM, which also requires more than usual attention to technical and procedural detail. The range of proteins identifiable in clinical material by immunoEM is given in Table 5.5.

One of the simplest forms of immunoEM is to dewax and process a light microscopy immunohistochemically-stained section from a glass slide. This is technically challenging and tends to give poor structural preservation. Sometimes also, identifying the immunostain, which is electron-dense as a result of having been exposed to osmium tetroxide, can be less than straightforward. The best techniques use a specific antibody labelled with colloidal gold particles. The gold particles

Table 5.5 Applications of immunoEM in clinical/pathological settings

- Hormone content in neuroendocrine granules in tumours
- Immunoglobulins and complement deposits in plasma cells, lymphoma, renal disease and crystalloidal keratopathy; amyloid in plasmacytoma
- Cytoskeletal proteins (smooth-muscle actin, α-actinin, cytokeratin, vimentin, desmin and neurofilament protein) in non-neoplastic and tumour cells
- Fibronectin at the surface of myofibroblasts
- Laminin and type IV collagen in basement membranes
- Intercellular adhesion molecules (e.g. ICAM-1, CD44) in reactive and neoplastic cells
- Cell surface molecules (CD4, CD8, CD56) in acute graft versus host disease
- The vasopressor and vasoconstrictive protein, endothelin-1, in adrenal gland
- The differentiation antigen, urokinase receptor, in neutrophils
- The anti-apoptotic protein, BCL2, in thyroid tumours
- von Willebrand factor in Weibel–Palade bodies in endothelium
- Lysozyme and mucins in glandular epithelial lesions
- Lactoferrin and lysozyme in myelomonocytic leukaemia
- Myeloperoxidase in myeloid leukaemia
- Charcot–Leyden crystal protein (lysophospholipase) in basophils
- Cathepsin D in lysosomes in vascular smooth-muscle cells in arterio–venous anastomoses
- Nitric oxide synthase in the human seminal vesicle
- Rotaviruses in human faecal extracts

are mostly 5, 10 or 20 nm diameter and, once localised on tissue sections, are very readily identified on the electron microscope screen by their sharply delineated contour, which also makes for ease of focusing and photography (Figure 5.8b).

Care needs to be taken to enhance antigen preservation. Proteins vary considerably in the preservation of their immunoreactivity and the extent, therefore, to which they can be demonstrated by immunoEM. Tissue available fresh should be fixed in newly prepared paraformaldehyde solution. Many antigens will survive histological formalin, though, and tissue can be retrieved from the main histological specimen. Heavy metal fixatives are not used, to avoid further protein denaturation, and dehydration is often not taken beyond 70% ethanol before embedding in a hydrophilic resin such as LR White$^{®}$. This is subjected to minimal thermal polymerization before cutting ultrathin sections and applying the appropriate gold-bearing reagents. Lowicryl$^{®}$ is an alternative hydrophilic resin, with, some claim, superior ultrastructural preservation, and, given that it is a low-temperature hydrophilic resin, better antigen preservation. The most demanding form of immunoEM uses frozen ultrathin sections (cryoultramicrotomy). ImmunoEM can also be carried out on ultrathin sections from epoxy resin-embedded tissue conventionally processed for TEM, often using reagents which etch the resin and expose antigenic sites.

Ultrastructural histochemistry

Ultrastructural histochemistry (electron histochemistry) is analogous to classical light microscopy histochemistry but provides information on the chemical or biochemical nature of cells and tissues at the ultrastructural level. In order to achieve this, the techniques require an electron-dense marker, usually a compound containing electron-scattering metal atoms. A wide range of substances in cells and tissues, including enzymes, have been identified by ultrastructural histochemistry (Table 5.6). Rather like immunoEM, the published studies demonstrating these substances lie in the field of research, rather than having a true routine value in diagnostic histopathology. However, as with immunoEM, individuals or laboratories with special interests, experience or research links are likely to find diagnostic applications for these techniques.

Handling techniques vary considerably, depending on the substance being demonstrated. For enzymes, such as platelet peroxidase, specialized fixatives (e.g. one containing tannic acid, formaldeyhyde and a low concentration of glutaraldehyde) may be required. For glycogen,

Table 5.6   Ultrastructural histochemistry: applications in clinical material

- Uranaffin reaction (uranyl acetate) for neuroendocrine granules
- Modified uranyl acetate–lead citrate for selective staining of nucleic acids
- Grimelius stain (silver stain) for neuroendocrine granules
- Warthin–Starry technique for melanin
- L-DOPA reaction modified for EM for tyrosinase and melanosomes
- Platelet peroxidase in the differential diagnosis of leukaemias
- Ethanolic phosphotungstic acid for synapses
- Osmium-potassium ferrocyanide procedure for glycogen
- Imidazole-buffered osmium tetroxide for lipid
- Acid phosphatase for lysosomes (e.g. in large granular lymphocytes)
- Ruthenium red, cuprolinic blue, silver methenamine, iron diamine for polysaccharide moieties

the osmium tetroxide fixative can be modified by the addition of potassium ferrocyanide, while for lipids, which are lost during typical TEM processing, an imidazole-buffered osmium tetroxide solution can be used. By contrast, in the Uranaffin reaction for neuroendocrine granules (Figure 5.9a), glutaraldehyde is preferable to histological formalin, since molecules may be lost from tissue retrieved from formalin, leading to a weak reaction.

The Uranaffin procedure is a useful EM stain for neuroendocrine granules, given that these show ultrastructural heterogeneity and can sometimes be difficult to distinguish from primary lysosomes, small lactational secretion granules and small serous granules. The technique is based on the hypothesis that the neuroendocrine granule core consists of a complex of hormone, core protein and nucleotides (Payne, 1993). The negative charges of the latter bind the positively charged uranyl ions to provide electron-density. All free phosphate needs to be washed out after aldehyde fixation, before steeping the tissue in concentrated uranyl acetate solution (for up to 2 days), and no other electron-density-imparting stains should be used. Ribosomes and nuclear chromatin, by virtue of their nucleotide content, can act as positive internal controls. Silver-staining techniques at the ultrastructural level are also available for neuroendocrine granules and melanin (Figures 5.9b, c).

X-ray microanalysis and electron diffraction

One of the interactions of electrons with the atoms of a physical specimen leads to a re-arrangement of energy levels in the electron shells around the atoms, resulting in the emission of X-rays. These are characteristic of the atomic number, and thereby establish the chemical, elemental nature of the material under investigation. A variety of elements can be identified with clinical significance using this technique, most important being respiratory particulates, including the various forms of asbestos fibre (Ingram *et al.*, 1989; Cameron and Toner, 1998). Often, it may be necessary to digest tissue to release fibres for analysis.

The technique of electron diffraction is potentially useful in demonstrating a periodicity and therefore the crystalline nature within an electron-exposed object, as a result of which diffraction patterns consisting of precisely spatially arranged spots of high intensity are observed. This information can discriminate substances of different chemical composition.

Freeze-fracture/freeze-etching

In the freeze-fracture/freeze-etching technique, tissue is rapidly frozen and then fractured by impacting a sharp edge on to it in a specifically designed and commercially available instrument. The fracture plane passes through or over membrane systems and provides a surface for observation following metal-shadowing. Metal-shadowing can be delayed following etching, to reveal larger areas of true membrane surfaces in addition to the surfaces of cleaved membranes. There are no truly diagnostic applications, but the technique has been applied to human cells and tissues to provide new information on cell membrane organization: e.g. exocytosis of neuroendocrine granules from cells and altered gap and tight junctions in human thyroid oncocytic tumours (Cochand-Priollet *et al.*, 1998).

Summary

This chapter has had the objective of conveying a sense of the contemporary value of electron microscopy in routine diagnosis in the field of pathology. Some of the scientific theory of these practical ultrastructural techniques has been given to facilitate the interpretation of electron micrographic images. In spite of the continual development of new techniques, especially in immuno-histochemistry and molecular biology, electron microscopy continues to be valuable in the diagnosis of lesions that are found to be problematical at the clinical or light microscopical levels of investigation. It is a matter of direct experience on the part of those who practise electron microscopy that lesions continue to be encountered where clinical and immunohistochemical findings conflict or are non-contributory, to the extent of giving an imprecise diagnosis: this can, in some circumstances, be refined by electron microscopy (and this despite the technique's own major sampling limitation). In the field of tumour diagnosis, some of these difficulties are due to limitations of immunohistochemistry, upon which the tumour pathologist currently relies heavily: this is a technique which, unlike electron microscopy, has not yet evolved to the stage of technological stability. In the larger field of non-neoplastic conditions—renal and neuromuscular disease, infectious organisms, ciliary diseases, dermatopathology, to mention perhaps the main ones—electron microscopy exerts a stronger influence in being less dependent on immunohistochemistry: here, electron microscopy can identify a multiplicity of structural changes within a given cell or tissue which can be related to distinct diseases.

By far the majority of applications are in transmission electron microscopy for morphology. Several other specialized techniques exist, however, which have contributed to enhancing our understanding of the structural cell biology of human tissues and lesions, but they harbour far fewer truly diagnostic applications.

Finally, electron microscopy is an essential contributory technique to the comprehensive diagnostic analysis of human lesions. In this context, it needs to be emphasized that while the analysis of gene expression is going to be fundamental to understanding disease, that understanding will be the more complete if we accept that the lesions we see in the H&E or ultrathin section result not only from gene expression but also from post-genomic activities: these activities can most effectively be demonstrated by phenotypic techniques, such as the immunohistochemical demonstration of functional proteins and their elaboration into functional cell structures by electron microscopy.

Acknowledgements

I would like to thank the following colleagues for their invaluable assistance in the preparation of this chapter: Dr Alan Curry (Manchester Royal Infirmary), Dr Liz Curtis (Queen Elizabeth Hospital, Birmingham), Ann Dewar (Royal Brompton Hospital, London), Dr Jill Moss and Ian Shore (Charing Cross Hospital, London), and Bart E Wagner (Northern General Hospital, Sheffield), for providing electron micrographs; and Paul Chantry and Elizabeth White (both Christie Hospital) for drawing Figure 5.1 and for assistance with literature searching and photographic printing, respectively. I am indebted to Dr Jill Moss, Dr Alan Curry and Professor Peter Toner for valuable comments on the manuscript, and I acknowledge the importance of the original chapter by Dr Stuart Cameron and Professor Peter Toner as the starting point for this work.

References

Al-Sarraj S, King A, Martin AJ *et al.*, Ultrastructural examination is essential for the diagnosis of papillary meningioma. *Histopathology* 2001; **38**: 318–324.

Cameron CHS, Toner P. Electron microscopy in pathology. In *The Science of Laboratory Diagnosis*, Crocker J, Burnett D (eds). 1998: Isis Medical Media, Oxford, 45–66.

Cochand-Priollet B, Raison D, Molinie V *et al.*, Altered gap and tight junctions in human thyroid oncocytic tumors: a study of 8 cases by freeze-fracture. *Ultrastruct Pathol* 1992; **22**: 413–420.

Dar AUH, Hird PM, Wagner BE, Underwood JCE. Relative usefulness of electron microscopy and immunohistochemistry in tumour diagnosis: 10 years of retrospective analysis. *J Clin Pathol* 1992; **45**: 693–696.

Eyden B. Electron microscopy in tumour diagnosis: continuing to complement other diagnostic techniques (part of "Expert Opinion" Feature: Electron microscopy for tumour diagnosis: is it redundant?). *Histopathology* 1999; **35**: 102–108.

Eyden B. Electron microscopy in the diagnosis of tumours. *Curr Diagn Pathol.* 2002; **8**: 216–224.

Hashimoto K. Diagnostic electron microscopy in dermatology. *Dermatol Clin* 1994; **12**: 143–159.

Kandel R, Bedard Y, Fan Q-H. Value of electron microscopy and immunohistochemistry in the diagnosis of soft tissue tumors. *Ultrastruct Pathol* 1998; **22**: 141–146.

Lloreta-Trull J, Ferrer L, Ribalta T *et al.* Electron microscopy in pathology articles: a retrospective appraisal. *Ultrastruct Pathol* 2000; **24**: 105–108.

Mierau G. Electron microscopy for tumour diagnosis: not redundant—resurgent! (Part of "Expert Opinion" feature: Electron microscopy for tumour diagnosis: is it redundant?). *Histopathology* 1993; **35**, 99–102.

Payne CM. Use of the uranaffin reaction in the identification of neuroendocrine granules. *Ultrastruct Pathol* 1993; **17**: 49–82.

Pearson JM, McWilliam LJ, Coyne JD, Curry A. Value of electron microscopy of renal disease. *J Clin Pathol* 1994; **47**: 126–128.

Tucker JA. The continuing value of electron microscopy in surgical pathology. *Ultrastruct Pathol* 2000; **24**, 383–389.

Further reading

Dickersin GR. *Diagnostic Electron Microscopy. A Text/Atlas*, 2nd edn. 2000: Springer Verlag, Heidelberg.

Erlandson RA. *Diagnostic Transmission Electron Microscopy of Human Tumors.* 1994: Raven, New York.

Eyden B. *Organelles in Tumor Diagnosis: an Ultrastructural Atlas.* 1996: Igaku-Shoin, New York and Tokyo.

Ghadially FN. Ultrastructural pathology of the cell and matrix, 4th edn. 1997: Butterworth-Heinemann, Boston, MA.

Griffiths G. *Fine Structure Immunocytochemistry.* 1993: Springer-Verlag, Berlin.

Ingram P, Shelburne JD, Roggli VI. *Microprobe Analysis in Medicine.* Ultrastructural Pathology Publication Series. 1989: Hemisphere, New York.

King R. *Atlas of Peripheral Nerve Pathology* 1999: Arnold, London.

Lewis PR, Knight DP. *Cytochemical Staining Methods for Electron Microscopy.* Elsevier Science, Amsterdam.

Maunsbach AB, Afzelius BA. *Biomedical Electron Microscopy. Illustrated Methods and Interpretations.* 1999: Academic Press, San Diego, CA.

Papadimitriou JM, Henderson DW, Spagnolo DV. *Diagnostic Ultrastructure of Non-neoplastic Diseases* 1992: Churchill-Livingstone, London.

Polak JM, Priestly JV. *Electron Microscopic Immunocytochemistry. Principles and Practice.* 1992: Oxford University Press, Oxford.

Schröder JM. *Pathology of Peripheral Nerves.* 2001: Springer-Verlag, Heidelberg.

Society of Ultrastructural Pathology Handbook Committee. *Handbook of Diagnostic Electron Microscopy for Pathologists-in-training.* 1996: Igaku-Shoin Medical Publishers, New York and Tokyo, in conjunction with the Society for Ultrastructural Pathology.

Special issues of journals devoted to or containing electron microscopy articles

- *Curr Diagn Pathol* 2002; **8**(4): contains a mini-symposium on diagnostic electron microscopy.

- *Semin Diagn Pathol* 2002; **20**(1) is devoted to electron microscopy of tumours.

- *Hum Pathol* 1998; **29**(12) contains an electron microscopy symposium on tumours.

- *Ultrastruct Pathol* 1992; **16** contains articles on specialized EM techniques, including immunoelectron microscopy, ultrastructural *in situ* hybridization, the 'pop-off' technique, ultrastructural morphometry.

Articles on specialized ultrastructural techniques

Techniques and procedures such as those listed in Table 5.3 can be found in specialized journals such as *Ultrastruct Pathol, J Submicrosc Cytol Pathol* and *Med Electron Microsc*.

6

Light microscopy

Brian Boullier

Introduction

The light microscope has come a long way since Hans and Zacharias Janssen created the first 'compound' microscope in 1590. Unlike a simple magnifying glass, it consisted of a tube with a separate lens at each end. Clinical scientists have subsequently benefited from radical improvements in microscope design, construction and technique, particularly during the past 100 years.

The compound light microscope is the standard workhorse of every modern clinical laboratory, with specimens most commonly observed using brightfield illumination. However, the rapidly increasing availability of diagnostic tools, such as fluorescently-labelled monoclonal antibodies, has required the clinical scientist to become routinely proficient in a broader range of microscope techniques in recent years.

This chapter will introduce the basic concepts of microscope design, briefly explain the rationale behind the most common procedures currently encountered in the clinical laboratory, and discuss various areas of application. The reader may wish to consult additional references (Bradbury and Bracegirdle, 1998; Determan and Lerpusch, 1988; Lacey, 1999) for a more extensive description and fuller explanation of each technique.

Basic microscope design

At its simplest, the compound microscope consists of two lens systems, the objective lens, which forms a real image of the specimen, and the eyepiece, which forms an image at infinity that can be viewed by the operator.

The overall magnification is the product of the magnification of these two groups of lenses. In practice the typical laboratory microscope contains additional lens groups, prisms and beam splitters, which may or may not affect overall magnification but which invariably improve the optical performance of the instrument and/or convenience of operation (by slanting the eyepieces towards the operator, for example).

Microscope performance is more correctly described in terms of resolving power—the capability of the microscope to discriminate between two points separated by a minute distance. At best, the unaided human eye can resolve two points as close as $150\,\mu m$ apart. The wavelength range of visible light and the numerical aperture of microscope lenses together combine to constrain the maximum theoretical resolution of the light microscope to $0.22\,\mu m$, irrespective of maximum magnification.

Most modern microscopes are modular in construction. This offers several benefits to the user, including the facility to expand the capabilities of the microscope to meet future demands. Perhaps more importantly, this allows the initial purchase budget to be biased towards obtaining the highest quality optics possible—after all, a fully-featured microscope is only as good as the quality of its lens systems. Future upgrades might include alternative sources of illumination and associated optical systems or perhaps the addition of a personal computer, software and digital still or video camera—the integration of personal computers with optical microscopes facilitates both the automated optimization of microscope settings and convenient image acquisition as well as affordable data storage and powerful image analysis.

The Science of Laboratory Diagnosis, Second Edition   Edited by David Burnett and John Crocker
© 2005 John Wiley & Sons, Ltd

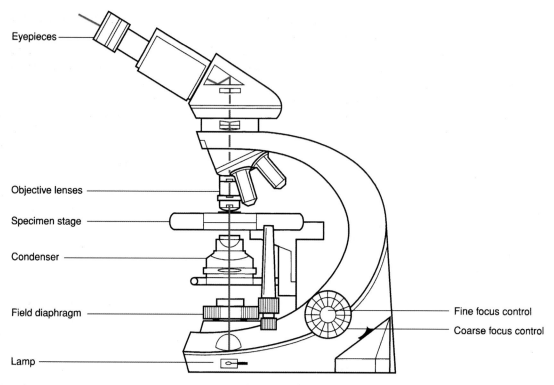

Eyepieces

Objective lenses

Specimen stage

Condenser

Field diaphragm

Fine focus control

Coarse focus control

Lamp

Figure 6.1 Cross-sectional diagram of a typical laboratory microscope (Courtesy of Leica UK Ltd)

Figure 6.1 illustrates the major parts of the typical laboratory microscope. Several parts deserve explanation, viz. the objective lenses, eyepieces, condenser, field diaphragm and light source(s).

The *objective lenses* are the most important part of the microscope, determining the various magnifications possible and defining the optical quality achievable to the rest of the instrument. Typically ×10, ×40 and ×100 objective lenses are attached to a rotating turret. This gives overall magnifications of ×100, ×400 and ×1000, respectively, when ×10 eyepieces are used.

The properties of each objective lens are usually inscribed on the lens barrel. Markings can include:

- The manufacturer's name.

- 'Fluotar', 'Fluor', 'Neofluar' or 'UV', which mean that the lens will transmit ultraviolet light and is therefore suitable for fluorescence microscopy.

- 'Phaco', 'Phase' or 'Ph', which indicates the presence of a phase ring and that the lens is suitable for phase contrast microscopy (an accompanying number, e.g. Ph 2, specifies the phase contrast condenser aperture to use).

- 'Plan', which means that the lens produces a 'flat field' image in which everything is in focus across the whole field of view.

- 'Apo' which means that the lens is highly corrected for chromatic aberration, which otherwise produces visible colour fringing around fine points in the image.

- Lens magnification and numerical aperture (essentially the light-gathering power of the lens), e.g. '40×/ 0.85'.

- Tube length (which is the effective distance between the eyepiece and the objective, and is usually 160 mm) and required coverslip thickness (in mm), e.g. '160/ 0.17'.

- 'Oel', 'Imm' or 'Oil', which means that the lens is designed for use with immersion oil between the final lens element and the cover-slip.

- 'DIC', which means that the lens is specifically designed for Nomarski 'differential interference contrast'.

The *eyepieces* further magnify the image produced by the objective lenses, usually by a factor of x10. The image they produce is focused at infinity, which allows the operator to comfortably view the image as if in the distance. 'High eyepoint' eyepieces are useful for spectacle wearers because they are designed to allow the full image to be viewed from several centimetres above the eyepiece.

The *condenser* is an important part of the illumination system. When correctly adjusted, it focuses a uniform cone of light onto the specimen (at low magnifications a 'swing out' lens above the condenser may have to be removed from the light path to ensure that the whole field of view is illuminated). Correct adjustment of the condenser diaphragm ensures an optimal balance of image resolution, contrast and depth of field.

The *field diaphragm* is centred and its aperture adjusted so that only the observed region of the specimen is illuminated. This minimizes unnecessary light scatter otherwise produced within the unobserved outer regions of the specimen.

The most commonly used *light source* in modern laboratory microscopes is a low-voltage tungsten/halogen bulb. This provides stable and intense illumination in the visible spectrum. The bulb may be housed within the body of the microscope or within an external lamp housing. Fluorescence microscopy usually exploits the more suitable spectral characteristics of the high-pressure mercury arc lamp, which emits strongly in the ultraviolet (UV) region of the spectrum. Lasers provide a high-intensity monochromatic light source, ideally suited to confocal microscopy as well as to various research techniques such as photobleaching and total internal reflection fluorescence.

Types of microscopy

Brightfield illumination remains the most commonly used form of microscopy in the clinical laboratory. Other methods including fluorescent, phase contrast and, increasingly, darkfield, polarized light and Nomarski microscopy are finding varied application in laboratory diagnosis. The cost and relative complexity of the confocal microscope, however, has largely restricted its application to research applications. Each of these types of microscopy will now be discussed in turn.

As its name suggests, *brightfield illumination* presents the observer with an image of the specimen set against a bright background. To work effectively, the specimen must absorb sufficient light to produce an acceptable degree of contrast. Stains are commonly employed to increase specimen contrast and reveal further structural detail.

Köhler illumination, introduced early last century by August Köhler, has become the universally used form of brightfield illumination because of the quality of image produced. However, optimum image quality requires regular adjustment of the microscope. Unfortunately, many instruments are not used to their full potential because of a disregard for the need to readjust the microscope when changing objective lenses and general ignorance of the required technique.

In Köhler illumination two sets of light rays contribute to the final image, one set called the 'illuminating rays' and the other called the 'image-forming rays'. Both are derived from the incandescent lamp filament (in practice, a ground glass filter is usually fixed in front of the lamp filament to provide a more even source of illuminating rays).

Figure 6.2 illustrates the separate paths followed by illuminating rays and image-forming rays in a microscope correctly set up for Köhler illumination. Most notably:

1. The illuminating rays are parallel at the specimen plane to provide the desired wide area of illumination.

2. The illuminating rays are finally focused on the eye lens before diverging to provide a wide area of illumination on the retina.

3. The image-forming rays converge on the specimen plane and results in a magnified but inverted image of the specimen at the primary image plane below the eyepiece.

4. The eyepiece lenses invert the specimen image-forming rays again before they enter the eye and are focused on the retina to produce an image of the specimen.

In this way, Köhler illumination provides a large, evenly illuminated field of view on the observer's retina, together with a focused and magnified image of the specimen.

Fluorescence microscopy takes advantage of the property of molecules called fluorochromes to emit light of a particular wavelength when excited by incident light of shorter wavelength. These fluorochromes may be native to the specimen under study, but more commonly the specimen is treated either directly or indirectly with fluorescing dyes. For example, the

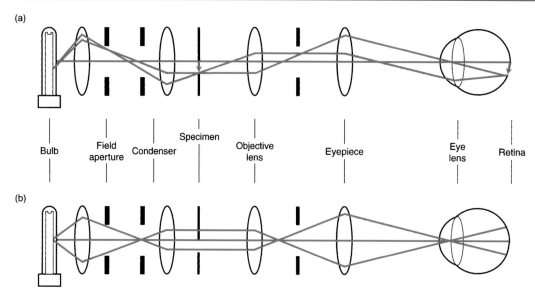

(a)

Bulb | Field aperture | Condenser | Specimen | Objective lens | Eyepiece | Eye lens | Retina

(b)

Figure 6.2 The compound microscope set-up for Köhler illumination: (a) paths of image-forming rays; (b) paths of illuminating rays

DNA-specific 4′,6-diamidino-2-phenylindole (DAPI) may be used directly to reveal the extracellular presence of DNA-containing mycoplasma which frequently contaminate cell cultures. Cellular components, e.g. the cytoskeleton, may be stained indirectly using highly specific probes created by conjugating fluorochromes, such as fluorescein isocyanate with monoclonal antibodies.

Fluorescence microscopy requires relatively simple upgrading of the conventional light microscope. High-pressure mercury arc lamps are commonly used to provide intense illumination in the ultraviolet (UV) region of the spectrum, which excites fluorescence in many important fluorochromes. The use of UV also requires the use of special objective lenses capable of UV transmission. This is because in the typical fluorescence microscope configuration, the objective lenses also serve to focus the illuminating rays onto the specimen. Because the illuminating rays pass through the objective and are incident on the specimen (rather than being transmitted through it from below) this technique is known as epi-illumination.

An appropriate combination of excitation filter, chromatic beam splitter and barrier filter must be used for each of the fluorochromes in use (Figure 6.3). The excitation filter is located in front of the mercury lamp and is chosen to allow transmission of a narrow range of wavelengths of light, which includes the wavelength required to excite fluorescence.

The chromatic beam splitter must reflect excitatory wavelengths of light onto the specimen and stop reflec-

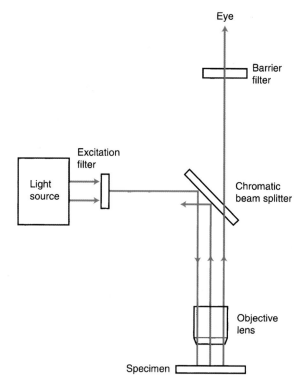

Figure 6.3 Light path in an epi-fluorescent microscope

ted incident light reaching the eyepieces. As its name suggests, the barrier filter ensures that only light emitted by the fluorochrome reaches the eyepieces (UV light can damage the eyes and unprotected skin).

Phase contrast microscopy allows unstained biological specimens with little inherent contrast—which includes living specimens—to be studied. The technique exploits the phase differences which arise between light passing through a biological specimen and light that passes uninterrupted through the surrounding medium—in biological materials this difference is about $1/4\lambda$. The phase contrast microscope requires a special condenser with a series of annular apertures at their front focal plane and matched objective lenses with phase rings at their rear focal plane (Figure 6.4). This arrangement

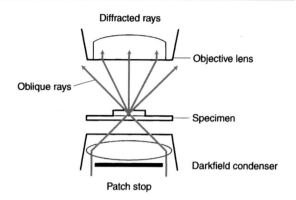

Figure 6.5   Light path in darkfield microscopy

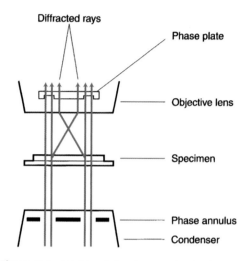

Figure 6.4   Light path in phase contrast microscopy

introduces a further relative phase shift of $1/4\lambda$ to the light already diffracted through the specimen, resulting in a total $1/2\lambda$ phase retardation relative to the background light. The destructive interference produced results in refractive specimen details appearing darker than the background, an effect known as 'positive phase contrast'. Conversely, 'negative phase contrast', in which specimen details appear brighter than the background, results when constructive interference is produced by retarding the background light by $1/4\lambda$.

Phase contrast microscopes are excellent for observing living specimens with minimal disturbance, including cultured animal cells in closed, sterile containers and motile spermatozoa in Petri dishes.

Darkfield microscopy reveals structural details as bright objects on a dark background. A special condenser is used to provide oblique illumination which, if unaltered by the specimen, fails to enter the objective lens. Only those parts of the specimen that deflect light into the objective lens present an image at the eyepieces. Two types of condenser facilitate darkfield illumination. A

simple 'patch stop' may be used to obscure the central portion of the illumination provided by a conventional condenser, leaving only oblique rays incident on the specimen (Figure 6.5). Special 'mirror condensers' provide the best image quality, but are only suitable for darkfield illumination.

Darkfield microscopy does not provide a fully representative image of the specimen—many intracellular structures may not be evident. However, the method is useful for revealing further details of fine line structures which are difficult to observe using brightfield illumination because of their lack of contrast. Furthermore, since staining is unnecessary (as with phase-contrast and Nomarski microscopy), this method of illumination is useful for observing live specimens—spermatozoa and flagellated protozoa offer fascinating images when observed in this way.

Polarized light microscopy represents another modification of the conventional light microscope. The light emanating from a light source may be thought of as many sine waves oscillating in any one of an infinite number of planes around a central axis—in other words, it is not polarized. The polarization microscope includes two polarizing filters: first, the 'polarizer', which can usually be rotated, is located between the lamp and the condenser and hence provides illuminating rays to the specimen which oscillate in only one plane; and second, the 'analyser', which is usually fixed, and is located between the objective lens and the eyepiece. Assuming that no specimen is in the light path, then there will be a single position of the polarizer where the transmitted planes coincide and the image will appear brightest. Conversely, at 90° to this orientation the two transmitted planes are crossed, resulting in the extinction of light reaching the eyepieces.

The polarizing microscope exploits the property of 'birefringent' specimens to split the polarized incident light into two components, which oscillate in planes parallel to the two directions of refractive index. The two components are retarded differently within the specimen, which introduces a phase difference. Since these components do not share the same plane, this does not lead to interference. However, on reaching the analyser, only the components that are parallel to the analyser are transmitted and, since they now share the same plane, they can interfere. Rotating the specimen stage allows the amount of constructive interference to be varied, resulting in a consequent change in the brightness of birefringent structures under observation.

Objects of known birefingence, called 'compensators', which include quartz and the 'first-order red plate' filter, can be inserted into the light path and used to calculate the birefringent properties of unknown structures, so assisting in their identification. The polarization microscope also benefits from the use of specialized 'strain-free' objective lenses, which minimize the amount of bifringence introduced by the optical system itself. Polarizing microscopy has found application in differentiating between sodium acid urate and calcium pyrophosphate dihydrate in synovial fluid, for example. Generally, however, the applications for polarizing microscopy in laboratory diagnosis are limited and infrequent.

Nomarski differential interference contrast microscopy (DIC) represents a combination of polarization and phase contrast microscopy and is best suited to thin unstained transparent specimens. Successful application requires a specially designed instrument, which includes crossed polarizer and analyser filters and two Wollaston prism beam splitters. In combination with the phase differences introduced by the beam splitters, the additional light retardation imposed by the specimen produces an image in which the background is grey, left hand edges are bright, central areas are grey and right hand edges are dark. This gives objects in the light path an almost three-dimensional appearance, with organelles such as mitochondria and nucleus being clearly defined. DIC microscopy is ideally suited to the study of living organisms. It has also found favour in the routine study of wet specimens such as urinary sediment.

No discussion of modern microscopical technique would be complete without at least brief reference to *confocal microscopy*, which represents an important modification of epi-fluorescent microscopy. The major difference between confocal microscopy and previously discussed methods is that it relies on point illumination rather than field illumination. This is provided by a finely focused laser beam, which is scanned through the specimen at a specific depth (Figure 6.6). The image produced is a computer-generated composite built up from

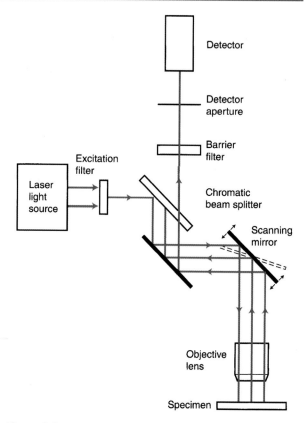

Figure 6.6 Light path in a confocal laser scanning microscope

the differing intensities of light emitted by different regions of the specimen. Thus, image quality is finally dependent on the light sensitivity and resolution of the electronic camera as well as the quality of the microscope optical elements and instrument set-up. Confocal microscopy can provide very sharp images devoid of the out-of-focus blur associated with conventional fluorescence observation and from within relatively thick (<100 μm) specimens.

Photomicrography

Good photomicrography remains something of an art in scientific laboratories, and is dealt with in more appropriate detail in several texts (Bradbury and Bracegirdle, 1998; Smith, 1990; Rost and Oldfield, 2000; Olympus Microscopy Resource Centre, November 2004). The ability to create a permanent and convenient record of microscope-derived images is important in many fields of diagnostic pathology and consequently most laboratories possess one or more photomicroscopes. For example, photomicrography is particularly useful for recording fluorescently-stained specimens, which tend to fade with time. Suitable instruments range from basic laboratory microscopes with a conventional 35 mm camera body attached by means of a simple adapter, to microscopes with sophisticated light-metering systems and one or more integral cameras. Recent improvements in the light sensitivity, resolution and affordability of electronic cameras, both traditional tube-type and charge-coupled device (CCD) and complimentary metal oxide semiconductor (CMOS) cameras, have made them increasingly popular for this purpose. Furthermore, the ready availability of powerful personal computers and specialized software easily meet the needs of even the busiest clinical or research laboratory with respect to microscope automation, digital image processing and analysis, as well as data management.

Despite increasingly affordable digital systems, many clinical laboratories still rely on conventional film cameras. The quality of conventional photomicrographs is dependent upon several factors. The recorded resolution is obviously affected by the quality of the optical components of the microscope, but also depends on the size of the film 'grain', which determines the sharpness of the photographic image. Unfortunately the light sensitivity or 'speed' of photographic film is inversely related to grain size, making the correct choice of suitable film a compromise between these two parameters. The accurate rendition of specimen colour requires careful consideration, primarily because the spectral sensitivity of photographic emulsions differs from that of the human eye. Hence, careful selection of colour-compensating filters with regard to the 'colour temperature' of the illuminating light (which varies as the lamp voltage is adjusted) is also necessary to record a faithful representation of the original specimen's appearance.

Digital photomicrography and video microscopy are increasingly finding a place in remote consultation, education and research between geographically distant sites. At its simplest, *telepathology* involves the one-way transmission of data, including digital images, between sites, perhaps via electronic mail. However, the afore-mentioned developments in microscope automation, together with affordable and accessible high-bandwidth Internet connections, mean that truly dynamic tele-pathology, involving the interactive control of a remote microscope (including specimen position, focusing, magnification, illumination, etc.) and simultaneous live videophone links is becoming an exciting reality in routine clinical pathology.

Further reading

Bradbury S, Bracegirdle B. *Introduction to Light Microscopy.* 1998: Bios Scientific, Oxford, UK.

Determan H, Lerpusch F. *The Microscope and Its Application.* 1988: Wild Leitz, Wetzlar

Lacey AJ. *Light Microscopy in Biology*, 2nd ed. 1999: IRL Press, Oxford, UK.

Smith RF. *Microscopy and Photomicrography.* 1990: CRC Press, Boca Raton, FL.

Rost F, Oldfield R. *Photography with a Microscope.* 2000: Cambridge University Press, Cambridge, MA.

Olympus Microscopy Resource Centre: http://www.olympusmicro.com/ (accessed November 2004).

7

Quantitative methods in tissue pathology

Peter W Hamilton and **Derek C Allen**

Introduction

The practice of measurement is central to nearly all aspects of scientific investigation as it provides a means to compare observations in an objective, reproducible and reliable fashion. Diagnostic pathology, from its outset, has been largely based on the visual assessment of tissue morphology by microscopy, the use of visual diagnostic clues to classify disease and the use of descriptive, linguistic criteria to convey how this process can be achieved. While enormous advances have been made in identifying clinically relevant morphological clues in histology and cytopathology, diagnostic pathology remains a subjective process, which often results in poor reproducibility in diagnostic classification, both between different pathologists and even by the same pathologist on different occasions.

The grading of early malignancy, such as dysplasia, provides such an example. Studies have demonstrated κ (kappa) values as low as 0.15 in the grading of cervical dysplasia, 0.27 in oral dysplasia and 0.55 in pre-invasive lesions of the bronchus. κ is a measure of agreement between different observers and ranges from 0 (no agreement) to 1 (perfect agreement). In cervical cytology, error rates of 2% have been quoted with κ values as low as 0.46 and the grading of cervical intraepithelial neoplasia from tissue sections has shown disagreement in up to 36% of cases. These results highlight the difficulty that exists in being able to accurately and consistently grade morphological changes using the naked eye. There are therefore opportunities to explore novel approaches to diagnosis that provide the objectivity, consistency and reproducibility that is desperately needed.

It has long been recognized that the measurement of histological and cytological features can provide objective data which can significantly improve our ability to make diagnostic decisions in pathology. Measurement in pathology has been called many different things, including morphometry, quantitative microscopy, quantitative pathology, image analysis and mathematical morphology Measurement in pathology has a number of distinct advantages. It allows us to describe in numerical terms the morphological changes we see with the naked eye. This provides us with quantitative data which are objective, reproducible and can be used to test statistically certain hypotheses about changes in tissue morphology. In addition, measurement allows the detection of subtle, 'subvisua' features, not readily apparent to the naked eye. In both instances, measurement can be an invaluable tool for the objective interpretation of morphological abnormalities and for the quantitative classification of human disease.

Methods

There are a variety of methods available that allow us to extract quantitative information from microscopy. Simple linear measurements can be made using an eyepiece graticule—a flat piece of glass on which is engraved a microscopic ruler or grid of defined dimensions that can be inserted into the ocular tube of any microscope. This overlays the image of the specimen and can be used to extract quantitative data (see Figures 7.1 and 7.11). In a simple setting this can be used to measure linear distances of depth or thickness (see Figures 7.11 and 7.12).

The Science of Laboratory Diagnosis, Second Edition   Edited by David Burnett and John Crocker

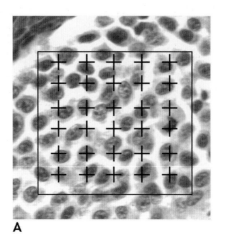 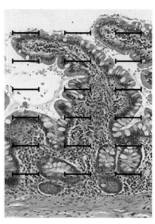

Figure 7.1 (A) The use of a point grid graticule to determine the percentage of area occupied by nuclei. The grid consists of 30 points, 14 of which fall within nuclei, giving a value of 47%. This approach is adopted in stereology to extract 2-D and 3-D measurements from microscopic images. (B) Shows a line graticule for extracting villi surface area from a small intestinal biopsy

A   **B**

Stereology, on the other hand, is an approach that uses point or line probes which overlay the image (see Figure 7.1). It is an old and well-established technique which, although simple, still has considerable value for extracting three-dimensional measurements (e.g. volume, surface area, length) from two-dimensional images (i.e. tissue sections). These methods are rarely applied in pathological research and practice any more. The reason for this is not because they are ineffective, but rather that the drive for automation and the analysis of large numbers of samples has established the computer as the central instrument for measurement in pathology. This has been further enhanced with the ubiquity of standard personal computers which, with the appropriate software, are more than capable of measuring linear, stereological and more complex morphological parameters from microscopic images of tissue and cell samples.

Computers

Computers have had a major impact on many aspects of medical practice and research. In pathology, computers now form an important part of the laboratory infrastructure, as patient information systems, for pathology report generation, specimen identification and digital photomicroscopy. Computers have also become the main tool for tissue and cell measurement in light microscopy. When presented with the profile coordinates of a tissue or cell structure, software can very rapidly compute a variety of measurements relating to that profile, such as area, perimeter, maximum diameter, minimum diameter, shape factor, etc. This information can be electronically stored in a database and analysed statistically to compare

diagnostic groups, tissue samples from patients with different prognosis and morphological changes following treatment. Two types of computer-based technique can be broadly defined.

Computer-aided interactive measurement

This approach completely relies on the human user to trace or mark the boundaries of tissue or cell structures that are to be measured. It consists of a computer with an attached drawing device, which could be the mouse or a more specialized digital pen and drawing tablet. By tracing the boundary of a given object, the x, y coordinates are registered by the system (Figure 7.2). These can be used to measure features of size and shape or to define the boundary within which densitometric measurements can be computed. One can trace boundaries from simple photomicrographs, from live images relayed to the computer screen using a video camera or from digitally stored images (see next section). Most desktop computers can be easily set up to act as interactive measuring devices. Software to facilitate measurement is available commercially. Free software, developed by the National Institutes of Health, is also available from Scion Imaging (www.scioncorp.com). This approach is therefore cheap, easy to implement and has been used in a wide variety of applications.

Digital images in pathology

Being able to record microscopic images digitally has had a major impact on our ability to electronically store large numbers of images in a convenient and

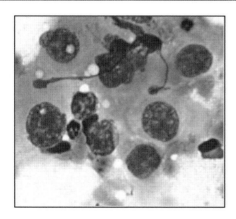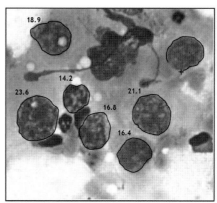

Figure 7.2 Interactive tracing of nuclei from live microscopic image. The left panel shows the original image. The right panel shows how the surface profile of each nucleus is traced using the mouse and used to compute the nuclear area. The nucleus on top right is in the process of being traced. These nuclear values can be stored and used to rapidly calculate a range of statistical measures on the sample, including mean, standard deviation and variation of nuclear size. This approach has been shown to be very useful in characterizing subtle changes in nuclear size and shape associated with malignancy

manageable form and also rapidly extract numerical information from these images for quantitative evaluation. Still digital cameras can be easily attached to a microscope using a standard adapter. Here the camera records the image to an internal memory card, which is subsequently transferred to a computer for processing and analysis. Alternatively, digital or analogue video cameras can be attached to a microscope and images digitized directly by the computer via a specialist image digitizing card. Either approach works well, although for specialist applications, control over camera settings such as shutter speed, gain and colour temperature is vital.

Most digital still/video cameras sample images in excess of three megapixels. Some specialist image capture equipment can record single images up to six megapixels.

Two factors determine the resolution of the image: the spatial resolution and the colour resolution. The spatial resolution is determined by the number of pixels that represents a defined area of the field. Each pixel (derived from 'picture element') represents a box which defines a point on the image. The more pixels that an image is composed of, the higher the spatial resolution (Figure 7.3).

While the number of pixels in an image determines its spatial resolution, we also need to determine how many values we allow for density or colour representation. In Figure 7.4, we see that each pixel can be represented by a single grey value. The more grey values used, the better the resolution of the image. As the human eye can only reliably distinguish about 64 grey values, 256 grey values usually gives a precise representation of the original image. Here, each pixel can be allocated any of the 256 possible grey values depending on the density of that point in the original image, where $0 = $ black and $255 = $ white. A digital image is therefore simply a matrix of numbers which can be stored and retrieved for display on a computer monitor.

Colour images are made of pixels with different intensities of the primary colours: red, green and blue. Again the number of possible values available to represent the red, green and blue contributions to a given colour, determines the colour resolution of the final image. As with a grey level image, each colour can be represented

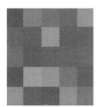 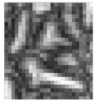 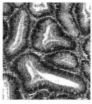 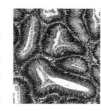

5x5 (25 pixels) 25x25 (625 pixels) 100x100 (10,000 pixels) 500x500 (250,000 pixels)

Figure 7.3 The same image with different spatial resolutions. It can be seen that the higher the pixel resolution, the better the definition of the image and its structures

Figure 7.4 The same image with different grey value resolutions. Normally, 256 grey values represents the maximum number of densities used to represent an image

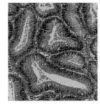
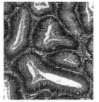
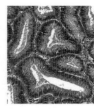

2 grey values   4 grey values   16 grey value   256 grey values

Figure 7.5 Each colour image is made of three grey value images, representing the red, green and blue components. Each grey value determines the contribution of that colour to a given pixel

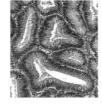
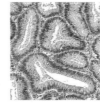
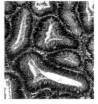
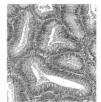

Full colour   Red channel   Green channel   Blue channel

by values in the range 0–255, giving a possible combination of over 16 million colours [256 (red) × 256 (green) × 256 (blue)]. Each colour image can therefore be split into three grey level images, each representing the red, green and blue components of the colour image (Figure 7.5).

Automatic image segmentation

Having a digital representation of a histological image allows us to carry out numerous procedures not possible with an analogue image. By drawing a grey level frequency histogram of the image, we obtain a summary of density information within the image. By setting a threshold on this histogram, we can select out all those pixels which fall above or below the threshold. This is called grey level thresholding and allows us to specifically identify objects within the image that have certain density characteristics, e.g. nuclei (Figure 7.6). The identification of objects in this way is called segmentation. The computer can automatically derive the profile boundary of the objects it segments and from these morphometric features can be derived.

The setting of a single grey level threshold does not always result in the accurate segmentation of all nuclei. In Figure 7.6, we can see that some nuclei that have been lying close together have been identified as a single object. If the area of these objects were to be automatically measured by the computer, the results would be inaccurate. However, since we have the information stored in a digital format, there are a variety of proce-

dures that can be used to resolve this problem. Each suspected nuclear profile can be examined independently for its morphometric (size, shape, etc.) characteristics. If these fall within defined limits, then the object can be accepted as a nucleus. If, however, the object features fall outside the defined range, it can be processed further to determine whether a better segmentation result can be obtained. For example, we can search the profile of the object for sharp transitions in direction (termed 'cusps'). If two are found to occur on opposite sides of the object, a splitting function can be called and the object divided (Figure 7.7). An extensive library of image-processing algorithms is available which allow us, in most circumstances, to reliably segment objects or structures within a histological or cytological image.

The ability to identify important image components using computer algorithms and to rapidly measure morphological characteristics and use these to classify a given case, begs the question whether this can be done in an automated fashion. Automation has developed rapidly in other laboratory disciplines, such as haematology and clinical biochemistry, but has been slow in pathology. The lack of automation in diagnostic pathology to date is not altogether unjustified. Diagnostic pathology requires direct visualization of complex tissue and cellular structures using the standard light microscope, making the process of automation extremely difficult in comparison to the use of biochemical tests or cell counts. However, with developments in computerized image analysis and machine vision, automating the task of morphological interpretation and diagnostic classification is theoretically possible. The major effort in this field has been in

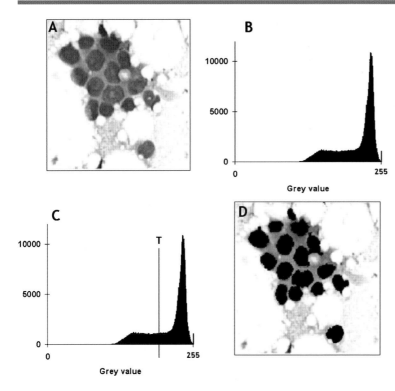

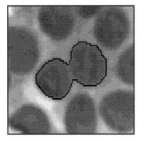

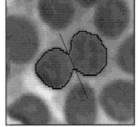

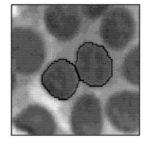

Figure 7.6 The use of histogram thresholding to identify objects within the image. (A) The original grey level image. (B) The grey level histogram for the image, showing the range of pixel grey values of 0–255. (C) A threshold is defined which instructs the computer to select all pixels with values to the left of the threshold line. (D) Image showing segmented regions which, due to their higher density (lower grey values), are mainly nuclei

Figure 7.7 Splitting algorithms for the accurate segmentation of nuclei

the development of automated cervical screening devices (discussed later) but techniques are now being extensively explored in tissue histology.

Of course, the development of a completely automated machine vision system such as this is time consuming and an alternative approach, used by many, is to use a combination of image segmentation algorithms and interactive tracing to ensure that all components of the image are accurately identified.

Densitometry and texture

As we have seen, when images are digitally recorded, quantitative information is stored on the density of each

pixel within the image. In pathology, this information can be used effectively to quantify the optical density (OD) of a given staining reaction. This is achieved by measuring the grey value of a series of OD filters and drawing a calibration curve to convert grey value to OD. While geometric information is easier to standardize and does not need sophisticated image-capture equipment, densitometric measurements require standardization and control of light levels from one image to the next, and this requires careful microscope calibration and all automatic gain, colour temperature and shutter settings on the camera to be switched off. Measurement of OD is most effective when the staining reaction is stoichiometric, i.e. when the density of the stain is proportional to the substrate being measured. This is found when

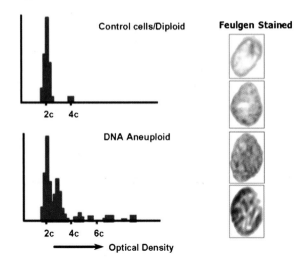

Figure 7.8 DNA cytometry. By measuring the optical density of nuclei stained for DNA, a quantitative measure of DNA content (ploidy) can be obtained. By comparison with control cells where the status is known to be DNA diploid (e.g. lymphocytes), deviations from normal DNA ploidy values can be identified and measured. This is generally called 'DNA aneuploid' and is particularly evident in neoplasia

using the Feulgen reaction to label DNA, where the measurement of integrated nuclear optical density by densitometry provides a quantitative measure of DNA content. As DNA content is disturbed, particularly in malignant disease, this measurement has been extensively explored as a useful quantitative clue in diagnosis and prognosis. The identification of disturbed distributions of DNA content (Figure 7.8) tends to be associated with chromosome instability which increases in malignancy and is generally associated with poor prognosis. Other methods, such as flow cytometry, allow a more rapid measurement of DNA content and ploidy alterations in clinical samples. However, DNA cytometry

using computerized imaging allows for a more specific analysis of defined populations of cells within a tissue section or smear.

In conventional diagnosis, the distribution of nuclear chromatin or chromatin phenotype is a visual clue that provides vital information on the biological behaviour of a cell. Using the numerical information provided to us through digital imagery, we can quantify chromatin organization by assessing the spatial distribution of grey values within a nucleus (Figure 7.9). Since the nucleus is digitally represented by a matrix of numbers representing the density of each pixel, a set of statistical features can be extracted which measures the spatial distribution of grey values within the nucleus (Figure 7.9). This set of features is collectively termed 'texture' and provides an objective measure of chromatin phenotype. As well as providing quantitative support for visually apparent changes in chromatin organization, these measures have been shown to illustrate chromatin characteristics that are not apparent to the naked eye. These features have been used extensively in the identification of malignancy associated changes (MACs), which are discussed later.

Conventionally, texture analysis has been carried out on nuclei stained specifically for DNA using the Feulgen reaction. More recently, however, haematoxylin has been used for the measurement of nuclear texture and shown to be very effective. This stain is easy to apply and is the common stain used in routine diagnostic pathology. However, it does not provide a stoichiometric reaction and does require careful standardization and control.

Nuclear spatial measurements

Nuclear crowding, the distances between nuclei and the patterns they form within tissues provide unique clues to

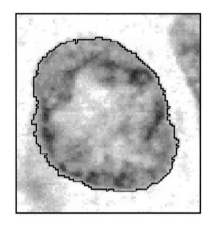
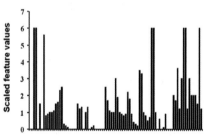

Figure 7.9 The analysis of nuclear chromatin texture involves the examination of the spatial relationships of grey values within a stained nucleus. This can be used to generate a nuclear chromatin signature, which provides subtle but very sensitive clues to the underlying pathobiology of the cell

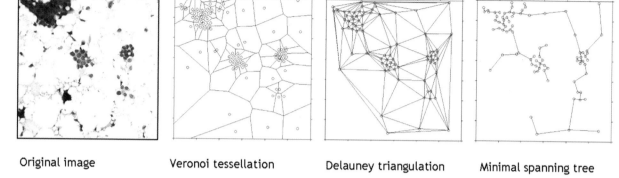

| Original image | Veronoi tessellation | Delauney triangulation | Minimal spanning tree |

Figure 7.10 Nuclear spatial measurements generated from breast fine needle aspiration cytology. Nuclear positions are identified and used as points on a graph. Spatial measurements generated from these graphs provide quantitative data on cell cohesion

the extent of the underlying disease and in particular the severity of pre-invasive lesions. A variety of approaches can be used to measure nuclear spacing, most of which are based on graph theory, which determines the spatial characteristics of a set of points in two-dimensional space. Collectively, the techniques are termed 'syntactic structure analysis' or 'cellular sociology'. There are a number of methods available for syntactic structure analysis, including Voronoi's tessellation, Delaunay triangulation and minimum spanning tree. A Delaunay triangulation is defined where triangles are formed between every possible set of points, accepting only triangles in which the circumcircle contains no other points than the triangle points (Figure 7.10). The complementary tessellation of the Delaunay graph is the Voronoi tessellation. From these graphs, a variety of measurements can be extracted, including number of points, average triangle line length, total length of lines, mean, standard deviation, skewness, kurtosis and entropy of line lengths, triangle area, enclosed object areas, etc. The minimum spanning tree (MST), on the other hand, is a graph without loops and connects all points where the sum of the length of the lines connecting the points is minimal. As before, a variety of measurements can be extracted from this graph, which reflects underlying changes in the crowding structure of nuclei. Examples of these three methods are illustrated in Figure 7.10. Applications for the role of this type of approach to quantitative morphology has been shown in grading colorectal dysplasia, in assessing gastric atrophy and to define nuclear distribution patterns in endometrial cytology samples.

Applications of measurement in diagnostic pathology

Diagnostic pathologists regularly use quantitation in daily practice. Simple linear measurements of tumour diameter determines pathological staging in the international tumour/nodes/metastases (TNM) classification and also gives prognostic information in various common cancers, e.g. breast cancer. Tumour clearance of surgical margins is important in predicting the possibility of local tumour recurrence and in selecting patients for postoperative adjuvant chemo-or radiotherapy in breast and colorectal cancer. Optimal treatment of cutaneous malignant melanoma and carcinoma is by complete surgical excision and margin clearance, and must be determined in the pathology specimen. Basic techniques are appropriate, such as use of the microscopic stage Vernier scale, an eyepiece graticule or ruler. Glass or Perspex dome magnifiers incorporating a linear scale are particularly helpful. Semi-quantitative estimates of percentage tumour involvement in prostatic needle biopsy cores is a good indicator of overall tumour volume and the likelihood of cancer having spread beyond the gland.

Various standard applications are detailed below but some more recent potential developments include:

- Quantitation of the pathology of neurodegenerative disorders, e.g. Alzheimer's disease.

- Separation of benign and malignant melanocytic lesions, using a combination of quantitative S100 protein immunoexpression, nuclear area and DNA cytometry.

- Quantitation of cell populations and tissue distribution in haematological disorders in bone marrow biopsies.

- Analysis of tissue architecture in pulmonary and hepatic fibrosis.

Breslow's measure of melanoma thickness

This represents one of the most commonly used measurements in diagnostic histopathology and is the measure of the depth of melanoma invasion below the granular cell layer of the skin (Figure 7.11). This

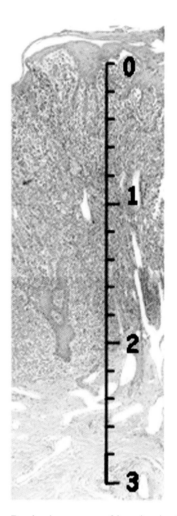

Figure 7.11 Breslow's measure of invasion in skin melanoma. Shows eyepiece graticule (major units in millimetres) overlying tissue section of melanoma

method and its prognostic value was defined by Breslow. Measurements can be made with an eyepiece graticule and it has now become accepted practice to define malignant melanoma as being thin (<0.76 mm), of intermediate thickness (0.76–1.5 mm) or thick (>1.5 mm), with the percentage disease-free survival being 100%, 70% and 40%, respectively.

Bone biopsy

Morphometric analysis can provide extremely valuable data for the diagnosis of metabolic bone disease. Bone biopsies are taken from the iliac crest and analysis carried out using undecalcified sections and microscopy with transmitted, cross-polarized and ultraviolet light. Measurements of trabecular and osteoid volume, osteoid and mineralized surfaces, and osteoid thickness can be made and used to diagnose osteoporosis and osteomalacia (Figure 7.12). These can be made using point/line

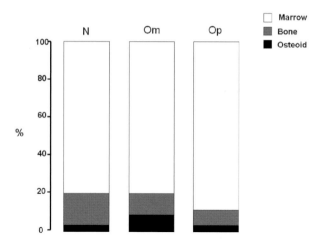

Figure 7.12 Quantitative estimation of bone, osteoid and marrow in bone biopsies allows the identification of normal bone (N), osteomalacia (Om) and osteoporosis (Op)

grids and stereological procedures. The use of computerized image analysis is now becoming a more attractive means of measuring these features.

Muscle biopsy

The assessment of muscle fibre characteristics in longitudinal and transverse sections is central to the diagnosis of neuromuscular disorders, including congenital, metabolic and destructive myopathies and muscular

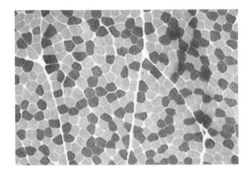

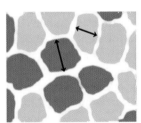

Figure 7.13 Muscle biopsy morphometry in the assessment of neuromuscular disorders. The left image shows a biopsy stained with ATPase reaction to distinguish Type I and Type II muscle fibres. Not only can the number of fibres be counted, but the lesser aspect of the muscle fibre can be measured (right) to determine fibre hypertrophy and atrophy

dystrophy. The morphometric measurement of muscle fibre size and number is carried out on transverse sections, stained differentially for fibre type using the myosin APTase reaction (Figure 7.13). Fibre atrophy and hypertrophy is determined by the measurement of fibre size, which is conventionally taken as the muscle fibre diameter across the lesser aspect of the profile.

Breast cancer

The Bloom and Richardson method of grading breast cancer was an attempt to introduce simple 'semi-quantitative' criteria into histopathological diagnosis. This requires the subjective grading of nuclear pleomorphism, an estimation of the percentage of the tumour showing tubule formation and counting the number of mitoses per 10 high-powered fields. The number of mitoses appears to be particularly relevant in predic-

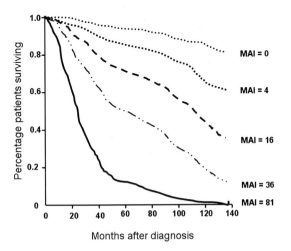

Figure 7.14 This figure illustrates the role of mitotic counts in predicting survival in patients with breast cancer. As the mitotic activity index (MAI = number of mitosis per 10 high-powered fields) increases, the percentage of patients surviving for longer periods within that group decreases

ting prognosis in patients with breast cancer (Figure 7.14). It has been shown in large-scale clinical trials that the calculation of a multivariate prognostic index based on mitotic counts, tumour size and lymph node status can provide a valuable measure of prognosis in breast cancer, particularly in premenopausal women. The quantitative analysis of duct architecture and epithelial pattern assessment can also provide useful data on the discrimination of intraductal hyperplasia and ductal carcinoma *in situ*.

Endometrium

The measurement of nuclear size and shape is of value in the discrimination of normal endometrium, atypical hyperplasia and endometrial carcinoma. These benefits can be supplemented by the quantitative analysis of architectural features which, in combination, allow the identification of cases of atypical hyperplasia that progress to cancer. A multivariate morphometric scoring system has been shown to correlate strongly with depth of myometrial invasion and to be more specific than subjective classification schemes such as the Kurman classification. In The Netherlands, morphometric analysis of endometrial curettings or hysterectomy specimens is carried out routinely in an attempt to reduce overtreatment of these lesions. It has been estimated that this could save approximately $15 million per year in USA. The combination of the mean shortest nuclear axis, DNA ploidy and depth of myometrial invasion has also been shown to have significant prognostic value, particularly in FIGO (International Federation of Gynecology and Obstetrics) stage I endometrial cancers.

Automated cervical cytology

Automated cervical cytology represents one of the major efforts over the past 30 years to introduce automation into a visually demanding diagnostic process.

The motivation for this came from the significantly reduced mortality from cervical cancer after the introduction of cervical cancer screening programmes and the demanding workload that this initiated. It was clear that overworked cytotechnicians and clinical cytologists could misdiagnose difficult cases. Work on the development of computer-based scanning devices began in the late 1950s but only recently have we seen the commercial release of systems with automated capabilities in this area.

These systems mostly work on the same principle, where slides are mechanically fed into an imaging microscope, mechanically scanned, sequential images of the smear are digitally recorded, cells are identified and segmented and are then subjected to quantitative analysis

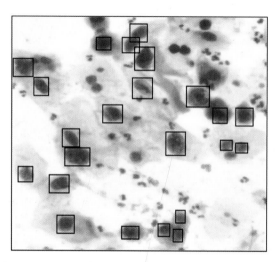

Figure 7.15 Automatic identification of cervical cell nuclei from a smear preparation. Quantitative characterization allows classification of cell type and identification of malignant cells

(Figure 7.15). A variety of features are recorded, including nuclear size, shape, density, texture, etc. Each nucleus is then classified as normal or potentially abnormal. This information can then be handled in a number of ways. Some systems are designed to store all images of the abnormal events, which must then be reviewed by the cytologist at a later date to confirm a diagnosis of malignancy. This retains human expertise in the final decision-making process but significantly reduces the workload, as suspicious fields are automatically selected by the machine.

Alternatively, the system can arrive at a diagnostic classification independently from human intervention. This totally automated classification of cervical smears can be used for a number of purposes.

Quality control

Cervical cytology screening demands an assessment of quality by the systematic re-screening of at least 10% of slides or rapid re-screening of all slides. This is conventionally carried out by experienced individuals within the cytology team and is a time-consuming process. An automated cervical screening system can be used to re-examine a proportion of slides, relieving the cytologist from this task. Discrepancies between human and machine classification of the same case will be highlighted and an explanation requested. Given that the machine will have a defined classification accuracy, this will ensure that the quality of diagnostic procedures will be maintained above this level.

Pre-screening

Up to 95% of cervical smears are normal. Automated systems could potentially select out a large proportion of perfectly normal smears leaving the more visually complex samples to be assessed by the human cytologist. This again could represent a significant reduction in the workload of a given laboratory, while at the same time enriching the job of screening by providing the cytologist with the more challenging cases.

Full automation

Completely automated devices, which provide a definitive diagnosis on all presented smears, have been advocated for many years and are now a possibility. There are medico-legal issues to be overcome but full automation could have a part to play in providing cervical screening services in countries where no screening programme currently exists.

The use of automated imaging systems in diagnostic cytology of the cervix and other sites is likely to develop rapidly over future years. Such systems have already been introduced in some laboratories as quality control devices and are currently being promoted as pre-screening systems. With advances in computer technology, machine vision and classification procedures, it is likely that fully automated systems will perform at levels that exceed the best human screeners.

Chromatin phenotype and malignancy-associated changes (MACs)

The quantitative characteristics of chromatin phenotype have been shown in many settings to provide unique clues to underlying cell behaviour and can be used as an objective means for classifying disease and, more importantly, in predicting clinical outcome. Chromatin texture analysis seems to have a major role in the diagnosis, grading and prognosis of bladder neoplasms. In addition, evidence suggests that analysis of the measurement of chromatin phenotype prior to treatment can be used to predict response to chemo- and radiotherapy in bladder cancer. Nuclear chromatin texture also can be used to discriminate between hormone-sensitive and hormone-resistant prostate carcinomas and has been shown to be useful in predicting prognosis in metastatic prostate cancer.

Subtle alterations in nuclear chromatin organization have been demonstrated not only in malignant cells but also in apparently 'normal' cells from patients with a malignant tumour. These changes have been termed 'malignancy-associated changes' or MACs. They can be reliably measured using computerized texture analysis of nuclei (Figure 7.16) and often highlight nuclear characteristics that are not apparent to the naked eye. For example, in cervical cytology, it has been shown that

in an analysis of only 30 normal appearing cells per sample, 70% of samples with moderate or severe dysplasia could be identified. This advocates their role in automated cervical screening devices and many of the current systems employ nuclear texture as a diagnostic feature. MACs have also been demonstrated in the colon, bladder, breast and lung (Figure 7.16). It is unclear whether these changes in apparently normal cells indicate a primary pre-malignant change in the cell or are secondary changes due to exposure of surrounding cells to tumour-related factors. The fact that MACs can disappear after the removal of a tumour suggests the latter, at least in some tissues. Recent work has suggested that MACs can be used as a potential method for the screening of lung cancer. Analysis of MACs in histologically normal lung biopsies allowed the correct identification of over 80% of cancer patients. In addition, the identification of textural disturbances in normal-appearing cells from sputum samples has been advocated in the screening of patients for lung cancer.

Automation in tissue histology

The automated analysis of cytology preparations is a demanding task. Even more difficult is the automated interpretation and analysis of histological scenes due to the complexity of the imagery. Until recently, automated analysis of histological imagery was considered an insurmountable task, except in the most simple applications. However, with development in computer processing power and the use of expert system methodology, the development of machine vision systems for complex imaging tasks is now possible. This requires the definition of knowledge concerning the components which comprise the image and their relationships to each other. These are defined in a knowledge file and are used to drive the actions of a scene segmentation expert system. Objects are accepted or rejected as histological components on the basis of defined quantitative criteria. Rejected objects can be selected for further image processing to facilitate their identification. Once all objects are identified, the histological scene is reconstructed, allowing the measurement of relevant histometric features. This methodology has now been applied successfully in colon, prostate and breast (Figure 7.17).

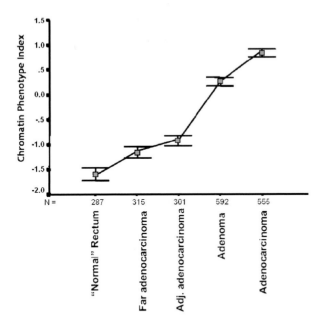

Figure 7.16 This graph shows the chromatin phenotype index, measured using texture analysis in normal mucosa at a distance (Far) from and adjacent (Adj.) to colorectal adenocarcinoma. It can be seen that there is a monotonic trend with increasing abnormalities as we move closer to the cancer. This highlights malignancy-associated changes (MACs) in chromatin organization in normal cells surrounding a malignant lesion. The graph also shows the major alterations in chromatin organization within adenomas and adenocarcinoma

Quantitative immunohistochemistry

One of the major advances in diagnostic pathology over the last 30 years has been the microscopic

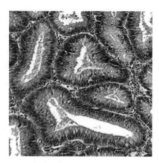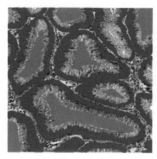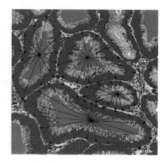

Figure 7.17 Automation in tissue histology. Using expert system guided machine vision, colorectal glands and their constituent parts can be automatically identified, segmented and measurements made which can be used to objectively measure the degree of colorectal dysplasia

visualization of proteins using immunocytochemical methods (see Chapter 4). However, the assessment of the staining reaction remains subjective, not only for assessing the number of immuno-positive cells but also in determining the intensity of the labelling reaction. Most visual approaches are based on a numerical scoring system for both percentage of positive cells and intensity, which are added to provide an overall immuno-score for a given case. Even this well-defined approach suffers from poor reproducibility when comparing the score generated by one expert compared to another expert on the same tissue sample. For this reason, many instrument manufacturers are now marketing image analysis equipment, which can extract quantitative immunohistochemical data through the analysis of densitometric information from colour digital images. As the primary reporter molecule has a specific colour, it is important that the imaging system is capable of identifying this colour in cell preparations and distinguishing it from any counterstain that may be present.

There are also issues over standardization and quality control in quantitative immunocytochemistry and the use of on-slide controls of defined immunoreactivity are recommended. The main focus in the development of quantitative immunohistochemistry has been for the quantitative evaluation of oestrogen and progesterone receptors and HER2/neu positivity in breast cancer. Automation is also the major driving force, with many commercial systems aimed at fast throughput analysis of tissue microarrays for the identification of potential immunocytochemical biomarkers of diagnosis, prognosis and response to therapy.

The digital slide

Recent advances in digital imaging now provide the capability to scan and digitally record an entire microscopic slide (Figure 7.18). This can be carried out at high magnification, so that the microscopic detail of the

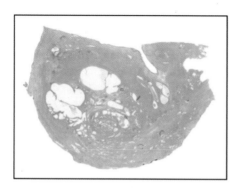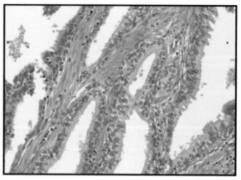

Figure 7.18 The digital slide. On the left is a scan of an entire prostate tissue section. The original tissue section was 27 × 9 mm. Scanned at ×40, this generated a digital image of 58 877 × 42 336 pixels in 24-bit colour. The final image was 456 megabytes in size. The small box in the middle of the image can be enlarged electronically to show the detail at which the image was recorded (right)

sample is retained and the slide can be viewed at any magnification by digitally enlarging or reducing the image on-screen. The sheer dimensions of the image would have made this an impossible task just a few years ago. Now, with fast processing, software has been developed which allows the rapid navigation and examination of these megapixel images. This potentially allows pathology cases to be distributed between centres digitally, rather than on glass slides. The scanning of entire slides also facilitates the automated analysis of tissue and cell features using machine vision, and this is becoming increasingly important in the assessment of tissue microarrays. Analysis of entire images in this way is still computationally demanding but, as this can be done in the absence of human intervention with automated handling of numerous slides, it has huge potential in facilitating automated analysis in pathological research and practice.

have adopted these approaches. This is often due to the financial and time constraints imposed on pathologists, prohibiting the additional effort necessary to generate numerical data from patient samples. The few institutions that do offer measurement in routine pathology (mainly in The Netherlands and the USA) charge for this additional service. This charge is either passed on to the patient, the health care insurer or the health care provider, and measurements are mainly made by technical staff. The drive by equipment manufacturers and the introduction of more automated approaches, in combination with the need to quantify new markers developed by pharmaceutical companies, might be the defining issues in the future of measurement in routine diagnostic pathology. This could significantly influence how pathology is practised and will complement the diagnostic ability of the pathologist, providing valuable objective support in diagnostic decision making and prognostication.

Conclusion

Measurement in pathology clearly enhances conventional visual interpretation. However, the incorporation of techniques into routine practice has been, and continues to be, slow. A number of factors are responsible, not least of which are the lack of large-scale clinical trials to test the efficacy of measurement in given diagnostic problems. Most studies have been carried out on relatively small numbers of cases under semi-controlled conditions. Even when large-scale studies have been carried out that have illustrated the clinical value and cost-effectiveness of tissue sample measurement, few centres

Further reading

Baak JPA, Janssen E. Expert Opinion: DNA Ploidy analysis in Histopathology. *Histopathology* 2004; **44**: 603.

Bartels PH. Future directions in quantitative pathology: digital knowledge in diagnostic pathology. *J Clin Pathol* 2000; **53**: 31–37.

Grohs HK, Husain OAN. *Automated Cervical Cancer Screening.* 1994: Igaku-Shoin, New York.

Hamilton PW, Allen DC (eds). *Quantitative Clinical Pathology.* 1995: Blackwell Science, Oxford.

Marchevsky AM, Bartels PH (eds). *Image Analysis. A primer for pathologists.* 1994: Raven Press, New York.

8

Proliferation markers in histopathology

Cheryl E Gillett and **Diana M Barnes**

Introduction

It is well recognized that in human tumours the rate at which cells are proliferating has a significant effect on prognosis. Since proliferative activity was first crudely estimated by measuring the change in size of a mass over a period of time, the whole subject of proliferation and how to measure it has flourished and there are now hundreds of publications on the subject. There is a continuous stream of papers introducing new markers, combining established markers, varying the demonstration techniques and advocating novel approaches to evaluation. Such a mass of information is a daunting prospect to the inexperienced person who wants to measure proliferation, and usually prompts the question "what's the best way of doing it?"

Before describing some of the different ways of measuring proliferation, it is important to have a basic understanding of the cell cycle, as all markers demonstrate a particular aspect. The cycling or 'growth fraction' stage has four phases, Gap 1 (G_1), DNA synthesis (S), Gap 2 (G_2) and mitosis followed by cytokinesis (M). During the cycling stage, the cell sequentially produces the necessary proteins to allow replication of its DNA and subsequent nuclear and cell division. Checkpoints exist at all phases of the cycle to assess the condition of the cell before entering the next phase. Normally only cells in which the DNA is in perfect condition are allowed to progress to the next stage. Cells that are defective in some way are either arrested until the DNA has been repaired or are directed towards programmed cell death (apoptosis). All cells can enter a stage of non-proliferation or non-cycling, which is known as Gap 0 or (G_0). Here the cells retain their viability and can move back into the cycle as required.

The term 'proliferation rate' is frequently used to describe the 'amount' of a proliferation marker in clinical material. These measurements are usually made on a piece of tissue at one given point in time, thus the term 'rate' is inappropriate. Proliferative 'activity' is a more accurate expression of this kind of evaluation and the term 'rate' should be reserved for methods which measure change over time.

Proliferation markers

The number of so-called proliferation markers continues to grow. Outlined below are those that are reasonably well established and have been shown to provide prognostic information.

Mitotic count (MC) or mitotic activity index (MAI)

Mitoses are the only proliferative marker that can be identified and quantified on a conventional haematoxylin and eosin (H&E)-stained tissue section (Figure 8.1). However, they are not always easy to recognize and can be confused with either hyperchromatic nuclei or nuclei in the early stages of apoptosis. Inadequate fixation, poor section cutting and overstaining can all lead to difficulties in the recognition of mitoses, and may even affect the number of mitoses identified.

The Science of Laboratory Diagnosis, Second Edition   Edited by David Burnett and John Crocker
© 2005 John Wiley & Sons, Ltd

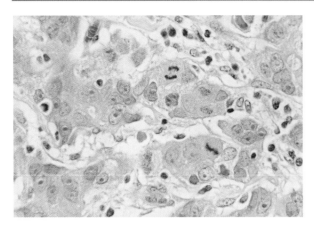

Figure 8.1 Mitotic figures in a conventional haematoxylin and eosin (H&E)-stained section (×400)

Estimating the proliferative activity of a piece of tissue according to the number of mitoses present may, at first, appear to be a straightforward task. However, several different methods of evaluation have been developed over the years and, despite the well-recognized value of mitoses as markers of proliferation, there remains as much debate as ever over the 'correct' method of evaluation. A mitotic 'count' was the first formal method of evaluation used, a step-up from an overall estimate or the 0, +, ++ system used by so many pathologists. A mitotic count literally counts the number of mitoses present in a number of high power fields (HPFs) and presents the results as the mean number of mitoses per HPF. In order to make the method more reproducible, refinements have been made, including evaluating the cells at the periphery of the lesion, making the count in consecutive fields and defining the area of the HPF. The mitotic count is an integral part of grading infiltrating mammary carcinomas, using the modified Bloom and Richardson criteria, and is also used to determine the diagnosis and prognosis of soft tissue sarcomas.

To overcome some of the inconsistencies associated with a mitotic count, the mitotic activity index was introduced. With this method of evaluation the number of mitoses is expressed as a proportion of the number of interphase cells. The total number of interphase cells and mitotic figures are counted in consecutive HPFs until the section has been sufficiently well sampled. As the MAI measures the proportion of mitoses in the lesion, it is not related to or affected by the area of the HPF. It also takes into account variations in both the cellularity of the lesion and the cell size. A mitotic activity index takes approximately 10 minutes longer than a mitotic count

but it is a more accurate way of comparing the proportion of mitoses present between tumours.

Another way of identifying mitotic figures is to use antibodies such as MPM2. These methods are aimed at reducing the chances of including apoptotic bodies in a mitotic count as well as lending themselves to automated analysis.

Nucleolar organizer regions (NORs)

NORs are the sites of rDNA genes and are present in groups or loops on a number of specific chromosomes. By having several sites of transcription, the cell can keep up with demand for ribosomes whenever necessary. The NOR-associated proteins, as the name implies, lie in very close proximity to the NORs and it is these proteins that are demonstrated as markers of proliferation. The NOR-associated proteins are argyrophilic and are demonstrable using a silver technique, and are thus referred to as AgNORs. They can be seen as small black dots within the nucleus (Figure 8.2). The number

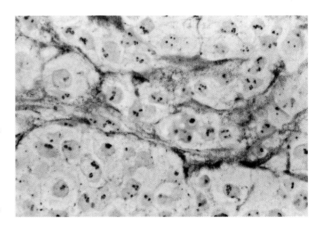

Figure 8.2 Nucleolar organizer region-associated proteins— AgNORs, demonstrated using a silver technique (×1000)

of AgNORs present is considered to reflect ribosome production and hence protein synthesis within the cell. The resultant AgNOR assessment has been portrayed as not only a marker of proliferative activity but also a method of distinguishing between benign and malignant lesions, a measure of tumour ploidy and grade of malignancy.

AgNORs are extremely laborious to count and some earlier authors also endeavoured to describe their pattern within the nucleolus, referring to 'clusters' and 'satellite AgNORs'. Evaluation was not reproducible, which accounted for much of the variation reported in their prognostic value. There have been a number of publications describing the use of image analysers to quantify the presence of AgNORs, and many of these have shown that the mean area occupied by AgNORs within the nucleus provides prognostic information.

Immunohistochemical demonstration of proliferation

The first antibody to be widely recognized as a marker of proliferative activity was monoclonal Ki67 (mKi67). The functional significance of Ki67 protein remains elusive, despite being well studied at the molecular level. However, it is well established that the protein is expressed during all phases of the cycling cell but not during the non-cycling stage. mKi67 has been used in many studies and the resultant measure of proliferative activity compares well with other established markers of proliferation, including mitotic counts and thymidine labelling index (Figure 8.3a,b). However, the drawback with mKi67 antibody is that the area of the antigen which it recognizes is very fixation-sensitive, and antigenicity is lost following standard formaldehyde fixation, paraffin-embedding procedures. Prognostic studies using mKi67, therefore, could only be undertaken prospectively using fresh frozen tissue.

The potential of mKi67 as a proliferation marker provided the impetus to produce similar antibodies to proteins which were functional during the cell cycle but were robust enough to survive formalin fixation and paraffin processing, thus giving the marker a far wider application. When an antibody to proliferating cell nuclear antigen (PCNA) was developed, it was hailed as the fixative-resistant equivalent of mKi67 (Figure 8.4). However, after the initial excitement, PCNA (also con-

fusingly known as cyclin in some papers) was found to have a role in both DNA replication and DNA repair. This duality has led to considerable variation in claims as to its value as a proliferation marker. Its expression appears to be related to proliferation in tissues which have active stem cells, but the relationship is less clear-cut in epithelial lesions. The protein also has a long half-life and therefore it continues to be detected long after its functional time slot within the cell cycle. Another antibody, KiS1, was initially considered to have been raised against the Ki67 antigen and was considered to be a fixative-resistant equivalent of mKi67. However, subsequent evaluation of the antibody has shown that it detects topoisomerase IIα, one of the enzymes controlling single- and double-stranded breaks in DNA during replication and transcription, Despite this new finding, KiS1 has still being used as a marker of proliferative

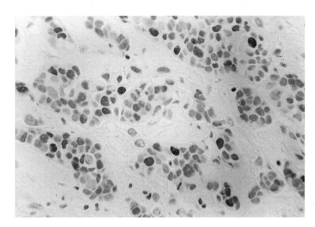

Figure 8.4 Proliferating cell nuclear antigen detected by PC10 antibody in formalin-fixed, paraffin-embedded tissue ($\times$400)

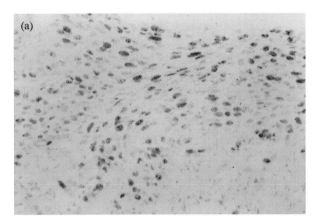

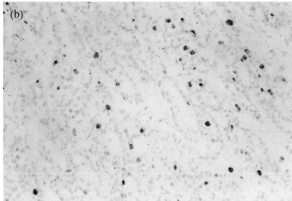

Figure 8.3 Ki67 antigen detected using monoclonal Ki67 antibody in frozen tissue from a rapidly proliferating (a) and slowly proliferating (b) tumour ($\times$200)

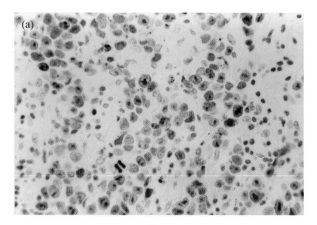

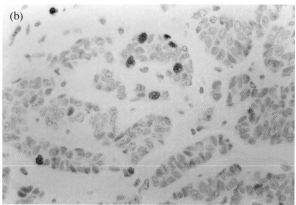

Figure 8.5 Topoisomerase IIα detected using KiS1 antibody in formalin-fixed, paraffin-embedded tissue from a rapidly proliferating (a) and slowly proliferating (b) tumour (×400)

activity as it is expressed in all phases of the cycling cell (Figure 8.5a,b). However, KiS1 is slightly less specific than mKi67, as it still detects some level of protein after the cell has completed the cycle and is in a non-cycling stage. There has been a steady flow of publications using these antibodies with modifications to both the method and the evaluation procedure, which are claimed to provide more accurate and reproducible proliferative information.

The most established antibodies for detecting Ki67, and thus proliferating cells, are polyclonal Ki67 (pKi67) and monoclonal MIB1. Both recognize part of the Ki67 structural protein and can continue to bind to the antigen following fixation and paraffin embedding (Figure 8.6). Both MIB1 and pKi67 expression have proved to be closely associated with mKi67 antibody and their proliferative activity information correlates well with other established proliferation markers. Coupled with the development of these antibodies have been the recent improvements in antigen retrieval methods beyond that of proteolytic digestion. Heat-mediated antigen retrieval is essential for the use of both antibodies in formalin-fixed paraffin-embedded material. Even mKi67 can be used in paraffin-embedded material following antigen retrieval, although the results are not as consistent as either pKi67 or MIB1.

Thymidine (TLI) and bromodeoxyuridine labelling index (BrdULI)

Both of these techniques involve the incorporation of a nucleotide during S-phase which can then be demonstrated. In the case of TLI, the thymidine is tritiated and

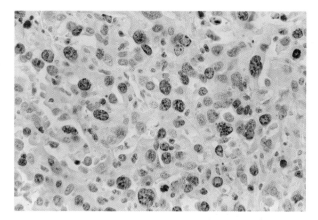

Figure 8.6 Ki67 antigen detected using MIB1 antibody in formalin-fixed, paraffin-embedded tissue from a rapidly proliferating tumour (×400)

its uptake is demonstrated using autoradiography (Figure 8.7). For BrdU, uptake is demonstrated using immunocytochemistry with an anti-BrdU antibody (Figure 8.8). A disadvantage is that both methods need viable material in order to incorporate the nucleotides into the DNA. Furthermore, detection of radiolabelled thymidine brings with it the problems of balancing accuracy with speed of development of autoradiographs and with safety aspects of the technique. However, results are good when carried out by experienced practitioners and provide an accurate evaluation of the proportion of cells in S phase. These are specialized techniques and are not easily introduced into histopathology laboratories with any degree of reliability.

BrdU labelling, in combination with flow cytometry, has more recently been used to measure proliferation

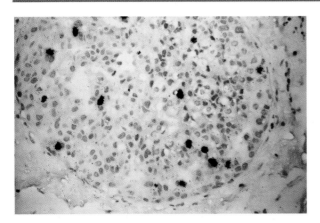

Figure 8.7   Autoradiographic detection of thymidine incorporated into the nuclei of proliferating cells (×200)

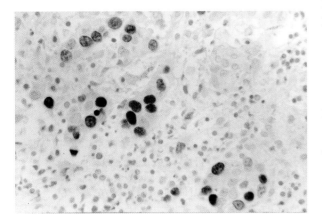

Figure 8.8   Immunohistochemical detection of bromodeoxyuridine incorporated into the nuclei of proliferating cells (×400)

in vivo, providing a true measure of proliferation 'rate'. Patients are injected with BrdU, which becomes incorporated into cells during DNA synthesis. The lesion is biopsied several hours after injection and from this tissue both the presence of BrdU incorporation and DNA content can be measured for individual cells. The relationship between the time between injection and sampling, BrdU uptake and DNA content allows the rate at which the cells in the lesion are proliferating to be determined.

Flow cytometry

Flow cytometry is one of the most reliable and reproducible methods of measuring proliferative activity and can be used on cytological, fresh or fixed, paraffin-embedded material. By measuring the amount of DNA in individual nuclei that have been disaggregated from a piece of tissue, a histogram can be generated showing the numbers of cells with similar amounts of DNA. Computerized analysis of these histograms allows the proportion of cells in each phase of the cell cycle to be calculated. As far as proliferative activity information is concerned, it is the proportion of cells in S-phase or the S-phase fraction which is of most interest.

Flow cytometry is one of the most objective methods of assessing proliferative activity but, as the tissue has to be disaggregated before analysis, the results cannot be related to morphology and the sample may include normal, benign and non-specific elements of the tissue under study. Furthermore, when using paraffin-embedded material, a substantial piece of tissue is needed and even then the number of incomplete or poorly preserved nuclei in the sample means that about a quarter of the histograms cannot be interpreted with any degree of accuracy. The capabilities of the flow cytometer have developed considerably since the early days of measuring a single parameter, DNA content. It now has facilities for multiple measurements and its use has become even more specialized. The measurement of DNA content is more likely to be carried out in conjunction with the measurement of one or more immuno-fluorescent detected proteins, providing information on the relationship between phase of the cell cycle and protein expression. The technique of flow cytometry and computerized analysis of the results suggests a more 'scientific' approach to assessing proliferation; however, a number of studies have shown that similar information can be obtained by careful counting of mitoses, Ki67 positivity and MIB1 positivity, all of which can be carried out in histopathology laboratories without special equipment.

Other markers

There continues to be a steady flow of potential markers of proliferation; many of these are antibodies raised against proteins which have an increased level of expression during the cell cycle. In a similar fashion to Ki67 and PCNA, it has been assumed that if an antigen is present during a specific phase or phases of the cell cycle, then its detection means that it can be used to identify cells which are proliferating. Amongst these putative markers have been different members of the cyclin family and their associated cyclin-dependant kinases (cdks) and retinoblastoma protein (pRb). Other proteins associated with DNA replication have also been identified as potential markers, including minichromosome maintenance proteins (Mcm). These Mcm proteins (of which there are six, Mcm 2, 3, 4, 5, 6 and 7) are involved in both the initiation of DNA replication and the prevention of re-replication in a single cell cycle.

Unfortunately, many of these cell cycle-associated markers have an altered expression in malignant cells, because of changes in the regulatory pathway of proteins controlling the cell cycle, and are not suitable markers of proliferative activity. As a consequence of the high level of interest in identifying proteins which control the cell cycle, novel antibodies are being developed and marketed at a great rate. This is outstripping the pace at which their potential as proliferation markers can be fully evaluated. Consequently, care must be taken when using any new antibody to ensure that it has been adequately validated before being accepted as a proliferation marker. Nevertheless, many of the antibodies are of interest as therapy-related targets to specific biological therapies, rather than tools for measuring proliferation.

In situ hybridization has also been used to demonstrate proliferative activity. Expression of histone 3 (H3) mRNA has been recognized as such a marker for a number of years and compares well with other markers that provide prognostic information. Histones are the major protein component of chromatin and have a role in packaging strands of DNA into a compact form, the nucleosome. As histones are so closely associated with DNA, they also have to be manufactured during DNA synthesis. Hence, detection of increased levels of H3 mRNA in S-phase reflects the prolferative activity of the tissues. Levels of H3 mRNA are known to rapidly decrease during G_2 and no synthesis occurs once the cell enters G_0, which makes it one of the most specific markers of proliferative activity. However, this method is not widely used, primarily because the *in situ* hybridization technique required to detect mRNA is not readily available in most laboratories; also, the results are not significantly better than other markers that do not require a specialized detection method. *In situ* hybridization techniques, and particularly the non-isotopic ones, are gradually being introduced into more laboratories, so perhaps proliferative information will be more frequently obtained using H3 mRNA in the future.

Figure 8.9 shows how the different markers of proliferative activity relate both to each other and to the different phases of the cell cycle.

Practical use of markers

The choice of method of measuring proliferative activity very much depends upon the type of material being assessed. If a retrospective study is being undertaken using paraffin-embedded material, methods such as TLI, BrdULI and mKi67 cannot be used.

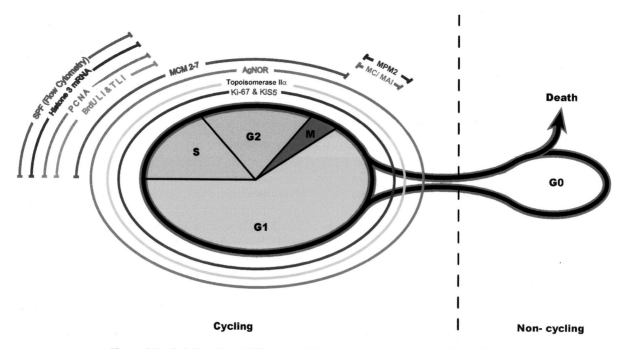

Figure 8.9 Relationship of different proliferation markers to phases of the cell cycle

Tissue preparation points to consider include the type of fixative used, since this influences all markers, and the effect that a delay in fixation may cause. Mitotic figures are very difficult to distinguish from apoptotic bodies in some alcohol-based fixatives; likewise, AgNORs can also be difficult to identify. Antigen expression is reduced and even lost in some fixative solutions, despite the use of heat-mediated antigen retrieval. Even in flow cytometry the nuclear dyes are unable to bind to the chromatin when a metal-containing fixative has been used. Some studies have shown that a delay in fixation reduces the number of mitoses in the tissue and would, therefore, underestimate the proliferative activity. Finally, section thickness is usually not considered to have a significant effect on the demonstration and evaluation of markers. Nevertheless, as well as altering the quality of staining, both mitotic and AgNOR counts will vary according to the thickness of the section and in immunohistochemistry the resultant staining will vary in intensity, an important factor if this is included as part of the evaluation. All sections that are to undergo a heat-mediated antigen retrieval step must be put onto adhesive-coated slides and baked on, otherwise the sections will lift and some become totally detached.

Method of evaluation

Once the most suitable proliferation marker has been selected and the method carried out, the next question is, "How do I count it?" This is often considered to be the final and easiest stage of the whole technique, but it requires a methodical approach to obtain consistent and reproducible results. It is at this stage where flow cytometry has a distinct advantage over the other markers, as thousands of cells can be quickly assessed with a satisfactory degree of consistency between samples. All of the other methods in which a proliferation marker is demonstrated in a histological section have a number of similar criteria which must be met.

First, the time taken to carry out the evaluation must be balanced against the value of the information being obtained. It would be pointless to spend 20 minutes carrying out a formal count on a section, when similar prognostic information can be obtained using a semi-quantitative method which takes a fraction of that time. Second, whatever method of evaluation is used, it must be both reliable and consistent.

Most methods of evaluation used with the markers discussed here are conventional counts or estimates, but there are an increasing number of image analysis-based systems coming onto the market which have a different method of evaluation. Using manual methods, a number of criteria have to be met in order to reduce subjectivity associated with the evaluation, thereby allowing comparisons to be made between both samples and evaluators. The following points should always be considered before undertaking any assessment and must not be deviated from during the course of the study.

Which area of the section should be evaluated?

Traditionally, the 'growing edge' of a tumour is considered to be the most appropriate area for evaluation. This tends to be the most proliferative and is often the area in which the mitotic count for a histological grade is calculated. An alternative is to use the 'worst' or most poorly differentiated area, which potentially provides the poorest prognostic characteristics. Selecting the growing edge is virtually impossible in some forms of tissue preparation, such as needle core biopsies or trans-urethral resections of prostate. Moreover, both TLI and BrdULI methods require that fresh tissue be cut into very small pieces to allow access of the nucleotides to the nucleus. Again, it is almost impossible to be certain that the 'growing edge' is being evaluated.

If a *formal count* is being made, then a sufficient number of cells must be evaluated to be representative of the section as a whole, thus reducing the effect of area selection, whereas if an *estimate* of the frequency of the marker is being made, then the entire section is assessed. Automated systems have the benefit of making a formal evaluation on selected areas across the whole section.

Which method of assessment should be used?

It is no longer appropriate to carry out an assessment of proliferation without defining the criteria used to reach the end result. It is important to decide whether intensity of staining is an important feature. Obviously, this will not be a consideration for evaluating either mitoses or AgNORs, but with immunohistochemical-based markers it may represent an increase in protein expression above its usual base level, such as in the case of PCNA. If intensity of staining is relevant, then it should be combined with either a count or an estimate of the proportion of stained cells.

Accurate quantification of any marker requires a formal count to be made of both the cells that are expressing the marker and those that are not, thus providing a 'proliferative index'. A quick look at the publications where a count has been undertaken reveals the considerable variation in the total number of cells evaluated. To be statistically correct, sufficient numbers of cells must be evaluated in order to reduce the counting error to an acceptable level; this is usually considered to be less than 5%. If only a few cells are evaluated, the result could considerably either overestimate or underestimate the true proliferative activity. As the number of cells included in the evaluation is increased, this error is gradually reduced. A universal figure for the number of cells to count cannot be applied to all of the different markers and different types of tissue. In general, counts need to be increased, both in heterogeneous tissues and when the incidence of demonstration of the marker is low. For example, MIB1 detects cells in all phases of the cell cycle except G_0, whereas a mitotic index 'detects' events only in a limited part of the cell cycle. Hence, in any given piece of tissue, the proportion of cells expressing MIB1 will be much higher than those undergoing mitosis. Therefore, in order to achieve the same acceptable level of error for both markers, the total number of cells evaluated for the mitotic activity index would need to be much more than for the MIB1 count.

There has been little published work directed at comparing counting methods, but in general counts in excess of 1000 cells appear to reduce the counting error to an acceptable level. Sometimes counting as many cells as this can be a problem in very small samples, such as needle core biopsies or when the lesion of interest forms only a small part of the tissue being examined, e.g. mammary ductal carcinoma *in situ* or other intra-epithelial neoplasms. In such cases it may be necessary to evaluate multiple levels of the tissue in order to get an accurate record of the proliferative activity.

As previously mentioned, it is important to balance the time spent evaluating a proliferative marker with the amount of information it provides. Although assessing more cells increases accuracy, it is often not practical and it will certainly not endear the technique to a busy histopathologist. Semi-quantitative assessments which have defined criteria are proving popular because of their relative speed of assessment and because they have been shown to correlate well with markers assessed more quantitatively. For many years mitoses have been counted and expressed per high-power field, which is in itself a semi-quantitative assessment. Prognostic information for both breast and smooth muscle tumours has improved with a more stringent approach to counting mitoses, whilst retaining the use of high-power fields. There are now guidelines on how many HPFs to examine and which area of the section to assess. The considerable variation in size of HPFs between different microscopes

has also been noted, so it is important to quote the area of the HPF which was used to make the mitotic count. By following these general guidelines, a considerable reduction in inter-observer variability has been achieved.

If a semi-quantitative assessment is used, it is important to remember that it is only an estimation and that the results should not be too precise; the use of quartiles is usually sufficient. The advantage with this type of evaluation is that it can be done quickly enough for the whole of the section to be assessed, thus removing the need to define which area of the section has been examined. If appropriate, a measure of intensity of staining can be combined with the proportion of cells staining, to give a total score.

A direct comparison of the different methods of evaluation and how long both the technique and the evaluation take for the established markers is shown in Table 8.1.

Controls

As with any technique, it is important to have controls throughout the procedure. Not only are methodological control sections required but also checks should be done to ensure consistency in both demonstration and evaluation of markers between samples.

Control material must always be included when demonstrating a proliferation marker. The same control sections should be used throughout a study in order to monitor inter-assay consistency. Internal controls, when the staining patterns of specific tissue elements are known, are also very useful to check on the quality of demonstration. They can also be used to make adjustments to the 'score' when the sections are thicker (and hence the staining is more intense), or when the method of fixation is sub-optimal.

Reproducibility of the evaluation procedure should also be included as part of the 'quality control' aspect of any study or individual case. If either a new marker or a new evaluation method is being introduced, or someone has not assessed proliferative activity before, then the assessment should also be carried out by an experienced 'evaluator'. Comparison of the data from both assessors provides a guide to the inter-observer variability. Any discordant values can be re-examined with joint consultation. Evaluator skills tend to improve with practice, therefore that have been assessed early on in a study, should be repeated at the end, to ensure that the result is the same and the method of evaluation has remained consistent.

Table 8.1 Comparison of time taken to demonstrate and evaluate different markers of proliferative activity

Marker	Method of evaluation	Time for technique	Time for evaluation (minutes)
Counting methods			
Mitosis	Mitosis/10 HPF	5 minutes	5
	Mitoses/2000 cells	5 minutes	15
pKi67/mKi67/MIB1/KiS5	Positive nuclei/1000 cells	2 hours	5–10
KiS1	Positive nuclei/1000 cells		
PCNA	Strong positive nuclei/2000 cells	2 hours	15–20
TLI	Labelled nuclei/2000 cells	10–14 days	15–20
BrDULI	Positive nuclei/2000 cells	3 hours	15–20
Histone 3 mRNA	Positive nuclei/2000 cells	24 hours	15–20
AgNOR	Mean number/100 cells	15–45 minutes	20–35
Automated methods			
S-phase fraction (flow cytometry)	Quantity of nuclear staining/ cell in > 10 000 cells	2–3 hours	>5
Image analysis methods			
pKi67, MIB1	Percentage of positive staining in relation to all non-positive in selected area	2 hours	15–20
AgNORS	Mean area of AgNORs occupying nucleus in 150 cells	15–45 minutes	15–20

There are now a number of computer-aided image analysis systems commercially available, with software specifically designed to detect and measure Ki67-associated proliferation markers. Moreover, these can be adapted for use with any immunohistochemically detected nuclear antigen. Evaluation of proliferation markers can potentially be more accurate and reliable with the aid of computerized systems, and the evaluation of AgNORs in particular has benefited from semi-automated analysis. AgNORs are extremely difficult to count with any degree of reliability and their proliferative value has been hotly disputed. Measuring the mean total area of silver deposition per nucleus by image analysis has shown a consistent association with proliferative activity measured by other means and has considerably improved the credibility of the AgNORs.

Recognition of individual cells in a histological section remains a difficult task for an image analyser, and discerning a weakly positive immunostained cell from a negative cell, whilst appearing easy to the human eye, proves difficult for an analysis system. If a slice is taken through a sphere, as when a nucleus is sectioned, then the internal edges of the sphere will be less dense than more central areas. If this is considered in the context of an immunohistochemically stained nucleus, then the nucleus will have reduced colour intensity at the periphery, which can be difficult to distinguish from the non-staining cytoplasm. Unfortunately, programmes that can recognize the various characteristics associated with nuclei undergoing mitosis are still not generally available.

One of the main problems that must be overcome with the move towards the use of automatic methods of evaluation is the need to break away from the idea that image analysis should provide information in an identical format to that of a visual assessment. In a number of studies, where immunohistochemical 'markers' have been shown to be prognostically useful, the image analysis systems have compared areas of colour. For example, in each HPF or specifically marked area, the analyser compares the total area of brown, which denotes DAB demonstration of a bound proliferation-associated antibody, with the total area of blue, which denotes the haematoxylin-stained nuclei. These parameters are measured within these selected areas and the resultant proliferative activity is shown by the ratio of total area of the proliferation marker to total area of nuclei. With the proviso that only groups of malignant cells are selected, some analysis systems transform the results so that they are presented in a conventional form, i.e. as a percentage of positive cells.

In conclusion

The initial confusion which greets most novices in the measurement of proliferative activity can be easily remedied by looking at one aspect of the procedure at a time. First of all, some of the markers, such as TLI or mKi67 may be discounted if the tissues of interest are fixed and embedded in paraffin. The choice of marker is also dependent upon the facilities available in the laboratory. Specific projects, with a limited number of cases, can often be undertaken in conjunction with a laboratory with specialized facilities. This would enable methods like flow cytometric analysis or autoradiography for thymidine labelling to be carried out. However, if measuring proliferation is an ongoing need, then the type of method used for detecting proliferating cells should be suited to the individuals' own laboratory. For this reason there is a tendency for the more conventional 'morphometric' methods, such as mitoses and AgNORs or immunohistochemical methods, to be used in histopathology laboratories.

The best methods of measuring proliferative activity in histological sections are still by examination of the proportion of either mitoses or MIB1-expressing cells. Both have been well documented in a variety of disorders, are technically easy to demonstrate and, provided that the sections are well prepared, are relatively easy to assess. They also give reproducible results which compare well with other more laborious or machine-dependent methods, such as TLI and flow cytometry. There remains great discussion as to how valid both mitoses and MIB1 are as markers of proliferative activity. Mitoses obviously only demonstrate a relatively short part of the cell cycle, and from the resultant mitotic count or activity index no inferences can be made about the rest of the cell cycle; however, there are certainly no problems with lack of specificity with this marker. MIB1 identifies a protein that is present virtually throughout the cell cycle, although some cells do not express the antigen early in G_1, and this effect would falsely underrepresent the proliferative activity in these particular tissues. As with the detection of many proteins expressed during the cell cycle, MIB1 can also be detected if the cell has recently left the cell cycle. Attempts have been made to develop new markers, and in particular antibodies, to overcome some of the problems with specificity. These novel markers would have to provide proliferative and prognostic information beyond that provided by mitoses or MIB1 if they are to be accepted as viable alternatives. A recent development is that most cell cycle-associated antigens which at one time would have been evaluated as proliferative markers are now being examined for their potential as therapy-related targets.

The evaluation debate looks set to continue for some time to come. For example, mitoses have been recognized as proliferative markers for decades and yet new 'improved' methods of evaluation are still being promoted. However, it must not be forgotten that once some of the evaluation criteria have been applied, and regardless of which method of assessment is chosen, the 'golden rule' is to be consistent from one case to the next. Automated analysis certainly improves accuracy and consistency in measuring some proliferation markers, but it is still not suitable for all. Until that time comes, sufficiently accurate results can be obtained by using either a formal count or a semi-quantitative evaluation, provided that a consistent approach is taken and adequate controls are used.

Further reading

Baak JPA. Mitosis counting in tumors. *Hum Pathol* 1990; **21**: 683–685.

Rüschoff J, Plate KH, Contractor H *et al.* Evaluation of nucleolus organizer regions (NORs) by automatic image analysis: a contribution to standardization. *J Pathol* 1990; **161**: 113–118.

Cattoretti G, Becker MHG, Key G *et al.* Monoclonal antibodies against recombinant parts of the Ki67 antigen (MIB-1 and MIB-3) detect proliferating cells in microwave-processed formalin-fixed paraffin sections. *J Pathol* 1992; **168**: 357–363.

Quirke P. Flow cytometry in the quantitation of DNA aneuploidy and cell proliferation in human disease. In JCE Underwood (ed.) *Current Topics in Pathology—Pathology of the Nucleus.* 1990: Springer-Verlag, New York, 215–256.

SECTION 2

CYTOLOGY

9

Cytopathology

Adrian T Warfield

This chapter is intended to provide a synoptic overview of the general principles of diagnostic cytopathology. This is largely a visual subject and therefore plentiful examples and illustrations are included as appropriate. It is by no means a technical or diagnostic treatise on the subject. For systematic, detailed coverage, the interested reader is encouraged to consult one of the many works of reference, some of which are listed at the conclusion of this chapter.

Introduction

Cytology is the scientific study of the structure and function of cells. Cytopathology is a branch of laboratory medicine concerned with the examination of cells in health and disease for screening, diagnostic and research purposes. Screening involves the examination of samples from asymptomatic individuals to detect premalignant or early malignant changes. Diagnostic work involves the assessment of material from patients with established signs or symptoms of disease.

It is a basic premise that the content of a cytology specimen should accurately and reproducibly represent the cell population of the target tissue or lesion. In reality, a number of confounding variables sometimes militate against this assumption to a greater or lesser degree.

A careful cytomorphological assessment by light microscopy is fundamental to the practice of diagnostic cytopathology and much information has traditionally been derived from the direct comparison of cell samples with corresponding histological sections. Certain limitations, however, are inherent in such extrapolation studies, even in adequately sampled, optimally preserved and well-stained material.

Cell culture utilizes immortalized cell lines to detect viral cytopathic and other toxic effects. This and novel, specialized microscopy, microsuction and microdissection techniques enable insight into the dynamic physiology of living protoplasm. At present, however, these are considered peripheral to mainstream diagnostic cytopathology and are encountered more commonly in viral diagnostic or research work.

Types of cytology specimen

Most clinical cytology specimens are obtained by one of the following processes.

Exfoliation

Cells sampled are shed (exfoliated) naturally from an epithelial surface. Examples include cells present in sputum (expectorated), urine (voided or via catheter or cystoscope) and nipple discharge (expressed) (Figures 9.1, 9.2). Spontaneously exfoliated cells differ in appearance from those forcibly denuded by mechanical means, tending to be disaggregated and individually disposed

The Science of Laboratory Diagnosis, Second Edition   Edited by David Burnett and John Crocker
© 2005 John Wiley & Sons, Ltd

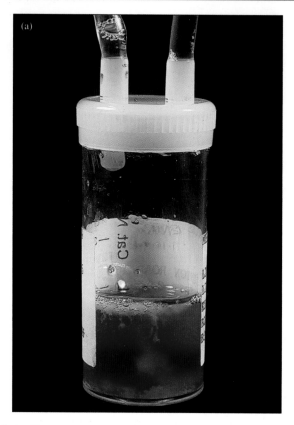

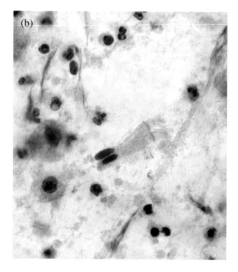

Figure 9.1   Sputum sample. (a) Mucoid, blood-stained sputum obtained by direct suction aspiration ('sputum trap'). This gives less contamination by oropharyngeal secretions than an expectorated sample. (b) Bronchial epithelial cells and pulmonary alveolar macrophages here indicate lower respiratory tract sampling. Terminal bars and surface microvilli can be seen at the apices of the bronchial cells amidst a sparse mucoinflammatory background (Pap ×250)

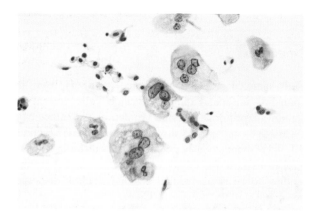

Figure 9.2   Normal superficial transitional cells in urine. These exfoliated uroepithelial cells show variable multinucleation corresponding to 'umbrella cells' in histological sections. Note the uncluttered ('clean') background (Pap ×100)

or in small clusters. Such cells often assume a spherical form, dependent upon such factors as the rigidity of the cell membrane, inherent cytoskeletal forces, surface tension, the nature of the local micro-environment and the time since shedding. They are susceptible to a series of degenerative changes involving both the cytoplasm and the nucleus, as outlined later.

Abrasion

Cells sampled result from denudation by physical force (abrasion). Examples include brushings (e.g. bronchus, cervix), scrapings (e.g. nipple, skin, cervix) or lavage (e.g. bronchus), where isotonic saline is insufflated and the fluid re-aspirated is submitted for examination. In contrast to naturally exfoliated cells, these cells tend to be better preserved, often in larger groups or cohesive aggregates.

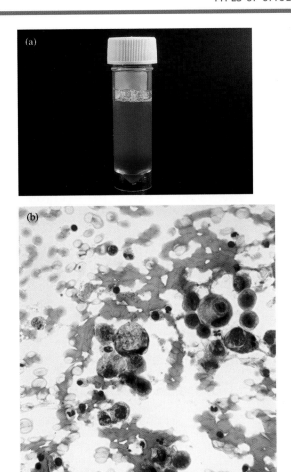

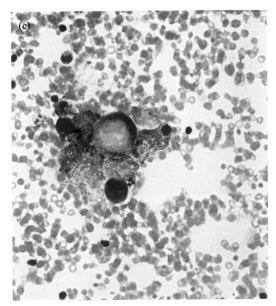

Figure 9.3 Malignant pleural aspirate. (a) Bloodstained sample from a unilateral pleural effusion in a patient who had undergone mastectomy for breast carcinoma. Microscopy (b and c) shows dyscohesive pleomorphic adenocarcinoma cells, many possessing a 'signet ring' morphology with abundant intracytoplasmic mucin indenting the peripheral nucleus (b, Pap ×100; c, MGG ×100)

Aspiration

There are few organs or sites in the body which are not readily accessible by needle to yield some sort of cellular material for examination. Radiological imaging techniques may assist in localizing small, deep, mobile lesions that are otherwise difficult to palpate. Cells are obtained through a needle, with or without suction, from a fluid-filled cavity or solid tissue. Examples include tumours, pericardial, pleural or peritoneal fluid (paracentesis), cerebrospinal fluid (lumbar or cisternal puncture) and vitreous humour (Figures. 9.3, 9.4).

Fine needle aspiration utilizes a fine bore needle (19–25 gauge) firmly attached to a syringe, which is introduced into a lesion. The syringe plunger is partially withdrawn, thereby creating a vacuum and aspirating lesional cells. Several passes through a lesion in different directions whilst maintaining suction may be attempted to increase the cellular harvest. Once completed, the plunger is released to equalize the pressure prior to withdrawal of the needle from the lesion. Various 'pistol grip' attachments designed to facilitate single-handed manipulation of the syringe are commercially available, freeing the opposite hand for palpation (Figure 9.5). Needle sampling without suction is preferred by some for superficially located lesions. Fine needle aspiration has gained widespread popularity, largely because it is cheap, rapid, largely atraumatic and therefore well tolerated with few complications and few contraindications. Percutaneous lesions usually require no local anaesthesia. Transrectal, transvaginal, transpleural and transperitoneal routes via an endoscope may also be attempted.

Bone marrow aspirates are normally the province of the diagnostic haematopathologist.

Failure to obtain a satisfactory aspirate may not necessarily be attributable to poor technique. Desmoplastic, hyalinized or vascular lesions, extensive necrosis, cystic change or haemorrhage may all preclude adequate cell sampling (Figure 9.6).

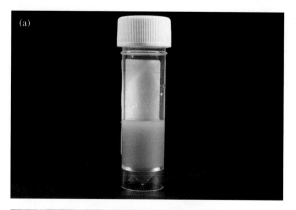

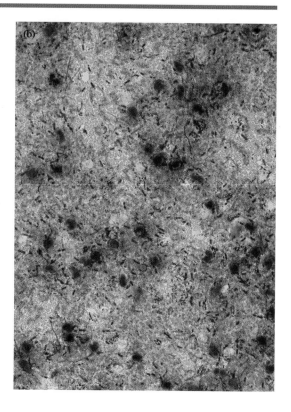

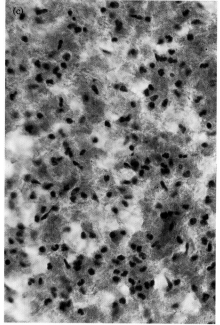

Figure 9.4 Ascitic fluid. (a) An aliquot of turbid, malodorous ascitic fluid aspirated from a patient with faecal peritonitis shortly prior to death. Microscopy (b) and (c) shows innumerable variform bacteria with pus cells. The debris and pigment are of stercoral origin (b, Pap ×100; c, MGG ×100)

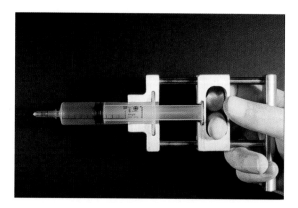

Figure 9.5 Pistol attachment for fine needle aspiration. Ready with loaded disposable syringe and 23 gauge needle, this allows single-handed manipulation of the syringe, freeing the other hand for palpation

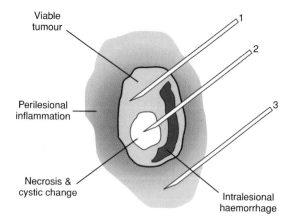

Figure 9.6 Schematic diagram of a tumour during fine needle aspiration. The viable solid portion of the tumour is pierced by needle 1 to yield potentially diagnostic material; needle 2, piercing areas of necrosis, haemorrhage or cystic change, and needle 3, sampling perilesional tissue, are unlikely to do so

Smearing techniques

The ideal smear should be evenly spread, uniformly thin and flat to enable rapid drying and fixation and to permit optimal penetration of stain. *Direct smear* techniques involve spreading fresh material across a slide, utilizing another slide, pick or spatula (Figure 9.7). *Indirect smear* techniques employ material suspended in fluid, e.g. saline or transport medium. A cell concentration procedure may be performed as an intermediary step to increase the yield from a hypocellular specimen.

Clot formation may sequester much of the cellular component of a specimen, preventing adequate transfer of material to a slide. If a clot cannot be dispersed by mechanical means, it should therefore be processed as a cell block or submitted for conventional histology and examined thoroughly (Figure 9.8).

Cell deposits from transudates, salinated washings and urine may not adhere well to glass slides. Adhesives, commonly of proteinaceous (e.g. bovine serum albumin) or ionic (e.g. poly-L-lysine) type, may enhance adherence, maximizing the cellular material for examination.

Other techniques less commonly employed include touch imprints, scrapings and squash preparations, the latter popular in peroperative neurosurgical diagnosis in preference to conventional histology on frozen sections.

Specimen fixation

Wet fixation

Wet fixation dehydrates protoplasm and coagulates protein, usually employing an alcohol-based fluid, either by immersion or coating. Such fixation induces a degree of cell shrinkage in the final preparation. Carnoy's fluid selectively lyses erythrocytes and may be helpful in heavily blood-stained specimens. Other fixatives, e.g. glutaraldehyde or formalin, may be preferred under certain circumstances. Polyethylene glycol in alcohol provides a protective waxy coating for postal despatch which should be thoroughly removed before subsequent staining.

Air drying

Air drying relies upon evaporation, which should be rapid and is best facilitated by forced air movement over the slide rather than passively. This method tends to flatten cells with apparent enlargement compared to wet fixation (Figures 9.9, 9.10). Air–dried preparations are almost invariably post-fixed in methanol after drying to prevent cross-infection hazards.

Material such as cyst fluid or needle washings following fine needle aspiration may be received in transport medium. It should be remembered that any fresh biological specimen constitutes a potential biohazard to laboratory personnel and recommended health and safety precautions should always be observed.

Cell concentration techniques

Centrifugation

This method is suitable for voluminous specimens such as serous effusions, urine or salinated lavage samples.

Cytocentrifugation

This utilizes small aliquots of fluid spun directly onto microscope slides to form a localized monolayer of cells (Figures 9.11, 9.12, 9.13). It is suitable for low-volume samples of modest cellularity. Some material is, however, inevitably lost into the filter card. Viscid or cellular specimens are unsuitable.

Membrane filtration

Positive pressure or vacuum filtration is employed by using various types of filter of predetermined pore size, e.g. cellulose acetate or polycarbonate. It is suitable for a wide range of large volume or hypocellular fluid specimens and may yield a greater cell capture than centrifugation methods.

Cell block preparation

Cells are aggregated into a tissue-like state enabling sections to be cut comparable to conventional histology. Methods include plasma thrombin clot utilizing plasma and agar cell block with hot agar. They are suitable for most cell suspensions and allow special staining including immunocytochemistry.

Liquid-based cytology

Refinement of the foregoing techniques of processing and preparation of cytology specimens has been gradual over a prolonged period. Increasing expectation in recent

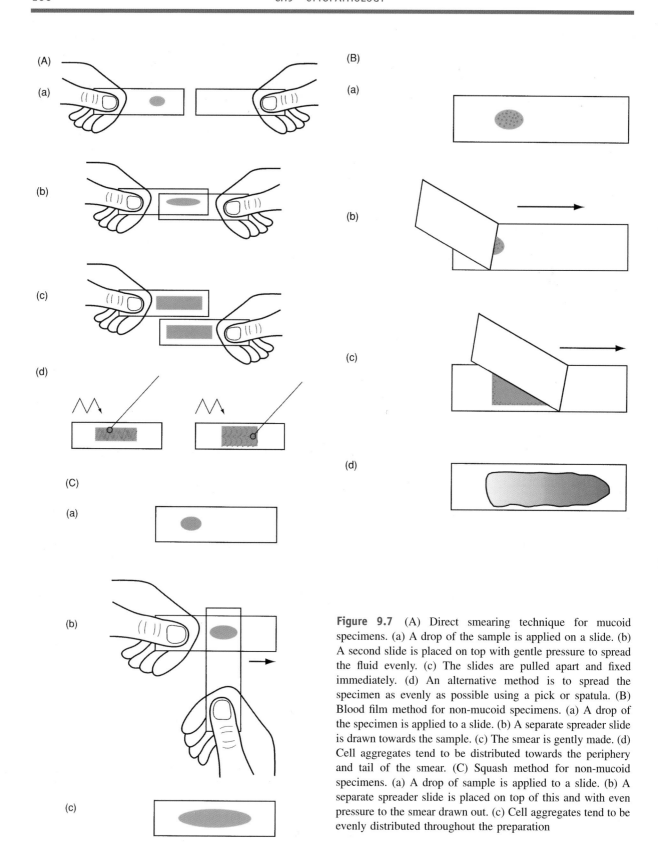

Figure 9.7 (A) Direct smearing technique for mucoid specimens. (a) A drop of the sample is applied on a slide. (b) A second slide is placed on top with gentle pressure to spread the fluid evenly. (c) The slides are pulled apart and fixed immediately. (d) An alternative method is to spread the specimen as evenly as possible using a pick or spatula. (B) Blood film method for non-mucoid specimens. (a) A drop of the specimen is applied to a slide. (b) A separate spreader slide is drawn towards the sample. (c) The smear is gently made. (d) Cell aggregates tend to be distributed towards the periphery and tail of the smear. (C) Squash method for non-mucoid specimens. (a) A drop of sample is applied to a slide. (b) A separate spreader slide is placed on top of this and with even pressure to the smear drawn out. (c) Cell aggregates tend to be evenly distributed throughout the preparation

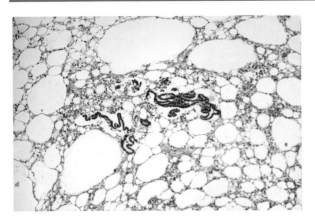

Figure 9.8 Benign mucinous tumour of ovary. This fibrin clot has sequestered virtually all of the aspirated epithelium from the fluid from this cystic ovary. The corresponding cytopreparations consisted almost exclusively of blood and, in isolation, were deemed unsatisfactory for diagnostic purposes. This illustrates the importance of examining any clot present in fluid aspirates (H&E ×25)

years, however, has led to critical re-examination of many aspects of the traditional methodology, in particular seeking ways of capitalizing upon the latest technological advancements.

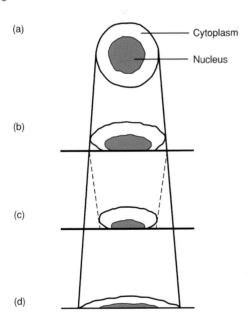

Figure 9.9 Effect of wet fixation and air drying on cells. (a) An unfixed cell in solution often assumes a spherical shape. (b) This settles onto a slide and partially flattens. (c) Wet fixation ultimately shrinks the cell somewhat. (d) Air drying causes flattening and spreading of the cell with apparent enlargement in its final state. A spherical cell may present a diameter twice its original size, whereas a mature squamoid cell will show little apparent increase in size

Liquid-based cytology has evolved out of a desire to augment the sensitivity and specificity of cytology as a screening and diagnostic modality. A number of proprietary systems are currently available, based upon manufacturer-specific manual, semi-automated or fully-automated protocols. The principles of operation are, nevertheless, broadly similar, with the aim of producing a homogeneous, cleaner, flatter sample covering a smaller area of the slide. This facilitates easier and quicker screening, with a concomitant reduction in the frequency of unsatisfactory specimens. The technology is being successfully adapted to both gynaecological and non-gynaecological applications.

Samples are generally collected in the usual manner and transferred into specified transport or preservation fluid to form a *cell suspension*. Some systems employ patented brushes or brooms, which are broken off into the fluid, thus ensuring capture of the whole specimen, whilst others utilize a rinsing procedure to harvest the target cell population. In the laboratory, the material is then processed to remove blood, inflammatory and proteinaceous exudate. An aliquot of the suspension is ultimately deposited as a thin, uniform layer onto a glass slide. The even dispersion, good cell preservation, consistent cell staining, enhanced microscopical detail and diminution in artefacts compare favourably with smears prepared by conventional techniques. Any cell sheets and groups tend to be smaller and there is less obfuscation by background elements.

The ThinPrep (*Cytyc Corporation*) method is centred around an open, disposable plastic tube lined by a filter. The specimen is collected in a methanol-based medium and centrifuged. A sample from the cell pellet is then transferred to a methanol-based preservative fluid. There are a further three main stages of preparation: first, *cell dispersion*, whereby the machine inserts the filter tube into the vial of cell suspension and agitates it to disperse mucus and any cell clumps; second, *cell collection*, where a slight vacuum pulse draws fluid into the tube through the filter, upon which a layer of cellular material is deposited. Some blood, inflammatory cells and cellular debris may pass through the filter and the flow of fluid is monitored to optimize cell capture; third, *cell transfer*, when the filter tube is inverted and gently pressed against an electrostatically charged slide. The slide is immediately immersed in fixative and is then ready for subsequent staining, either manually or by machine. The whole procedure is relatively swift at under 30 minutes and requires little technician time. The cell deposition area measures 1.9 cm in diameter and contains in the order of 100 000 cells.

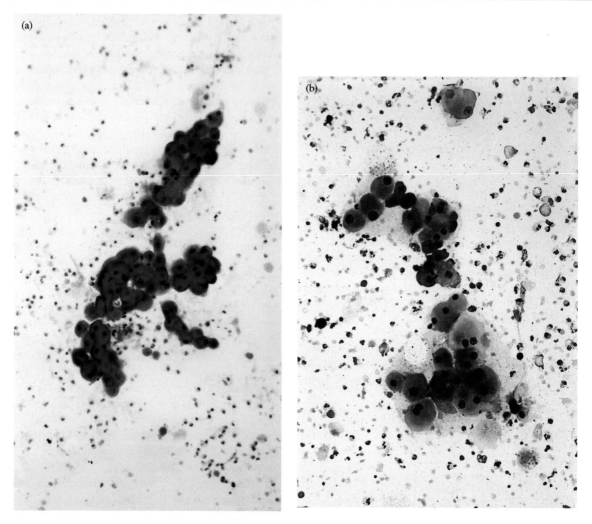

Figure 9.10 Metaplastic apocrine cells from a breast cyst. These benign epithelial cells were present in fluid from a breast cyst and illustrate the complementary nature of the Papanicolaou and May–Grünwald–Giemsa staining. The apparent disparity in the size of the cells at identical magnification is due to wet fixation and dry fixation, respectively (a, Pap ×50; b, MGG ×50)

The SurePath Prep (TriPath Imaging Inc.) method begins with collection of the sample into an ethanol-based medium. In the laboratory the vial is vortexed to disperse the cells and the suspension undergoes a stage of *cell enrichment* via density gradient centrifugation. This also removes blood and other contaminant debris. The supernatant fluid is removed, the cell pellet is re-suspended and centrifuged for a second time. An aliquot of the cell pellet is then robotically transferred to a settling chamber, where the cells are allowed to sediment under gravity to produce a thin layer on a poly-L-lysine-coated microscope slide. The machine subsequently stains the slides automatically. This process takes roughly 60 minutes and requires a degree of manual intervention. The circular deposit measures approximately 1.3 cm in diameter and includes around 100 000 cells.

The Cytoscreen method is a manual process relying upon photometry to evaluate the cellularity of the cell suspension prior to centrifugation onto a glass slide. The Labonard Easy Prep is another manual method, whereby an aliquot of sample fluid is loaded into a separation chamber attached to a glass slide, which contains absorbent paper. The cells settle in a thin layer and the preparation is stained using normal laboratory procedures.

Liquid-based cytology does not utilize the entire sample, thus affording the opportunity for ancillary test procedures, e.g. *in situ* hybridization or hybrid capture techniques to detect *Human papillomavirus* or other

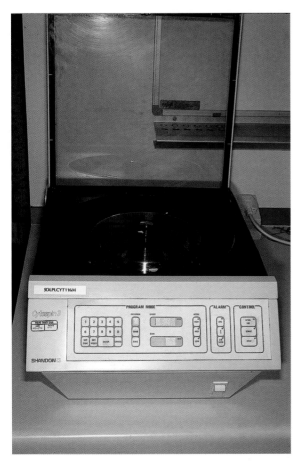

Figure 9.11 A modern cytocentrifuge machine

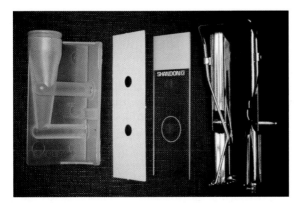

Figure 9.12 Cytocentrifuge chamber components. Suction chamber, filter card, glass slide and spring clip prior to assembly

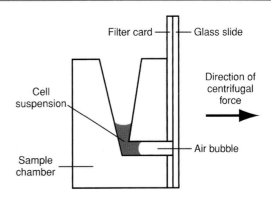

Figure 9.13 Schematic diagram of cytocentrifuge assembly. Centrifugal force drives the cell suspension through the filter card and onto the glass slide. This is unsuitable for mucoid specimens

infectious agents. The preparations are as amenable to other staining procedures, such as immunocytochemistry, as conventional techniques, with the advantage that the uncluttered background is less susceptible to spurious staining. In certain non-gynaecological specimens, where loss of background material and modulation of architectural features may be a problem, liquid-based procedures may be employed alongside traditional techniques as a helpful adjunct.

Staining methods

Many techniques applied to tissue sections may also be performed on cytopreparations. In general the Papanicolaou (Pap) stain is employed for wet-fixed material. The differential staining pattern is useful for both gynaecological and non-gynaecological specimens and permits prolonged periods of microscopy with minimal eye strain.

Romanowsky stains (May–Grünwald–Giemsa (MGG), Diff Quik, etc) are usually performed on air–dried preparations and are amenable both to automatic and rapid manual techniques. This method is employed predominantly for non-gynaecological material.

Haematoxylin and eosin staining is favoured by some more familiar with conventional histological sections.

A wide variety of ancillary histochemical stains may be performed as indicated. Examples include periodic acid–Schiff with or without diastase predigestion for neutral mucosubstances and glycogen, trichrome stains, Ziehl–Neelsen, Gram and Grocott methenamine silver stains, amongst others.

The repertoire of immunocytological techniques is comparable to that on tissue sections. Immunocytochemistry may be invaluable in ascertaining the presence of

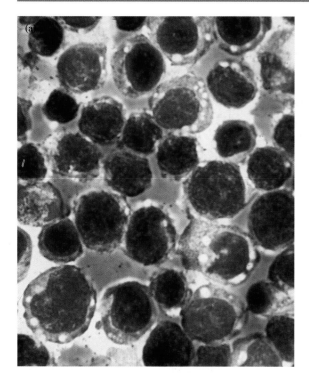

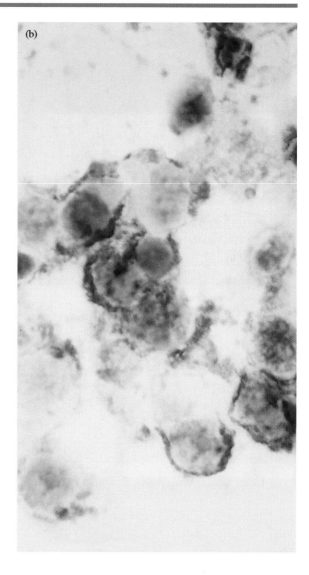

Figure 9.14 Low-grade non-Hodgkin's lymphoma. (a) This aspirate of vitreous humour from the eye contains innumerable, modestly pleomorphic, immature-looking lymphocytes with varying amounts of cytoplasm (MGG × high power). (b) Immunocytochemistry confirms widespread CD45 (leukocyte common antigen) reactivity (immunoperoxidase × high power)

microorganisms or in demonstrating tumour cell differentiation (Figure 9.14).

Cytodiagnosis

The cytodiagnostic procedure is a complex process. It cannot be overemphasized that reaching a final conclusion depends on many factors, including detailed site-specific knowledge coupled with experience of normality, familiarity with the manifold appearances of many disease processes, awareness of mimics and artefacts and cognizance of the limitations of the technique, in conjunction with patient-specific details and the clinical context (see Table 9.1). Abundant, well-preserved mate-

rial as ever affords the best opportunity of reaching a definitive diagnosis. Without this background information the cytopreparation is in danger of becoming a two-dimensional, brightly-stained artefact which may be as misleading as it can be potentially helpful. In some instances it may be better to reach an initial 'blind' morphological diagnosis from first principles to avoid preconceived bias. This may then be modified, taking into account such variables as appropriate, before a diagnosis is proffered and any advice on patient management forthcoming.

A cytopreparation is usually a complex admixture of components in varying proportions, depending upon the tissue or lesion sampled. Normal and abnormal cells may be present and the cell content, disposition and

Table 9.1 Variables which might influence the final interpretation of a cytopreparation

Patient-specific details	Age and sex
	Hormonal status, e.g. pregnancy
	Clinical impression
	Previous treatment, e.g. radiotherapy, surgery
	Previous material, e.g. histology, cytology
	Other laboratory tests
Site-specific details	Knowledge of local anatomy
	Radiological features
	Awareness of pitfalls and mimics
	Limitations of technique
Cell population	Degree of cellularity
	Type of cells present, e.g. biphasic or single population
	Alien or native populations
	Normal or abnormal morphology
Cytomorphology	Background milieu
	Cell distribution and cohesion
	Individual cell morphology
Ancillary information	Electron microscopy
	Histochemical stains
	Immunocytochemistry
	Image analysis
	Flow cytometry
	Cytogenetics

distribution within a sample should be systematically assessed. Not all features will be relevant to any particular specimen.

Cytomorphology

Much of the diagnostic workload in most laboratories is concerned with discriminating between non-neoplastic, pre-neoplastic and neoplastic lesions. Normal cells are characterized by their morphological uniformity. The nuclear morphology reflects the state of proliferation of a cell and its reproductive capacity. The cytoplasm of a cell generally gives an indication of its origin, functional state and degree of differentiation.

Increased cell activity may be physiological, such as *hyperplasia*, due to hormonal modulation, or reparative and regenerative in response to damage. An abnormal, uncontrolled proliferative state implies neoplasia.

Decreased cell activity may also be physiological due to atrophy, involutional changes secondary to hormonal influence, senescence or degenerative, as in apoptosis.

There is no single cytomorphological criterion or limited set of criteria which in isolation allows a reliable distinction between biologically benign and malignant conditions under all circumstances. The cytonuclear differences between regenerative or hyperplastic cells and low-grade neoplastic cells may be subtle and on occasion indistinguishable. Post-radiotherapy, post-chemotherapy, viral and other changes may induce appearances which mimic closely those seen in neoplasia (Figure 9.15).

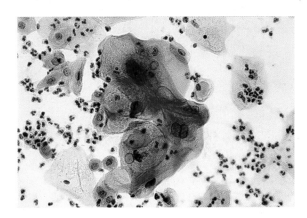

Figure 9.15 Radiation atypia in a vaginal vault smear. Abnormal giant squamous cells ('macrocytes') following radiotherapy. Similar bizarre changes may follow chemotherapy, accompany vitamin B12 or folate deficiency and may occur in viral condylomata. Note the multinucleation and increase in both nuclear and cytoplasmic area. Background inflammatory cells and superficial squamae are useful reference features (Pap ×100)

Specimen cellularity

The number and type of cells present give important information about the target tissue. Both are subject to lesional and non-lesional factors, particularly the sampling method employed. In general, hypercellularity raises the index of suspicion for a proliferative process, either hyperplasia or neoplasia. Conversely, however, paucicellularity is not necessarily a reassuring feature, as an absence of abnormal cells by no means excludes serious pathology. Low-grade neoplasms may exfoliate sparsely and yield cells showing minimal deviation from normality. A poverty of adequate material may be a crucial limiting factor in the degree of confidence in interpretation of a sample.

Cytoarchitectural pattern

Many of the architectural clues present in conventional histological sections are often absent in cytopreparations. Larger collections of cells (microbiopsies), if present, often recapitulate the histological pattern of the target tissue (Figure 9.16). Normal epithelium from

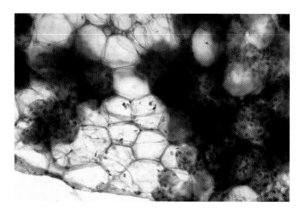

Figure 9.16 Normal parotid gland. This fine needle aspirate contains a 'microbiopsy' comprising adipose connective tissue intimately admixed with normal acinar secretory tissue from a middle-aged patient (Pap ×80)

many sites is characterized by retained cell polarity and intercellular cohesion. Glandular epithelium yields regularly arranged, monolayered sheets which when viewed *en face* give a 'honeycomb' appearance and in profile a palisaded 'picket-fence' pattern (Figures 9.17a,b).

Hyperplastic and benign neoplastic epithelia generally also retain cohesion but may exhibit an unusual outline, such as a papilliform, rosette or morular configuration. Syncytium formation with ill-defined cell boundaries and some malorientation is suspect of neoplasia. Malignant epithelical cells (carcinoma) usually present as poorly polarized, overlapping cells, sometimes in three-dimensional clumps (proliferation spheres) with a tendency towards dyscohesion and disaggregation. Normal lymphoid cells display poor intercellular cohesion, as do their neoplastic counterparts (lymphoma), and the dispersed cell pattern of poorly differentiated carcinoma and high-grade lymphoma may on occasion be indistinguishable without resort to ancillary techniques. Normal, reactive or neoplastic stromal cells (mesenchyme) may be apparent and adipocytes, capillaries or other connective tissue fragments often emanate from a perilesion site. Benign stromal elements usually manifest as ovoid or fusiform, loosely cohesive cells or bare nuclei (sentinel or bipolar cells), depending on the precise circumstances. Malignant stromal cells (sarcoma) show a similar pattern but with superimposed abnormal nuclear and cytoplasmic features.

Nuclear features

Abnormalities of nuclear morphology are termed *dyskaryosis* and may be graded as mild, moderate a severe or as high-grade and low-grade with increasing deviation from normality. In the normal end-differentiated (mature) cell the nucleus is relatively small compared

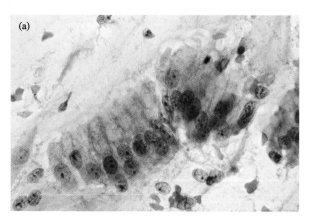
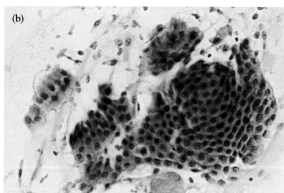

Figure 9.17 Normal gastric glandular epithelium. (a) Tall columnar glandular epithelial cells give a regular palisaded or 'picket-fence' appearance when viewed in profile. Note the preserved polarity and round, evenly-spaced nuclei with one or two small nucleoli (Pap ×80). (b) A monolayer of cohesive, well-orientated, isomorphic glandular epithelium displays a 'honeycomb' pattern when viewed en face. Again, the regularly spaced nuclei with occasional small nucleoli and rounded nuclear contour are well demonstrated (Pap ×40)

to the overall volume of the cell, usually of round or ovoid shape with a smooth nuclear contour, evenly distributed, with finely granular chromatin and little variation between cells of similar type (isomorphic or monomorphic).

In a two-dimensional cytopreparation the nuclear size is proportional to the relative nuclear area and may be expressed as the cytonuclear index, nuclear:cytoplasmic ratio or quantified as a percentage. Poorly differentiated cells usually possess enlarged nuclei (karyomegaly or nucleomegaly) and for the same absolute cytoplasmic volume therefore exhibit elevated nuclear:cytoplasmic ratio.

Most normal cells show reasonably homogeneous nuclear chromatin with a finely granular distribution and modest affinity for nuclear dyes. Increased nuclear DNA content results in greater density of nuclear staining (hyperchromasia). Irregularly distributed chromatin with a coarse, clumped texture and thickened nuclear envelope is termed *karyotheca*. Variation in size and shape of nuclei between cells is termed *anisokaryosis* or *anisonucleosis* and with increasing abnormality the nuclear membrane may become irregular in contour with grooving, indentation or crenation. The constellation of abnormal variation in size, shape and intensity of nuclear staining is termed *nuclear pleomorphism* (Figure 9.18).

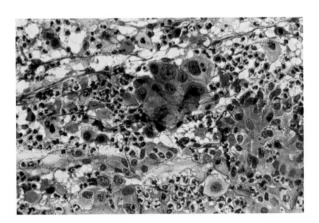

Figure 9.18 Poorly differentiated squamous cell carcinoma. These malignant cells from bronchial brushings are highly pleomorphic, poorly polarized and demonstrate karyotheca with macronucleolation. Keratinization was more conspicuous in the accompanying bronchial biopsies (Pap ×100)

Normal nuclei may contain small, discrete nucleoli composed of RNA and associated proteins. Multinucleolation and macronucleoli are observed in proliferation states, both neoplastic and non-neoplastic. Degenerative

chromatin may appear as a dense, contracted mass (*karyopyknosis*), as dense fragments (*karyorrhexis*) or may undergo dissolution (*karyolysis* or *chromatolysis*). Cytolysis may yield naked or bare, often hypochromatic, nuclear remnants and inherent nuclear membrane fragility of some cells results in nuclear streaming or smearing artefact. This often affects lymphoid cells or may be a feature of small cell, anaplastic carcinoma

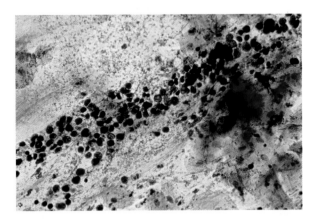

Figure 9.19 Anaplastic small cell carcinoma in sputum. Loosely cohesive, largely degenerate 'oat cell' carcinoma cells lie within a streak of mucus. In some the finely dispersed ('salt and pepper') chromatin is just discernible as is focal nuclear moulding. They possess minimal cytoplasm with hyperchromatic, karyopyknotic nuclei for the most part. Superficial squamae, erythrocytes and lymphocytes give an indication of relative size (Pap ×100)

(Figure 9.19). This may be closely mimicked by *vorticose* damage when cells are forcibly ejected through a fine bore needle onto a slide.

Most cells possess a single nucleus although some, undergoing regenerative or reparative activity, e.g. hepatocytes and chondrocytes, may be *binucleated*. Osteoclasts and syncytiotrophoblast are normally polynucleated. Multinucleation may be a feature both of inflammatory and neoplastic conditions. (Figures 9.20, 9.21).

It is unusual to encounter mitoses in cyto-preparations. An increased number of mitoses implies cell proliferation and abnormal spindle forms (tripolar, tetrapolar, etc.) are not usually seen in benign conditions.

Cytoplasmic features

Variation in the size and shape of similar cells is termed *anisocytosis*. The cytoplasmic volume of an abnormal

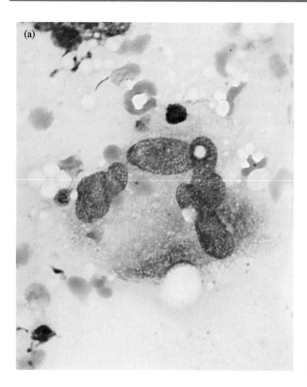

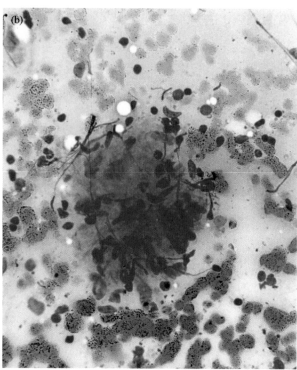

Figure 9.20   (a) Langhans' giant cell in tuberculosis. This multinucleated giant cell in a fine needle aspirate is of histiocytic origin. The peripheral 'horseshoe' orientation of the nuclei is typical. Other types of giant cell may be observed in a multitude of inflammatory and neoplastic conditions (MGG ×250). (b) Epithelioid cell granuloma in tuberculosis. This tightly clustered group of ill-defined epithelioid histiocytes from the same fine needle aspirate is evidence of a granulomatous response. Fibrillogranular necrosis was apparent elsewhere and acid/alcohol-fast bacilli were cultured from a similar specimen (MGG ×100)

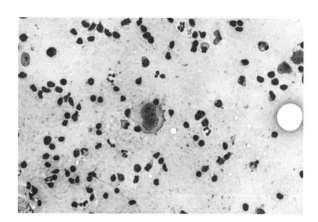

Figure 9.21   Hodgkin's lymphoma. Central Reed–Sternberg cell showing 'mirror image' binucleation with conspicuous 'owl's eye' macronucleoli. The variform background of eosinophil and neutrophil polymorphs, lymphocytes, plasma cells and histiocytes is characteristic of this condition (MGG ×100)

cell may be larger or smaller than its normal counterpart, thereby influencing the nuclear : cytoplasmic ratio, irrespective of any accompanying nuclear changes. The ultrastructural composition of the cytoplasm, namely the concentration of Golgi apparatus, ribosomes, endoplasmic reticulum, mitochondria and any products of metabolism, exert a major influence on the affinity of various tinctorial staining reactions. Storage products, e.g. mucin, lipid, carbohydrate, hormones or crystalloids, may be highlighted by special stains as appropriate. Mucin globules, foamy microvacuolation, microvillus brush borders and cilia may be discernible in normal or well-differentiated cells. Keratinization indicates squamous differentiation and bizarre elongate or caudate (*non-isodiametric*) cells may be apparent rather than the more usual round or polygonal (*isodiametric*) shapes (Figure 9.22).

Adjacent cells may demonstrate cytoplasmic moulding or in extreme cases apparent cell engulfment

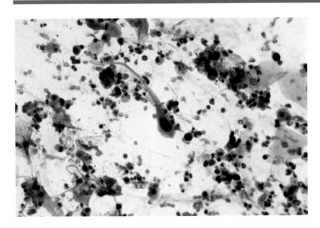

Figure 9.22 Squamous cell carcinoma. This elongated, bizarre squamous cell (caudate, 'tadpole' or 'comet' cell) possesses an enlarged, hyperchromatic nucleus and lies amidst tumour diathesis and degenerate, dyskeratotic squamous cell remnants. Strap-like ('fibre' or 'snake' cell) and brightly orangeophilic ('carrot' cell) forms may sometimes be seen (Pap ×100)

(*embracement* or '*cannibalism*') (Figures 9.23a,b). This is seen both in benign and malignant conditions, but is more common in the latter.

Degenerative cytoplasmic changes include swelling or hydropic change, vacuolation and loss of integrity of the plasma membrane with spillage of cell contents (*cytolysis*).

Background milieu and artefacts

The background content of a cytopreparation may include material of both cellular and non-cellular deriva-tion. This may be either helpful in reaching a diagnosis or a nuisance. Intensely blood-stained material or a vigorous inflammatory response, for example, often obscure the cytonuclear details of any epithelial cell population, limiting the amount of information available.

In addition to the connective tissue stromal components noted earlier, basement membrane material, ground substance, mucus, crystals, fibrinopurulent exudate, colloid, protein-rich fluid or even chondroid tissue microbiopsies may be discernible (Figure 9.24). Mineralization may manifest as amorphous calcium deposits or sometimes as *psammoma bodies* (Figure 9.25).

Invasive tumour may be associated with blood, necroinflammatory and degenerate debris (*tumour diathesis*) (Figure 9.26).

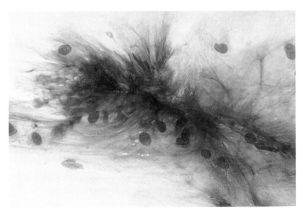

Figure 9.24 Ground substance from a benign salivary pleomorphic adenoma. The epithelial cells are almost obscured by fibrillary ('feathery') Giemsaphilic mucomyxoid ground substance which was much less inconspicuous on Papanicolaou staining (MGG ×125)

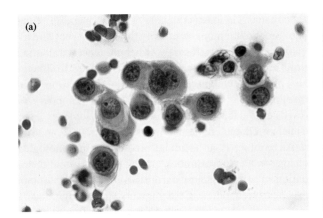 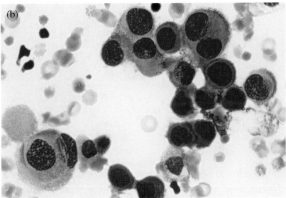

Figure 9.23 Reactive mesothelial cells arranged both individually and as small groups. Microvillous brush borders are just appreciable around some cells. Empty intercellular spaces ('windows') are a typical feature. Nuclear moulding and apparent cell engulfment (embracement or 'cannibalism') can be seen (a, Pap ×250; b, MGG ×250)

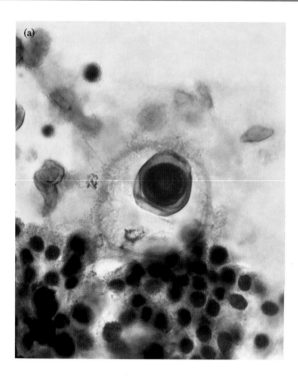

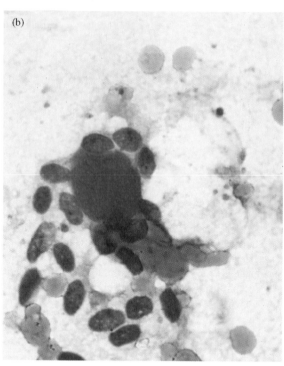

Figure 9.25 Psammoma body. (a) Central psammocalcification exhibiting a typical concentrically laminated, slightly refractile appearance amidst a background of lymphocytes and red blood cells (Pap ×250). (b) Epithelial-myoepithelial carcinoma of parotid gland. Loosely cohesive, modestly pleomorphic epithelial cells surround densely stained globules of basement membrane material, recapitulating the histological appearances. Similar patterns may be seen in a variety of tumours of salivary and non-salivary gland origin, both benign and malignant (MGG ×250)

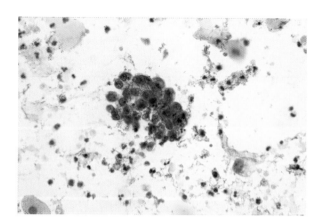

Figure 9.26 Transitional cell carcinoma of bladder. A loosely cohesive, poorly polarized clump of pleomorphic uroepithelial cells. There is nuclear hyperchromasia, an irregular nuclear contour and macronucleolation. Biopsy confirmed a high-grade transitional cell carcinoma. Note the cytolytic and inflammatory ('dirty') background (Pap × medium power)

A search for microorganisms or parasites is sometimes indicated. Commensals include *Lactobacillus* in cervicovaginal smears and *Candida* in oropharyngeal specimens. Pathogens include viruses, bacteria, fungi and protozoa amongst others. Some may be directly visible by light microscopy, whereas most viral infections are implied by their cytopathic effects. Koilocytosis in *Human papillomavirus*, multinucleation with 'ground glass' nucleoplasm in *Herpes simplex* and 'owl's eye' nuclear inclusions in *Cytomegalovirus* infections are characteristic examples (Figures 9.27, 9.28).

An artefact is an artificial product or morphological change in a cytopreparation arising from physical degradation of a specimen or during sampling, transportation or smear preparation. Contaminants are 'foreign bodies' introduced during these processes. Their importance is due mainly to the fact that they may cause difficulties in accurate interpretation of microscopical appearances. These may be classified as *intrinsic*, arising from an

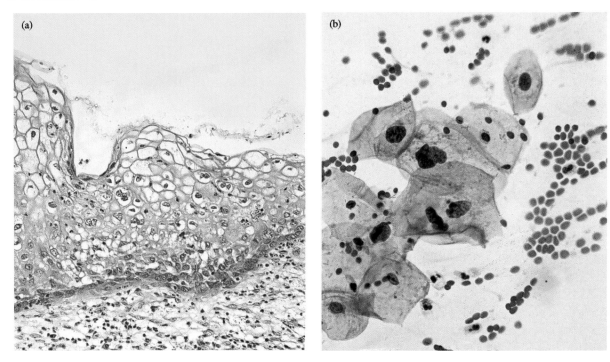

Figure 9.27 Human papillomavirus cytopathic effect. (a) Histology shows multinucleation with clear halos surrounding hyperchromatic, irregular nuclei (koilocytosis) (H&E × medium power). (b) Similar koilocytes present in a cervical smear. Note again the multinucleation, perinuclear clearing of cytoplasm and faint peripheral cytoplasmic condensation (Pap ×100)

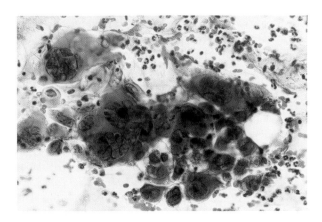

Figure 9.28 Epithelial cells in a cervical smear demonstrating Herpes simplex viral cytopathic effect. The overall appearance with nuclear enlargement, crowding, overlap, moulding, plurinucleation and areas of ground glass karyoplasm has been likened to pomegranate seeds

Figure 9.29 Rhomboidal cholesterol crystals aspirated from a benign thyroid cyst. Such deposition may be a consequence of previous haemorrhage (MGG ×50)

endogenous source, e.g. vegetable or meat fibres and cholesterol crystals (Figure 9.29), or *extrinsic*, e.g. stain deposits and talc or starch granules from surgical gloves (Figure 9.30). Poor fixation, particularly initial air drying of subsequent alcohol-fixed, Papanicolaou-stained preparations, xylene artefact and air bubbles all give typical appearances (Figure 9.31). Non-organic elements, e.g. asbestos fibres, are occasionally encountered (Figure 9.32).

Transfer of cellular material (*cross-contamination, 'carry over' or 'floaters'*) from one specimen to another during transport, fixation or staining procedures constitutes a potentially important source of false-positive

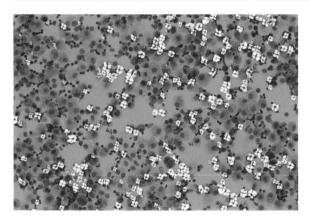

Figure 9.30 Numerous starch granules contaminating this bronchiolo-alveolar lavage specimen most likely emanate from surgical glove powder. Their characteristic Maltese cross morphology is best appreciated when transilluminated by cross-polarized light (MGG ×50 polarized)

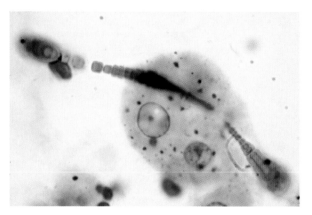

Figure 9.32 Ferruginous body in sputum. A multinucleated pulmonary alveolar macrophage partly engulfs a refractile ferruginous body. The brown beaded appearance is due to encrustation of iron pigment upon a colourless fibre, most likely asbestos. The dark intracytoplasmic granules comprise a mixture of anthracotic and haemosiderotic pigment (Pap ×1000)

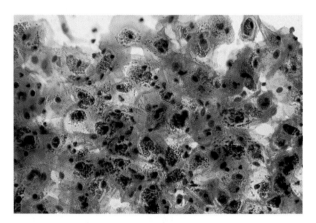

Figure 9.31 'Cornflake' cells in a cervical smear. A brown, faintly refractile deposit overlies the nuclei and cytoplasm of these squamous cells. This is most commonly seen in cervical smears and is believed to result from air trapping on the surface of cells during mounting. It is rarely so extensive as to render a smear completely uninterpretable (Pap ×100)

diagnosis of malignancy and should be avoided at all costs. It is usually preventable by rigorous technique and good laboratory hygiene.

Spurious environmental contamination is usually of waterborne or airborne origin and may be of biological or non-biological nature (Figures 9.33, 9.34).

Accuracy and limitations of cytology

Some measure of the reliability and accuracy of diagnostic cytology in various circumstances is useful for comparison and is often expressed statistically (see Table 9.2). Sensitivity (*true positive rate*) is a measure of how successfully a test detects patients with the disease process under consideration. Specificity (*true negative rate*) indicates how well a test excludes those individuals without the disease. *Positive predictive value* and *negative predictive value* give an indication of how accurately the test ascertains the presence or absence of the disease, respectively. A *false-negative result* is where the test fails to detect subsequently proven disease. This may be due to errors of screening or difficulties in interpretation. A true false negative is when retrospective review of the material confirms adequacy of the specimen and corroborates a genuine negative result. Possible explanations for this include perilesional rather than lesional sampling or the onset of disease following performance of the test procedure (*interval disease*). The sensitivity of a test decreases as the number of false negatives rises. A *false-positive result* is where the test is reported as positive but the disease cannot subsequently be demonstrated. This may result from difficulties in interpretation or where the appearances of certain conditions may closely resemble each other. The specificity of a test decreases as the number of false positives increases. The *efficiency* of a test is a measure of how well it correctly classifies those patients who should receive treatment and those for whom treatment is unnecessary.

The absolute statistical values for a particular test may be modulated by the inclusion or exclusion of inadequate

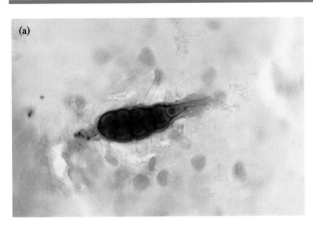

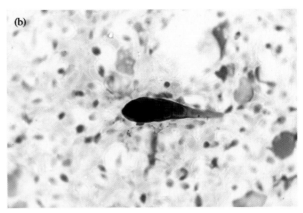

Figure 9.33 Aerial contaminants. These internally segmented fungal condia ('snow shoes') were present at the edge of a smear. They are consistent with Alternaria spp. and are presumed aerial contaminants (a, Pap ×250; b, MGG ×250)

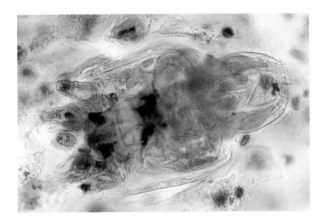

Figure 9.34 A free-living mite discovered as an exogenous contaminant in a cervical smear. It is of no clinical consequence (Pap ×250)

Table 9.2 Some of the more useful parameters measuring the accuracy of cytology and how they are calculated

	Disease positive (a + c)	Disease negative (b + d)
Test positive (a + b)	True positive (a)	False positive (b)
Test negative (c + d)	False negative (c)	True negative (d)

$$\text{Sensitivity} = \frac{a}{a + c}$$

$$\text{Specificity} = \frac{d}{b + d}$$

$$\text{Positive predictive value} = \frac{a}{a + b}$$

$$\text{Negative predictive value} = \frac{d}{c + d}$$

$$\text{Accuracy} = \frac{a + d}{a + b + c + d}$$

$$\text{Likelihood ratio of a positive test} = \frac{\text{sensitivity}}{1 - \text{specificity}}$$

$$\text{Likelihood ratio of a negative test} = \frac{1 - \text{sensitivity}}{\text{specificity}}$$

or unsatisfactory specimens. Inclusion of these gives an overall indication of the clinical effectiveness of the test, whereas excluding these more accurately reflects the laboratory performance.

Gynaecological cytopathology and cervical screening

Cytology specimens from the female genital tract form a major proportion of the routine throughput of most diagnostic laboratories, largely as a result of cervical screening. The prime objective of the cervical smear ('Pap') test is the detection of squamous cell carcinoma and its precursors in asymptomatic women. It is also used in the investigation of women suffering gynaecological symptoms and as part of the monitoring process following treatment. Of secondary importance are the detection of glandular lesions of the cervix or other gynaecological sites, the recognition of a variety of inflammatory and infective conditions and the assessment of hormonal status.

Cervical screening has been demonstrated to be effective in reducing the mortality and morbidity of cervical carcinoma in several countries, albeit not by means of randomized controlled trials. A cervical screening

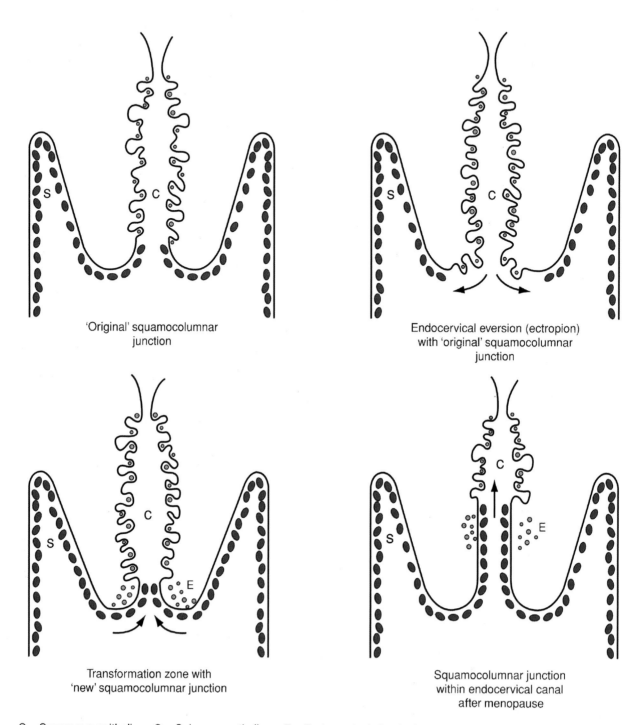

'Original' squamocolumnar
junction

Endocervical eversion (ectropion)
with 'original' squamocolumnar
junction

Transformation zone with
'new' squamocolumnar junction

Squamocolumnar junction
within endocervical canal
after menopause

S = Squamous epithelium C = Columnar epthelium   E = Endocervical glands deep to metaplastic squamous epithelium

Figure 9.35   Schematic diagram of the anatomy of the cervix. This illustrates the changing morphology of the cervical transformation zone and squamo-columnar junction with advancing years

programme has been in operation in the UK since 1964. Systematic call and recall of the population was introduced in 1988 under the auspices of the NHS Cervical Screening Programme (NHSCSP) with establishment of a national coordinating network. This encourages the uniform classification of abnormalities, standardization of terminology, follow-up of abnormal smears, implementation of quality control mechanisms, evaluates the effectiveness of the Programme via multidisciplinary audit and monitors training of health care professionals.

When all aspects of the screening process are performed optimally, the test is a very sensitive method for the detection of precursors of squamous cell carcinoma, less so for invasive carcinoma. It should be remembered, however, that as a screening test it has a low but significant diagnostic error rate. The ultimate goal of eradication of cervical carcinoma has yet to be realized by this route.

The aim of a cervical smear is to representatively sample the cervical transformation zone bordering the squamo-columnar junction, which is the site at greatest risk of neoplastic change (Figure 9.35). It is ultimately the responsibility of the smear taker to visualize the cervix and ensure that its entire circumference has been sampled, whatever the cellularity or cell content of the smear (Figure 9.36). Indicators of probable transformation zone sampling include immature metaplastic squamous cells and/or endocervical glandular epithelium with mucus. There are no reliable indicators of transformation zone sampling in atrophic smears.

The normal cervical smear

The cytomorphology of superficial, intermediate and parabasal squamous cells largely recapitulates the histological structure of mature stratified squamous epithelium (Figure 9.37). Mucosal thickness and glycogen content depend upon hormonal activity. Superficial cells usually exfoliate naturally and there is normally no keratinization. They tend to be dyscohesive and individually disposed. Endocervical glandular cells show a wide variation in appearance, depending upon their preservation and orientation. They tend to retain cohesion and may show cytoarchitectural patterns comparable to other glandular sites. Subcolumnar reserve cells are generally present as bare, isomorphic nuclei. Metaplastic squamous cells are a normal constituent of a smear during the reproductive years. Whilst immature they do not exfoliate spontaneously and when removed by abrasion they often exhibit cytoplasmic projections

('*spider cells*'). Once fully mature they are indistinguishable from the squamous cells of the original ectocervix. Endometrial stromal cells, glandular cells and histiocytes ('*exodus*') may be observed from the beginning of menstrual flow until day 12 of the menstrual cycle. Outside this interval they are considered abnormal and such hyperexfoliation may be caused by menstrual irregularities and intra-uterine contraceptive devices in addition to polypi, hyperplasia and neoplasia. Polymorphonuclear leukocytes are invariably present, most conspicuously around menstruation. Lymphocytes, eosinophils, mast cells and plasma cells are usually scanty. The mere presence of inflammatory cells does not necessarily imply infection. Spermatozoa may persist for several days after sexual intercourse. Trophoblast and deciduoid stroma may be shed during pregnancy or abortion and pseudodeciduoid cells may be the result of hormonal therapy.

Abnormal keratinization (*hyperkeratosis*) yields anucleate, deeply orangeophilic squamae in Papanicolaou preparations. *Parakeratosis* shows spikes ('*sprigs*') or '*pearls*' of similar squamae possessing pyknotic nuclei. Both patterns may be seen in inflammatory and neoplastic conditions. A variety of contaminants, including helminths, lice, fungi, pollen and lubricant jelly, may be encountered.

Hormonal cytology

Cytohormonal evaluation is based upon the maturation of vaginal squamous epithelium in response to circulating gonadotrophic hormones in combination. The epithelium is thin and immature when deprived of oestrogen and progesterone. Unopposed oestrogen promotes growth and maturation. Progesterone causes desquamation and exfoliation with cytolysis and '*navicular cells*'. Androgens stimulate partial maturation to intermediate cell level in atrophic epithelium with a reciprocal effect in mature epithelium.

Characteristic patterns are recognizable in the postnatal period, during puberty, sexual maturity, pregnancy, post-parturition, lactational, pre-menopausal and established post-menopausal states, modulated by exogenous hormonal influences or abnormal endogenous hormonal sources, e.g. ovarian tumours.

Various indices may be used to report hormonal changes, including the maturation index, maturation value, karyopyknotic index, eosinophilic index and the folded cell index.

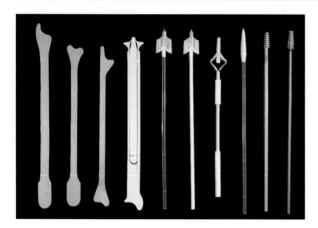

Figure 9.36 Cervical sampling devices. The spatulae, particularly the extended tip type (Aylesbury), give a better cell yield and are recommended for screening. Brush devices for endocervical sampling may be of benefit in addition following an abnormal smear. Sampling technique and visualization of the cervix are of paramount importance, irrespective of the design employed

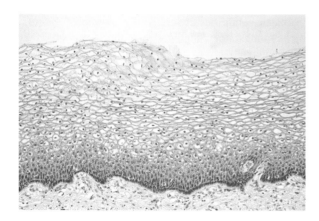

Figure 9.37 Normal mature ectocervical squamous epithelial maturation. Note the ordered polarity from stratum basalis to superficial squamae and the absence of surface keratinization (H&E × medium power)

Inflammation and regenerative changes

Inflammation in the female genital tract sometimes has an infective origin and may be of acute, chronic or granulomatous pattern. It is a dynamic process wherein degenerative and regenerative changes are observed synchronously.

Commoner infections include follicular cervicitis strongly associated with *Chlamydia* spp., *Lepthothrix*

spp. often accompanying *Trichomonas vaginalis*, bacterial vaginosis associated with *Gardnerella vaginalis*, *Actinomyces* spp., *Neisseria gonorrhoea*, *Mycobacterium tuberculosis*, *Treponema pallidum*, *Candida albicans*, *Herpes simplex virus* and *Human papillomavirus*, many of which are sexually transmissible (Figures 9.38, 9.39).

Iatrogenic influences include laser ablation, thermal damage, surgery, radiotherapy, hormonal replacement or

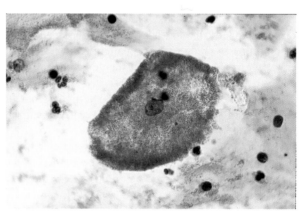

Figure 9.38 'Clue cell' in bacterial vaginosis. Coccoid overgrowth imparts a granular appearance to a superficial squamous cell ('clue cell') in a cervical smear. It is usually due to mixed bacterial flora including Gardnerella vaginalis. Their presence is not necessarily an indication of clinical symptoms (bacterial vaginosis) (Pap ×250)

manipulation and intrauterine contraceptive devices. These may result in various hyperplasias and metaplasias, further complicating accurate interpretation of a cervical smear.

Dyskaryosis, CIN and cervical carcinoma

Invasive squamous cell carcinoma of the cervix is preceded by a prodrome of precancerous changes (*dysplasia*) of the epithelium of the cervical transformation zone, termed cervical intraepithelial neoplasia (CIN). This is a continuous biological spectrum which is arbitrarily subdivided or graded in histological sections into CIN 1, CIN 2 and CIN 3 with increasing severity of dysplasia (Figures 9.40, 9.41). Each stage harbours the potential for progression of regression. These categories correspond to mild, moderate and severe squamous cell dyskaryosis in cervical smear preparations (Figure 9.40). The Northern American Bethesda system uses slightly different nomenclature for the same cytomorphological

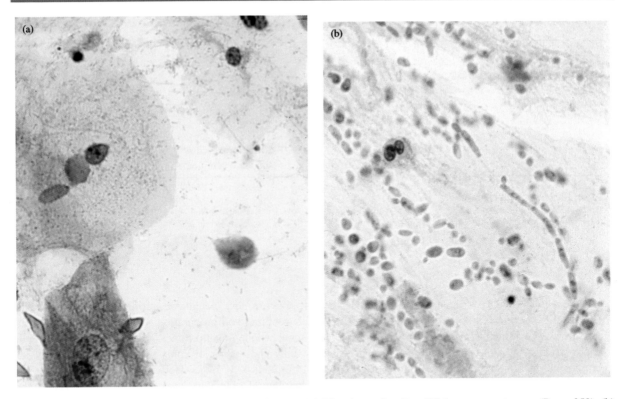

Figure 9.39   Trichomonas and Candida in a cervical smear. (a) Binucleate, flagellate Trichomonas protozoon (Pap ×250). (b) Candidal blastospores and pseudohyphae (Pap ×250)

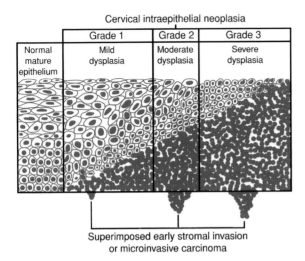

Figure 9.40   Precursors of invasive squamous cell carcinoma of the cervix. Schematic representation of potential progression of cervical intraepithelial neoplasia to invasive cervical carcinoma

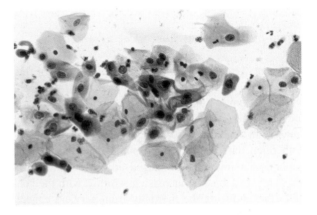

Figure 9.41   Moderate squamous cell dyskaryosis. Note disproportionate nucleomegaly, the nucleus occupying up to two-thirds of the cytoplastic area, nuclear hyperchromasia, irregular nuclear contour and angulated cell borders (Pap ×100)

Table 9.3 Broad comparison of the most recent terminologies applied to abnormal squamous cells in cervical cytology

Histological counterpart	WHO, 1973	BSCC, 1986[*]	Bethesda, 1991
		Borderline	ASCUS
CIN I	Mild dysplasia	Mild dyskaryosis	Low-grade SIL
CIN II	Moderate dysplasia	Moderate dyskaryosis	High-grade SIL
CIN III	Severe dysplasia	Severe dyskaryosis	High-grade SIL
	Carcinoma *in situ*		
Invasive carcinoma	Epidermoid carcinoma	Severe dyskaryosis	Squamous carcinoma
		?Invasive carcinoma	

WHO, World Health Organization; ASCUS, atypical squamous cells of uncertain significance; BSCC, British Society of Clinical Cytology; SIL, squamous intraepithelial lesion.
[*]Amendments proposed by the BSCC in 2002 to employ a simplified two-tier classification (i.e. low-grade dyskaryosis and high-grade dyskaryosis) in preference to the current three-tier stratification of dyskaryosis (i.e. mild, moderate and severe) have yet to be fully ratified in the UK.

appearances (see Table 9.3). The more severe the degree of abnormality, the greater the statistical risk of progression to invasive carcinoma.

Early stromal invasion, microinvasion and invasive squamous cell carcinoma proper indicate transgression of basement membrane to varying degrees, the latter with tumefaction. This is best assessed by histological examination as the severe dyskaryosis of CIN 3 may be cytomorphologically indistinguishable from the severe dyskaryosis seen in invasive carcinoma. Bizarre dyskeratotic cells and tumour diathesis may be helpful distinguishing features but are neither pathognomonic nor universally present.

Screening programmes to detect breast carcinoma in asymptomatic women have been established in several countries and initial results appear encouraging.

Liquid-based cytology in cervical screening

In recent years, alongside acknowledgement of the efficacy of cervical smear testing, there has also been wider recognition of some of the limitations of the process. The accepted sensitivity of a single cervical smear is in the order of 50–60%, which contrasts sharply with often unrealistically high public expectation. The methods employed have changed little over many decades and are subject to increasing scrutiny, with the goal of further reducing the mortality from cervical cancer. Only a minor proportion of false-negative smears are believed to be the consequence of human observational or interpretative error during microscopical assessment by laboratory personnel. More significant confounding

factors are now recognized during the preceding stages of sampling and preparation. For example, the conventional wooden spatula does not sample abnormal cells evenly and it typically only transfers anything between 10% and 60% of collected cells onto a slide. The distribution of material may, therefore, be patchy and non-representative. This and any mucus, inflammatory or other obscuring component may be detrimental to fixation, resulting in artefact, poor staining and loss of cytonuclear detail, contributing to an overall inadequate smear rate of roughly 10%.

Liquid-based cytology (LBC) techniques minimize many of these problems. As of October 2003 the National Institute of Clinical Excellence (NICE) has recommended to the NHS in England and Wales that liquid-based cytology is introduced as the primary means of processing samples in the NHSCSP. It is anticipated that it will take approximately 5 years for this to be fully implemented. This decision follows evaluation of two different, commercially marketed systems, called ThinPrep (Cytyc Corporation) and Sure-Path Prep (TriPath Imaging Inc.). These products gained similar approval from the US Food and Drug Administration (FDA) several years previously. Other commercial products are likely to compete for official validation in due course. The pilot studies variously predict enhanced clinical effectiveness (greater sensitivity and specificity, fewer borderline smears), improved cost-effectiveness (fewer inadequate smears, quicker consultation times and better laboratory productivity) and better acceptability (to both the public and health care professionals) compared to conventional cervical smear techniques.

Automated screening and image analysis

High resolution *image analysis* systems may be semi- or fully automated and linked to powerful neural network computers. The goal of obviating the subjectivity of manual assessment and the potential for autonomous machines to reduce human error during the screening process are attractive. The requirement for optimum quality, uniform specimens has to a large extent driven the advancement of liquid-based cytology. Several commercial packages have been developed and marketed at one time or another, most short-lived. To date, however, there seems little prospect of wholesale replacement of skilled cytologists and the cost-effectiveness of such technology remains to be established.

Computer-assisted microscopy devices have been used as an adjunct to the training of cytologists and to record quality control data but they are yet to become routinely employed in most laboratories.

Telepathology and *teleconferencing* capitalize upon real time links between multiple, geographically remote users, allowing interactive consultations for training, peer or expert review and quality assessment.

Ancillary techniques

Cytomorphological assessment is at times a highly subjective process and therefore susceptible to differences in intra-observer and inter-observer reproducibility. Attempts to refine and quantify this more rigorously have been undertaken, with varying degrees of success.

Flow cytometry involves the automated assessment of cells in suspension, usually for DNA analysis or immunophenotyping purposes. Microfluorimetry enables focus on individual cells in a field to assess the amount of fluorescent activity within labelled nuclei.

Cytogenetic analysis detects chromosomal abnormalities, some of which are characteristic of certain tumours, e.g. t(x:18) in synovial sarcoma, t(11:22) in Ewing's tumour. The majority of neoplasms, however, do not show such typical consistent translocations.

Silver-stained nucleolar organizer regions (AgNORs) are increased in most malignant nuclei. Unfortunately, the overlap between benign and malignant conditions is often considerable.

Scanning and *transmission electron microscopy* may identify helpful ultrastructural details not discernible by light microscopy, which enables more precise classification of cell differentiation, e.g. dense core neurosecretory granules, tight junctions, tonofilaments, etc.

In situ hybridization techniques may be used to identify viral nuclear material and detect oncogene activation in tumours.

Confocal laser scanning microscopy processes digital images, which may be manipulated further to reconstruct the three-dimensional microtopography of cells. It is particularly suited to thick preparations and fluorescent products may be quantified.

Laser scanning cytometry is a hybrid technique combining features of flow cytometry with static image analysis of cells labelled by multicolour fluorochromes. It can assess DNA ploidy and incorporate fluorescent *in situ* hybridization (FISH) methods, using both conventional and liquid-based cytopreparations.

Laser capture microdissection techniques enable the selection of a relatively pure subpopulation of chosen cells from a cytology or histology slide. A low-energy infra-red laser is used to extend a proprietary plastic adhesive onto the selected cells of interest, which are then gently lifted off for further study.

Quality assurance in diagnostic cytology

The purpose of a quality assurance programme is to evaluate the diagnostic process as it is practised. Internal quality control indicates a series of procedures within a particular laboratory. This encompasses continuing education, training, review of laboratory procedures and their implementation, rescreening, double screening and audit. External quality assurance indicates performance evaluation against an external peer group, either regionally or nationally, and this may be as part of an accreditation scheme, either voluntary or compulsory.

Further reading

Atkins KA. Liquid-based cytological preparations in gynaecological and non-gynaecological specimens. In *Progress in Pathology*, vol 6, Kirkham N, Shepherd NA (eds). 2003: Greenwich Medical Media, London, 101–114.

Coleman DV, Chapman PA (eds). 1989: *Clinical Cytotechnology*. Butterworths, London.

Gray W, McKee G (eds). 2003: *Diagnostic Cytopathology*, 2nd edn. Elsevier Science, London.

Woods AE, Ellis RC (eds), 1994: Cytopathology. In *Laboratory Histopathology—a Complete Reference*. Churchill-Livingstone, New York.

Young JA (ed.). 1993: *Fine Needle Aspiration*. Blackwell Scientific, London.

SECTION 3

MICROBIOLOGY—BACTERIOLOGY

10

Microscopy in bacteriology: application and sample preparation

Dugald R Baird

Introduction

In the late seventeenth century the Dutch draper and amateur scientist Antonie van Leeuwenhoek ground small lenses of extraordinary quality and visualized microorganisms for the first time. Since then microscopy has continued to play a fundamental role in clinical bacteriology. Microscopical examination of a clinical specimen may help to assess the adequacy of the specimen (see section on Sputum, below), and may by itself immediately suggest the likely nature of the bacterial pathogen in normally sterile sites such as cerebrospinal fluid (CSF) or blood cultures. Methods in a diagnostic clinical laboratory include both light and fluorescence microscopy; specimens may be unstained or stained, depending on the application.

Light microscopy

Light microscopy may be employed in three ways—ordinary transmitted light (brightfield), darkfield and phase contrast microscopy, of which the first is by far the most commonly used. A modern microscope is capable of achieving a magnification of 1000 times and a resolving power of approximately 0.2 μm. Most microscopes are designed so that the observer looks through the eyepieces, which are slanted at a convenient angle, down on to the stage containing the object to be viewed. An alternative arrangement (the inverted plate

microscope), is designed to examine the subject from below. *Darkfield illumination* effectively increases the resolving power of the light microscope to below 0.2 μm. Specimens are illuminated indirectly, scatter the light and appear bright against a dark background. Using this technique one can visualize bacteria such as spirochaetes, which have a diameter of approximately 0.1 μm. *Phase contrast microscopy* allows examination of the fine internal structure of living unstained bacteria and tissues, the different structures appearing in various shades of grey.

Fluorescence microscopy

Fluorescence occurs when a molecule is struck by light of a particular wavelength and emits light of a longer wavelength. Fluorochromes (fluorescent dyes) absorb non-visible UV light and emit visible light. A fluorescent microscope uses a mercury vapour lamp which emits high-intensity ultraviolet light (*excitation light*) and a mirror directs this on to the specimen from above. Bacteria stained with a fluorochrome absorb this short wavelength light, emit longer wavelength light, and appear as glowing yellow or green objects against a dark background. Fluorescence microscopy allows the use of lower power objectives and hence a much larger area of specimen can be scanned rapidly. This is important, for example, when searching for mycobacteria in a specimen in which they may be very scanty.

The Science of Laboratory Diagnosis, Second Edition   Edited by David Burnett and John Crocker
© 2005 John Wiley & Sons, Ltd

Specimens for microscopy

These are of two main types: (1) dried smears of fluid specimens or swabs, or of bacterial cultures, spread over an area of 1–2 cm diameter onto standard 3 × 1 in glass slides and fixed by heat ('films'); and (2) 'wet preparations' of fluids, examined under a coverslip or in special chambers. Swabs contained in transport medium are moist and can be rubbed directly onto the surface of a slide, while films of fluid specimens such as pus, aspirates, CSF, etc., are made by taking up a loopful and spreading this thinly. Tissue samples are either pressed on to the surface of slides to form imprints, or may be ground up in a small volume of peptone water. Colonies of bacteria growing on solid media are examined by touching the colony with a loop and emulsifying this in a drop of saline on the slide, aiming for a very light suspension so that individual cells can be distinguished clearly.

Examination of unstained specimens by transmitted light

Examination of fluid specimens in a *counting chamber* or on a slide with a coverslip is routinely used to assess the presence of clues to infection or inflammation in normally sterile body fluids such as urine, CSF and joint aspirates, and peritoneal dialysis effluents. Transmitted light is used, with or without phase contrast, and the sample examined using the ×25 objective for white and red blood cells, organisms, casts or crystals, as appropriate to the specimen. Cell counts may be expressed quantitatively if a counting chamber is employed, or semiquantitatively (e.g. 'per high power field').

Bacteria growing in liquid culture media may be examined for *motility* using a ×50 objective. Lowering the condenser increases the contrast and makes the organisms easier to see; alternatively, phase contrast microscopy may be used.

Examination of tissue culture cell monolayers for cytopathic effects is mainly the province of virology, but has an application in bacteriology in the detection of *Clostridium difficile* cytotoxin in faecal extracts or culture supernatants.

Cerebrospinal fluid (CSF)

CSF is normally sterile, and contains not more than five white cells per mm^3, predominately lymphocytes. The first step in its examination consists of microscopy of uncentrifuged fluid to quantitate the number of cells present and their type. A counting chamber is used, commonly the modified Fuchs–Rosenthal. This is a glass slide containing a well, the floor of which is etched with a grid of nine large squares, each 1 mm^2 in area. Each of these squares is subdivided in turn into 16 small squares. When a coverslip is applied over the counting chamber and fluid run in using a Pasteur pipette, the depth of fluid is 0.2 mm. The volume of fluid overlying five large squares is thus 1 mm^3.

A coverslip is applied to the slide to make a firm uniform seal over the counting chamber, by pressing gently at its edges until the colours of the rainbow are seen uniformly around the sides of the coverslip (Newton's rings), confirming that close and even contact has been made between the coverslip and chamber. CSF is introduced into the chamber using a fine Pasteur pipette applied carefully to the edge, so that fluid runs in to completely fill the chamber, without air bubbles.

After allowing a few minutes to settle, cells are counted using a ×40 objective, the number of squares being examined depending on the number of cells present. CSF containing very large numbers of white cells or that is heavily bloodstained, either as a result of intracerebral haemorrhage or due to accidental puncture of small blood vessels during lumbar puncture, may have to be diluted before an accurate cell count can be performed. A fluid containing dilute acetic acid and crystal violet is used for this purpose: this lyses erythrocytes and stains the nuclei of the white cells, making them easier to see. Identification of cell types is facilitated by centrifuging an aliquot of the CSF and making a film, which is stained using a differential stain such as Leishman's.

Urine

Not all laboratories perform microscopy as a routine on specimens of urine. In specimens taken from patients via catheters (catheter specimens of urine, CSU) this is justifiable, since the absence of pus cells in such samples does not exclude infection. In samples collected cleanly from patients without catheters (mid-stream urine, MSU), however, the absence of pyuria suggests that the significance of an isolate is at best uncertain; it may be a contaminant, and repeat sampling is advised. Microscopy is also useful to detect red cells, casts and crystals, all of which may be of diagnostic significance. The information that can be obtained from urine microscopy is thus valuable, and it should be done whenever possible.

Microscopy is performed on fresh uncentrifuged urine. The visualization of organisms in such preparations is of secondary importance, since it is quantitation of bacterial growth that is important in assessing the significance of isolates from a urine specimen. Neutrophils are excreted in variable numbers in healthy urine, and only numbers above 10^4/ml can be considered abnormal in MSUs. Red cells are found as contaminants in the urine of healthy younger females, associated with menstruation, but may also indicate serious renal tract pathology such as calculi, neoplasm or glomerular disease. In the latter case, the morphology of the red cells may be abnormal (dysmorphism), the cells exhibiting fragmentation, crenation or other bizarre shapes.

Laboratories handling small numbers of urine specimens may examine them in counting chambers, as described for CSF, but most use a semiquantitative method. These include simply using an ordinary glass slide and a coverslip, commercially produced disposable counting chambers or an inverted plate microscope. The latter allows batching of many samples in flat-bottomed wells in a plastic plate. A ×40 objective is used and if the area of the field ('high-power field') and the depth of the urine is known, the number of cells visible can be translated into counts/ml, although in practice many laboratories simply express the findings as scanty, moderate or numerous.

Other specimens

The techniques described for urine may be applied to other normally sterile fluids, such as aspirates from joints (where examination for crystals such as uric acid is also important), serous fluids and peritoneal dialysis effluent. Microscopy of faeces is employed for the diagnosis of parasitic infections, but has no place in the diagnosis of bacterial gastroenteritis.

Examination of unstained specimens using darkground illumination

This has one application in clinical bacteriology, namely in the examination of material taken from a suspected primary chancre for the presence of the causal organism of syphilis, *Treponema pallidum*. Material is taken from the suspect lesion and a wet film made under a coverslip, which is examined immediately for motile treponemes.

Staining of specimens

Using transmitted light, since the refractive index of bacteria is similar to that of their background, it is necessary, when using transmitted light, to increase the contrast by the use of stains. The most widely used method of staining bacteria remains that introduced by Christian Gram in 1884. Although not a stain, but a staining *method*, the term 'Gram stain' is used universally; it exploits the differences in cell wall structure that exist between various classes of bacteria. The material to be stained may be a clinical specimen, a broth culture or a light suspension in saline of an organism taken from an agar plate. In all cases a thin smear is made on a glass slide and allowed to dry naturally or with very modest heat, after which the smear is fixed to the slide, either by passing the slide quickly three times through a Bunsen flame or by the use of a heated plate. *Gram's staining method*, which has several modifications, involves treating the smear successively by: (a) a basic positively charged dye, usually crystal violet; (b) mordanting with aqueous iodine; (c) decolorizing with acetone; and (d) counterstaining with carbol fuchsin or safranin.

Most bacteria are initially stained by the crystal violet and iodine which form insoluble complexes within the bacterial cell. Those bacteria which possess thick layers of peptidoglycan in their cell walls, and hence retain the stain after treatment with acetone and so appear purple, are defined as *Gram-positive*; those with thinner peptidoglycan layers, which readily lose the complex with acetone and hence stain with the pink counterstain, are called *Gram-negative*. Examples of both are given in Table 10.1. Some bacteria stain only poorly with the Gram stain (e.g. *Legionella* species), some are inconsistent in their staining behaviour (*Gram-variable*; e.g.

Table 10.1 Some examples of bacterial genera classified according to morphology and Gram staining

Shape	Gram-positive	Gram-negative
Cocci (spheres)	*Staphylococcus* *Streptococcus* *Peptococcus*[*]	*Neisseria* *Moraxella* *Veillonella*[*]
Bacilli (rods)	*Bacillus* *Listeria* *Corynebacterium* *Clostridium*[*]	Enterobacteriaceae *Pseudomonas* *Haemophilus* *Bacteroides*[*]

[*]Anaerobic genera

Gardnerella vaginalis) and others do not stain at all (e.g. mycobacteria).

Special staining methods are required for mycobacteria due to the peculiar composition of their cell walls, which contain high concentrations of mycolic (fatty) acids. The Ziehl–Neelson stain involves treatment of the film with hot carbol fuchsin, followed by successive decolorization steps with concentrated sulphuric acid and with alcohol, finally counterstaining with malachite green or methylene blue. Mycobacteria appear red against a green or blue background (Figure 10.1).

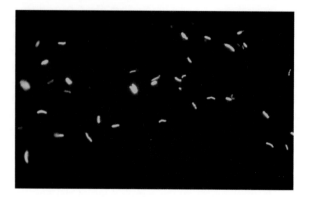

Figure 10.2 Sputum stained with phenol-auramine and viewed under ultraviolet light, showing mycobacteria glowing with a green-yellow fluorescence (×400). Courtesy of Dr B Watt

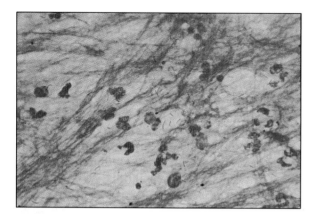

Figure 10.1 Sputum stained by Ziehl–Neelson's method, showing mycobacteria (red) against a blue background (×1000). Courtesy of Mr J Winning

The other staining method employed for mycobacteria is phenol-auramine. This involves treating dried and heat fixed smears of the specimen (usually sputum, pleural and ascitic fluids, early-morning urine, CSF, pus, etc.) with phenol-auramine, decolorizing with 1% hydrochloric acid in industrial methylated spirit, followed by a dilute solution of potassium permanganate. Films are viewed under ultraviolet light using the ×40 objective, and mycobacteria glow green-yellow against a dark background (Figure 10.2). This technique allows rapid screening of a smear, and is useful when numbers of bacteria in the specimen are small.

Two other staining methods are employed in fluorescence microscopy work—acridine orange and fluorescein–antibody conjugates. Staining with acridine orange is a useful method for demonstrating bacteria that may not show up clearly in a Gram stain (as in blood cultures; see below). Under UV light, bacteria appear orange.

Two main *immunofluorescent* techniques using fluorescein–antibody conjugates are available, direct and indirect fluorescent antibody tests (DFAT and IFAT,

respectively). The DFAT utilizes a fluorochrome, commonly fluorescein isothiocyanate, conjugated to a specific antibody which binds directly to bacterial surface antigen. The IFAT is a two-stage procedure: the specific antibody (e.g. prepared in a rabbit) binds to the antigen and is itself detected by a conjugated antibody (e.g. antirabbit). The advantage of the IFAT is that a single conjugated antibody can be used to detect a whole range of specific antibodies.

In clinical bacteriology the major uses of these immunofluorescence techniques are (a) in the detection of *Legionella* species, which are fastidious and slow to grow but can be rapidly visualized in sputum, bronchoalveolar lavages and lung tissue (fresh or formalin-fixed), using either DFAT or IFAT; and (b) for the direct demonstration of chlamydia in genital or respiratory specimens.

Some further examples of the use of microscopy of stained preparations in clinical microbiology are given below.

Specimens from normally sterile sites

It is with these specimens that microscopy can be a powerful tool in predicting the likely causal pathogen. The finding of organisms in cerebrospinal fluid, joint aspirate, or peritoneal dialysis effluent, for example, especially when accompanied by an infiltrate of pus cells, is a certain indicator of infection, and the appearance of the bacteria alone may be diagnostic. A very thorough search for bacteria may have to be made, as they are sometimes very scanty in such specimens, which are examined by centrifuging (e.g. at 3000 rpm for 10 minutes), discarding the supernatant, and making a film of the deposit, which is then stained by Gram's method, and also by auramine or Ziehl–Neelson if the clinical situation suggests possible mycobacterial infection.

Most laboratories now use some form of semi-automated *blood culture* system, and examination of a Gram-stained drop of broth from a bottle registering positive growth is the first step in the identification of the organism. Microscopy may by itself be diagnostic: e.g streptococci in the blood of a patient with fever and a heart murmur would support a clinical diagnosis of infective endocarditis (see Figure 10.3). On the other

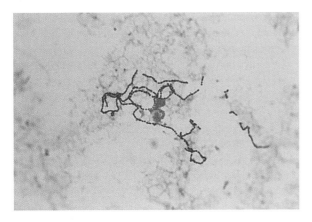

Figure 10.3   Gram stain of a blood culture showing gram-positive cocci in long chains. The organism turned out to be *Streptococcus sanguis*, and the patient had infective endocarditis (×1000). Courtesy of Dr A McLay

hand, Gram-positive cocci in clusters are usually staphylococci, but *Staphylococcus aureus* cannot be distinguished by microscopy from the many coagulase-negative species and, since the latter, being skin organisms, are the commonest contaminants of blood cultures, the significance of staphylococci seen in a blood culture usually has to await further identification. Gram-negative organisms in blood cultures are sometimes difficult to see against the general background pink staining, and when no organisms are visible it is often useful to perform an acridine stain.

Specimens from sites with a normal resident bacterial flora

Oral swabs

Microscopy is the only method of diagnosing Vincent's angina (anaerobic stomatogingivitis), since the causal

organisms (which act synergistically to produce the infection) cannot be cultured artificially. Films of oral swabs show many pus cells and large numbers of spirochaetes and fusiform (spindle-shaped) Gram-negative bacilli.

Sputum

All sputum specimens are regarded as potentially hazardous to the operator, since they may contain tubercle bacilli, and preparation of films is performed in a safety cabinet housed in a Category 3 containment laboratory. Although sputum originates from the normally sterile lower respiratory tract, it is inevitably contaminated before collection by flora from the upper respiratory tract. Care is needed in interpreting Gram films of sputum, and only rarely can one confidently predict the causal organism of pneumonia on the basis of microscopy alone. Gram films are nevertheless useful in that specimens of 'sputum' which show fewer than 10 neutrophils per squamous epithelial cell are probably saliva rather than sputum, and indicate that culture may be misleading. When mycobacterial infection is suspected, auramine-stained films are examined, and positives confirmed by making fresh films and staining by the Ziehl–Neelson method.

The disadvantages of sputum are largely overcome by performing bronchoalveolar lavage, a procedure increasingly employed in the diagnosis of pneumonia in patients who are very ill, or are immunosuppressed. Specimens obtained are free of contaminating upper respiratory tract flora, and can be examined by Gram, auramine and Ziehl–Neelson stains, and by immunofluorescence techniques for *Legionella* species and a wide range of protozoal, fungal and viral pathogens.

Skin lesions

Swabs of skin lesions are rarely of diagnostic value, due to the presence of a normal skin flora, with one important exception. This is the microscopical examination of material scraped from the purpuric lesions associated with meningococcal infection, in which the presence of Gram-negative cocci in pairs, with their characteristic morphology, is diagnostic.

Pus and wound swabs

The value of microscopy of these specimens is variable, depending on a number of factors beyond the control of the laboratory. Pus or pus swabs from such sites as skin or soft tissue infections may suggest infection with staphylococci, streptococci or anaerobes, whereas similar specimens from intra-abdominal sites may show a highly mixed picture, not always easy to correlate with what is subsequently obtained on culture. In many of these cases, prior antibiotic administration may account for the discrepancies. However, it is often useful to be able to give a provisional report that a pus sample or swab is likely, for example, to be staphylococcal in origin or, alternatively, that it is composed of mixed organisms of probable faecal origin.

High vaginal swabs

Gram films are used to ascertain whether pus cells are present, and also the presence of epithelial cells covered with small Gram-variable bacilli (clue cells). The finding of the latter is a pointer to the condition known as bacterial vaginosis. In genitourinary medicine, urethral and endocervical swabs are examined for the presence of pus cells containing intracellular Gram-negative cocci in pairs, *Neisseria gonorrhoeae* (see Figure 10.4).

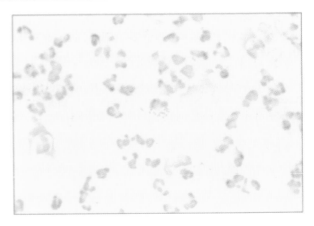

Figure 10.4   Film of urethral discharge showing numerous intracellular Gram-negative cocci, *Neisseria gonorrhoeae* (×1000). Courtesy of Mr J Winning

Further reading

Bishop BJ, Neumann G. The history of the Ziehl–Neelsen stain. *Tubercle* 1970; **51**: 196–206.

Larson HE, Price AB. Pseudomembranous colitis: presence of clostridial toxin. *Lancet* 1977; **2**: 1312–1314.

Preston NW, Morrell A. Reproducible results with the Gram stain. *J Pathol Bacteriol* 1962; **84**: 241–243.

11

Culture media in bacteriology

Eric Y Bridson

Culture media in microbiology

The history of plagues and pestilences from the first records of mankind to the early twentieth century has been written by Bulloch. Although the terms 'contagion' and 'infection' were used in mediaeval times, the role of minute infectious agents could not be proved until the work of Louis Pasteur (1822–1895). Much of Pasteur's work involved demolishing Galen's theories of infectious disease and that of the spontaneous generation of microscopic life.

The father of culture media, however, was Robert Koch (1843–1910; Figure 11.1), who created methods for the cultivation, isolation and identification of bacteria. Pasteur first showed that bacteria caused infection of humans, animals and food but it took Koch's work to confirm that specific organisms caused specific diseases. The basis of Koch's work was to move away from liquid cultures, with their painstaking dilutions and frequent contamination, to a simple but powerful technique using 'solid' media. By adding gelatin, later agar, to his meat extract broth, he created the streak plate with its isolated colonies. He later demonstrated how thorough mixing of suspected material into the molten medium and pouring the plate yielded a quantitative assessment of bacterial numbers, a technique now widely used as the pour plate. Richard Petri, one of Koch's assistants, replaced Koch's glass plate under a bell jar with the Petri dish. This elegant design has remained unchanged for over 100 years.

Koch was aware that a universal medium for pathogenic bacteria was unlikely. He showed that *Mycobacterium tuberculosis* would not grow on his meat-infusion

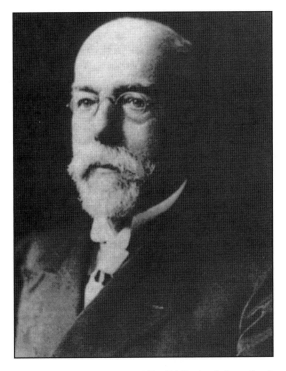

Figure 11.1   Robert Koch (1843–1910), the father of culture media

agar medium. For this organism he used coagulated serum, egg or sliced potato. By the end of the nineteenth century a textbook of medical bacteriology would list about seven media. The most important addition to Koch's meat infusion broth was peptone, a peptic digest of protein which was suggested by Loeffler. He also incorporated 0.5% w/v sodium chloride and his nutrient

The Science of Laboratory Diagnosis, Second Edition   Edited by David Burnett and John Crocker
© 2005 John Wiley & Sons, Ltd

medium has remained the bedrock of undefined complex culture media for chemo-heterotrophic organisms (i.e. those requiring organic carbon compounds for utilization, as opposed to autotrophic bacteria, which can synthesize carbon compounds from carbon dioxide).

Many more formulations of culture media arose in the first decades of the twentieth century, when enrichment, selection and indicator media were designed for organisms isolated from areas outside medicine, e.g. agriculture, food and drink manufacture, pharmaceuticals, etc. By 1930 a survey of published media described 2540 formulations, many of them small variations of previously published media. The number has grown enormously since but no similar survey has been repeated.

Formulation of culture media

The formulations used for different media may contain as few as three ingredients (Loeffler nutrient broth) to ten times as many in media for fastidious organisms. The number of ingredients has little relationship to its growth performance. 'Simple' culture may be highly complex and totally undefined. A common structure of culture media for chemo-heterotrophic organisms is as follows:

- *Amino-nitrogen base* (peptone, protein hydrolysate, infusion or extract of protein). Few organisms can utilize coagulated proteins, and pre-digested or acid-hydrolysed derivatives are provided. The peptides and amino acids can be transferred into the cell and used as carbon sources for energy or polymerized into functional proteins.

- *Supplemental growth factors* (blood, serum, yeast extract, nucleotides, vitamins). Microorganisms described as nutritionally fastidious, e.g. *Neisseria, Bordetella, Legionella*, demand extra growth factors. The considerable benefit of whole blood to these organisms was once attributed solely to the extra growth factors supplied. It is now considered that the major role of whole blood is to protect vulnerable organisms from toxic oxidation processes.

- *Energy sources, other than peptides* (sugars, alcohols and complex carbohydrates). These substances are usually added to indicator media to enhance pH changes by those organisms that can ferment the energy source. Many other organic molecules can be metabolized by chemo-heterotrophic organisms to provide energy.

- *Buffer salts* (phosphates, acetates, citrates). Buffers are commonly added to high carbohydrate formulations (e.g. containing soya peptone) to prevent excessive changes in pH levels. Unfortunately, many buffers have a tendency to chelate essential metals and they must be used carefully. Peptides and amino acids can act as buffering agents through the zwitterion effect of the NH_2/COOH groupings.

- *Mineral salts and metals* (phosphates, sulphates, Ca^{++}, Mg^{++}, Fe^{++}, Mn^{++}, trace metals). These substances may be added separately in macro- or micro-quantities, where particular demands are evident. It is important that the metals are in soluble form and are not complexed into insoluble forms during heat processing. It is usually assumed that hydrolysed animal or plant tissues contain sufficient minerals and metals for optimal growth.

- *Selective agents* (chemicals, antimicrobials and some aniline dyes). As the name implies, these agents are added at sufficient concentration to inhibit unwanted organisms but to allow the selected organisms to multiply. Extreme care is required to determine the optimum concentration in the medium. All selective agents exhibit some toxicity towards the selected species and can often fail to suppress all unwanted organisms. A general rule is that any increase in nutrients to the medium requires an increase in selective agent and vice versa. Selective agents may interact with each other to enhance or diminish their selectivity, e.g. bile salts diminish the toxicity of dyes. Selective agents can also be affected by substances (e.g. most buffers) which chelate cations, e.g. certain dyes and bile salts can become more toxic. This effect can be reversed by the addition of cations (Mg/Ca).

- *Indicator dyes* (phenol red, neutral red, bromocresol purple). These dyes indicate changes in pH value following fermentation, deamination or decarboxylation. Chromogenic culture media developed to indicate colonies producing specific enzyme activities are commonly mixtures of indicator dyes. All dyes require careful titration to avoid selective inhibition.

- *Gelling agents* (agar, gelatin, alginate, silica gel). Agar, extracted from species of the seaweed genus *Gelidium*, is the most common gelling agent for chemo-heterotrophic organism growth. Although the quality of agar has improved a great deal from its early beginnings, it cannot be considered to be an inert polymer gel. It contributes metals, minerals and pyruvates which can influence the growth of organisms. Not all agars are similar: differences in agarophyte source and the industrial processes of extraction may cause significantly different growth performance and antibiotic diffusion.

The above eight categories of materials cover almost all the variations in published culture media formulations. Further details on these materials and manufacture can be found elsewhere.

Enrichment and selection in fluid media

The procedures of enrichment and selection in fluid media are not mutually exclusive. Enrichment is generally described as a process of increasing the numbers of an organism from less than 10 cells to detectable levels. Enrichment broths may have supplemental growth factors added to reduce the lag phase of distressed or low numbers of organisms. Blood culturing is the most common example of such an enrichment procedure.

The term 'enrichment' is also used, in a mixed microbial population, when one species is selected for preferential growth. This is arranged by the use of preferential formulations, including selective or elective chemicals, pH adjustment or favourable temperature of incubation. It is seldom possible in fluid media to specifically enhance the desired organism and to suppress all other organisms present. The dynamics of growth of mixed cultures of organisms in broth are usually complex. Undesired organisms may be retarded for an initial period but they may later overgrow the desired organisms.

Although fixed periods of incubation and subculture are usually set by the working hours of the laboratory, they may not be ideal for the successful recovery of particular organisms. The most important function of enrichment broth is to raise the number of the desired organisms to a level that is sufficient for one loopful of subcultured broth to produce a detectable number of recognizable colonies on selective agar plates. Probably 10^4 organisms/ml in the broth is the minimal figure for detection by this method.

It must be remembered that the function of enrichment broths is usually judged by the results of subculture to a solid selective medium. The interaction of selective chemicals in the broth and those present in the agar plate could be inhibitory to small numbers of organisms. Tetrathionate broth subcultured to MacConkey agar

can yield greater numbers of salmonellae or shigellae than when subcultured to deoxycholate-citrate agar.

In summary, the following factors significantly affect the successful enrichment of particular organisms from liquid media: (a) the formulation of the medium and its selective agents; (b) the inoculum size of the desired organism; (c) the competitor-organism numbers and the variety of competitors; (d) the presence/absence of organic material in the broth; (e) the temperature of incubation; (f) the period of time before subculture; (g) the interaction of enrichment broth components with the selective agar plate used for subculture.

It is not surprising that much conflicting opinion has been published on this subject, when the complexity of variation possible in the end results is taken into consideration.

Chemically defined culture media versus complex undefined media

Until the middle of the twentieth century, medical microbiologists accepted the fact that culture media were prepared more as culinary works of art than as scientific formulations. Practically all the ingredients used were undefined, variable natural materials. Growth performance varied widely and this generated a desire for synthetic or chemically defined media, which should yield standard performance. During 1950–1975, microbiologists attempted to put together selected amino acids, nucleotides, vitamins, minerals and metals which would grow chemo-heterotrophic organisms at the same speed and with the same characteristics as on undefined media. Microbiological journals of this period contained hundreds of published culture media formulae, but they all showed growth performances that were inferior to undefined media or were restricted to a few species only. Not one could be recommended as a general-purpose enrichment medium for medical microbes. The sheer difficulty of designing and testing defined media, together with the disappointing results obtained, eventually caused a loss of interest in this ambition. One factor was the replacement of laboratory-prepared raw material media with commercially prepared dehydrated equivalent products. The benefits of better raw material specifications, large-scale controlled manufacture and stringent quality control testing overcame the major problems of media performance variation. More recently, commercially prepared ready-to-use media has replaced much of the culture media preparation that previously took place in microbiological laboratories.

Paradoxically, in 1966, a new undefined blood agar medium was published under the name of Columbia agar. It contained a deliberate mixture of peptones from different protein sources, hydrolysed by different enzymes, thus creating a broad spectrum of peptides from the largest possible [molecular weight (MW) = 5000] to single amino acids (MW = 100). One g starch, 5 g sodium chloride and 12 g agar made up the formula. Columbia agar, a complex undefined medium, has become the most widely used enrichment medium, in broth and agar forms, for recovering a wide variety of fastidious pathogenic organisms. This appeared to be a triumph of reality over hope for those who wished to replace such media with synthetic or defined formulations.

The dilemma of defined versus undefined media still remains unanswered. It appears that protein hydrolysates and growth factors are the two most likely groups of materials to cause difficulty. It would seem that mixtures of amino acids cannot replace a complex mixture of peptides. It is possible that a wide selection of various growth factors may be required to ensure recovery of stressed or naturally exigent organisms. It is unlikely that a defined medium comparable to Columbia agar can be developed or justified on a cost–benefit basis.

Growth environmental factors

The presence of essential growth nutrients does not by itself guaranteed optimal growth of desired organisms. All culture media are susceptible to oxidation if exposed to light, heat and air; this is called photo-, thermo- and chemo-oxidation. It was once considered that chemo-heterotrophic aerobic and facultative anaerobic organisms were little affected by oxidation processes and only obligate anaerobes suffered. It is now evident that all, except a few well-protected species, are vulnerable to oxidation effects. Toxic oxygen radicals (superoxide, singlets, hydroxyls) formed from captured extra electrons can damage nucleic acids and enzymes. Organisms attempt to protect themselves by producing protective enzymes that can neutralize these toxic radicals. Catalase, superoxide dismutase and peroxidases are examples. Some amino acids are effective scavengers of toxic oxidants. Protective agents can be added to culture media for the same purpose, e.g. whole blood, charcoal, pyruvate, reduced iron salts. It may be essential to include these agents for organisms which are particularly vulnerable, e.g. *Neisseria, Bordetella, Campylobacter, Legionella.* Sulphydryl compounds, such as thioglycol-late and cysteine, are added to anaerobic media to reduce the oxidation–reduction potential (Eh) with –SH groups, which will neutralize toxic oxidizing agents. Some media auto-oxidize on autoclaving, particularly media containing cysteine, glucose, phosphates and some metals.

Water activity (a_w)

Microorganisms must have 'free' water in which to grow and this especially applies to agar plates. The transfer of nutrients to the colony and the efflux of toxic waste from it depend on free water present in the agar. Water can be 'bound' or complexed so tightly with proteins or polymers that organisms cannot utilize it. Ice is one form of bound water and other forms are often described as 'quasi-ice'.

The biological range of water activity is from 0.97 (1.00 is pure water) to 0.61 (the surface of dried salted fish). Only xerophilic moulds can grow (slowly) at the lowest figure. Fluid media are generally suitable for the growth of all organisms, unless solutes have been added to the medium (sodium chloride or glycerin) to lower the water activity and make it selective for staphylococci or moulds.

Freshly prepared agar plates have satisfactory levels of free water but on storage evaporation reduces the water activity of the agar surface. Overdried or overlong-stored agar plates become inhibitory, demonstrate small colonies and fail to recover 'stressed' inocula (Figure 11.2).

Storage of culture media

A good basic rule is that freshly prepared media are better than stored media. However, it is seldom possible to prepare media just prior to use and some form of storage is inevitable. Stored media should be used strictly in rotation to avoid overlong storage. All containers of media should be dated and batch-numbered.

Culture media should be stored away from light to prevent photo-oxidation. All liquid media should be stored in closed tubes or bottles, preferably using screw-capped closures. Store at 2–8°C, except thioglycollate broth, which is better kept at 15–22°C. Liquid media, without antibiotics or other labile ingredients, can be stored for many weeks in the cool and away from light.

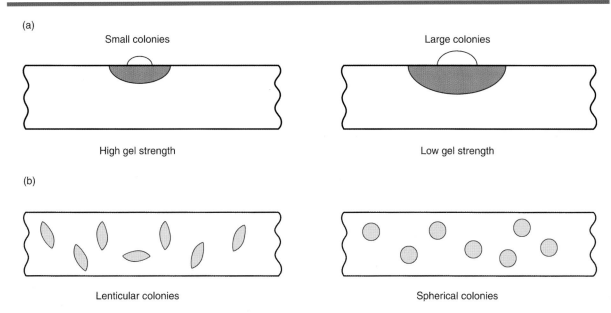

Figure 11.2 The effect of water loss from agar plates: (a) reduction of size of surface colonies; (b) changes in shape of immersed colonies from spherical to lenticular

Poured plates should be stored at 2–8°C, wrapped in shrinkfilm. This is preferable to polythene bags which trap all the moisture in the form of pools of liquid in each bag. The shelf-life of prepared plates depends on the formulation and on the conditions of storage and transport to the laboratory. With plates wrapped in semipermeable film and stored in expanded polystyrene boxes at the correct temperature, claims have been made of shelf-lives of many months. No-one should keep or attempt to use plates of this age. A useful check is to measure the loss of water during storage. A 5% weight loss suggests that the plates have reached a terminal state.

Quality tests

The great majority of microbiological laboratories purchase culture media in dehydrated or prepared form. The responsibility for quality testing has largely fallen on the manufacturers and they should provide details of their testing protocol and results to individual purchasers. It must be appreciated, however, that these tests would have been carried out on freshly manufactured media and that storage time, both before and after delivery, may reduce the quality of the medium.

The increased use of media preparators has protected agar culture media from the complex, unpredictable oxidative effects of autoclaving undissolved culture media. Falling pH values and darkening in colour indicate overheating, which causes carbohydrate–peptide complexes to form.

When testing purchased culture media, three selected strains of appropriate organisms should be sufficient. Standard strains of organisms can be purchased and a quantitative assessment of growth should be undertaken. Selective media should be tested for inhibition of unwanted organisms as well as enrichment of selected strains.

If a new media supplier is being chosen, or a large contract is being placed, then more extensive testing may be appropriate, using a control medium inoculated in parallel. Use small inocula and include some stressed organisms in the test. Snell *et al.* (1991) provides more information on this subject.

The recovery of stressed organisms in culture media control testing is increasingly being studied. Clinical microbiological isolates are often stressed, as are organisms isolated from heated/processed foods. The very stressed *viable but not culturable* (VNC) organisms represent an extreme form of stress. Stephens *et al.* (1997) used laboratory-stressed *Salmonella* and showed that the recovery of these organisms varied between the same formulation of culture media from different manufacturers. This work showed a very broad distribution of lag times between different brands of the same medium, when single cell inocula were used, with some lag times in excess of 20 hours. In the past, media manufacturers used a mixture of clinical isolates and standard NCTC/ATCC strains of organisms to test batches of culture media. The use of clinical isolates has been stopped in industry and only standard strains of organisms are commonly used. These organisms are not stressed when properly reconstituted and they can hide deficiencies in batches of culture media. The use of standard strains, stressed in the laboratory by high or low temperature exposure, is being increasingly studied and they could replace the loss of clinical isolates.

The future of culture media

The Koch agar plate, which is cheap, simple and highly versatile, is a very powerful amplifier of small inocula. Properly prepared, it will grow all expected and many unsuspected organisms from samples. Modern diagnostic devices that are forecast to replace conventional microbiology are expensive, complicated and very specific. It is likely that conventional microbiology will continue well into this century.

Undoubtedly, there will be improvements to the methodology, e.g. semi-automatic labelling, inoculation and signalling, using film technology with confocal laser microscopy for early detection of growth and built-in identification markers for specific enzyme activity. There will be better recovery of damaged organisms at the lag phase of growth. These improved recovery procedures will throw doubt on some existing sterilization kinetics theories and will solve some of the mysteries surrounding 'viable but non-culturable organisms'. The old bacteriological axiom of 'What does not grow, does not exist' will vanish. It is unlikely that microbiology will be taken over by automation in similar fashion to biochemistry or haematology. Much of the activity in microbiology consists of matching images of colonies or microscope fields with the data bank held in the microbiologist's head. The human brain is incredibly better at this than any computer.

Quantal microbiology

Large populations of microbes obey the rules of taxonomy but the individual cells exhibit uncertainties caused by mutation and adaptation to local environments. Such cells are variants that may be the forebears of the next selected population. Mutations are quantal processes involving molecules that are pushed over an energy barrier from one stable configuration to a different stable configuration. Complex chemical substances obey the laws of quantum mechanics, and the science of individual microbial cells can be called 'quantal microbiology'. There is an analogy between classical physics/quantum mechanics and classical microbiology/quantal microbiology. Now we need a system to study individual cells.

Further reading

Barer MR, Harwood CB. Bacterial viability and culturability. *Adv Microb Physiol* 1999; **41**: 94–138.

Bridson EY. *The Development, Manufacture and Control of Microbiological Culture Media.* 1994: Oxoid Ltd, Basingstoke, UK.

Bridson EY, Gould GW. Quantal microbiology. *Lett Appl Microbiol* 2000; **30**: 95–98.

British Standard BS EN 12322. *In Vitro Diagnostic Devices. Culture Media for Microbiology—Performance Criteria for Culture Media.* 1999. British Standards Institution London, UK.

Brock TD. *Robert Koch—A Life in Medicine and Bacteriology.* 1988: Science Tech Publishers, Madison, WI.

Bulloch W. *The History of Bacteriology.* 1938: Oxford University Press, Oxford. Reprinted 1984: Dover Publications, New York.

QA for Commercially Prepared Microbiological Culture Media, 2nd edn. Approved Standard: NCCLS M22-A2, vol 16. 1996: Villanova, PA.

Stephens PJ, Joynson JA, Davies KW, Holbrook R, Lappin-Scott HM, Humphrey TJ. The use of an automated growth analyser to measure recovery times of single heat-injured *Salmonella* cells. *J Appl Microbiol* 1997; **83**: 445–455.

12

Identification of bacteria

Andrew J Hay

Introduction

The ability to identify bacteria quickly and accurately is a skill requiring many years of experience at the laboratory bench to master. The purpose of this chapter is to demystify the approached adopted by UK clinical laboratories in the identification of common bacteria of medical importance. It is hoped that the reader will gain a basic insight into the process, and be able to consult the excellent detailed texts with more confidence.

Bacteria can be identified directly in patient samples, or more commonly following growth of the organisms on culture. Although considered separately, these two approaches may be combined.

Direct identification

Microscopy

Bacteria can be directly visualized in clinical samples by microscopy and the use of stains. Although useful, this on its own rarely permits full identification. The Gram stain is the most widely used differential staining procedure in clinical bacteriology laboratories today. There are many modifications, but the principle is the same. A solution of methyl violet followed by an iodine solution is applied to a heat-fixed preparation of bacteria on a microscope slide. After washing, the preparation is exposed to a decolorizer (alcohol or acetone) for a few seconds, before a red counterstain (e.g. safranin) is applied. Gram-positive bacteria are not decolorized by alcohol or acetone and stain purple. Gram-negative bacteria are decolorized, allowing the cells to take up the red counterstain. This reaction depends upon differences in the structure of the cell wall between Gram-positive and Gram-negative bacteria. The size and shape of the bacteria are also taken into account, e.g. round (cocci), rods (bacilli).

However, there are many bacteria that stain poorly or not at all with Gram's stain, e.g. mycobacteria such as *Mycobacterium tuberculosis* require stains for 'acid-fastness', such as Ziehl–Neelsen. These stains rely on the fact that certain bacteria can, after being stained with warm solutions of carbol fuchsin, resist the decolorizing action of hydrochloric acid and alcohol. Modifications of these stains can visualize other bacteria, e.g. *Nocardia* spp.

In the past, fluorescent antibody stains were used to detect specific bacteria such as *Legionella*, but poor performance precludes their use in routine bacteriology today.

Antibody and antigen detection

These tests are useful for bacteria which are not routinely cultured on solid media, including the spirochaetes, and the obligate intracellular pathogens *Rickettsia, Coxiella* and *Chlamydia*. Infections caused by these genera are usually diagnosed by antibody detection in serum (serology) or, in the case of *Chlamydia* genital infection, antigen detection.

Antigen detection can be used for the rapid diagnosis of serious bacterial infections, e.g. in meningitis cases, bacterial antigens in cerebrospinal fluid (CSF) can be detected using latex agglutination.

The Science of Laboratory Diagnosis, Second Edition   Edited by David Burnett and John Crocker
© 2005 John Wiley & Sons, Ltd

A variation is the detection of a bacterial product, e.g. the use of an enzyme immunoassay to detect the toxin of *Clostridium difficile* in faeces, a cause of antibiotic-associated diarrhoea.

Molecular methods

Since the last edition of this book, significant developments have occurred in the field of diagnostic molecular bacteriology. Although it is still true that few of these techniques have made the transition from research and reference laboratory to clinical bacteriology laboratory, the growth in the number of commercially available test kits make this a distinct possibility in the near future, particularly if the relatively high cost of these molecular methods can be addressed. Some examples are given below.

The polymerase chain reaction (PCR) and gene probes have shown promise in the rapid identification of *Mycobacterium tuberculosis* in clinical samples. This slow-growing organism usually takes several weeks to identify by conventional methods. Similarly, nucleic acid amplification tests, such as PCR or ligase chain reaction, are recommended for the diagnosis of genital *Chlamydia trachomatis* infection. In faeces samples, PCR is used to detect genes encoding verotoxins produced by vero-toxin-producing *Escherichia coli* (VTEC), e.g. *E. coli* O157. Simultaneous detection of *Neisseria meningitidis, Streptococcus pneumoniae* and *Haemophilus influenzae* DNA in CSF or whole blood by multiplex PCR is proving invaluable in rapid diagnosis of bacterial meningitis. Commercial systems have also been developed for the rapid (less than 3 hours) detection of methicillin-resistant *Staphylococcus aureus* (MRSA) and vancomycin-resistant *Enterococcus* spp., using real-time PCR (Roche Diagnostics, Mannheim, Germany). These methods should enable early initiation of effective antimicrobial chemotherapy and infection control precautions, thus improving clinical outcomes. See other chapters for a fuller discussion of the methods themselves.

Identification following culture

Pure culture

The first step in identifying a bacterium is to establish a pure culture. Failure to do this is a common error, leading to delayed or misleading laboratory reports.

Clinical material should be plated on primary isolation media in such a way that much of the growth consists of well-isolated colonies (Figure 12.1). The colonies thus obtained should be examined carefully with a magnifying hand-lens under good lighting, and single colonies for investigation picked and transferred to a non-selective medium using a straight wire and a steady hand! If this process fails to yield adequate growth of a pure culture, it should be repeated. Short-cuts taken at this stage will delay identification, waste reagents and possibly produce misleading results, to the frustration and aggravation of bacteriologist and clinician, and potentially the wrong treatment for the patient.

Note that a non-selective medium must be used at this stage, as selective or inhibitory primary isolation media often interfere with subsequent biochemical and other identification techniques.

The art of identification

When faced with a primary isolation plate that may contain up to a dozen or so different species of commensal bacteria, and the knowledge that almost any bacterium can cause disease, the novice bacteriologist must despair of producing a meaningful report before retirement! However, experience in examining these plates, combined with knowledge of site sampled, clinical picture, likely pathogens and commensal flora will yield a reasonably accurate idea of the organisms that require identification and sensitivity testing. This approach allows the bacteriologist to choose the initial range of tests that are likely to lead to rapid identification of the pathogen.

If this fails to confirm the most probable causal organism, the investigator must proceed with an open mind and widen the investigations. This method, termed the progressive method, requires the establishment of a few fundamental characteristics of the organism, and from these, subsequent sets of tests are chosen according to tables until the organism is identified.

Finally, if all else fails, the blunderbuss method may be adopted where every conceivable test is done and compared with those listed in standard texts of systematic bacteriology. This is rarely necessary, but will be required, for example, to verify a new species.

Preliminary identification

The ability of bacteria to grow under aerobic or anaerobic conditions, their growth requirements, colonial morphology, effect on the medium (e.g. haemolysis on blood agar), motility in liquid medium, ability to form spores

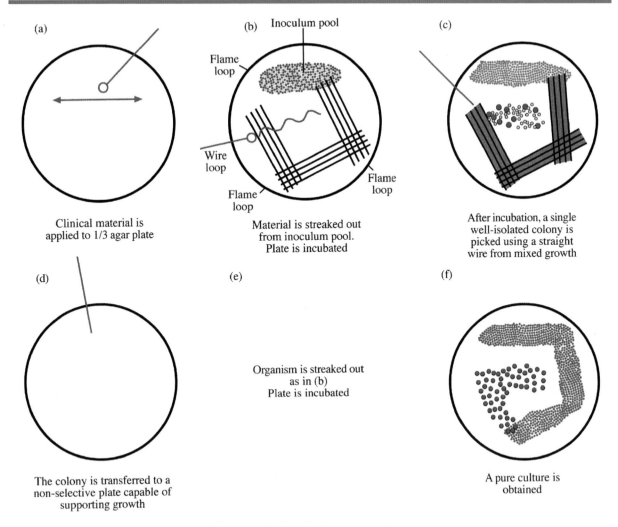

(a) Clinical material is applied to 1/3 agar plate

(b) Inoculum pool
Flame loop
Wire loop
Flame loop
Flame loop
Material is streaked out from inoculum pool. Plate is incubated

(c) After incubation, a single well-isolated colony is picked using a straight wire from mixed growth

(d) The colony is transferred to a non-selective plate capable of supporting growth

(e) Organism is streaked out as in (b) Plate is incubated

(f) A pure culture is obtained

Figure 12.1 Establishing a pure culture

and appearance and reaction on Gram staining allow a preliminary identification to be made. Subsequent application of a few simple, rapid tests will then indicate which further tests (if any) are required to complete identification.

After the Gram stain—the bacteriologist's toolbox

Like a master craftsman, the skilled bacteriologist selects the tools required to complete identification based on the results of colonial morphology and Gram stain. These tests may be grouped into the broad categories listed below. They may be performed sequentially or simultaneously, depending on the organism to be identified. They must be carefully controlled each time

they are performed, e.g. by using control strains with known reactions.

Enzyme detection

The ability of a bacterium to produce an enzyme is tested by exposing it to a substrate and detecting the resulting product. Common tests are:

1. *Catalase test.* Catalase-producing organisms, when exposed to hydrogen peroxide, produce visible bubbles within 30 seconds. This test may help differentiate staphylococci, which are catalase-positive, from streptococci, which are catalase-negative.

2. *Oxidase test.* This tests for the presence of cytochrome oxidase. Oxidase-positive bacteria, such as

Pseudomonas can oxidize the reagent tetramethyl-*p*-phenylenediamine dihydrochloride to produce a colour change. Enterobacteriaceae are oxidase-negative.

3. *Urease test.* Certain species produce a powerful enzyme that splits urea to ammonia, which can be detected by a colour change using a pH indicator incorporated into the growth medium. This test helps differentiate urease-positive *Proteus mirabilis*, a gut commensal, from urease-negative *Salmonella* spp. and *Shigella* spp., which important intestinal pathogens.

4. *Coagulase test.* *Staphylococcus aureus* possesses an enzyme that coagulates plasma *in vitro*. Other staphylococci are negative.

This list is not comprehensive. Many other tests exist, and these are often incorporated into commercial kits.

Antigen detection

Detection of cell antigens by specific antisera is used widely in bacteriology to speciate and type organisms. Two examples are:

1. *Lancefield grouping.* A cell wall group antigen is extracted from β-haemolytic streptococci by an enzyme. The antigen is then detected by agglutination with antisera bound to latex particles.

2. *'O' and 'H' typing.* Cell wall (O) antigens and flagellar (H) antigens are detected on Gram-negative bacilli such as *Salmonella*, by mixing suspensions of the organisms with specific antisera on a slide or in a test tube. A positive reaction is noted by the clumping of organisms.

Carbohydrate metabolism

The ability of an organism to utilize certain sugars such as glucose, oxidatively (aerobic) or fermentatively (independent of oxygen), or other carbohydrates, e.g. starch, is a useful characteristic commonly used in identification. The test requires a defined medium containing the carbohydrate, and a detection system for the metabolic product, often a pH indicator.

Sugar utilization may be incorporated into primary isolation media, such as MacConkey agar, which differentiates lactose-fermenting Enterobacteriaceae from Enterobacteriaceae which are non-lactose-fermenters, and thiosulphate citrate bile sucrose agar (TCBS), which identifies sucrose-fermenting *Vibrio cholerae* from other species. Other tests detect the ability of the organism to use a carbohydrate as a sole carbon source, e.g. citrate utilization. Panels of carbohydrates can be conveniently tested simultaneously in commercial kits.

Growth factors

The absolute requirement of defined compounds for bacterial growth on a particular medium is utilized as an identification tool, e.g. *Haemophilus* species differ in their requirements for two factors present in blood, X (haematin) and V (diphosphopyridine nucleotide), for growth on nutrient agar. Only *Haemophilus influenzae*, the most important pathogen of the genus, requires both.

Protein metabolism

The ability of a bacterial species to metabolize a protein or an amino acid to a defined product is tested. Detection systems for the product and the need for a defined medium are similar to those required for carbohydrate utilization, e.g. different species of the Enterobacteriaceae will vary in their ability to: (a) liquify gelatin; (b) decarboxylate or deaminate amino acids; (c) produce hydrogen sulphide from sulphur-containing amino acids; and (d) produce indole from tryptophan. These tests are often performed in commercial kits.

Susceptibility tests

The susceptibility of a species to a compound may be used not only to help decide on antibiotic treatment, but also to aid in identification. Two commonly used examples are given, both tested by placing a filter paper disc containing the compound onto a culture plate, incubating, then observing for a zone of inhibition.

1. *Optochin test.* *Streptococcus pneumoniae* is sensitive to optochin (ethylhydrocupreine hydrochloride). Other streptococci which resemble it on blood agar are resistant.

2. *Metronidazole sensitivity.* True anaerobes are almost always sensitive to this antibiotic. Aerobes which can grow anaerobically are invariably resistant.

Toxin production

This important characteristic may help differentiate pathogenic from non-pathogenic species. Examples:

1. *Elek test.* This test is used to differentiate toxin-producing (therefore pathogenic) strains of *Corynebacterium diphtheriae*, the cause of diphtheria, from non-pathogenic strains. A filter paper strip containing diphtheria antitoxin is laid onto a defined medium. The organism is streaked onto the agar at right angles to the strip. After incubation, precipitin lines representing antigen (toxin)–antibody (antitoxin) complexes may be seen.

2. *Cytotoxin.* A cytotoxin produced by strains of *Clostridium difficile* associated with antibiotic-associated diarrhoea may be detected by antitoxin neutralization in cell culture.

Commercial identification systems

The development of commercial systems for the rapid identification of pathogenic bacteria has greatly simplified the life of the clinical bacteriologist. Prior to their introduction, each biochemical test had to be set up individually in a test tube or glass bottle, leading to impressive displays of laboratory glassware! Commercial systems allow many biochemical tests to be performed simultaneously from a pure culture. The pattern of test results obtained is then compared with patterns derived from known bacteria held in a computerized data bank. Statistical tests are used to determine the likely identity of the clinical isolate. The data bank may also suggest additional tests if identification is in doubt. Commonly used systems in the UK are the API system and Vitek, both made by Bio Merieux (Bio Merieux UK Ltd, Basingstoke, England), BD Phoenix (B D Diagnostic Systems Europe, Le Pont de Claix, France) and Mastascan elite (Mast Group Ltd, Bootle, Merseyside, UK).

1. *API (appareils et procedes d'identification) identification system.* This system consists of plastic cupules containing a variety of substrates and indicator chemicals held on a plastic strip. Each cupule comprises a different biochemical test. The addition of a standard inoculum of the test organism to each cupule in the strip, after incubation, results in a series of colour changes that can be read by the naked eye. The pattern of results obtained can be readily decoded by the data bank. Customized strips with panels of tests exist for the identification of staphylococci, streptococci, coryneform bacteria, Enterobacteriaceae, anaerobes and non-fermenting Gram-negative bacteria.

2. *The Vitek and BD Phoenix systems.* These systems employ similar principles. The biochemical tests are performed simultaneously in wells encased in a plastic card (Vitek) or strip (BD Phoenix). The wells are filled with the bacterial suspension by vacuum suction (Vitek) or pouring (BD Phoenix). After incubation, the cards are read by a customized, computer-controlled reader and the results interpreted by computerized expert systems. A range of cards are produced to identify common bacteria of medical importance, often within 4–6 hours. The advantages of these systems include their ability to perform antibiotic susceptibility testing, semi-automation requiring reduced operator time, and an enclosed system for greater laboratory safety.

3. *Mastascan elite.* This system employs multipoint inoculation of identification media in Petri dishes. Following incubation, the plates are analysed in a reader which automatically reads and interprets the identification tests incorporated in the test media. The system also permits antibiotic susceptibility testing, and direct inoculation of plates with urine samples, thus eliminating the need for primary culture of urine.

All systems require strict adherence to the manufacturer's instructions if errors are to be avoided. Failure to start with a pure culture is a common source of error. This can be avoided by inoculating a purity plate from the suspension used to inoculate the card or strip. If the plate shows a mixed growth, the tests are repeated. Inexperienced bacteriologists often accept the results from these systems without question, regardless of how improbable they may be clinically. Experienced workers will interpret the results in their clinical context, and will confirm or repeat unlikely or unusual identifications.

New developments

Molecular techniques

As already discussed, molecular methods are useful in detecting slowly growing and uncultivatable pathogens in clinical samples. In addition, these methods have been widely adopted for the typing of bacteria by research and reference laboratories, and for the characterization of new species.

Particularly exciting is the development of DNA chip technology, e.g. DNA microassays, in which thousands of oligonucleotides, located on a solid support (chip), are produced. These can be used to sequence PCR products. Intriguingly, under development are bioelectronic chips which use electrical fields to move samples to different analytical areas on a chip, realizing the ultimate goal of a 'lab on a chip'. For further discussion, see Nolte and Caliendo (2003).

Mass spectrometry

Developments in mass spectrometry techniques have stimulated research into their application in the field of bacterial identification. For example, matrix-assisted laser desorption ionization time-of-flight mass spectrometry (MALDI–TOF–MS) of intact organisms has been shown to produce, within minutes of removal of a colony from a culture plate, characteristic mass spectral finger-

prints which permit identification. Although time will tell whether this technique makes it to the routine clinical laboratory, it is certainly an interesting development.

Identification of bacteria of medical importance

The following is a brief introduction to the identification of bacteria of medical importance. For further information, please see the reading list.

Gram-positive cocci

The ability of a Gram-positive coccus to produce catalase is a useful rapid test differentiating catalase-positive genera, such as *Staphylococcus* and *Micrococcus* from catalase-negative genera, viz. *Streptococcus* and *Enterococcus*. Subsequent identification proceeds according to Figure 12.2.

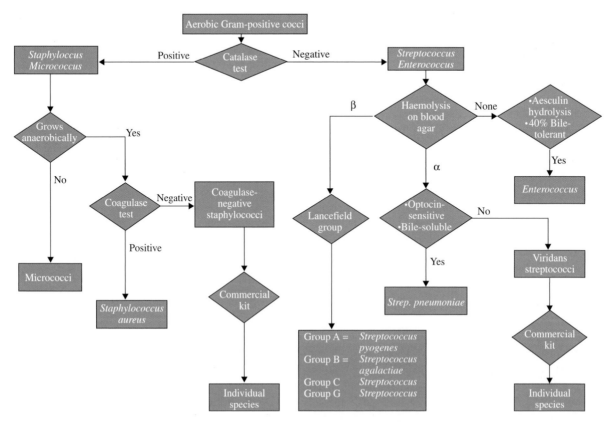

Figure 12.2 Identification of aerobic Gram-positive cocci of medical importance

Staphylococcus and Micrococcus

These catalase-positive genera characteristically produce cells arranged in clusters when grown in liquid medium. Staphylococci may be differentiated from micrococci by their ability to grow under anaerobic conditions.

Staphylococcus aureus, a common cause of skin, wound and lung infection can be differentiated from other staphylococci which are skin commensals by its ability to coagulate plasma and produce a thermostable DNAase enzyme. Coagulase activity is detected within a few hours, providing a rapid, reliable identification. Coagulase-negative strains of staphylococci may be speciated by commercial kits.

Streptococcus and Enterococcus

In liquid medium these catalase-negative genera produce cells arranged in pairs or chains. On blood agar, they produce colonies 0.1–1.0 mm diameter after 24 hours of incubation, and the type of haemolysis observed around the colonies provides a useful initial classification.

β-Haemolytic streptococci are best demonstrated in cultures grown anaerobically. Strains producing complete clearing of the blood-containing growth medium around the colony (β-haemolysis) comprise several important pathogenic species which are differentiated by Lancefield grouping. This can be performed by commercial tests in less than 1 hour. Generally, this is sufficient to complete identification, although commercial biochemical test kits may be used in cases of doubt.

α-Haemolytic streptococci produce partial haemolysis (α-haemolysis), a greenish discolouration of the blood-containing growth medium around the colony. The most important pathogenic species is *Streptococcus pneumoniae*, the pneumococcus. It is differentiated from other α-haemolytic species by its colonial appearance (draughtsman colonies), optochin sensitivity and the solubility of its colonies in bile salt solution. Other α-haemolytic species are found as commensals in the upper respiratory tract, but may occasionally cause serious sepsis, e.g. subacute bacterial endocarditis. They may be speciated by commercial kits.

Enterococci are typically non-haemolytic on blood agar, although individual strains can show α- or β-haemolysis. Enterococci, unlike most streptococci, can grow on medium containing 40% bile and can hydrolyse aesculin, and these properties are used to identify them in the clinical laboratory. They often carry Lancefield group D antigen, and may be speciated, if required, by commercial kits.

Gram-positive bacilli

The medically important genera are initially identified by their colonial morphology, spore-forming ability and requirement for aerobic or anaerobic growth conditions (Figure 12.3).

Bacillus and Clostridium

These spore-forming genera may be differentiated by catalase and conditions required for growth. *Clostridium* species are catalase-negative and strict anaerobes. Bacilli are catalase-positive and all grow aerobically. *Clostridium perfringens*, the cause of gas gangrene, may be provisionally identified by the Nagler test, which detects a specific enzyme, lecithinase, produced by this species. Both genera may be speciated by biochemical tests.

Listeria and Corynebacterium

These aerobic, non-spore-forming genera can be confused with each other on primary isolation media. *Listeria monocytogenes*, a cause of sepsis and meningoencephalitis, shows characteristic 'tumbling' motility in broth culture at room temperature but not at 37°C, can hydrolyse aesculin and is often β-haemolytic on blood agar. *Corynebacteria* spp. comprise skin commensals, opportunist pathogens and several major pathogens. Few species are β-haemolytic. The most important pathogen is *Corynebacterium diphtheriae*, which can be isolated from throat swabs on selective media containing tellurite. Toxigenic strains are detected by the Elek test.

Gram-negative cocci

There are three major human pathogens in this group: *Neisseria gonorrhoea* (the gonococcus), the cause of gonorrhoea; *Neisseria meningitidis* (the meningococcus), a cause of septicaemia and meningitis; and *Moraxella catarrhalis*, a cause of chest and eye infections. They must be distinguished from each other and other species which are common human commensals by growth characteristics and biochemical tests (Table 12.1). They are oxidase- and catalase-positive.

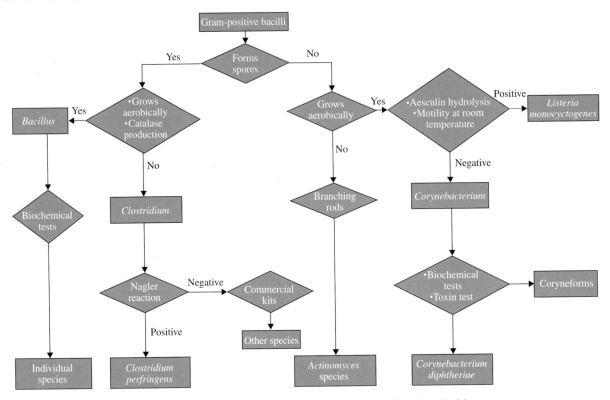

Figure 12.3 Preliminary identification of Gram-positive bacilli of medical importance

Aerobic gram-negative bacilli

Simple growth requirements

Commercial systems have greatly simplified identification for this group. However, a few simple tests are still required to screen out commensal flora from potential pathogens, and to help choose the correct test card or strip (Figure 12.4). The oxidase test is a useful preliminary investigation that takes seconds to perform. Oxidase-negative genera comprise many species that are commensals and pathogens of the gastrointestinal tract (Enterobacteriaceae). Lactose fermentation is usually noted on MacConkey agar which supports growth of these organisms on primary isolation. Non-lactose fermenters may be screened by a urease test or a

Table 12.1 Identification of aerobic Gram-negative cocci of medical importance

	Neisseria gonorrhoea	Neisseria meningitidis	Commensal Neisseria species	Moraxella Catarrhalis
Acid from[*]				
Glucose	+	+	v	−
Maltose	−	+	v	−
Lactose	−	−	v	−
Sucrose	−	−	v	−
Grows on nutrient agar	−	−	v	+
Tributyrin[**]	−	−	−	+
DNAase	−	−	−	+

v = Variable, depending on species
[*] = Test performed on serum-free medium
[**] = Detects ability of bacterium to split glyceryl tributyrate

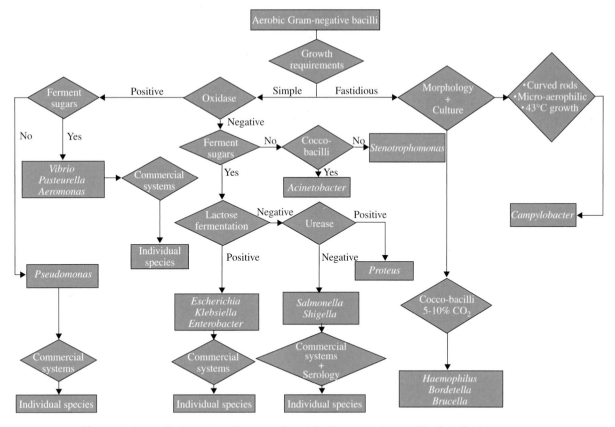

Figure 12.4 Preliminary identification of aerobic Gram-negative bacilli of medical importance

commercial kit for the possible presence of *Salmonella* and *Shigella*, which are then confirmed by further biochemical tests and 'O' (*Salmonella* and *Shigella)* and 'H' (*Salmonella* only) agglutination. Oxidase-positive genera may be differentiated into those which ferment sugars, e.g. *Vibrio* and *Aeromonas*, and non-fermenters, e.g. *Pseudomonas*. Different commercial test strips and cards may be required for fermenters and non-fermenters.

Fastidious growth requirements

Within this group, *Campylobacter* spp. are most readily identified by their morphology and their ability to grow in a micro-aerophilic atmosphere at 42°C but not in air at 37°C.

Haemophilus, *Bordetella* and *Brucella* are small, mainly non-motile Gram-negative bacilli which grow comparatively poorly on blood agar and poorly, or not at all, on MacConkey agar. This allows them to be readily differentiated from *Pseudomonas* and Enterobacteriaceae. They require enriched, blood-containing media

for primary isolation, and the addition of 5–10% CO_2 enhances growth.

Haemophilus spp. are commonly isolated from respiratory specimens. They are speciated by their differing requirements for X and V factors for growth on nutrient agar. *Bordetella* may be identified initially by agglutination with specific antiserum. *Brucella* may be speciated (usually by reference laboratories for health and safety reasons), by susceptibility to the dyes fuchsin and thionin, requirement for CO_2, and H_2S production.

Anaerobes

Strict anaerobes are differentiated by their inability to grow in the presence of oxygen and sensitivity to metronidazole, detected by a disc placed on the primary isolation plate. They may be speciated by commercial kits or by detection of their products of metabolism by gas–liquid chromatography. However, this is rarely undertaken in clinical laboratories unless the anaerobe has been isolated from a sterile site, e.g. blood or soft tissue. Gram-positive genera include *Peptostreptococcus* (cocci), and *Clostridium* and *Actinomyces* (bacilli). Common Gram-negative genera include *Bacteroides*, *Fusobacterium, Prevotella, Porphyromonas* (anaerobic bacilli), and *Veillonella* (cocci).

Further reading

Barron GI, Feltham RKA. *Cowan and Steel's Manual for the Identification of Medical Bacteria*, 3rd edn. 1993: Cambridge University Press, Cambridge.

Bright JJ, Claydon MA, Soufian M, Gordon DB. Rapid typing of bacteria using matrix-assisted laser desorption ionisation time-of-flight mass spectrometry and pattern recognition software. *J Microbiol Methods* 2002; **48**: 127–138.

Collins CH, Lyne PM, Grange JM. (1995). *Collins and Lyne's Microbiological Methods*, 7th edn. 1995: Butterworth-Heinmann, Oxford.

Gill VJ, Fedorko DP, Witebsky FG. The clinician and the microbiology laboratory. In *Mandell, Douglas and Bennett's Principles and Practice of Infectious Diseases*, 5th edn, Mandell GL, Bennett JE and Dolin R (eds). 2000: Churchill Livingstone, Philadelphia, PA, pp 184–221.

Nolte FS, Caliendo AM. Molecular detection and identification of microorganisms. In *Manual of Clinical Microbiology*, 8th edn, Murray PR, Baron EJ, Jorgensen JH, Pfaller MA, Yolken RH (eds). 2003: ASM Press, Washington, DC, pp 234–256.

Stokes EJ, Ridgway GL, Wren MDW. *Clinical Microbiology*, 7th edn. 1993: Edward Arnold, London.

13

Automated tests in bacteriology

Paul C Boreland

Automation: the use of automatic equipment to save mental and manual labour. *The Concise Oxford Dictionary.*

Introduction

Although automated instrumentation was first introduced into the clinical microbiology laboratory over 30 years ago, many microbiologists have been reluctant to embrace the concept fully. This has been due in part to a conservative attitude among microbiologists, which perpetuates the use of methods for detecting growth which were developed at the end of the nineteenth century. Other relevant factors include the variety and complex nature of the specimens submitted to the laboratory, the greater complexity of microbiological tests, the difficulty of integrating an instrument into the existing laboratory regime, together with the fact that many of the earlier machines did not perform adequately. However, recent improvements in technology and bi-directional interfacing between instruments and laboratory computer systems have now made automation a practical and cost-effective alternative.

Today, instruments are the integral part of many clinical microbiology laboratories and automated equipment is available for the detection of positive blood cultures, the antimicrobial susceptibility testing and identification of microorganisms, the screening of urine samples for bacteria, and the isolation and antimicrobial susceptibility of *Mycobacterium tuberculosis* in clinical samples. The automated systems described in this chapter are not totally inclusive of all the systems currently on the world market, or some which have come and gone, but represent those most commonly encountered in clinical microbiology laboratories within the UK.

Blood culture systems

The rapid detection of microorganisms in a patient's blood is of diagnostic and prognostic importance. Blood cultures, therefore, are essential in the diagnosis and treatment of the aetiological agents of septicaemia. As septicaemia constitutes one of the most serious infectious diseases, the rapid detection and identification of blood-borne bacterial pathogens is a major function of the clinical microbiology laboratory. Consequently, automated blood culture systems have been developed and refined over the past 30 years. The first semi-automated instrument to be used, the BACTEC 460 (Johnston Laboratories Inc.), detected radioactive carbon dioxide metabolized by microorganisms growing in a liquid medium with ^{14}C incorporated. This soon gave way to the non-radiometric BACTEC 660/730, using infra-red detection of carbon dioxide.

Subsequently a number of fully automated instruments have emerged, each of which is comprised of three basic units; an incubator, a detector and a computer. The inoculated blood culture bottles or vials are placed in racks and may or may not be agitated. Each bottle is continuously monitored for growth every 10–15 minutes, the computer analyses the data by means of a predetermined algorithm and indicates when a culture

The Science of Laboratory Diagnosis, Second Edition   Edited by David Burnett and John Crocker
© 2005 John Wiley & Sons, Ltd

is positive. When a positive bottle is identified, it can be removed from the system for isolation and identification of the microorganism. Importantly, unlike the older instruments, microbial growth is measured non-invasively. Most detection methods are based directly or indirectly on the production of gases (mostly carbon dioxide), or the resulting pH changes, following growth of microorganisms in broth culture.

The *BACTEC 9000* series (9240, 9120, 9050) of blood culture instruments (Becton Dickinson) are designed for the rapid detection of microorganisms in clinical specimens. The sample to be tested is inoculated into a vial, which is entered into the instrument for incubation and periodic reading. In the base of each vial is a pH-sensitive sensor containing fluorochemicals which respond to carbon dioxide, embedded in a matrix. Carbon dioxide, produced by microorganisms metabolizing nutrients in the culture medium, diffuses through the matrix, causing a decrease in pH which is detected by the fluorochemicals. The instrument's photodetectors specifically measure the level of fluorescence emitted from the sensor every 10 minutes, an increase in which is proportional to the increasing amount of carbon dioxide or the decreasing amount of oxygen present in the bottle. The measurements are interpreted by the computer software according to pre-programmed positivity parameters.

The *BacT/Alert 3D* system (bioMerieux) incubates, agitates and continuously monitors the growth of microorganisms in blood cultures. Bonded into the base of every blood culture bottle is a colorimetric sensor covered by an ion-exclusion membrane, which is permeable to carbon dioxide but impermeable to free hydrogen ions, the components of media and whole blood. When carbon dioxide is produced by the growth of microorganisms, it diffuses across the membrane, lowers the pH and initiates a change in colour of the sensor from green to yellow. This colour change is detected by reflecting light from a red light-emitting diode off the sensor onto a photodiode (Figure 13.1). The voltage signal produced is proportional to the intensity of the reflected light and thus the concentration of carbon dioxide in the bottle. The data obtained by the computer is plotted as a growth curve of reflectance units versus time.

Antimicrobial susceptibility testing and identification systems

The identification and antimicrobial susceptibility testing of bacterial isolates are two of the most important tasks in the clinical microbiology laboratory. A number of systems are currently available, from semi-to fully automated instruments and most offer identification of organisms as well as antimicrobial susceptibility testing with a choice of conventional or rapid incubation and analysis times. Some instruments have strips which can be inoculated either automatically or manually, incubated externally and then placed in a reader, which interprets colour reactions and growth end-points. With fully automated systems, microdilution trays or cards are incubated within the instrument which continually monitors and interprets growth or biochemical reactions.

Each system requires an inoculum standardization step, usually performed using a densitometer, to measure bacterial density, which may be expressed in McFarland units. For the detection of colour changes or growth in liquid medium containing either substrates or dilutions of antibiotics, most automatic readers employ a combination of three methods of light measurement: (a) the transmission of light in four regions of the spectrum—*colorimetry*; (b) the intensity of transmitted light, which is inversely proportional to the amount of bacterial growth—*turbidimetry*; and (c) the intensity of scattered light at 30°, which is directly proportional to the amount of bacterial growth—*nephelometry*. Light measurements are easily converted into electrical impulses, and then quantified.

A few instruments use fluorogenic substrate hydrolysis to detect bacterial growth and can provide results within 4–5 hours. All the systems are equipped with a computer and software capable of interpreting results from the reader, producing algorithm-derived minimum inhibitory concentration (MIC) or breakpoint values, identifying organisms from a database containing

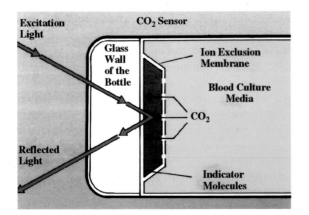

Figure 13.1 Detection of accelerating carbon dioxide production from microbial growth. Reproduced with kind permission from bioMerieux

several biocodes and performing statistical and epidemiological analyses.

The *Vitek* system (bioMerieux) uses plastic credit card-size reagent cards containing small quantities of growth medium and either antibiotics or biochemical test media in test wells. Cards are available for the identification of 300 species of bacteria and yeasts and a range of 17 antibiotics as either Susceptible (S), Intermediate (I) or Resistant (R) or giving MIC results. Each identification card has 30 reaction wells containing a range of biochemical tests, which do not require the addition of reagents. The susceptibility card has 45 reaction wells containing a range of 17 antibiotics, each present over a range of concentrations. Specific tests for the detection of resistance mechanisms are also included in this card. The system includes a filling and sealing module for the inoculation and hermetic sealing of the cards, and a combined incubator and reader in which the cards are held in a carousel and where biochemical colour changes and optical density are photometrically measured every hour. The system uses turbidometricially determined kinetic measurements of growth in the presence of antibiotics to perform linear regression analysis and, ultimately, to determine algorithm-derived MICs.

Results are usually available within 4–18 hours, with the identification and antimicrobial susceptibility of an individual microorganism being derived from computer analysis of the data.

The *Vitek 2* is a more automated version of the Vitek System, with automated front-end sample processing, including initial inoculum dilution, density verification and card-filling and -sealing steps. The instrument automatically transfers cards to the reader-incubator and ejects them into a disposal bin at the completion of testing. The system allows kinetic analysis by reading each test every 15 minutes. The optical system combines multichannel fluorimeter and photometer readings to record fluorescence, turbidity and colorimetric signals. The Vitek 2 system uses a 64-well card and allows for the testing of up to 20 antibiotics.

The *Phoenix* Automated Microbiology System (Becton Dickinson) uses a sealed, self-filling moulded plastic tray with inoculation ports at the top for filling, and contains 136 microwells. This is for use with the instrument for either microorganism identification (ID) or antimicrobial susceptibility testing (AST), or a combination of both.

For bacterial identification, the ID portion of the Phoenix panel utilizes a series of conventional, chromogenic and fluorogenic biochemical tests in 51 wells. Both growth-based and enzymatic substrates are employed to cover the different types of reactivity within the range of taxa. The tests are based on microbial utilization and degradation of specific substrates detected by various indicator systems. Acid production is indicated by a change in phenol red indicator when an isolate is able to utilize a carbohydrate substrate. Chromogenic substrates produce a yellow colour upon enzymatic hydrolysis of either *p*-nitrophenyl or *p*-nitroanilide compounds. Enzymatic hydrolysis of fluorogenic substrates results in the release of a fluorescent coumarin derivative. Microorganisms that utilize a specific carbon source reduce the reazurin-based indicator. In addition, there are other tests that detect the ability of an organism to hydrolyse, degrade, reduce or otherwise utilize a substrate.

The *Phoenix* AST method is a broad-based microdilution test, using a redox indicator for the detection of organism growth in the presence of an antibiotic. Continuous measurements of changes to the indicator, as well as turbidity, are used in the determination of bacterial growth. Each AST panel configuration contains several antibiotics with a wide range of two-fold doubling dilution concentrations. Microorganism identification is also used in the interpretation of MIC values of each antibiotic.

The *Sensititre ARIS* (AccuMed International Ltd) detects bacterial growth by means of compounds known as fluorophores. They consist of different substrates, such as peptides and esters, linked to the fluorescing compounds 4-methylumbelliferone (4MU) and 7-aminomethylcoumarin (7 AMC). Normally these complexes are non-fluorescent, but during bacterial growth specific enzymes are produced which cleave the substrates from the fluorophores, allowing the 7 AMC or 4 MU to fluoresce under UV light. Susceptibility to a specific antibiotic is recorded as absence of fluorescence, i.e. no growth, and resistance is recorded as fluorescence due to enzyme production by actively growing bacteria. Results usually take only 4–5 hours but may require overnight incubation. The system comprises an inoculator, an incubator, a fluorimeter reading fluorescence at 450 μm and a computer. Tests are performed in wells in prepared microtitre trays and the software contains an algorithm that can interpret the signals and produce breakpoint or MIC results. The identification system works similarly, with only those biochemical tests that can produce fluorescence or are non-fluorescent being included. The microorganism is identified from a computer database.

The *Mastascanelite* (Mast Group Ltd) is a unique modular system that uses multipoint technology to inoculate agar dilution antimicrobial susceptibility tests, both breakpoint and MIC, and biochemical identi-fication tests. It consists of a scanner module containing a colour video camera, a multipoint inoculator 'multi-pointelite' and a computer. Predosed, freeze-dried pel-lets of antibiotics are used to prepare breakpoint and MIC plates, and a range of culture media are used for bacterial identification. Agar plates are inoculated with up to 96 different microorganisms, incubated, and growth is seen as 19 or 36 macrocolonies. They are then placed in the scanner module and inspected at predetermined points by the video camera. The quantity of each of the three basic colours, red, blue and green, is sent as an electrical signal to the microcomputer, which converts the signals to numbers. For breakpoint and MIC plates, where susceptibility or resistance is defined as growth or no growth, the three-colour signals combine to produce the equivalent of a black and white signal. When biochemical identification agar plates are exam-ined, details of the colours measured are used to define positive or negative results from the different microor-ganisms tested. The multipoint technology can also be used for urine screening.

The increasing need for standardized and quantitative methods of AST, such as are recommended by the British Society for Antimicrobial Chemotherapy (BSAC) or the National Committee on Clinical Labora-tory Standards (NCCLS), has encouraged several man-ufacturers to produce semi-automated instruments based on disc diffusion technology, which requires the accurate measurement of inhibition zone diameters. These instru-ments, *Aura Image* (Oxoid Ltd), *BIOMIC* (Giles Scien-tific Inc.), *Mastascanelite* (Mast Group Ltd), *Osiris* (Sanofi Diagnostic Pasteur) and *Sirscan 2000* (i2a Mont-pellier), are all image analysis systems that use a video camera to measure the inhibition zone diameter and interpret the results for disc diffusion susceptibility agar plates. The agar plate is placed on a motorized sliding tray and a clear image with fully calculated diameters appears on the video screen. A zone of inhibition is interpreted as S, I, R by reference to BSAC/NCCLS antibiotic tables.

Most systems have a user-programmed rule-based expert system and a comprehensive epidemiological database.

Urine screening systems

The investigation of urine samples for the presence of bacteriuria and pyuria represents a significant proportion of the workload and cost of running a clinical micro-biology laboratory. Only 20–30% of these specimens yield clinically significant results, and consequently various attempts have been made to automate the pro-cess in order to screen out negative urines. The require-ment has been for an instrument that has the ability to detect bacteria and other particles in urine, such as erythrocytes and leukocytes, can process specimens

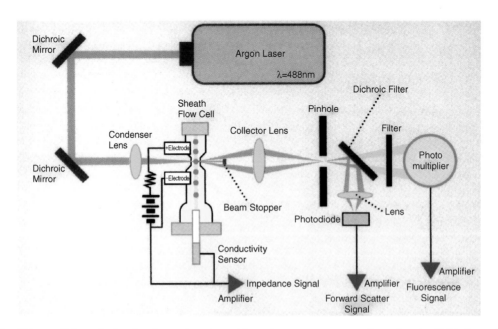

Figure 13.2 Urine particle analysis using flow cytometry and impedance measurement. Reproduced with kind permission from Sysmex UK Ltd

rapidly, and has a high negative predictive value. There is currently only one such instrument which employs the technology of particle counting and fulfils these criteria.

The *UF-100* (Sysmex UK Ltd) combines flow cytometry together with impedance detection to directly identify and count cells and microorganisms in urine (Figure 13.2). Each urine sample is mixed with a diluent, and a two-part fluorescent stain with affinity for both DNA and RNA is added. The stained sample is then guided into a flow cell, which is irradiated by an argon laser. The laser beams are scattered by the cells in the sample, and forward-scattered light (fluorescent and non-fluorescent), which is proportional to the cross-sectional area of the cells, is measured by a photodiode. The fluorescence emitted, which indicates the degree of nucleation of the cell, is measured by a photomultiplier. Using five signals of fluorescent and non-fluorescent height and width plus impedance measurements, the instrument differentiates the three-dimensional cell structures into their appropriate cell types and numbers, and counts numbers of microorganisms. The cell distribution can be displayed on scattergrams and histograms, using the Adaptive Cluster Analysis computer software.

Identification and antimicrobial susceptibility testing systems for mycobacteria

The remergence of tuberculous and the increasing incidence of outbreaks of multiple-drug-resistant strains of *Mycobacterium tuberculosis* has brought into sharp focus the need for automated systems for the rapid detection, identification and antimicrobial susceptibility testing of mycobacteria. Most of the systems currently available have been developed from existing blood culturing technology and use similar instrumentation. All instruments have safety features designed to protect the operator and prevent environmental contamination.

The *BACTEC 460 TB* (Becton Dickinson) was the first semi-automated instrument used for the rapid detection of mycobacteria. It is a radiometric method, using vials of Middlebrook 7H12 broth medium containing radiolabelled palmitic acid as the substrate and five antimicrobial agents to reduce contamination. Radiolabelled carbon dioxide is released into the headspace of the vial by mycobacteria in the inoculated specimen, metabolizing palmitic acid. The radioactivity in the carbon dioxide is measured by a scintillation counter and converted to a growth index (GI) value. A GI value of 10 or

more indicates the presence of mycobacteria. The *M. tuberculosis* (MTB) complex may be differentiated from other mycobacteria by inoculating an aliquot from a positive vial into a BACTEC vial containing nucleic acid phosphate (NAP test). No increase or a decrease in the GI value indicates the presence of the MTB complex. The system may also be used for antibiotic susceptibility testing of MTB complex isolates.

The *BACTEC 9000 MB* System (Becton Dickinson) is designed for the rapid isolation of mycobacteria from clinical specimens and uses fluorescent technology to detect mycobacteria growing in liquid culture medium. Each culture vial contains a fluorescent sensor, which responds to the concentration of oxygen present. When microorganisms are present, nutrients in the vial are metabolized, resulting in a depletion of oxygen in the medium. Photodetectors in the instrument measure the level of fluorescence, which corresponds to the amount of oxygen consumed. Analysis of the rate of oxygen decrease, as measured by increasing fluorescence, enables the instrument to determine whether the vial is instrument positive. The vials are arranged in six racks, each of which holds up to 40 vials. The racks are continously incubated at 37°C and are agitated at 10 minute invervals for maximum recovery of microorganisms. The vials are tested every 10 minutes by light-emitting diodes (LEDs) which activate the fluorescent sensors. A positive determination indicates the presumptive presence of viable mycobacteria and is flagged by an indicator light on the front of the instrument and displayed on the monitor.

The *BacT/ALERT 3D* (bioMerieux) module for the growth, detection and susceptibility testing of mycobacteria has a detection system identical to that for blood cultures. A sensor on the base of each bottle detects carbon dioxide as an indicator of growth, with the change in colour from green to yellow being continuously monitored by a reflectometer in the detection unit. The incubation module has four drawers of 60 wells each, and each of the drawers has an independent shaking mechanism to allow for static or shaken cultures within the same system.

The *BACTEC MGIT 960* System (Becton Dickinson) is a high-capacity, fully automated, continuously monitoring instrument that can test up to 960 7 ml MGIT tubes for the presence of mycobacteria, using the same fluorescence technology as used by the *BACTEC 9000MB* system. The culture tubes contain a fluorescent sensor that responds to the concentration of oxygen in the culture medium. The instrument's photodetectors measure the fluorescence in each tube every 60 minutes. The level of fluorescence corresponds to the amount of oxygen consumed by the microorganisms, which, in turn, is proportional to the number of bacteria present.

The instrument can also use the *BACTEC MGIT 960 SIRE* kit as a rapid qualitative procedure for susceptibility testing of *Mycobacterium tuberculosis* from culture to streptomycin, isoniazid, rifampicin and ethambutol.

Comment

It is inevitable that, in order to perform 'real-time' microbiological tests, i.e. to send meaningful clinical diagnostic information from the laboratory to the physician, microbiologists must increasingly turn to automated instrumentation. This will also help to alleviate the pressure caused by shrinking budgets, staff reductions and an ever-increasing workload.

The many advantages of automated tests include: the release of skilled staff from repetitive work to perform more demanding complicated tasks, thus enhancing the overall quality of the work of the laboratory; improved turnaround times; better standardization of tests by eliminating subjectivity and human error; and cost-effective performance of tests by screening out negative specimens which require no further processing. It is difficult to imagine the disappearance of the agar plate and the wire loop after over a century of use; however, the time may be swiftly approaching when they are not the first tools the clinical microbiologist reaches for.

Further reading

Reimer LG, Wilson ML, Weinstein MP. Update on detection of bacteremia and fungemia. *Clin Microbiol Rev* 1997; **10**: 444–465.

Ferraro MJ, Jorgensen JH. Susceptibility testing instrumentation and computerized expert systems for data analysis and interpretation. In *Manual of Clinical Microbiology*, 7th edn, Murray PR, Baron EJ, Pfaller MA, Tenover FC, Yolken RH (eds). 1999: ASM Press, Washington, DC, pp 1593–1600.

Miller JM, O'Hara CM. Manual and automated systems for microbial indentification. In *Manual of Clinical Microbiology*, 7th edn, Murray PR, Baron EJ, Pfaller MA, Tenover FC, Yolken RH (eds). 1999: ASM Press, Washington, DC, pp 193–201.

Langlois MR, Delanghe JR, Steyaert SR, Everaert KC, De Buyzere ML. Automated flow cytometry compared with an automated dipstick reader for urinalysis. *Clin Chem* 1999: **45**, 118–122.

Watterson SA, and Drobniewski FA. Modern laboratory diagnosis of mycobacterial infections. *J Clin Pathol* 2000; **53**: 727–732.

14

Bacteriology molecular techniques: sample preparation and application

Richard E Holliman and **Julie D Johnson**

The need for molecular methods

To justify the significant resources required to develop and perform molecular diagnostic methods, a bacterial infection must satisfy a number of basic criteria. First, the infection must represent a significant clinical problem in terms of numbers of cases, morbidity and mortality. Second, early diagnosis of the infection should improve the prognosis for the patient; usually specific, efficacious therapy will be available. Finally, the existing diagnostic approach based on traditional methods of microscopy, culture and serology, should produce a sub-optimal performance. There is little clinical justification in developing a molecular-based diagnostic method for a bacterial infection that can be readily identified and tested for antimicrobial susceptibility in the routine laboratory. The application of advanced molecular methods should be targeted on bacteria that are fastidious and difficult to grow in culture; bacteria that are sublethally damaged; that cannot be readily distinguished from similar non-pathogenic bacteria; those that cannot be reliably assessed for antimicrobial susceptibility; and species that cannot be separated with sufficient discrimination by existing typing methods. This chapter will concentrate on molecular methods dealing with bacterial nucleic acids.

Sample preparation

The success of any technique employed in studying bacterial nucleic acids initially relies upon the release and purification of the target nucleic acids. As yet there is no universally accepted method for the preparation of clinical specimens but there are many interrelated factors which must be taken into account. Once the target organism has been selected, the type of clinical specimen examined will be dictated by the pathogenesis of the disease. To maximize the chance of detection, the bacterial load within the specimen (the number of organisms per specimen volume) should be considered. Optimally, where the bacterial load is low, the largest convenient sample volume should be screened; however, molecular techniques often use volumes of $<100\,\mu l$. Ultimately concentration of the target organism into a small volume is required. This will require a high level of concentration in specimens such as sputum for *Mycobacterium tuberculosis* and blood for bacteraemia, but low levels in specimens such as urine for *Chlamydia* in order to achieve the required sensitivity. Large sample volumes require complex target extraction techniques, such as ethanol precipitation and nucleic acid target capture, which result in decreased sensitivity of the assay employed. Large sample volumes may

The Science of Laboratory Diagnosis, Second Edition   Edited by David Burnett and John Crocker

also contain higher levels of non-specific nucleic acid from extraneous DNA, which may compromise the assay. The specimen type and how it is processed during and after collection is of relevance. Specimens such as cerebrospinal fluid (CSF), urine and sputum may contain inhibitors. Haem (at 0.8 µM) and its metabolic products are known inhibitors of DNA polymerases, due to binding of haem and/or porphyrin to the amplification enzyme. Acidic polysaccharides, components of glycoproteins in sputum, are also inhibitory. Additional steps may be necessary for the removal of inhibitors from specimens such as sputum and blood compared to urine or CSF (Woodford and Johnson, 1998).

For the detection of sexually transmitted diseases such as *Chlamydia trachomatis, Neisseria gonorrhoeae* and *Trichomas vaginalis*, novel self-administered sampling techniques using tampon-collected specimens have proved more sensitive by PCR than urine analysis (Tabrizi *et al.*, 1998).

Amplification enzymes are also inhibited by reagents used in specimen collection, such as EDTA and heparin. If the target is present in abundance, dilution of the specimen may eliminate the inhibitory effect whilst maintaining the nucleic acid at a level at which the frequency of sampling zero copies is low. In contrast, enzymatic or chemical destruction of the nucleic acid will reduce the effective number of amplifiable nucleic acid targets. The target organism and the durability of its cell wall will have a significant effect upon the extraction procedure, e.g. the cell wall of *M. tuberculosis* is particularly resistant to lysis, whereas that of *Mycoplasma* spp. will lyse spontaneously. It is also important to protect laboratory personnel employing molecular techniques when pathogens such as *M. tuberculosis* are the target organism. It may therefore be necessary to include sterilization steps within the extraction procedure. Minimal sample handling and robust protocols are required with the reduced requirement for specialized equipment. Broad-range amplification of bacterial DNA requires sample processing which releases DNA from an array of target organisms and washes out inhibitory factors. For enhanced detection of organisms with difficult-to-lyse cell walls, DNA purification with glass fibre filter columns with an additional sonication step have proved to be as good as standard phenol–ether DNA extraction (Rantakokko-Jalava & Jalava, 2002). Sample preparation procedures contribute to the reliability of target detection within clinical specimens; numerous commercial kits exist and it is strongly recommended that DNA extraction techniques should be carefully selected with particular regard to the specimen type. Commercial kits have proved superior for extraction of

DNA from faecal samples (McOrist *et al.*, 2002) and for the rapid DNA extraction for molecular epidemiological studies of *Plasmodium falciparum* (Henning *et al.*, 1999); yet the non-commercial wash/alkali/heat lysis has proved to be the most sensitive and simple method for the extraction of bacterial, yeast and fungal DNA from blood culture material (Miller *et al.*, 2000). Some workers have modified commercial kits to maximize the recovery and purity of extracted DNA, particularly with intestinal protozoa (da Silva *et al.*, 1999). If sample preparation is inefficient, false negative results may be generated (Table 14.1).

Amplification

Nucleic acid targets may be either DNA or RNA, double- or single-stranded, and must be stabilized against degradation once isolated. RNA is more difficult to stabilize than DNA. It is a requirement of the isolation of RNA that no contaminating DNA is present. Selective extraction or destruction of DNA or RNA allows one to target the appropriate nucleic acid. rRNA may be stabilized in chaotrope solutions for months at room temperature. Pathogens that have an RNA and a DNA stage in their life cycle are problematic. Reverse transcription polymerase chain reaction (RT-PCR) commonly detects mRNA but also detects DNA unless steps are taken to destroy this target (Dilworth & McCarrey, 1992). Nucleic acid sequence-based amplification (NSABA) may also be used to detect mRNA; this is an isothermal reaction not requiring a thermal cycler. More recently, reverse transcriptase-strand displacement amplification (RT-SDA) has also been used as an indicator of bacterial viability (Keer & Birch, 2003). Amplification methods such as self-sustaining sequence replication (3SR) that are theoretically capable of using solely RNA templates should not amplify DNA unless a denaturation step is included as part of the extraction technique. It is important to determine whether single-stranded DNA actually interferes with this RNA-specific approach. Analogously, PCR would detect only DNA unless a reverse transcription step precedes the PCR. Investigations of blood and semen stains in forensic pathology have shown that DNA and RNA may be simultaneously isolated from the same specimen for analysis using ethanol precipitation acid phenol/chloroform extraction (Bauer & Patzelt, 2003). Amplification methods that target stable nucleic acids can detect dead, dormant and replicating organisms. Detection of all forms of the organism may be advantageous when viability is rapidly lost during transport or storage or if the organism

Table 14.1 Problem solving in sample preparation

Clinical context	Problem	Solution
Large-volume samples	Large amounts of extraneous DNA compared to small processing volume	Stringent DNA extraction Maximize amplification sensitivity
Range of clinical specimen types	Variable levels of enzyme inhibition	Individualize extraction techniques
Chemicals used in specimen collection	Enzyme inhibition	Dilution Chelating agents Positive controls
Range of pathogens to be detected	Variable target stability	Rapid specimen processing Optimal storage/transport conditions
Partially treated patients	Presence of viable or non-viable pathogens	RT-PCR
Presence of clinical samples and previous amplification products in the laboratory	Contamination of samples generating false positive reactions	Positive displacement/plugged pipettes Dedicated pre- and post-PCR workstations Dedicated equipment

cannot be cultured. However, discrimination of dead from viable organisms would present a problem if non-viable or dormant organisms remain once active infection has cleared.

Quality control

Once isolated, the target must be placed into an aqueous environment compatible with amplification. Amplification enzymes are inhibited by many reagents used in molecular biology for the purification of nucleic acids; these include detergents such as sodium dodecyl sulphate (SDS), or chaotropes such as guanidinium HCl, used to solubilize cell membranes or inactivate nucleases, particularly in the extraction of bacterial and yeast DNA from blood products (Golbang *et al.*, 1996). Additional steps must be taken to remove or neutralize such reagents. Quality control of reagents and equipment in clinical molecular biology techniques is of paramount importance. With techniques as powerful and sensitive as PCR, the risk of false positive reactions due to contamination and of false negatives due to reaction inhibitors have led to scrupulous avoidance procedures, which make the technique relatively expensive and the domain of those who can afford to dedicate the necessary time, facilities and expertise. Of particular importance in diagnostic microbiology is the use of insert controls for avoidance of false negatives, i.e. intrinsic

DNA controls of a low copy number of a control sequence can be spiked into the clinical specimen. If the control does not amplify, it can be assumed that the specimen is inhibitory. Special equipment requirements include plugged tips or positive displacement pipettes, separate workstations, thermocyclers and detection-based equipment. All require a large initial financial outlay. Due to lack of validation and standard protocols, along with variable quality of reagents and equipment, molecular techniques are still, as yet, the tool of reference laboratories and research units. The European Commission has approved research into validation and standardization of the use of diagnostic PCR for the detection of pathogenic bacteria in foods (Malorny *et al.*, 2003) and it is hoped that similar future developments in clinical diagnosis may eventually lead to more general usage.

Current practice

In the early 2000s an increasing number of bacterial infections are subject to molecular diagnostic methods in the course of routine clinical practice. A larger number have been investigated in the research laboratory and some of these may find a clinical role in the future. Routine laboratory methods are used in a number of distinct functions in the process of diagnosis; these comprise detection of the organism in a clinical sample,

Table 14.2   Clinical application of molecular methodology

Function	Bacteria	Conventional methods	Molecular methods
Pathogen detection	*Neisseria meningitidis*	Microscopy Culture on agar media Antigen detection	PCR amplification and DNA probing of amplification products
Identification of isolates	*Staphylococcus* spp.	Examination of phenotypic characteristics, e.g. coagulase enzyme production	PCR amplification using species-specific primers for 16S rRNA gene sequences
Antimicrobial susceptibility	*Mycobacterium tuberculosis*	Culture on/in media containing antibiotics	Electrophoresis of PCR products to detect genetic differences associated with resistance
Typing	*Streptococcus pyogenes*	M protein serotyping	PCR amplification of 16S rRNA and examination of restriction enzyme fragments of the product

identification of the isolate, susceptibility testing and epidemiological typing. Molecular methods have been applied to each of these four functions and representative examples are listed in Table 14.2. From the clinical perspective, molecular methods are used in the diagnosis of bacterial infections of the respiratory tract, soft tissues, urogenital system, gastrointestinal tract and central nervous system (Mandell *et al.*, 2000).

Respiratory tract

A number of bacteria causing infection of the respiratory tract are difficult to grow or identify in culture. Consequently, these infections are suited for the application of advanced molecular methods. *Mycoplasma pneumoniae* can be detected in throat swabs using PCR, while *Legionella pneumophila* can be detected in deep lung secretions by PCR and DNA probes (Mandell *et al.*, 2000). A single-tube nested PCR incorporating an EIA-based detection system has been developed for the diagnosis of *Chlamydia pneumoniae* infection (Clewley, 1996). Isolates of the *Mycobacterium avium* intracellular complex grown on slopes or in liquid media can be rapidly identified by hybridization with specific DNA probes. Molecular methods can be used to detect *Mycobacterium tuberculosis* in clinical samples, identify isolates grown *in vitro*, assess susceptibility, monitor the response to therapy (by quantifying mRNA levels) and distinguish strains in epidemiological studies.

Soft tissues

Established methods for the identification of staphylococcal species are based on phenotypic characteristics. Such methods can be unreliable due to variable expression of these phenotypic factors. The 16S rRNA gene has conserved and variable regions. By designing PCR primers for specific sequences within the gene it has been possible to speciate staphylococcal isolates with greater accuracy (Clewley, 1996).

Group A streptococci (*Streptococcus pyogenes*) isolates can be genotyped by analysis of the restriction enzyme pattern of 16S rRNA—a process known as ribotyping. The pyrogenic exotoxin gene can be detected by PCR amplification. A further typing scheme is based on PCR amplification and restriction enzyme digestion of the virulence regulon, a gene cluster comprising virulence factors such as complement inactivating factor and antiphagocytic activity under the transcription control of a virulence gene [Clewley, 1996). Molecular examinations of skin samples have achieved a sensitivity of up to 68% for the diagnosis of Lyme disease.

Urogenital system

Chlamydia trachomatis can be detected in genital specimens by ELISA, immunofluorescence tests and DNA probes, but these methods have proved to be less sensitive than conventional cultures. In contrast, PCR amplification appears to be more sensitive than

Chlamydia culture while retaining high specificity, and can be applied to urine samples as well as endourethral swabs.

The diagnosis of gonorrhoea remains based on isolation of the bacterium by conventional culture. However, DNA probing or amplification by PCR or ligase chain reaction may be of value when isolation is impractical due to difficulties in specimen transport or lack of immediate access to a laboratory with culture facilities. DNA probes to *Neisseria gonorrhoeae* have a sensitivity limit of approximately 10^3 organisms per sample. Precision of amplification methods many equal or even exceed that of culture but clinical experience is restricted (Mandell *et al.*, 2000). Molecular methods have been described for the diagnosis and epidemiological study of *Haemophilus ducreyi*, *Treponema pallidum* as well as pathogens associated with bacterial vaginosis.

Gastrointestinal system

In general, molecular methods are of limited value for the diagnosis of gastrointestinal infection. Although conventional methods of microscopy and culture are relatively insensitive and time consuming, most patients require only supportive treatment and a specific diagnosis will often not affect management. A possible exception is *Campylobacter* infection, where current identification methods are based on unreliable biochemical factors. PCR primers specific for the genus *Campylobacter* and species within the genus, e.g. *C. upsaliensis*, *C. helveticus*, *C. fetus*, *C. hyointestinalis* and *C. lari*, are based on the conserved and variable regions of the 16S rRNA gene. Restriction enzyme digestion of the amplified products can be used to develop a typing scheme for following the spread of strains in outbreaks (Mandell *et al.*, 2000). Molecular amplification has also found a role in the detection of *Escherichia coli* 0157: H7.

Central nervous system

DNA probes have not been able to provide a clinically useful level of sensitivity when used for the detection of bacteria in the CSF. DNA amplification methods has been more successful. PCR for *Neisseria meningitidis* in CSF samples has achieved levels of sensitivity and specificity of over 90% compared to conventional cultures. This technique may be of particular value when the patient has been given antibiotic therapy prior to lumbar puncture and represents a significant advance over antigen detection methods. Molecular studies of the diversity of the meningococcus have identified hyper-invasive lineages and assisted the introduction of new vaccines. PCR has also been used to detect *Listeria monocytogenes* in immune-suppressed patients with meningitis and *Treponema pallidum* in the diagnosis of symptomatic neurosyphilis. The sensitivity and specificity of these applications is not yet established (Mandell *et al.*, 2000).

16S rRNA amplification and sequencing

Universal primers for the amplification of 16S rRNA genes, with subsequent sequencing of the products, can be used for the identification of bacterial isolates and the detection of pathogens in clinical samples. This approach has been used in the diagnosis of infective endocarditis and the examination of CSF samples in suspected meningitis. The major advantage of universal primers is the elimination of the need to aliquot clinical samples when searching for a range of pathogens, thus conserving sample volume and avoiding errors associated with pathogen-specific assay selection. This technology is currently used to search for previously unrecognized infective causes of clinical illness, such as multiple sclerosis. The cause of bacillary angiomatosis, *Bartonella henselae*, was identified in this way.

DNA/RNA microarrays

Given that partial or complete genomic sequences of many bacterial pathogens are now established, application of microarray technology can be used to measure transcript levels and to detect sequence polymorphisms. DNA probes are immobilized on a solid support and used to detect target DNA or RNA following PCR amplification. Low-density chips are more suitable for routine clinical applications due to their simplicity, easy data management, enhanced reproducibility and low cost. Microarrays can be developed to detect a range of pathogens in a single clinical sample (e.g. CSF) or to rapidly establish antibiotic resistance and susceptibility in a single isolate. At present, such applications are restricted to research laboratories but are likely to enter diagnostic use in the near future.

Molecular detection of antimicrobial resistance

Traditionally, antimicrobial resistance is determined by attempting to grow a bacterial pathogen in the presence of appropriate concentrations of selected therapeutic agents. Unfortunately, the variable growth rates of bacteria result in an inherent time delay, so that results are only available many hours after initial isolation of the pathogen. The increasing understanding of the genetic basis of resistance has allowed the development of molecular methods to rapidly detect genomic changes found in resistance phenotypes. This approach has been applied to the identification of the methicillin resistance-encoding Mec A gene in staphylococci, penicillin-binding protein in *Streptococcus pneumoniae* and the various rifampicin resistance determinants in *Mycobacterium tuberculosis*. However, molecular methods have certain limitations; unrecognized or novel resistance mechanisms may be missed and, when the number of different genes resulting in resistance is large, molecular methods become costly. As a result, phenotypic assays remain the method of choice for testing most bacteria.

Epidemiology and typing

Conventional typing methods applied to bacteria include phage typing and serotyping. Such methods often show low discrimination power and poor reproducibility, particularly when applied to slow-growing organisms such as *Mycobacterium tuberculosis*. The repeated DNA sequence IS 6110 shows sufficient polymorphism to allow a typing scheme based on PCR amplification of the insertion sequence and Southern blotting of the restriction enzyme fragments. Strains carrying only a single copy of the insertion sequence cannot be separated by IS 6110 typing. Such isolates may be investigated using another repetitive element, the DR sequence (Clewley, 1996). In each case the target gene consists of direct repeats separated by unique sequences. The variability of these unique sequences leads to different banding patterns after cutting with restriction enzymes—restriction fragment length polymorphism. The method developed to amplify and label DNA sequences in the DR region is known as spacer oligotyping or 'spoligotyping' (Marshall & Shaw, 1996). Such methods have revealed unsuspected microepidemics and shown the enhanced importance of recently acquired disease to the tuberculosis burden. Multilocus sequence typing (MLST) has provided insight into the routes of dissemination of individual types of multi-resistant *Staphylococcus aureus* (MRSA). MLST has advantages over pulsed-field gel electrophoresis (PFGE), which include ease of data entry into a database.

Problems with molecular methods

Although molecular methods have led to advances in the diagnosis and management of infection, significant problems remain to be addressed. The resource requirements of these techniques are often greater than that of the conventional methods they seek to replace. Specialized equipment and reagents, combined with the need for further operator training, has limited the application of molecular methods in routine diagnostic laboratories. The clinical significance of the enhanced sensitivity of assays based on DNA probing and, in particular, DNA amplification may be uncertain. For example, a smear positive sputum sample on routine microscopy must contain around 10^4 tubercle bacilli. Despite this relative lack of sensitivity, the findings are of great clinical value for predicting infectivity. In contrast, the significance of a positive PCR assay for *M. tuberculosis* performed on a sputum sample taken from a patient on appropriate therapy is less certain.

The danger of false positive reactions due to carryover in the performance of DNA amplification is well described. In contrast, the restricted test volumes used in these methods can result in false negative results, due to sampling error associated with non-uniform distribution of the pathogen in clinical specimens. Finally, first generation molecular methods were designed only to detect the presence or absence of a pathogen and gave no information as to the viability of the organism. Conventional techniques for determining viability rely on demonstration of cellular integrity or activity and the correlation between DNA detection and viability is poor. Molecular targets for assessment of viability include mRNA and rRNA. The longer half-life of rRNA species and their variable retention following a variety of bacterial stress treatments make rRNA a less accurate indicator of viability than mRNA targets (Keer & Birch, 2003). Although later assays have corrected this defect, they tend to be complex and more difficult to perform.

Future application

Molecular methods are likely to be developed for other organisms which are difficult to grow in culture, such as anaerobic bacteria, or conditions where antibiotic therapy has been given before specimens are taken for diagnosis, including respiratory tract infection and osteomyelitis. Molecular methods may provide useful information as to the likely virulence of clinical isolates of coagulase-negative staphylococci and α-haemolytic streptococci. Genotyping may assist studies into the spread of antibiotic resistance and mechanisms of cross-infection in hospitals. While molecular methods have not yet revolutionized the field of infectious diseases, the introduction of automated workstations will improve standardization, reduce costs and lead to wider application of molecular methods in the clinical laboratory.

Further reading

Bauer M, Patzelt D. A method for simultaneous RNA and DNA isolation from dried blood and semen stains. *Forens Sci Int* 2003; **136**(1–3): 76–78.

Clewley J. The work of the Molecular Biology Unit at Central Public Health Laboratory. *PHLS Microbiol Dig* 1996; **13**: 49–53.

da Silva AJ, Bornay-Llinares FJ, Moura IN, Slemenda SB, Tuttle JL, Pieniazek NJ. Fast and reliable extraction of protozoan parasite DNA from specimens. *Mol Diagn* 1999; **4**(1): 57–64.

Dilworth DD, McCarrey JR. Single step elimination of contaminating DNA prior to reverse transcriptase-PCR. *PCR Methods Applic* 1992; **1**: 279–282.

Golbang B, Burnie JP, Klapper PE, Bostock A, Williamson P. Sensitive and universal method for microbial DNA extraction from blood products. *J Clin Pathol* 1996; **49**(10): 861–863.

Henning l, Felger I, Beck HP. Rapid DNA extraction for molecular epidemiological studies of malaria. *Acta Trop* 1999; **72**(2): 149–155.

Keer JT, Birch L. Molecular methods for the assessment of bacterial viability. *J Microbiol Methods* 2003; **53**: 175–183.

Malorny B, Tassios PT, Radstrom P, Cook N, Wagner M, Hoorfar J. Standardization of diagnostic PCR for the detection of foodborne pathogens. *Int J Food Microbiol* 2003; **83**: 39–48.

Mandell GL, Bennett JE, Dolin R (eds). *Principles and Practice of Infectious Diseases*, 5th edn. 2000: Churchill Livingstone, New York.

Marshall BG, Shaw RJ. New technology in the diagnosis of tuberculosis. *Br J Hosp Med* 1996; **55**: 491–494.

McOrist AL, Jackson M, Bird AR. A comparison of five methods for extraction of bacterial DNA from human faecal samples. *J Microbiol Methods* 2002; **50**: 131–139.

Miller BC, Jiru X, Moore JE, Earle JA. A simple and sensitive method to extract bacterial, yeast and fungal DNA from blood culture material. *J Microbiol Methods* 2000; **42**(2): 255.

Rantakokko-Jalava K, Jalava. Optimal DNA isolation method for detection of bacteria in clinical specimens by broad-range PCR. *J Clin Microbiol* 2002; **40**(11): 4211–4217.

Tabrizi SN, Paterson BA, Fairley CK, Bowden FJ, Garland SM. Comparison of tampon and urine as self-administered methods of specimen collection in the detection of *Chlamydia trachomatis, Neisseria gonorrhoeae* and *Trichomonas vaginalis* in women. *Int J STD AIDS* 1998; **9**(6): 347–349.

Woodford N, Johnson A (eds). *Molecular Bacteriology: Protocols and Clinical Applications*, 1st edn. 1998: Humana Press, Totowa, NJ.

15

Other tests in bacteriology

Darrel Ho-Yen

Introduction

A major part of the work in a bacteriology diagnostic laboratory is the culturing of bacteria. Such identification of bacteria allows definitive diagnosis, especially when pathogenic organisms are grown; however, when commensal organisms are grown, their role may not be related to the patient's illness. Other problems with the culture approach to diagnosis is that some bacteria are difficult to grow (e.g. *Legionella pneumophila*, the cause of Legionnaires' disease), some cannot be cultured (e.g. *Treponema pallidum*, the cause of syphilis) and some are too dangerous to culture (such as *Brucella abortus*, the cause of brucellosis). Despite these limitations, bacterial culture has remained the mainstay of the diagnostic bacteriology laboratory.

This chapter will consider other methods of identification of bacteria as a potential cause of a patient's illness. Direct approaches to diagnosis are the identification of bacteria (antigen detection) or identification of specific antibodies to the presence of bacteria (antibody detection). With antibody detection techniques, the presence of IgM, four-fold rises of IgG antibody, low IgG avidity or high levels of IgA may indicate current infection. It is important to remember that although antibody results may indicate current infection, infection may not result in disease. Therefore, a sensitive specific IgM test for *Toxoplasma gondii* may be positive but this may not be related to the patient's symptoms, but simply represent past infection.

Immune complex formation is a natural process during any infection. Over many decades, there have been intricate and imaginative methods to attempt to identify specific microorganisms within immune complexes.

Success has been limited, but this area remains a great intellectual challenge for microbiologists. Lastly, indirect tests of bacterial infection are performed in many bacteriology laboratories. These tests fall into two groups. In the first, markers of a particular infection may be used to identify the organism (such as gas–liquid chromatography and breath tests). The second group involves general markers of infections and are not specific to any bacteria (such as C-reactive protein).

Tests for antibody

Although all body fluids can be tested for antibodies, in diagnostic bacteriology it is usually a serum sample that is tested. In immunocompetent patients, infection by bacteria will almost always produce specific antibody against that organism. Antibodies are proteins which occur in the serum (the cell-free compartment of blood) and which are complex molecules of different types (named immunoglobulins). Immunoglobulins take part in many different defence mechanisms against invading bacteria. There are five types of immunoglobulins in man but for diagnostic bacteriology, IgM and IgG are the most used, with IgA and IgE much less important. The IgM antibody is formed early in the course of infection (in the first week) and is usually diagnostic of current infection. IgG antibody is formed later in the infection (in the second week) and is usually indicative of past infection and immunity. IgG antibody also crosses the placenta and offers immunity to the newborn. IgA is the major mucosal immunoglobulin and IgE is mainly involved in allergic reactions; however, both are unable cross the placenta and can aid diagnosis in the newborn.

The Science of Laboratory Diagnosis, Second Edition Edited by David Burnett and John Crocker
© 2005 John Wiley & Sons, Ltd

IgM does not cross the placenta but a quarter of new-borns do not produce IgM. The rises and falls of all these immunoglobulins (IgM, IgG, IgA and IgE) in serum are different, and these differences can be used to time the onset of an infection, e.g. the diagnosis of infection during pregnancy.

Older tests

Agglutination tests

Specific antibodies present in a patient's serum are able to agglutinate bacterial particles or latex particles coated with bacterial antigens. An example of an agglutination test is the direct agglutination method for detection of antibody to *Brucella abortus*. In this test, a suspension of *B. abortus* is added to a series of dilutions of the patient's serum contained in test tubes. The tubes are incubated for an hour or longer, usually at 37°C, and the result is then read. To detect the weakest agglutination, the test can be incubated overnight to increase its sensitivity. Agglutination is read by tapping the tubes gently to disturb the cells which will rise in the fluid either as aggregates or, in the case of negative controls, as a fine wispy suspension. Agglutination tests can be easily adapted to use on slides and then these tests become quick and easy to perform.

Agglutination tests are particularly sensitive when IgM antibodies are present, as this class of immunoglobulin is better at agglutination than others. However, it must be remembered that IgM antibody does not always cause agglutination and false negative results can occur. One technical problem is the prozone effect, in which agglutination is not seen at the highest concentrations of antibody, due to steric inhibition of the antibody-binding sites, and only becomes obvious when the sample is diluted.

Red blood cells (e.g. from sheep) can also be coated with antigens from bacteria. The *Treponema pallidum* haemaglutination assay (TPHA) is used for the diagnosis of syphilis. These coated particle tests have the benefit that they do not suffer from autoagglutination, i.e. agglutination of the particles simply through protein adhesion effects, which are a frequent problem with bacterial suspensions.

Complement fixation tests

Patient's serum is first heated to 56°C to destroy the complement. In the second stage, the patient's serum in a range of dilutions is mixed with the organism or its antigens. A source of complement which is usually an aliquot of fresh guinea-pig serum is added and the mixture incubated. Antigen–antibody complexes formed between the bacteria and the patient's sample activate the guinea-pig complement and therefore remove it from the mixture. At the end of the incubation period, all the mixtures are removed to the third stage of the test, reagents for which are prepared from red cells of a suitable species which have been sensitized with antibody against the red cell antigens. Typically one uses sheep red cells which are sensitized with rabbit anti-sheep red cell antibody, so that the red cells are coated with antibody in the absence of complement. If complement is present in the second stage, the sensitized red cells will lyse. Lysis therefore indicates that patient's samples in the second stage of the procedure did not have any antibody present, whereas non-lysis indicates that antibody was present and that the complement was used up in that second stage.

Complement fixation tests have been frequently used for many purposes, e.g. the diagnosis of *Brucella* infection. There are potentially many problems with complement fixation tests. The reliability of the tests depends on the standardization of all the reagents in the test before the test is performed. Further, it is not uncommon to find substances in serum which have anti-complementary effects.

Precipitation tests

The principle is that antibody, particularly IgG, will precipitate soluble antigen. Precipitation can be carried out in aqueous solution in test tubes, but it is more frequently performed by the Ouchterlony method. This uses a plate (Petri dish) containing 1–2% plain agar, with wells punched out which are filled with antigen (from the organism of interest) or antibody (patient's serum). The general format is shown in Figure 15.1. Antigen and antibody diffuse towards each other through the agar and where they meet, a line of precipitation forms. Almost any antigen can be used, provided that it diffuses easily. By using an antibody of known specificity, the identity of an unknown antigen can be determined. Typically, this kind of test can be used with bacterial toxins such as those associated with tetanus and diphtheria.

Newer tests

The principle of these tests is that the patient's antibody in the serum binds to a substrate which is provided in the form of bacteria, or their products attached to a solid

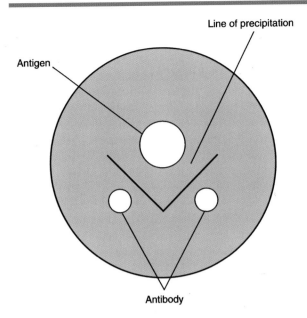

Antigen

Line of precipitation

Antibody

Figure 15.1 Format of Ouchterlony precipitin test

microscope. If the specimen contains antibody to the test organism, that antibody will have attached to it and reacted with the labelled anti-immunoglobulin to produce organisms that fluoresce bright green in UV light. By using a series of dilutions of the patient's serum, it is possible to quantitate the amount of antibody present. There are several problems with these tests, e.g. they are labour-intensive and the reading of the end result is subjective and dependent on the experience of the observer. Further, the UV light causes the fluorescence to fade, so observations must be fairly rapid. Generally, these tests work best for cell wall antigens, as the antibodies will not usually penetrate into the organisms to detect internal antigens. The test is not easy to use for IgM antibody measurement. Despite these difficulties, fluorescent antibody tests have been very useful, and are still used in the diagnosis of syphilis.

Enzyme-linked immunosorbent assay (ELISA)

This extremely popular method can be fully automated, but is usually semi-automated. Typically, 96-well plastic microtitre trays are used, which can carry large numbers of samples as well as controls and which can be machine-washed, centrifuged if necessary and the results generated and analysed by a reading machine. Many ELISAs are produced commercially. Samples are pipetted into the antigen-coated wells, incubated and washed, and anti-human immunoglobulin labelled with an enzyme is added. After further incubation and washing, a substrate for the enzyme is added. There is a change of colour of the substrate if the enzyme is present and this can be machine-read. The intensity of colour is proportional to the amount of antibody which is attached to the antigen. Therefore, the method is fully quantitative. However, it is important to remember that this will only be true if there is an excess of antigen attached to the plate and an excess of anti-human immunoglobulin is provided in the later stages. These conditions are guaranteed in commercial kits but it is important with in-house ELISAs to attend to these details.

The anti-immunoglobulin used can be anti-IgM, anti-IgG, anti-IgA, etc. and therefore the test offers an easy route to determine the type of antibody present at different stages of infection. The most valuable aspect of this is the measurement of IgM as an early marker of acute infection. ELISA methods are easy to use, cheap and less labour-intensive than many other serological methods. On a minor technical note, for in-house assays, it is important to recognize that the outside rows of ELISA plates are frequently unreliable as adsorbents.

surface. Next, unwanted serum proteins are washed from the substrate and a second antibody, usually raised in rabbits, sheep or goats, which is specific for human antibody and is labelled with an appropriate marker, is added in the second stage of the test. If the patient's antibody has attached to the substrate in the first stage, the second stage antibody will also attach. The marker, or label, varies but is usually something which is easily measurable. For example, in the fluorescent antibody technique, this label is fluorescein, which can be visualized in ultraviolet light, whereas in the enzyme-linked immunosorbent assay (ELISA), the label is an enzyme which can subsequently be made to act on a suitable substrate to produce a measurable colour change. The number of available labels is very large and includes radioactive labels, but the principle is the same for all of these tests.

Fluorescent antibody tests

Usually special Teflon-coated slides are used which have 10 'spots', so that several specimens can be examined on a single slide. A suspension of the test organism is dried onto the slide, fixed in acetone or ethanol, and patients' sera are added. After incubation (usually 30 min) the slide is washed and anti-human immunoglobulin (IgG, IgM or IgA), which has been labelled with fluorescein, is added. After further incubation and washing, coverslips are applied and the slide is examined under a UV

This problem can be easily overcome by using only the inner rows.

Radioimmunometric methods

These were the forerunners of ELISA and the principle is exactly the same. Generally carried out in tubes rather than wells, the only significant difference is that the anti-immunoglobulin added is radio-labelled, usually with ^{131}I or ^{125}I. Because of the potential hazards from radioactivity, these tests are used infrequently nowadays, although they do have greater sensitivity than ELISA, and they may have a place in some research work where meticulous measurement is required.

Tests for antigen

Tests for microbial antigen are becoming increasingly popular. The main reason for this is that antigen will be present early in the course of infection and therefore its detection will provide useful clinical information. A good example is the detection of antigens from *Legionella pneumophila* in the urine of patients with Legionnaires' disease. These tests are often positive when the patient is severely and acutely ill when other diagnostic procedures are not usually helpful.

There are, however, other good examples, one of which—the detection of antigens from *Neisseria meningitidis* is in cases of septicaemia or meningitis due to this organism—has been in use for many years. Originally, this method used a technique called counter-immunoelectrophoresis, which is a variant of precipitation methods discussed above. Essentially, serum from the patient is separated in an agar gel by passing an electrical potential through the gel, which causes human proteins and meningococcal antigen to migrate to different positions and to be separated. Then, a trough is cut longitudinally in the gel alongside the separated proteins and antibody specific for the microbial antigen of interest is added to the trough. Diffusion of the antibody towards the separated proteins will detect the presence of the microbial antigen if it is there.

As with other precipitation methods, counter-immunoelectrophoresis is relatively insensitive, and most attempts to detect and measure microbial antigen now utilize ELISA systems. The modification required to the ELISA is to use antibody specific for the antigen of interest on the surface of the microtitre plate. This antibody, often a monoclonal antibody, is used to 'capture' antigen from the patient's specimen. In a second

stage, antibody which is specific for the antigen and is enzyme-labelled is added and the remainder of the test procedure is carried out. It is generally accepted that the capture antibody and the detecting antibody should be different, although the test will work with the same antibody on both sides of the 'sandwich'. Whether one uses monoclonal antibodies for both purposes or whether a polyclonal and a monoclonal are used is essentially a question of trial and error.

This kind of approach has been particularly useful for the diagnosis of viral infections such as HIV and the hepatitis viruses. For bacteria, there has been a tendency to try to simplify the methods using latex particles in an agglutination test, the particles being coated with antibody against the antigen of interest. Like all agglutination tests, these are relatively insensitive and have not proved to be as useful as initially thought possible.

On a technical note, where specimens such as urine or sputum are used for antigen detection testing, it is often necessary to remove 'inhibitors'. The nature of these inhibitors is not well established but, generally, heating the specimen to boiling point for 2 or 3 minutes is sufficient to remove them. This usually does not have any deleterious effect on the antigen. There will probably be improvements in ELISA methods for antigen detection in the coming years. Particularly, there should be a move away from the use of these tests to simply detect antigen towards full quantitation of antigen, which the method is perfectly capable of achieving.

Antigen-specific immune complex testing

Figure 15.2 shows a theoretical analysis of the events which happen during an infection. It indicates that the growth of a microorganism will produce increasing amounts of microbial antigen, to which the infected host responds by producing specific antibody. Eventually, in a successful response the amount of antibody formed will suppress the growth of the organism. Several things are worth considering from this diagram. First, at an early stage there is more antigen available for measurement than there is antibody. Second, free measurable antibody only appears late in the course of infection. Third, throughout much of the infection, immune complexes are formed between antigen and antibody as represented by the hatched area on the diagram. As these immune complexes will contain antigens from the infecting organisms, their measurement provides a means towards diagnosis.

It has been known for many years that the majority of systemic microbial infections produce elevated levels of

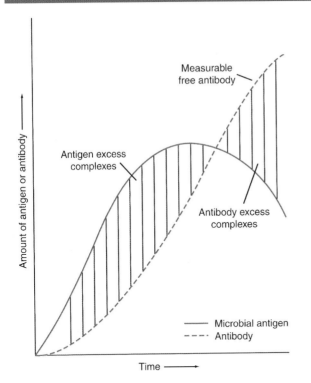

Figure 15.2 Diagram of the theoretical aspects of antigen and antibody interactions in an infection

immune complexes in the patient's blood. This recognition has rarely been exploited diagnostically, probably because the techniques for measurement of the complexes have in the past been difficult. In the last few years, methods for diagnosing pneumococcal pneumonia, infective endocarditis, Lyme disease, leprosy, tuberculous meningitis and *Hepatitis C virus* infection using immune complex assay have all been described. Some of the techniques used are discussed below.

Methods using polyethylene glycol

In these tests, complexes are precipitated from serum by the addition of polyethylene glycol. This works because the complexes have a different size from native immunoglobulin or antigen. The polyethylene glycol is allowed to work for several hours, usually overnight, and at the end of this time the serum sample is centrifuged vigorously and the precipitate removed for further analysis. The next stage of the test involves disrupting the complexes and detecting the antigen component. This can be done by heating (60°C for 30 minutes), by adding a low pH buffer (e.g. glycine/

HCl) or adding a high molarity buffer, such 1 M phosphate. After disruption of the complexes, the antigen is assayed using one or other of the methods described above, e.g. ELISA.

Direct ELISA measurement

These tests usually use monoclonal antibodies specific for the antigens of interest, attached to the wells of microtitre plates and used as capture reagents. The patient's sample is added and complexes present are captured. In a second stage, enzyme-labelled anti-human immunoglobulin is added, which will attach to any human antibody bound to the surface of the plate via an immune complex. This version relies on the high specificity of monoclonal antibodies to capture only the antigens of interest. It should also be noted that the diagnosis by this method is only *inferred*, not proved, in that it is argued that the patient's antibody cannot be present unless it is bound to the antigen which is captured on the ELISA plate.

Tests utilizing binding agents for immune complexes

There are many substances known to specifically bind immune complexes, e.g. separated and purified C1q (the first component of complement), rheumatoid factor (an antibody developed in some patients and directed against human IgG) and conglutinin (a bovine serum protein), all bind immune complexes. These substances can be attached to microtitre plates in the manner described for ELISA assays in general and thereafter these substances will capture any immune complexes present in the patient's sample, the nature of the complex then being determined by using an enzyme-labelled antibody against antigens of interest. Many of the reports on the use of this kind of assay are experimental at present but they offer speed and economy and are generally more sensitive than the other methods described above. They may become more frequently used in the future.

Other tests

Chromatography tests

As described above, the detection of antigen from microorganisms can be used as a marker of their presence in an infection. In the same way, the detection of metabolites from organisms has been used to signal the presence of the organism. The detection and identification of the metabolites is carried out by gas–liquid chromatography (GLC) or high-performance liquid chromatography (HPLC), although the former method accounts for the best-known diagnostic examples.

GLC is generally used to separate and identify volatile and non-volatile fatty acids by passing a sample through a suitable separating substance (e.g. Chromasorb), using a flow of carrier gas. Different fatty acids separate at different times. An early application was the identification of arabinitol in the serum of patients with systemic *Candida albicans* infection. It was initially thought that high levels of this metabolite were associated only with that infection but subsequent investigations proved that the measurement was an unreliable diagnostic marker. It is said that the presence of such organisms in pus and exudates can be determined directly, although it is not common practice to use the method on routine specimens. More successful has been the use of the method to identify and classify anaerobic bacteria, particularly Gram-negative organisms.

Breath tests

These non-invasive tests have been used to detect *Helicobacter pylori*, now recognized as the cause of duodenal ulcers. *H. pylori* has a powerful urease enzyme which is able to hydrolyse ingested radioactivity-labelled urea to release labelled CO_2, which can be measured in exhaled breath. For the test, two isotopes, ^{13}C and ^{14}C, have been used: ^{13}C is safer but more expensive than ^{14}C. The tests are semiquantitative and, as urea is distributed throughout the stomach, there is no sampling error. The sensitivity and specificity of these tests compare well with culture and histology. The tests may be used for the diagnosis of *H. pylori* or for monitoring the response to management.

Future developments

There are several challenges in the general area of serology. The first is to address the question of speed of results. A slow result (i.e. several days) is either of academic interest or useless in terms of diagnosing and treating a patient's infection. It will be clear that antigen or antigen-specific immune complex detection offers a faster route to diagnosis than antibody detection, and development of these assays is therefore desirable.

Further, both antigen and antigen-specific immune complex assays can be fully quantitative and, used properly with serial measurements, they should be able to assess the severity of any infection and the response to treatment. It is disappointing that these methods have usually been used qualitatively to date, and improvement in their performance will be more to do with a change in philosophy rather than a change of technology.

A real challenge for the future will be to apply some of the above methods to infections caused by commensal organisms. There are many instances, but the diagnosis and management of serious infection due to *Escherichia coli* serves as a useful example. Conventional techniques are frequently unhelpful and PCR methods, as used at present, have little to offer because they will only identify the presence of the organism. The challenge is to know what the organism is doing.

The future is therefore one of increasingly sophisticated quantitation of antigen, whether free or complexed, and it is likely that immunosensors or their equivalents will participate in this development. Given that most serological methods depend on antigen–antibody interaction and that this takes place within minutes, it is surprising that most available tests take several hours and have to use separated serum. Methods which can quantitate microbial antigen within 5 minutes, using whole blood or body secretions, are long overdue and their development offers a real challenge for the future.

Further reading

Collee IG, Marmion BP, Fraser AG, Simmons A (eds). *Mackie & McCartney's Practical Medical Microbiology*, 14th edn. 1996: Churchill-Livingstone, Edinburgh and London.

Korpi M, Leinonen M. Pneumococcal immune complexes in the diagnosis of lower respiratory infections in children. *Pediatr Infect Dis J* 1998; **17**: 992–995.

Laperche S, Le Harrec N, Simon N, Bouchardeau F, Defer C, Maniez-Montrecial M *et al*. A new HCV core antigen assay based on dissociation of immune complexes: an alternative to molecular biology in the diagnosis of early HCV infection. *Transfusion* 2003; **43**: 958–962.

16

Control of antimicrobial chemotherapy

Ian M Gould

Introduction

The modern age of chemotherapy can be said to have started over 100 years ago with the pioneering work of Robert Koch and others, who described the germ theory of disease and allowed concepts to develop about 'magic bullets' that would kill microbes while not harming the host. The first agents, derivatives of mercury, antimony and arsenic, proved too toxic for general use but found a limited role in the treatment of syphilis. While great advances have been made in most areas of antimicrobial chemotherapy, derivatives of these early agents are still used for certain parasitic diseases, such as leishmaniasis and sleeping sickness.

In the 1930s German industrialists and scientists worked together to create the first modern antimicrobials—the sulphonamides, which were derived from dyes. These were quickly followed by the discovery of naturally occurring antimicrobials (antibiotics) such as penicillin, (in fact discovered in 1928 by Alexander Fleming, but first used in a major way to treat infection during the Second World War). At first, penicillin was in such short supply that doctors would collect urine from treated patients to extract the 'miracle drug' to re-use in other patients.

Thus, the era of chemotherapy, as we understand it, had begun and during the 1940s, 1950s and 1960s great leaps were made in discovering new antibiotics, learning to synthesize them and, indeed, designing and synthesizing totally new agents, such as the quinolones.

The first principles of chemotherapy

As early as the 1940s it was realized that different antibiotics interacted with bacteria in different ways that might affect the optimum dosing regimen, and in the 1950s it became apparent that resistance to almost any antibiotic developed after prolonged use. The first clinical applications of these two founding principles of the science of chemotherapy were in the treatment of tuberculosis, a disease with an annual incidence and death rate both measured in millions.

The first principle of the control of therapy learnt in those early days was the application of knowledge on the dose–response parameters (the pharmacodynamics) of the antimicrobial–microbe interaction, which led to intermittent (twice-weekly) treatment with rifampicin and izoniazid. This was feasible due to the prolonged suppressive effect of these antimicrobials on growth of the tubercle bacillus long after the drugs had been excreted from the body, and allowed more user-friendly treatment regimens, allowing improved compliance. This prolonged suppression of growth is called the 'post-antibiotic effect'.

When the first anti-tuberculous drug, streptomycin, was released it was found that the initial response led to relapse after a few weeks, due to the surviving bacteria becoming resistant. In fact, it is now understood that simultaneous therapy with three active drugs (triple therapy) is essential for the cure of tuberculosis without the risk of development of resistant strains. This is the

The Science of Laboratory Diagnosis, Second Edition   Edited by David Burnett and John Crocker
© 2005 John Wiley & Sons, Ltd

second principle which is relevant to treatment of many infections with antimicrobials and illustrates the need for primary testing of sensitivity of isolates as a guide to successful therapy. Routine use of clinical diagnostic laboratories for such sensitivity tests started at this time (late 1950s, early 1960s) and is now in extensive, world-wide use.

The issue of compliance with therapy is another important principle of the control of chemotherapy learnt in those early days of treatment of tuberculosis and is particularly important for diseases where cure depends on prolonged therapy (6–18 months). Unfortunately, many of the sufferers of tuberculosis came from socially deprived backgrounds, which made compliance with therapy difficult. It was soon learnt that treatment was frequently unsuccessful in this situation, often due to the development of resistant organisms. Consequently, directly observed therapy became popular. Alternatively urine from patients can be checked for the excreted drugs. These basic lessons had to be relearned recently in New York, where cut-backs in social and medical services led to cessation of directly observed therapy and produced a large outbreak of multi-resistant tuberculosis with a high fatality rate.

Antibiotic resistance (Table 16.1)

Unfortunately, the very success of antimicrobial chemotherapy is leading to its downfall. Antimicrobials are seen by both doctors and patients as a panacea or cure-all, such that antimicrobials are frequently used undiscriminately. This over-use is linked inextricably with resistance in the form of a natural selection phenomenon, allowing survival of resistant strains. Although technically available only on prescription in many countries, the majority of the world's population can purchase antibiotics legally or illegally. They are a multi-billion dollar industry world-wide and there is a large black market in them. The economically deprived people of the Third World who need antibiotics more frequently because of their very high infection rates cannot afford the proper medical advice, laboratory tests or full treatment courses necessary to eradicate infections, so antibiotic resistance is a particular problem in those areas of the world, particularly in deprived inner-city areas. Even in the rich countries of Western Europe and North America, doctors frequently misuse antimicrobials and the last 10 years has seen very worrying trends in resistance. Misuse includes prescriptions where not indicated or the wrong agent, dose, duration or route of administration. While use exerts a cumulative pressure on selection of resistant strains (most commonly by mutation or acquisition of resistant plasmids) at both a patient and societal level, low doses for prolonged periods are more likely to select for resistance than the same total weight of drug administered as a higher dose for a shorter period. Many countries have now introduced public and professional educational campaigns. The one in the UK has been particulary successful in reducing community use of antibiotics, although hospital use probably continues to rise, continuing to drive the major resistance problems, such as multi-resistant *Staphylococcus aureus* (MRSA).

Table 16.1   Trends in resistance levels (%)

	1997		2003	
	UK	Southern Europe	UK	Southern Europe
Penicillin/pneumococci	10	50	5	50
Penicillin/meningococci	0	40	0	40
MRSA	5	75	40	75
Glycopeptide/enterococci	1	5	5	10
Ciprofloxacin/*E. coli*	2	15	8	30
Gentamicin/*Pseudomonas*	3	40	7	50
Ceftazidime/*Klebsiella*	1	20	10	40
Amoxicillin/*Haemophilus*	20	30	15	40
Amoxicillin/*Moraxella*	80	80	95	95
Ciprofloxacin/*Campylobacter*	1	40	10	60

General principles of laboratory control of chemotherapy

There are currently over 100 antibiotics licensed for clinical use in the UK and many more world-wide. The main role of the routine hospital-based diagnostic laboratory is to define the causative pathogens responsible for disease in individual patients from whom specimens are being processed and, where possible, to test the isolate(s) for sensitivity to relevant antibiotics. Normally, testing will only be performed on a limited, predetermined, battery of antibiotics which are clinically relevant for that patient's infection and which are thought to be active against the isolated pathogen.

The decision-making process about which antimicrobials will be tested and/or reported is complex and should take into account factors such as site and seriousness of infection, method of excretion or metabolism of the antimicrobial, function of the patient's liver and kidneys, toxicity, available routes of administration, cost, need for combination therapy, proven clinical benefit, current treatment with both antimicrobials and non-antimicrobials and drug interactions. Although there are over 100 licensed antimicrobials in the UK, these are made up from only some dozen different drug classes and it is often appropriate to test just one representative agent from each class.

Often patients will have been started on treatment empirically, before culture and sensitivity results are available, but hopefully only after appropriate specimens have been sent to the laboratory for processing. Nevertheless, it is still important to process specimens as quickly as possible, in case treatment needs to be modified in the light of culture and sensitivity results, e.g. to a more potent or less toxic agent. Similarly, it is important to have good transport of specimens and good communication to enable advice to be easily obtained and results to be disseminated quickly. It is also useful for the laboratory to publish summaries of sensitivities of various organisms to help doctors in choosing appropriate empirical therapy, and for the laboratories to take part in sentinel surveillance schemes to give early warning of the emergence of unusual or new resistance variants. This enables doctors and public health officials to use the information, both for appropriate treatment and also to contain the spread of these new resistant variants, which in the modern world of high speed travel can and do spread rapidly from country to country and continent to continent (Figure 16.1).

There are other ways in which the laboratory can usefully direct or control antimicrobial therapy. The

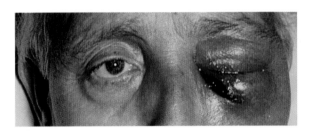

Figure 16.1 An example of a highly immunosuppressed patient, suffering Pseudomonas skin and eye infection with bloodstream spread after receiving cancer therapy which reduced his body's defences against infection. Once this type of infection commonly killed patients; now treatment with modern antibiotics is often successful. However, such patients are increasingly common as modern medicine becomes more successful and more aggressive. Consequently, more and more antibiotics are used, both in hospital and in general practice

most important is the measurement of blood and, occasionally, tissue levels of the drugs, to ensure adequate therapeutic levels are being achieved in critically ill patients and to ensure that toxicity is minimized or prevented. These measurements are not necessary in the majority of patients, only in those where it is thought necessary to use antimicrobials with a narrow therapeutic ratio, i.e. agents where doses needed to be effective approach those that may be toxic to the patient. The aminoglycosides and glycopeptides are the most obvious examples of such groups of antibiotics. The use of such particularly toxic drugs should be reserved for those serious infections where the choice of active agents is limited, often through problems of resistance.

Measurement of antimicrobial activity in the patient is not often performed but is most easily achieved by measuring the inhibitory or cidal activity of the antimicrobial in the patient's serum, usually taking samples before administration of a dose (the trough level) and approximately 1 hour after administration of a dose (the peak level). Distribution of the antimicrobial in the tissues is usually complete by then. Depending upon the pharmacodynamics of the antimicrobial and the disease state, it may be important to achieve high inhibitory or cidal levels in the peak sample, e.g. for aminoglycosides such as gentamicin, which have concentration-dependent activity. In contrast, the β-lactams are drugs where it is usually important to have activity during the whole dosing period, due to their lack of a post-antibiotic effect against many bacteria (time dependence).

In critically ill patients it is sometimes useful to assess potential benefits of combination therapy in the laboratory to try to predict the most active regimens. These tests can be useful, particularly in cystic fibrosis and in patients who are immunosuppressed or have infections such as endocarditis or meningitis, when it is necessary to achieve killing of the microbe by the antibiotics in order to cure the patient without the help of the host's immune system.

Sensitivity testing

The concept of sensitivity testing has remained remarkably constant since it was first introduced on a wide scale almost 40 years ago. Of necessity, tests are simple to perform as the average clinical laboratory serving a population of 250 000 will perform such tests on tens of thousands of organisms per annum. Despite the simplicity of the tests they have proved remarkably useful over the years in guiding therapy. This is all the more surprising when one considers the complexity of individual cases, where the microbe interacts with the host immune system in a set of conditions apparently remote from the test situation in the laboratory.

There are four methods of sensitivity testing in common use: (a) agar diffusion (Figure 16.2); (b) agar incorporation; (c) broth macrodilution; and (d) broth microdilution. The first is the one in most common use in the UK—in about 85% of laboratories as the routine method. In this method, carefully controlled amounts of antibiotics are contained in paper discs which are placed on an agar plate surface previously inoculated with a carefully controlled number of the bacteria to be tested. Normally up to six antibiotics are tested per plate. The plates are incubated in carefully controlled conditions for 18–48 h, depending on the rate of growth of the bacteria. The zones of inhibition of growth due to the diffused antimicrobial are measured and related to those of known sensitive and resistant control bacteria. Results are usually reported as simply 'sensitive' or 'resistant', based on knowledge about the specific pharmacokinetics of each antimicrobial, including achievable concentrations of the drug at the site of infection. Many laboratories in the UK have recently switched to more carefully standardized agar disc diffusion methods, with a view to allowing more exact comparability of results for surveillance purposes (British Society for Antimicrobial Chemotherapy and National Committee for Clinical Laboratory Standards; see Further Reading).

Alternatively, in agar dilution, pre-set concentrations of an antimicrobial are included in agar plates before they are poured and then, when they have set solid, the bacteria are 'spotted' on the surface. Up to 30 microbes

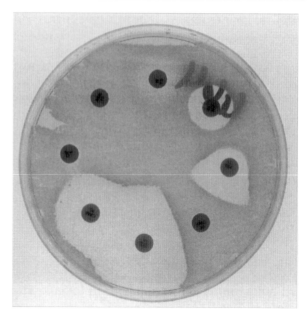

Figure 16.2 An example of disc sensitivity tests. This is the most common method of sensitivity testing used in the UK. The zone of inhibition of growth of the lawn of bacteria is determined by the concentration of antibiotic in each of the paper discs and the sensitivity of the bacterium. In this example the bacterium is completely resistant to four antibiotics. There are small zones of inhibition around two discs (the bacterium is still resistant) and large zones of inhibition around another two discs (sensitive). This example of a multiply-resistant organism is increasingly common. The odd, non-circular zone of inhibition of two discs is because the adjacent disc between them contains an antibiotic which is interacting with them, causing antagonism of action (cut-off) and synergy (bell shape), respectively

can be tested to a single agent per plate. The lowest concentration of antimicrobial that inhibits visible growth of the bacteria after incubation is the minimum inhibitory concentration (MIC).

Broth dilution tests of antimicrobial sensitivity are either carried out in test tubes (macrodilution) or in microtitre plates (microdilution). A carefully controlled inoculum of the test microbe which, unlike in agar tests, can be a virus (if a cell line is included) or certain fungi or protozoan parasites, such as malaria parasites, in addition to bacteria, is incubated with known concentrations of the antimicrobial. The MIC is the lowest concentration inhibiting growth (as assessed by turbidity to the naked eye). Normally it is adequate just to assess levels of the antimicrobial which will inhibit growth, the host's immune system allowing cure by killing most of the microbes after they have been brought under control by the antimicrobial.

Unlike with agar tests, the minimum bactericidal concentrations (MBC) can be assessed by sub-culturing the inhibitory concentrations to look for any survivors. The lowest concentration with 99.9% kill of the original inoculum is the MBC. For complicated infections it can be important to establish such values for individual organisms and make sure such levels of activity are achieved in the patient.

MIC and occasionally MBC tests are still performed in the treatment of difficult to treat infections, such as infective endocarditis and osteomyelitis.

Tests on microbes other than bacteria

The sensitivity testing of microbes other than bacteria is, by comparison, in its infancy. Very little work had been done until recently, probably because of the relative absence of effective antimicrobials for many of these microbes. This has meant that there was no alternative choice of therapy in the presence of resistance. There has, undoubtedly, also been a lack of perception of the problems of resistance. Now, however, there is an explosion of new agents, particularly anti-fungals and anti-virals, in response to increasing needs generated by new diseases such as HIV/AIDS. This disease not only requires antiviral therapy specific for the HIV virus but also therapy for many other viral, fungal, bacterial and protozoal infections to which the patients become more susceptible.

HIV patients are frequently given suppressive antimicrobial therapy over many months or years as, due to their severe immunosuppression, it is frequently impossible to eradicate the infecting microbes. This is a recipe for emergence of resistance analogous to the situation with tuberculosis, and lessons on the use of combination therapy to improve therapeutic efficacy and prevent emergence of resistance are having to be relearnt for the proper treatment of HIV/AIDS.

Resistance is a particular problem in the treatment of the primary viral infection of HIV/AIDS where, by the time disease is clinically apparent, there is a huge viral load with the potential for innately resistant mutants to exist that can survive therapy and multiply. Now that many new anti-HIV agents are being made available, detection of these strains will be important in the future, so that the best combination therapy can be individualized to each patient.

Recent developments have allowed the ascertainment of MICs of both bacteria and fungi on agar plates by the use of E tests®, which contain gradients of antimicrobials on plastic strips, and the inhibitory value can be

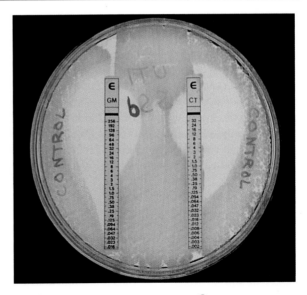

Figure 16.3 An example of 'E' test® sensitivity testing. Graduated concentrations of an antibiotic are contained in each of the plastic strips. A 'control organism' of known sensitivity is plated on the outside of each strip and a test organism on the inside. In this case the 'test' organism is very resistant. The level of resistance or MIC (see text) can be read off the strip

read off after incubation in much the same way that zones of inhibitions are measured in the classical agar disc diffusion test (Figure 16.3).

Automation

As automation becomes more widespread in laboratories, attempts have been made to adapt existing sensitivity testing methods. Broth microdilution tests are probably the most amenable for modification and pre-prepared plates are now available which can be read automatically by spectrophometry. Automated reading of inhibition zones in agar disc diffusion tests also holds some promise.

Newer methods of sensitivity testing are much more susceptible to automation and indeed often require it. These include nephilometry, bioluminescence, impedance or conductance monitoring and flow cytometry. While these 'direct' methods can give rapid results (within 1–2 hours) on inhibitory and also perhaps cidal activity of antimicrobials, they are, at the moment, research techniques only.

Many serum levels of antimicrobials are routinely measured by automated methods, such as EMIT® and TDX®, which utilize enzymatic reactions and fluorescence. Levels of newer antimicrobials can be assayed by high performance liquid chromatography (HPLC) or by traditional plate assay, where the patient's serum or tissue specimen takes the place of the antibiotic-containing disc in the agar disc diffusion test and the lawn of organism is a sensitive control strain. The concentration of drug in the serum (volume known) or tissue (weight known) and the size of the zone of inhibition can be used to calculate the concentration of drug. While assay of serum levels of certain antimicrobials is routine, assay of tissue levels is really a research technique.

Hospital control and clinical liaison

The knowledge base acquired from working in the laboratory can be utilized to coordinate the work of various groups of people concerned with infection who work in the community and hospitals. These people include the infection control team of nurses and doctors and the public health physicians concerned with control of infection in the community. By giving early warning, outbreaks can be controlled more effectively. Hospital-acquired infection is very common (probably about 10% of patients admitted to hospital) so any advice on its prevention and update on the latest epidemic organisms can prevent a lot of infections and limit the inappropriate use of antibiotics.

A knowledge of local sensitivity patterns is useful for all doctors to help them in the empiric treatment of infection, although rapid communication of individual patient results is also important to guide antimicrobial therapy from a rational base. Most hospitals and some general practices have written antibiotic policies and the sensitivity data available from the local laboratory forms a useful basis for designing these policies, allowing the local recommendations for empirical treatment to be the most appropriate. This is proven to save unnecessary

exposure to antibiotics, some of them costly and toxic, and to improve patient outcome.

The laboratory should also be a platform for education of doctors and the public on improved use of antimicrobials. Very little on the subject is taught to undergraduates and yet it is a complex field with an ever-expanding number of drugs which it is increasingly difficult for the average doctor to use properly. There are new initiatives on undergraduate and postgraduate teaching in antimicrobial therapy (www.bsac.org.uk). A policy of limited sensitivity reporting, either reducing the number of agents reported to those seeming most appropriate (perhaps two or three) or not reporting any sensitivities to isolates that are not clinically important, may be a further way of reducing antibiotic exposure. However, these strategies have not been properly assessed and rely heavily on appropriate information being given to the laboratory by the doctor submitting the specimens. Table 16.2 lists current strategies that are used to improve antimicrobial stewardship. The evidence base for such strategies is currently being reviewed, in both hospitals and the community (www.cochrane.org). It is important that efforts to limit inappropriate antibiotic use are redoubled. This is all the

Table 16.3 New antibiotics, 2003

Gram-positive	Respiratory
Synercid	Ketolides
Linezolid	Quinolones
Daptomycin	
Dalbavancin	*Broad spectrum*
Ortavancin	Tigecycline
Iclaprim	Ertapenem
Anti-PBP2′ cephalosporins	

Table 16.2 Antibiotic prescribing—types of intervention/stewardship

Educational	Regulatory	Organizational	Structural	Restrictive
Guidelines* (AGREE)	Reimbursement	Multidisciplinary teams	Computerized prescribing	Limited lists, formularies Therapeutic substitution (including switch)
Programmes Outreach/academic detailing* Audit/feedback* Interactive workshops*			Order forms	Cycling Limit susceptibility tests/reports Automatic stop dates

* = Cochcrane review

more important as a recent European meeting confirmed that several major pharmaceutical companies were ceasing or downgrading their antibiotic research capabilities. The pipeline of promising new antimicrobials is severely restricted compared with 30 years ago (Table 16.3) Only one completely new class of antimicrobial has been introduced in the past 40 years.

Conclusion

Pasteur or Fleming would have no trouble orientating themselves in a routine hospital diagnostic laboratory in 2005. There have not been the great advances in test procedures that one might have imagined from knowledge of current work in microbial genetics. This work has increased our knowledge base and understanding of resistant mechanisms tremendously and no doubt will have an impact on the way we test for resistance in the routine diagnostic laboratory in the next 10 or 20 years. Even now, larger laboratories can test directly by DNA probe for a small selection of resistant genes, such as the *mec A* gene that turns *Staphylococcus aureus* into a superbug, resistant to all β-lactam antimicrobials. Similarly, we routinely test for the presence of β-lactamase enzymes in some bacteria rather than assessing the phenotypic expression of these enzymes (which can be difficult by traditional sensitivity test methods). Certainly, direct genotypic tests are going to be much more widely used in the future, as they tell us the potential resistance profile of an organism, rather than just what it is resistant to at the time of testing under the rather artificial experimental conditions of the laboratory. On the other hand, progress to establish these new tests in routine diagnostic laboratories has been slow.

This is an optimistic although, I think, realistic view of the future role of the laboratory in this field. One cannot, however, help but be pessimistic about the potential of bacteria to become resistant to all antimicrobials unless we learn to use them much more carefully. The discovery of the ingenuity of microbes, as attested by their use of integrons, transposons, operons, regulons, synergons, etc., teaches us that microbes are supremely adaptable and usually at least one step ahead of us in the microbial–antimicrobial battle that we wage.

Further reading

British Society for Antimicrobial Chemotherapy. Antimicrobial susceptibility testing. BSAC Working Party Report. *Journal of Antimicrobial Chemotherapy* 2001; **48**: S1.

European Union Conference. The Microbial Threat: The Copenhagen Recommendations. September 1998: Danish Ministry of Health and Ministry of Food, Agriculture and Fisheries.

Finch RG, Greenwood D, Norrby SR, Whitley RJ. *Antibiotics and Chemotherapy*, 8th edn. 2003: Churchill Livingstone, Edinburgh.

Garrett L. *The Coming Plague*. 1995: Penguin Books, Harmondsworth.

Gould IM, van der Meer JWM. *Antibiotic Policies: Theory and Practice*. 2005: Kluwer Academic/Plenem Publishers, New York.

House of Lords Select Committee on Science and Technology 7th Report. The *Resistance to Antibiotics and Other Antimicrobial Agents*. 1997–1998: The Stationary Office, London.

Kucers A, Bennett NM. *The Use of Antibiotics*, 4th edn. 1987: Heinemann Medical, Oxford.

Levy SB. *The Antibiotic Paradox*, 2nd edn. 2002: Perseus, Cambridge.

Lorian V. *Antibiotics in Laboratory Medicine*, 4th edn. 1996: Williams & Wilkins, Baltimore, MD.

Performance Standards for Antimicrobial Susceptibility Testing, Twelfth Informational Supplement. 2002: NCCLS, 940 West Valley Road, Suite 1400, Wayne, PA 19087–1898, USA.

Standing Medical Advisory Committee Sub-group on Antimicrobial Resistance. The Path of least Resistance. 1998: Department of Health, London.

World Health Assembly Resolution. Emerging and Other Communicable Diseases: Antimicrobial Resistance. 16 May 1998: WHA 51.16.

World Health Organization. The current status of antimicrobial resistance in Europe. Report of a WHO workshop held in collaboration with the Italian Associazione Culturale Microbiologia Medica, Verona, Italy, 12 December 1997. WHO/EMC/BAC/98.1. WHO, Geneva.

World Health Organization. The medical impact of the use of antimicrobials in food animals. Report of a WHO meeting, Berlin, Germany, 1997. WHO/EMC/ZOO/97.4. WHO, Geneva, pp 13–17.

SECTION 4

MICROBIOLOGY
Virology, Mycology
and Parasitology

17

Microscopy in virology: application and sample preparation

Marie M Ogilvie

Introduction

Light microscopy has played a significant role in virology from its earliest use in examination of stained cell preparations or sections of tissue. Today on the virology bench of many microbiology laboratories no microscope is to be found, since diagnostic work at a district general level is based on the use of immunoassay kits for detection of virus antigen or antibody. Increasingly, even in the specialist virus diagnostic laboratory, microscopy is used less frequently as more sensitive methods of virus detection, based on nucleic acid amplification by the polymerase chain reaction (PCR), are introduced alongside existing culture and antigen detection methods. However, in the early years of this new millennium microscopes are still in daily use for diagnostic virology work, as cell cultures are examined for cytopathic effects due to virus growth and cells stained with fluorochrome-labelled reagents are screened for virus antigens.

Histopathology: inclusion bodies and multinucleate giant cells

The histopathologist who examines fixed stained cell smears or tissue sections observes the characteristic morphological changes that are associated with the presence of specific virus infections. The best known of these distinctive features are *inclusion bodies*—accumulated virus particles (as in the classical Negri body of rabies) or excess proteins synthesized during virus replication, and *multinucleate giant cells*. The latter form as a consequence of fusion between the plasma membranes of adjacent cells, and are a feature of infection with enveloped viruses, which possess a glycoprotein inducing pH-independent fusion at the cell surface, e.g. respiratory syncytial virus (RSV) and human immunodeficiency virus (HIV). Virologists use the term *syncytium* (from the Greek, *syn* = together) for such a cell. *Herpes simplex virus* (HSV) and *varicella-zoster virus* (VZV) produce multinucleate cells *in vivo* and *in vitro* ('in life' and 'in glass', i.e. in culture). Tzanck's name is still given to cell smears prepared by his method of taking scrapings from the base of an ulcer or vesicle, which are then stained and examined for the giant cells of herpes (HSV or VZV). (Figure 17.1).

The well-known 'owl's eye' inclusion body seen in cells infected with *cytomegalovirus* (CMV) is an intranuclear inclusion surrounded by a clear halo, within a considerably enlarged (*megalic*) cell, but there is usually only one nucleus. CMV can produce multinucleate giant cells *in vivo;* these are of endothelial origin and their presence in the circulation signifies serious systemic disease. Evidence of the intracellular location of CMV is important in confirming the pathological significance of finding this virus, which simple virus isolation cannot always provide.

The Science of Laboratory Diagnosis, Second Edition   Edited by David Burnett and John Crocker
© 2005 John Wiley & Sons, Ltd

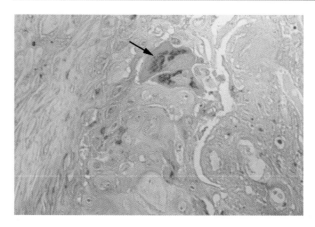

Figure 17.1 Section of an herpetic skin lesion, stained with haematoxylin and eosin. A multinucleate giant cell is indicated by the arrow. Courtesy of Dr K McLaren, Department of Pathology, University of Edinburgh

Virology

Success in the isolation of virus (by culture) or detection of viral antigens in cells from clinical material is very dependent on obtaining the correct sample, handling it appropriately, and using the range of cell cultures and immunofluorescent probes most suitable for detection of the virus(es) likely to be responsible for the patient's condition. Resources are not available for undirected screening for every possible virus, although inoculation of a range of cell cultures will allow any that can be cultured routinely to grow. Modern standard texts on diagnostic work should be consulted for fuller details of the aspects discussed below, and one such as that edited by Mahy and Kangro (see Further Reading) gives a good introduction for the research worker.

Sample collection and transport

Many infections are relatively short with respect to the period of active viral replication once symptoms have developed, so that samples containing infectious virus and antigen-expressing cells are best collected within the first 2–3 days of illness. Material should contain cells from the affected site: epithelial cells from the back of the nose and throat, or from the base of an ulcer. Respiratory secretions may be collected from infants by suction up a fine catheter, or washed out in older subjects, but cells collected onto a swab should be placed in a virus transport medium. Any buffered isotonic fluid containing stabilizing protein can be used to preserve infectivity and prevent cells drying out. Samples should *not* be frozen before processing, but transported to the virus laboratory as soon as possible, being kept chilled on ice or in a refrigerator if there is any delay. When the period between collection of a sample and its inoculation into cell culture is kept to a minimum, the isolation rate is increased and virus is detected sooner. If it is not possible to inoculate appropriate cells within the same day, a sample may be held at 4°C overnight. Longer storage to maintain viability has to be at very low temperatures—usually in an ultrafreezer running at −70°C. (The commoner laboratory freezers running at −18 to −20°C are *not* suitable for virus preservation; a considerable drop in infectivity occurs at that temperature range).

Sample processing and inoculation of cell cultures

Request forms accompanying samples should indicate clearly the nature of the current illness, the date of onset, the nature of the sample and the site from which it has been collected, and the age of the patient, in order that appropriate investigations may be undertaken. Sample processing for inoculation of cell cultures and/or preparation of cells for immunofluorescent staining is generally a standardized procedure, according to the nature of the specimen. Cultures have to be examined for any *cytopathic effects* (CPE: the morphological change in cells resulting from virus replication) on a daily basis for the first 5 days after inoculation so as not to miss any signs, although later 'reading' of the tubes on alternate days is usually sufficient to catch the more gradual changes of slower-growing viruses such as CMV and many adenoviruses.

Requirement for rapid diagnosis of virus infections

Few viruses can be identified in routine cell culture in less than 3 days—herpes simplex virus is the only regular one. For clinical management, control of infection within hospital wards, and specific antiviral therapy where available, the earliest confirmation of a clinical diagnosis or identification of an unsuspected infection is important. To this end, appropriate samples are examined directly for evidence of specific viruses—by immunofluorescence (IF) microscopy for respiratory, skin and other infections where infected cells are readily obtainable. Respiratory secretions must first be diluted and washed in a buffered saline to prepare respiratory epithelial cells (free of mucus) that can be deposited on slides. Several spots or wells are generally used, but a cytocentrifuge preparation is useful and quick if one is to test for a predominant virus first—as in an influenza epidemic or RSV season. Once air-dried, the slides are fixed by immersion in cold acetone for 10 minutes. This ensures that the cells remain on the slide, retain antigenicity and are permeable to antibody, but in most instances have no residual infectivity.

Immunofluorescence

Virus diagnostic laboratories in the 1980s and 1990s expanded their use of microscopy, particularly as an aid to rapid diagnosis of viral infections. The commercial availability of high-quality reagents in the form of monoclonal antibodies supports the application of immunofluorescence (IF) for a wide range of viral antigens. Specific antibody (or a pool of antibodies) conjugated to a fluorochrome dye may be applied to a cell preparation in a *direct immunofluorescence test* (DIF) for the target antigen. This is the most widely-used method for rapid diagnosis by light microscopy, particularly suitable for single samples as they arrive, but also applied to the daily influx of respiratory secretions from infants and children which constitutes a major part of the work of a virus laboratory serving a children's unit during the annual epidemic of respiratory disease.

The same reagents may also be useful for staining cells from cell cultures, either for *culture confirmation*, and *typing* in the case of HSV, or for screening for *early (pre-CPE) detection of antigens*, particularly useful for slower-growing viruses, such as CMV and adenoviruses. Examples of the range and applications are given below. Some *serological tests for viral antibodies* are still based on *indirect immunofluorescence*, commonly for antibodies to Epstein–Barr virus, *human parvovirus* (erythrovirus B19) or *human herpesvirus 6* (HHV6).

In virology the most commonly used fluorochrome dye is fluorescein isothiocyanate (FITC), which gives a bright apple-green fluorescence. It is helpful if a counterstain has been included, so that contrasting negative background cells are visible (stained dull red if Evans' blue dye is used). The appropriate antibody is applied to the well or slide bearing the cells to be examined; a smear or deposit of cells direct from a patient, cells from a culture, or a shell vial coverslip. An incubation period (averaging 15–30 minutes) in a humid chamber permits the antibody to react with any virus-specific antigen in the cells. Unbound excess antibody is removed by washing in buffered saline, before the slide is air-dried and mounted for viewing on a special microscope with a source of incident UV light. Mounting fluid consists of analytical-grade glycerol (50%) in phosphate-buffered saline at a pH optimum of 8.6 to maximize fluorescence. Fluorescence fades rapidly on exposure to UV irradiation, so prolonged viewing is not advisable and photographic records should be obtained promptly when required.

Respiratory viruses

Direct immunofluorescence is now the commonest IF procedure in diagnostic virology for the rapid detection of antigens, and may be the only test used to diagnose RSV infection in children, having become so reliable in experienced hands that parallel virus isolation is no longer considered necessary as a routine. Most infants become infected with RSV in their first winter season, and one in every 100 babies is admitted to hospital having developed the alarming condition of bronchiolitis. Since in the annual winter epidemic season RSV is by far the commonest respiratory pathogen in infants and children, a rapid test for RSV is a top priority. The characteristic appearance (intracellular globules staining apple-green) of a positive DIF test for RSV in respiratory cells in secretions from such an infant is shown in Figure 17.2. There is specific antiviral treatment for RSV infection in those at special risk of serious disease, and the DIF test (or an equivalent enzyme-labelled one) is often required as an urgent or on-call procedure.

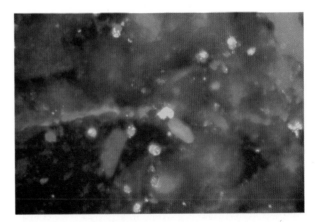

Figure 17.2 Direct immunofluorescence stain of respiratory epithelial cells from an infant with acute bronchiolitis. Bright apple-green staining of cells labelled with fluorescent antibody to RSV indicate infection with that virus; uninfected cells counterstained with Evans blue dye appear dull red in contrast

Skin or mucocutaneous cell preparations

Cells scraped from the base of vesicular skin lesions are frequently examined by DIF with antibodies specific to HSV-1, HSV-2 or VZV (if it is not obvious clinically which infection is present). Since specific antiviral therapy is available, and herpes infections are serious in immunocompromised hosts, rapid diagnosis is important. To be effective, antiviral drugs have to be given as soon as possible, and the dosage varies according to which virus is to be treated. The contagious nature of VZV is also a problem for control of infection—approximately 10% of young adults have not had chickenpox and are at risk if exposed to VZV.

Cells from culture

This is very similar to DIF on patient cells. The benefits of rapid confirmation of a presumed CPE are clinical and save laboratory time and resources. As HSV-1 and HSV-2 have different associations and vary in their tendency to cause recurrent disease at different sites, it is useful to know the virus type, and this can be done with type-specific antibodies. Monoclonal antibody to common group-specific antigens present in adenoviruses (hexon antigen) or enteroviruses (VP1 antigen), can be used to confirm the CPE produced by members of these groups, respectively.

Virus antigens produced early in the growth cycle

When CMV was recognized as a serious pathogen in transplant recipients who would require antiviral ther-

apy, it became essential to detect this virus much more rapidly than in the past. Gleaves (USA) and Griffiths (UK) established the value of looking for the CMV early antigens that appear after a few hours, compared to the days it takes for viral DNA and later antigens and a CPE to appear. The term 'shell vial' came from the USA, while in the UK the test was referred to as the DEAFF test (Detection of Early Antigen Fluorescent Foci). Early antigens of VZV are also sought occasionally. Wider use of the shell vial system has become popular in the USA and in mainland Europe, where many laboratories use it for respiratory virus detection particularly. Our own experience has shown it to be very useful in that regard, for early detection of adenovirus eye infections, and also for rapid and improved rate of isolation of VZV. Examples of shell vial IF are illustrated (Figure 17.3).

Microscopic examination of cell cultures

Although certain gross changes in cell culture are visible to the naked eye, as in the unfortunate case of turbidity or acidity due to growth of bacteria or fungi, microscopic examination is necessary before changes produced by virus growth can be detected. Serial observations are made over days and even weeks, and virus may have to be passed to fresh cultures for subsequent tests, so cultures are examined unstained. A rest holds the culture tube on the microscope stage, while the whole area of the cell monolayer is carefully scanned at low power (using ×4 or ×10 objectives) with the substage condenser lowered. Focal areas of altered cells are then inspected at higher magnification. It is not difficult to notice the difference between a complete healthy cell monolayer (uninoculated control tube from

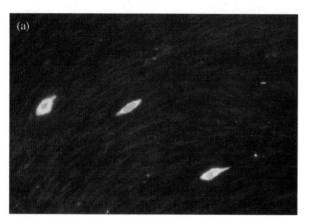

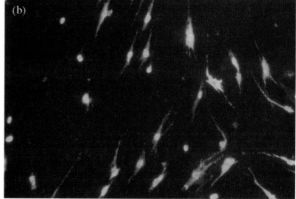

Figure 17.3 DIF staining of infected HEF shell vial cultures 48 hours post-inoculation with (a) a conjunctival swab, stained with adenovirus group-specific monoclonal antibody; (b) a throat swab, stained with influenza A group-specific antibody, showing nuclear staining and no spread of infection outside original cells infected

same batch of cells) and one in which holes have appeared as infected cells round up and fall off, or groups of cells form large clusters, but it takes a good deal of experience and careful, regular observation to develop real expertise in recognizing the characteristic cytopathic effect produced by specific viruses in different cell cultures.

Cytopathic effects in routine cell cultures

- *Degenerative CPE*: scattered areas with round, shrunken cells, which soon fall off the surface of the tube—seen with enteroviruses such as poliovirus, and rhinoviruses.

- *Round, refractile, swollen cells in clusters*: seen with adenovirus ('bunches of grapes' in HEp_2 cells) and HSV. HSV grows very fast, starting in a few patches ('plaques') the day after inoculation and spreading throughout the monolayer by next day. Small syncytia are seen, especially with HSV-2.

- *Cytomegalovirus CPE*: quite unique, progressing very slowly and exhibiting elongated foci of swollen (cytomegalic) cells in human fibroblast cultures.

- *Classical syncytial CPE*: the hallmark of RSV growing in fresh HEp_2 cells (Figure 17.4), but multinucleate giant cells are also seen with measles and VZV in sensitive cell lines. The features are different to the trained eye in each case.

HIV is not cultured routinely, but its growth may be recognized by the appearance of syncytia in the mononuclear blood cell cultures, which grow in suspension, not as monolayers. The *human herpesvirus type 6* (HHV6) was discovered in 1986 when it produced syncytial CPE in cultures of peripheral blood (Figure 17.5) and, on further examination, turned out to be not HIV but a previously unknown herpesvirus. The most recently famous CPE was that observed in the first cultures of the previously unknown human coronavirus associated with SARS.

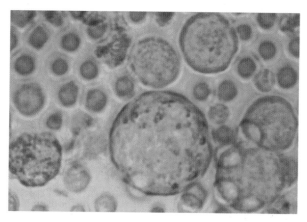

Figure 17.5 Large balloon-shaped syncytial CPE (unstained) produced by human herpesvirus type 6 (HHV6) in suspension culture of lymphoblastoid (JJhan) cell line

Non-cytopathic growth of viruses in cell culture

The virology microscopist is aware that there are some viruses that replicate in cell culture without producing obvious cytopathology. The best known example is of influenza viruses growing in monkey kidney cells, where the presence of virus may be revealed by *haemadsorption*. A glycoprotein (haemagglutinin) coded for by the virus and inserted into the cell plasma membrane is able to attach to red blood cells added to the surface. In the earliest stages of any virus replication, when only single cells are infected, a CPE is not obvious, but viral antigens will be present.

Further investigations of cytopathic agents

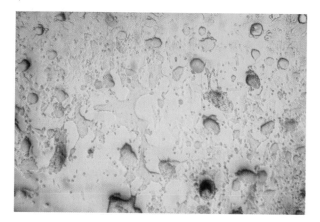

Figure 17.4 Classical syncytial cytopathic effect of RSV growing in HEp_2 cell culture (unstained), 5 days post-inoculation of patient's respiratory sample

The microscopist has not finished when a recognizable CPE is observed in an inoculated culture. Confirmation of the informed diagnosis is expected, and further identification may be indicated. The judgement of the microscopist, who will select the confirmation test based on the CPE, cell line, sample, and other factors, is critical in reaching a speedy diagnosis and saving resources. Confirmation and typing of HSV has already been mentioned. Adenovirus or enterovirus CPE can now be confirmed by IF of cells, but typing will require a *neutralization assay* because there are so many different types. This entails mixing aliquots of a well-grown isolate with separate pools of antisera covering common types, inoculating fresh cultures and observing which antiserum inhibits CPE, i.e. has neutralized the infectivity of the virus. These typing exercises seldom affect clinical management but are important for epidemiological studies.

Developments

The diagnostic virologist wishes to have the best of all approaches to identification of virus infections. Rapid detection is critical for the reasons outlined previously, and while IF microscopy may continue to be of use for individual samples, antigen-capture enzyme immunoassays or immunofiltration, less subjective methods, which can be automated, could be used for screening larger sample numbers and culture-amplified fluids. Molecular amplification of nucleic acid by the polymerase chain reaction (PCR) does provide the most sensitive means of detection of an ever-increasing range of viruses, and laboratories are moving more to this approach, reducing their use of classical isolation and microscopy. Parallel attempts at virus isolation will still be required in a laboratory offering a comprehensive service including epidemiological typing and antiviral susceptibility testing. Enhanced culture is used now, and there is a continuing search for sensitive cells, particularly for currently non-cultivable viruses. The emerging area of genetic engineering of cells may provide more novel approaches, such as enzyme-linked virus-inducible systems (ELVIS), already tested for HSV (Olivo 1996), which combine three strands (old and new) cell culture, antigen detection and recombinant DNA technology, including microscopy.

Acknowledgements

Thanks are expressed to the following in relation to figures used in this chapter: Figure 17.1, photography by Dr K McLaren, Consultant Histopathologist, University of Edinburgh; Figures 17.2–17.5, photography by AJ MacAulay FIMLS, Chief Biomedical Scientist in Clinical Virology Laboratory, Department of Medical Microbiology, University of Edinburgh; for all Figures, the copies submitted were prepared as colour prints by the Medical Photography Unit at the Royal Infirmary of Edinburgh, Little France.

Further reading

Lennette EH, Lennette DA, Lennette ET (eds). *Diagnostic Procedures for Viral, Rickettsial and Chlamydial Infections*, 7th edn. 1995: American Public Health Association, Washington, DC.

Mahy BWJ, Kangro HO (eds). *Virology Methods Manual*. 1996: Academic Press, London.

Olivo PD. Transgenic lines for detection of animal viruses. *Clin Microbiol Rev* 1996; **9**: 321–343.

Simmons A, Marmion BP. Rapid diagnosis of viral infections. In *Mackie & McCartney's Practical Medical Microbiology*, 14th edn, Collee JG, Fraser AG, Marmion BP, Simmons A (eds). 1996: Churchill-Livingstone, Edinburgh.

Zuckerman AJ, Banatvala JE, Pattison JR Griffiths PD, Schoub BD (eds). *Principles and Practice of Clinical Virology*, 5th edn. 2004 Wiley, Chichester.

18

Electron microscopy in virology

Hazel Appleton

Introduction

Viruses are regarded as malign agents that cause disease and suffering. When visualized in the electron microscope, however, a variety of elegant structures is revealed. Viruses from different virus groups look different, and it is this characteristic morphology that is the basis for their identification by electron microscopy. Electron microscopy provides the means for very rapidly detecting and identifying viruses in material taken directly from patients (Table 18.1). This rapid diagnosis can facilitate the management and treatment of patients. It also has public health implications in the management of outbreaks and controlling the spread of infectious diseases in the community. In the long term it has a role to play in epidemiological surveillance of infectious disease. Unlike many diagnostic tests, which select for one particular agent, electron microscopy is a 'catch-all' method that can be used to detect any virus or mixture of viruses present in the sample. It is particularly useful in the diagnosis and study of viruses that cannot be readily cultured *in vitro*. Use of electron microscopy has led to the discovery and identification of many new viral agents in recent years and it will continue to have a leading role in the study of newly emerging viruses.

Methods

Negative staining

This is the most widely used method for diagnostic virology and entails staining the background of the virus rather than the virus itself. Specimen preparation is simple and results can be obtained rapidly. The technique, however, does rely both on the presence of sufficient numbers of virus particles in the specimen (a minimum of 10^6 virus particles per ml specimen is usually required for detection) and on the structural integrity of the virus particles remaining intact so they can be recognized and identified. Enhanced sensitivity can sometimes be achieved by the use of immune sera (immune electron microscopy—IEM). Viruses that do not stand out clearly against the background material, e.g. parvoviruses, may be aggregated into clumps by mixing the sample with a specific antiserum and hence may be seen more easily. Alternatively, viruses may be attracted onto a grid by coating the grid with antiserum (solid phase immune electron microscopy—SPIEM). IEM methods can be used for antigenic typing of viruses. When a virus is detected by simple negative staining it is identified as a member of a virus group or family, but it is not usually possible to differentiate between members of the group without further tests, e.g. the herpesvirus causing chickenpox (varicella-zoster virus—VZV) is identical in appearance to the herpesvirus causing cold sores (herpes simplex virus—HSV).

Thin sectioning

Thin sectioning electron microscopy is useful for examination of specimens where there are insufficient numbers of virus particles present to be seen in negatively stained suspensions. Some viruses, such as retroviruses, have structures that are more easily identified in thin

The Science of Laboratory Diagnosis, Second Edition   Edited by David Burnett and John Crocker
© 2005 John Wiley & Sons, Ltd

Table 18.1   Viruses detected by electron microscopy

Specimens examined	Examples of viruses detected
Skin—vesicle fluids or scrapings of lesions[*]	Herpesviruses—herpes simplex, varicella-zoster virus Poxvirus—orf, molluscum contagiosum Papillomavirus (human wart)
Faeces[*]	Gastroenteritis viruses—rotavirus, adenovirus, astrovirus, norovirus, sapovirus (Hepatitis A and E, enterovirus)
Serum	Parvovirus B19 Hepatitis B
Urine	Polyomavirus BK Cytomegalovirus Adenovirus (haemorrhagic cystitis)
Liver	Hepatitis B
Foetal liver	Parvovirus B19 (hydrops fetalis)
Brain	Measles virus (SSPE) Polyomavirus JC Herpesvirus
Tumour	Epstein–Barr virus
Laboratory cell cultures for rapid identification of isolates[*]	Any virus that grows, e.g. influenza, parainfluenza, measles, mumps, adenovirus, polyomavirus, enterovirus, herpesvirus, retrovirus (Exotic viruses e.g. Marburg, Ebola)

[*]Current main uses of electron microscopy in diagnostic virology

sections than in negatively preparations. Although enhanced sensitivity can be achieved, it is not a rapid technique and has limited application in a diagnostic laboratory. It is useful in studying the pathogenesis of infection, and can be used for confirmation of diagnosis in biopsy and post-mortem specimens. Virus structures are resistant to cell lysis and poor tissue preservation, and positive results may be obtained from apparently unpromising material.

Scanning electron microscopy

Few diagnostic laboratories have access to a scanning electron microscope or even a scanning attachment to a transmission electron microscope. The scanning electron microscope is mainly used as a research tool for investigating virus attachment and pathogenesis, and so far has had little use in diagnostic virology. There has been some interest in solid phase immunoassays,

using latex beads coated with specific antibody. Virus attaches to the beads and is coated with gold. The technique appears to offer little advantage over negative staining IEM, and has the disadvantage that characteristic virus morphology is obscured and the reagents are expensive.

Uses of electron microscopy

Electron microscopy first came to prominence in diagnostic virology in the 1960s for the rapid diagnosis of smallpox. The skin lesions produced in smallpox and those caused by chickenpox can be clinically confusing. The alarming implications of smallpox infection made rapid differentiation of these infections essential. Skin lesions and particularly fluids from vesicles are normally rich in virus particles. By just mixing the sample with a drop of negative stain, the virus can readily be seen without the need for concentration. Smallpox is caused by a member of the poxvirus family, and chickenpox by the herpesvirus VZV. Poxviruses and herpesviruses have very different morphologies and can readily be distinguished in the electron microscope (Figures. 18.1 and 18.2). The smallpox virus, variola, and the vaccinia virus

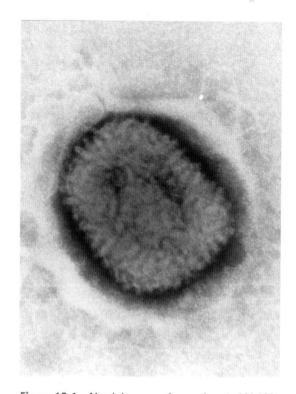

Figure 18.1   Vaccinia—an orthopoxvirus (×180 000)

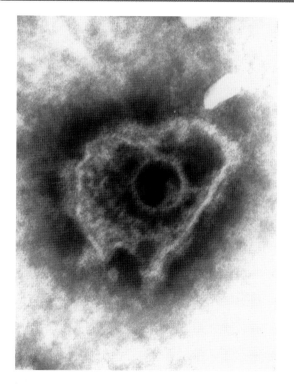

Figure 18.2   Herpesvirus from a skin lesion (×180 000)

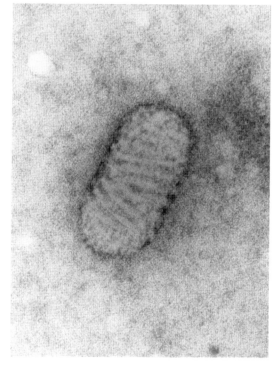

Figure 18.3   Orf—a parapoxvirus (×180 000)

used in the vaccine are indistinguishable and further, more complex, tests were required to differentiate between these two: this was usually by culture on the chorioallantoic membrane of fertile hens' eggs, which took 3 days. Detection of a herpesvirus avoided the need for all the public health measures that would have to be activated if there was a possibility of a case of smallpox.

Skin lesions

In 1980, the World Health Organization declared that smallpox had been eradicated, but electron microscopy has continued to have an important role in the rapid diagnosis of herpesvirus infection. It is particularly useful for immunocompromised patients, where the use of appropriate antiviral drugs can facilitate treatment. Furthermore, it can aid the management of patients on transplant units, where an outbreak of chickenpox could have very serious and sometimes fatal consequences. Electron microscopy is still used in the diagnosis of two other poxvirus infections, orf and molluscum contagiosum, neither of which can be readily identified by other means. Orf is a zoonotic infection acquired from sheep, caused by a parapox virus, which is smaller and more elongated than the orthopox viruses, such as vaccinia

and cowpox (Figure 18.3). Molluscum contagiosum is a human poxvirus that causes benign eruptions on the skin and is similar in appearance to the orthopox viruses. Electron microscopy is also occasionally used for the detection of the human papillomavirus (HPV) that causes warts.

Gastroenteritis

The discovery of viruses that cause gastroenteritis led to a massive expansion in the use of electron microscopy in diagnostic and public health laboratories in the 1970s and 1980s. Several different viruses can cause gastroenteritis and all were discovered by electron microscopic examination of faecal samples from patients. It was surprising that viruses could be visualized in such complex material, but in fact these viruses are excreted in vast numbers into the intestinal contents and can readily be detected if samples are collected at the appropriate time.

Gastroenteritis viruses do not grow in conventional cell cultures, and electron microscopy has been the main method for their detection and identification. Some gastroenteritis viruses, such as rotaviruses and adenoviruses, have such distinctive morphologies that only

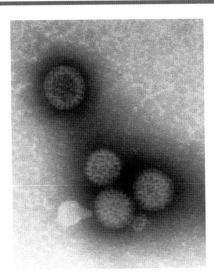

Figure 18.4 Rotavirus—a major cause of gastroenteritis in babies and young children. The typical 'spokes' can be seen around the particles. The centre particle has lost its outer capsid layer ($\times 180\,000$)

one or two particles need to be seen for positive identification (Figures 18.4 and 18.5). Samples can be so rich in virus that no concentration is necessary (concentrations of 10^{12} particles/g have been estimated). It is often sufficient simply to emulsify a small sample of faeces in a drop of distilled water, mix with negative stain and place on a grid. For other gastroenteritis viruses, such as astroviruses and noroviruses, identification is more difficult, and more particles may have to be examined to make an accurate identification (Figures

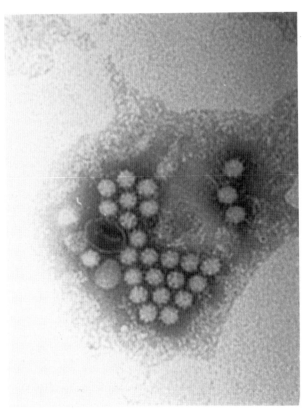

Figure 18.6 Astrovirus. Solid five- or six-pointed stars can be seen on the surface of some particles ($\times 180\,000$)

18.6 and 18.7). It is usually necessary to concentrate the virus from the specimen in these cases.

Commercial assays, such as ELISA, latex agglutination tests, PCR and even dip-stick tests, have been developed and are now used as the first approach in

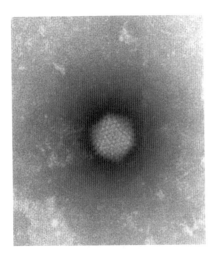

Figure 18.5 Adenovirus—largely associated with infections of the respiratory tract and the eyes. Two adenoviruses are associated with gastroenteritis, mainly infecting young children ($\times 180\,000$)

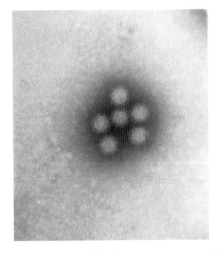

Figure 18.7 Norovirus. This virus causes many outbreaks of gastroenteritis in the community ($\times 180\,000$)

many diagnostic laboratories. This allows larger numbers of samples to be tested than is feasible by electron microscopy, and often with greater sensitivity. However, these tests have limitations in that they are selective for a specific virus type and do not detect all strains within a virus group. Samples giving negative or equivocal results may subsequently be examined by electron microscopy.

The Health Protection Agency Centre for Infections collects reports of the viruses detected in cases of gastroenteritis in England and Wales. This has enabled an epidemiological picture to be drawn up of the age groups affected by the different viral agents, seasonal distributions, patterns of excretion and modes of transmission. This information makes it possible to give appropriate advice on such factors as management of outbreaks, how long food handlers should be excluded from work and the optimum time for collection of specimens.

Rotavirus

The most well known and readily identified of the gastroenteritis viruses is the rotavirus (named from the Latin word *rota*, meaning wheel: the arrangement of capsomeres seen on the surface of the virus particles looks like the spokes of a wheel) (Figure 18.4). Rotavirus is a major cause of gastroenteritis in babies and young children. In the UK and other developed countries, it is responsible for the largest number of admissions to hospital in this age group, and in underdeveloped countries it is estimated to cause about half a million deaths per year. Infection mainly occurs over the winter months in temperate climates. Outbreaks are also seen among the elderly, presumable due to waning immunity.

Rotavirus was first found in thin sections of duodenal biopsies of children in Australia, but such invasive techniques are not necessary, as the virus can readily be seen in simple emulsions of faecal samples. Commercial kits for the detection of rotaviruses are widely used. These kits, however, only detect the commonest type of rotaviruses known as group A rotaviruses. Other types, such as group C rotaviruses, also infect humans, although they are seen less frequently. Group C rotaviruses infect all age groups and have been associated with a number of family and school outbreaks. In many laboratories, specimens are only examined by electron microscopy if the results of an ELISA or latex test are negative. Non-group A rotaviruses are usually detected when there is a discrepancy with a negative kit result and positive electron microscopy finding. Characterization is by PAGE analysis or PCR.

Adenovirus

The examination of faecal samples from children with gastroenteritis led to the discovery of two new adenoviruses. Adenoviruses had long been associated with respiratory and eye infections, and are routinely isolated in cell cultures. The two new adenoviruses, designated types 40 and 41, are associated specifically with gastroenteritis and cannot be readily cultured. Electron microscopy has limitations and can only indicate the presence of adenoviruses (Figure 18.5) and not specifically types 40 and 41, for which further tests are required. Common respiratory adenoviruses are sometimes isolated from faecal specimens, but this is regarded as an incidental finding. As for rotavirus, ELISA and dipstick kits are now readily available. Adenoviruses types 40 and 41 have a similar epidemiology to rotavirus in that they mainly infect young children and occur during the winter months.

Astrovirus

Another virus associated with gastroenteritis is astrovirus, a novel virus, so-named from the solid five-or six-pointed star seen on the surface of a proportion of particles (Figure 18.6). Astroviruses account for around 1–2% of gastroenteritis virus reports in the UK. Infection has mainly been reported in the very young, and outbreaks in newborn baby units have been described. However, it is suggested that infection in other age groups may be under-recognized. Like rotavirus, outbreaks occasionally occur in the elderly. On rare occasions, foodborne transmission has been implicated. Electron microscopy is still the main method of detection.

Norovirus

Noroviruses, previously known as Norwalk-like viruses or small round structured viruses (SRSV), are considered the most common cause of gastroenteritis in the community. They occur in all age groups and are frequently associated with outbreaks in hospitals, residential homes and schools. Gastroenteritis viruses are usually transmitted directly from person to person vial the faecal–oral route or in aerosol droplets. Occasionally some may also be transmitted via food or water, and in these situations it is noroviruses that are most frequently implicated. The first virus of the group was discovered by electron microscopy in 1972. It originated from an outbreak in the town of Norwalk in the USA and became known as the Norwalk agent. The term 'small round structured virus' or SRSV relates to the appearance of the virus in the electron microscope (Figure 18.7). Virus particles measure 30–35 nm in diameter and have an amorphous surface and ragged outline. Noroviruses are classified within the family *Caliciviridae*. There are many different strains and these form two broad genogroups. There is also a third, more distantly related genogroup, called sapoviruses, named from an outbreak in a nursery at Sapporo in Japan. Sapoviruses have the classical appearance of a calicivirus, with cup-like depressions seen on the surface of the virus particles. These cup-like depressions are not commonly seen on noroviruses. The differentiation of norovirus, calicivirus and also astrovirus by electron microscopy can be difficult and needs an experienced microscopist.

Noroviruses cannot be cultured and most diagnosis has been by electron microscopy. However, noroviruses are only excreted in numbers sufficient for detection for about 48 hours after onset of symptoms and hence it is often difficult to obtain appropriate specimens. Noroviruses tend not to be excreted in such great numbers as rotavirus and adenoviruses and, as they do not have such distinctive morphological features, they are technically far more difficult to detect and identify. Hence, noroviruses are grossly under-reported. Electron microscopy is not sensitive enough to be able to detect virus in food or environmental samples. PCR assays for noroviruses have been developed but are only available in specialized laboratories at present. These assays are very sensitive: they can detect virus in clinical samples for up to a week after the onset of symptoms and can be used for testing foods and environmental samples. However, they do not detect all strains of norovirus. In 2003, commercial ELISA kits that detect a wide range of genogroup 1 and genogroup 2 noroviruses became available. These have sensitivity similar to electron microscopy, but are much easier to use, can handle larger numbers of specimens and have had a significant impact on testing for noroviruses. There is great diversity within the norovirus group, however, and ELISAs do not detect all strains. Thus, electron microscopy will continue to have a role in diagnosis.

Other infections

Electron microscopy had a major role in the discovery of other viruses, particularly some of the hepatitis viruses, papovaviruses and parvovirus B19. Other tests have now largely superseded electron microscopy for diagnosis.

Hepatitis viruses

The virus causing hepatitis A was discovered in 1972 by immune electron microscopy of faecal specimens from patients involved in volunteer studies. However, it was quickly shown that most virus excretion occurs in the prodromal phase of illness, and diagnosis is now mainly by detection of hepatitis A-specific IgM antibody. Although not used for diagnosis, it was electron microscopy that revealed that the other enterically transmitted virus, hepatitis E, has the morphology of a calicivirus. Hepatitis E is not commonly seen in the UK, but has been associated with large water-borne outbreaks in developing areas of the world and infection is particularly severe in pregnant women.

It is in the diagnosis of hepatitis B infection that electron microscopy was most useful. Viral particles and viral antigens, particularly the hepatitis B surface antigen, are present in serum for prolonged periods. Diagnosis can readily be made if complete virus particles are detected, but often only 22 nm spheres of virus coat protein (surface antigen) can be seen. Surface antigen is difficult to distinguish from other background material in serum. To enhance sensitivity and ease identification, the patient's serum is usually mixed with a specific antiserum in an IEM test, which is not suitable for testing large numbers of specimens, and must be used selectively.

Parvovirus B19

It was while looking for hepatitis B by IEM that the serum parvovirus B19 was first discovered. B19 was subsequently identified as the aetiological agent of erythema infectiosum, a common childhood rash infection that is also often known as 'slapped face syndrome'. Infection in pregnancy can cause damage to the foetus. It can also cause severe aplastic crisis in patients with haematological disorders such as sickle cell anaemia. Laboratory confirmation of B19 infection may significantly influence the management of these patients. Although no longer used for routine diagnosis, conflicting results between tests for parvovirus B19 infection (e.g. a positive PCR but a negative IgM result) may be rapidly resolved by electron microscopy.

Brain

When antiviral drugs first became available for the treatment of herpes encephalitis, attempts were made to detect herpesvirus in negatively stained suspensions of brain material. Rapid and accurate diagnosis was important because early antiviral drugs were extremely toxic. Electron microscopy did not prove particularly sensitive, however, and was soon replaced by fluorescence microscopy and subsequently by PCR techniques. Paramyxovirus helix of measles virus has been detected in thin sections of brain tissue from patients with subacute sclerosing panencephalitis. The first human polymavirus, JC, was discovered in thin sections of brain tissue from patients with progressive multifocal leukoencephalopathy. Although electron microscopy was useful for establishing the aetiology of both these conditions, fluorescence techniques and PCR assays are more sensitive for examining brain material.

Urine

Attempts to find viruses in urine samples have had mixed success. Electron microscopy was responsible for the discovery of a second human polyomavirus known as BK virus. This virus commonly infects transplant patients and is excreted in urine. It is very slow-growing in cell cultures and electron microscopy has been extremely useful for diagnosis. PCR assays have been developed and are now the usual method employed diagnostically. Cytomegalovirus (CMV), a member of the herpesvirus group, is also excreted in urine, but is only detected by electron microscopy when very large numbers of virus particles are present. The symptoms of both CMV and BK virus infections can mimic organ rejection. Diagnosis of a viral cause results in better patient management, since inappropriate use of immunosuppressive drugs would actually prolong virus infection.

Virology laboratory

Apart from its primary diagnostic role, electron microscopy has many other functions in a virology laboratory. The electron microscopist provides support in the development of new, alternative diagnostic tests and frequently supports research projects. Electron microscopy is used for the rapid identification of viruses isolated in cell cultures, and can greatly reduce the time spent in trying to identify a cytopathic agent,

especially when more than one type of virus is present. It is used when conflicting, equivocal or even negative results are obtained from other tests, e.g. PCR assays and ELISAs for norovirus do not detect all strains and electron microscopy may provide positive results on apparently negative samples. Electron microscopy is also used to check viral antigens, such as measles virus and rubella virus, prepared for other tests, and is used for detecting naturally occurring viral contaminants of cell cultures, such as SV40 (Figure 18.8).

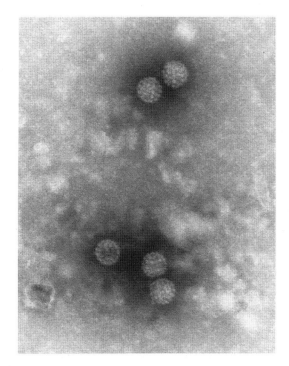

Figure 18.8 Polyomavirus found as a contaminant in a cell culture (×180 000)

Rapid emergency response

Current world events have led to a heightened awareness of the potential for bioterrorist activity and government agencies are continuously reviewing contingency plans to deal with any such event. Smallpox has been identified as a possible agent for deliberate release. Since electron microscopy is the most rapid method for detecting an orthopoxvirus, microscopists have been reviewing protocols and examining external quality assurance panels to ensure that they are in a position to respond. Following eradication, vaccination ceased and hence most laboratory staff are unvaccinated. Whilst the threat of infection remains very low, it is considered that the risks associated with vaccination may outweigh those of smallpox. To protect staff who may be unexpectedly faced with a possible smallpox specimen, inactivation of the specimen prior to processing is recommended. It is essential that any method chosen does not compromise the ability to identify both poxviruses and herpesviruses. A 5% solution of phosphate-buffered formaldehyde solution has been found to inactivate virus without masking the identifying morphological features. Glutar-aldehyde is frequently used as a fixative for electron microscopy. Some microscopists prefer to put the unfixed specimen and stain onto a grid and then dip the prepared grid into a drop of glutaraldehyde. How-ever, if the specimen is treated with glutaraldehyde prior to processing, the surface structure of any negatively stained virus is completely obscured. If an orthopoxvirus is detected by electron microscopy, further tests are required to identify it. This is now usually done by PCR in specialized laboratories. The most commonly occurring orthopoxvirus in the UK is cowpox, which is most usually acquired from domestic cats. In 2003 there was an outbreak of an illness with vesicular lesions in humans in the USA that caused concern and consider-able publicity. An orthopoxvirus was quickly detected by electron microscopy and was subsequently identified as monkeypox, which had been acquired from exotic pet rodents. Although monkeypox infection can be very severe, this poxvirus fortunately is not highly transmis-sible between humans.

Newly emerging viruses

New viruses continue to be discovered and electron microscopy continues to be at the forefront in the search and initial characterization of such agents. The ease of international travel means that new infections can be transmitted round the world to non-immune populations in a very short time. For instance, in the spring of 2003 the severe acute respiratory syndrome, SARS, originat-ing in the Far East, was identified as a new disease. There was a worldwide effort, coordinated by the World Health Organization, to identify the aetiological agent. Electron microscopy played a prominent role in rapidly identifying a new coronavirus as the cause (Figure 18.9).

Conclusions

Electron microscopy has an essential role in the rapid response to emergency situations where public health is

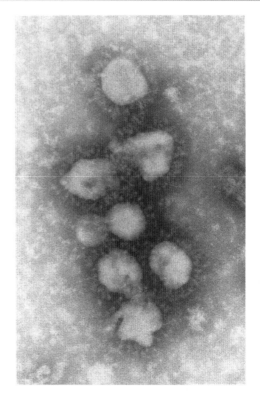

Figure 18.9   SARS virus (×180 000)

put at risk, whether this is from the deliberate release of a biological agent or from a naturally emerging new infection. Electron microscopy is often used as a primary diagnostic method in the early stages after a virus is first discovered until easier tests are developed. Electron microscopy is labour-intensive and is not suitable for examining large numbers of specimens. Consequently, if suitable alternative tests become available, electron microscopy tends to take on a more confirmatory role. The main emphasis for electron microscopy in virology appears to be moving more to research aspects, where it has always had an essential role. The initial cost of the equipment means that electron microscopy is not avail-able in all laboratories. Furthermore, a satisfactory service requires highly skilled and experienced staff and time spent in maintaining equipment in optimal working condition. As electron microscopy is currently declining in routine virology, it may be sensible to consider pooling resources by collaborating with elec-tron microscopists in other fields of pathology, so that a full range of electron microscopy techniques can be offered and expertise maintained. This could work well, provided that the different needs of all the users are catered for and there is convenient and easy access for all users.

Electron microscopy has been used widely for the detection of viruses in faecal specimens from patients with gastroenteritis, and particularly for the investigation of infants with diarrhoea. The introduction of newer commercial ELISA kits is likely to reduce the numbers of specimens examined by electron microscopy. These kits offer cheaper tests and the capability of testing large numbers of samples, but they do have limitations and are unable to detect all virus strains. Electron microscopy remains the most rapid method for the diagnosis of vesicular lesions caused by viruses, and has special relevance in the management of immunocompromised patients. Electron microscopy also has an important role in the rapid identification of viruses isolated from clinical specimens in cell culture.

Many new viruses have been discovered by the use of electron microscopy, particularly since the early 1970s. Electron microscopy has a major contribution to make in the discovery and characterization of new viruses in the future, alongside the recent advances in molecular virology. For instance, 40% of gastroenteritis infections still remain undiagnosed. There are hepatitis viruses and retroviruses that still require characterization by electron microscopy. Electron microscopy is still being used to look for viruses in tumours. It will continue to be used for gaining an understanding of the pathogenesis of viral infections and the role of viral antigens, which could lead to the development of effective treatments and vaccines. Such studies are being aided by the development of improved and more rapid automated preparation techniques for thin sectioning and scanning. Recent advances in electron microscope design, such as environmental scanning microscopes that do not require lengthy, complex drying procedures, mean that not only can specimens be processed more rapidly and easily, but shrinkage and distortion of specimens is avoided. As microscopes increasingly become more 'user-friendly', viral investigation by electron microscopy becomes easier.

Further reading

Appleton H, Field AM. The electron microscope and public health virology. *Microsc Anal* 1990; **20**: 7–9.

Caul EO, Appleton H. The electron microscopical and physical characteristics of small round human faecal viruses: An interim scheme for classification. *J Med Virol* 1982; **9**: 257–265.

Doane FW, Anderson N. *Electron Microscopy in Diagnostic Virology: A Practical Guide and Atlas*. 1987: Cambridge University Press, Cambridge.

Madeley CR, Field AM. *Virus Morphology*, 2nd edn. 1988: Churchill-Livingstone, Edinburgh.

Field AM. The contribution of the electron microscope. In *Public Health Virology: 12 Reports*, Mortimer PP (ed.). 1986: Public Health Laboratory Service, London.

19

Tissue culture

William L Irving and **Alan Pawley**

Introduction

Virus particles consist of genetic material (nucleic acid), plus a small number of proteins—hence the derivation of Sir Peter Medawar's memorable quote that 'viruses are trouble wrapped in a protein coat'. Some viruses, in addition, possess a lipid envelope. There are no internal organelles, such as mitochondria, ribosomes, or Golgi apparatus. Viruses are therefore *obligate intracellular parasites*, i.e. they can replicate only within living cells, usurping the host cell's energy-generating and biosynthetic machinery to do so. Isolation of viruses from clinical material thus presents a number of challenges quite distinct from those encountered in a bacteriology laboratory, where bacteria can be grown on inanimate media. The presence of living cells in one form or another is the first essential prerequisite for successful growth of viruses. For many years, viruses were grown in fertile hens' eggs. An alternative is to use whole experimental animals. Whilst both of these techniques may still be of value in specialized circumstances, they have been largely replaced in routine virus laboratories by the use of cell cultures derived from a variety of tissues, grown as monolayers on glass or plastic surfaces (i.e. tubes or flasks). In this chapter, the practicalities of running a cell culture laboratory for the isolation of viruses will be discussed and the advantages and disadvantages of this approach to the diagnosis of virus infection highlighted.

Choice of cell cultures

The first step in the replication cycle of any virus is that of attachment to its target cell. This is a very specific process, involving precise interaction between a ligand on the surface of the virus, and a receptor on the surface of the target cell. Thus, not all viruses will infect and grow in all cell types; cells that lack the appropriate receptor for a particular virus will be resistant to infection by that virus. This creates a problem for the diagnostic laboratory—to provide a comprehensive service for the isolation of all possible viruses would require the availability of a multitude of different cell types. In practice, most laboratories will run only two or three different cell types, each of which will support the growth of as broad a range of viruses as possible. The most commonly used cell cultures are listed in Table 19.1, which also indicates which viruses may grow in each. Although this list includes many of the common viruses encountered in clinical practice, some important viruses, (e.g. human immunodeficiency virus, (HIV), the hepatitis viruses, the viral causes of gastroenteritis, including rotaviruses and enteric adenoviruses, and Epstein–Barr virus (EBV)) are clearly missing, as are several others. Isolation of some of these viruses can be achieved by use of particular specialized cell culture techniques, such as organ culture. The differentiated properties of the tissue of origin can be maintained in organ culture, e.g. human fetal tracheal rings have

The Science of Laboratory Diagnosis, Second Edition   Edited by David Burnett and John Crocker
© 2005 John Wiley & Sons, Ltd

Table 19.1 Commonly used cell cultures

Type of culture	Viruses capable of growth
Primary/secondary cultures	
Monkey kidney cells	Influenza viruses, parainfluenza viruses, enteroviruses, mumps virus
Semi-continuous cell lines	
Human embryonic fibroblasts	Herpes simplex virus (HSV), varicella zoster virus, cytomegalovirus, enteroviruses, adenoviruses, rhinoviruses
Continuous cell lines	
Vero cells (derived from monkey kidney)	HSV, mumps virus
Hep-2 cells/HeLa cells	Respiratory syncytial virus, adenoviruses
Madin Darby canine kidney (MDCK) cells	Influenza viruses

functioning ciliated epithelial cells of the respiratory tract, able to support the replication of common cold viruses. Alternatively, specialized cell cultures may be used, e.g. HIV and EBV can be grown in human peripheral blood lymphocytes, and some of the hepatitis viruses will grow in primary hepatocyte cultures or hepatoma-derived cell lines. However, the difficulties involved in the provision of a regular supply of these more specialized cultures means that isolation of these viruses is usually restricted to reference or research laboratories. Yet other viruses (e.g. the human papillomaviruses, hepatitis C virus) are so exacting in their requirements for growth that isolation in cell culture has proved to be virtually impossible. Diagnosis of infection with these viruses must of necessity rely on approaches other than isolation in cell culture.

Preparation of cell cultures

Efficient functioning of a diagnostic virology laboratory requires the availability of (a) stock cells grown up on a large scale, and (b) mature cells in small numbers ready and waiting in a receptacle (usually a tube, but cell culture 'microtitre' plates are an alternative) ready for inoculation with appropriate clinical material, as and when that material arrives in the laboratory. As these tubes are used up, they are replaced by fresh tubes prepared from the stock cultures.

All of the standard cell types listed in Table 19.1 grow as adherent cells, rather than as cell suspensions. This means that they will attach themselves to a flat surface (usually plastic cell culture flasks) and then multiply and divide, provided that the culture medium contains the necessary nutrients, until the whole surface is covered. At this point, most cells will stop dividing due to contact inhibition. This process is known as *growing to confluence*. Once a cell sheet is confluent, the cells can be stripped off the surface using a proteolytic enzyme such as trypsin, diluted in culture medium, and poured back into a number (e.g. 3 or 4) of new flasks, where they will then once again grow to confluence. This process is known as *passaging* of cells, and in this way, the number of cells available can be rapidly expanded. Alternatively, the cells from a confluent flask may be distributed in low cell concentrations into a rack of cell culture tubes, which, once the cells have settled down and reached confluence, will then await inoculation with clinical material.

Cells differ in their ability to be repeatedly passaged. *Primary cultures*, i.e. those established directly from tissue (e.g. monkey kidney cells) do not survive more than two or three passages *in vitro*. This is a major drawback to their use, as continual supply of fresh primary cultures is expensive and inconvenient. Indeed, there is considerable concern that the supply of monkey kidney cells may cease for a number of reasons. These cells traditionally have been replied upon for isolation of circulating influenza viruses, and there has been a great deal of effort to find alternative cell substrates for these viruses. By comparison, tumour cell lines (e.g. Hep-2 cells, Hela cells) are able to divide indefinitely when passaged *in vitro*, and are therefore referred to as *continuous cell lines*. In between these two extremes, diploid cells derived from human embryonic tissue (e.g. human embryonic fibroblasts) can be successfully grown for 30 or 40 passages before finally petering out, and are therefore known as *semi-continuous cell lines*.

Cells are cultured in culture flasks under sterile conditions. Preparation is often done in vertical laminar flow cabinets, but can be performed on an open bench with a bunsen burner and appropriate aseptic technique. Medium added to the flasks must be isotonic and of suitable pH (e.g. 7.2–7.4) and is usually based on physiologically balanced salt solutions. The exact composition of the medium may vary according to cell type—detailed recipes are available in practical guidebooks. It is useful to add an indicator dye to enable recognition of cell metabolism by colour change (healthy and growing cells produce an acid medium). For growth, essential amino acids and protein are necessary, and these are usually provided in the form of serum derived from fetal calves. Antibiotics are often added to the growth medium as an added precaution against bacterial or fungal contamination, the main sources of which are water-borne bacteria, yeast from the carbon dioxide source, and *Mycoplasma* species from contaminated reagents or from the operator. The latter will severely reduce the ability of the cells to support virus growth.

Once confluence is reached, cells can be stripped using physical means with a sterile silicon rubber scraper (known as a 'rubber policeman') or, more usually, by treatment with trypsin and EDTA, which disrupt the binding of cells to the plastic surface, and cause the cells to round up and detach. The cells can be counted in a haemocytometer at this stage, and the appropriate volume for resuspension (to give the optimum seeding concentration) calculated. However, with experience, a rough guess of the necessary volume will suffice.

If the cells are not to be further passaged, e.g. those in tubes ready for inoculation, then once they have reached confluence, the growth medium is replaced by maintenance medium, the difference being that in the latter the concentration of serum is dramatically reduced. Confluent cells in cell culture tubes in maintenance medium will survive for several days, but eventually they will slowly decay despite medium changes, at which point they must be discarded.

Cells being propagated for virus investigations may, when surplus to requirements, be preserved as seed pools frozen in liquid nitrogen. The cells are suspended in medium containing dimethyl sulphoxide, which prevents ice crystal formation destroying the cells. With renewed need or in the event of bacterial contamination of cells in use, frozen cells may be rapidly thawed and fresh cultures prepared.

Clinical specimens for virus isolation

There are no restrictions on the nature of clinical material that can be inoculated into cell culture for virus isolation. Fluid samples (e.g. cerebrospinal fluid, CSF, saliva, urine, vesicle fluid, nasopharyngeal aspirate, bronchoalveolar lavage fluid, blood, diarrhoeal faeces) can be sent to the laboratory in a sterile container and added to appropriate cell culture tubes, either neat or after dilution in maintenance medium. Swabs (e.g. conjunctival, throat, base of ulcer, cervical, rectal) must be broken off into viral transport medium (isotonic fluid plus antibiotics to inhibit microbial overgrowth), as viruses will not survive on dry swabs. After vortexing

the bottle to release as much cellular material as possible from the swab into the medium, the transport medium is inoculated onto the cell sheets. Tissue biopsies (e.g. brain, bowel, lung) should also be placed in viral transport medium. The tissue can be finely minced and both cellular and supernatant material inoculated into culture.

Identification of virus growth

Once a clinical specimen has been inoculated into cell culture tubes, the tubes are incubated under conditions which most resemble those from where the material was obtained. Most cultures are held at 37°C, but some viruses, most notably those from the upper respiratory tract, will grow better at a slightly lower temperature, e.g. 33°C, and in the presence of 5% carbon dioxide. Cultures may be slowly rotated on a roller drum, which improves the aeration of the cell sheet, or held stationary. The challenge for the microbiologist is now to determine whether or not a given cell culture contains cells in which a virus is replicating. There are a number of options available to achieve this goal.

Cytopathic effects

When viruses replicate within cells, the cells may undergo morphological changes, e.g. swelling due to alteration of membrane permeabilities, shrinkage due to cell-death, giant multi-nucleate cell formation due to the presence of a fusion protein encoded by the virus. These changes in cellular morphology, visible under the light microscope, are referred to as a *cytopathic effect* (CPE) and viruses that induce these changes are said to be cytopathogenic. Thus, the presence of a virus within a cell culture may be determined by regular examination (e.g. every other day) of the culture under the low-power lens of a light microscope for the development of a CPE.

The exact appearance of a CPE is variable, according to which virus is responsible, and in which cell type it is occurring. The cells may balloon in size, shrivel up or fuse into syncytia (giant multinuclear cells). The effect may be widespread throughout the whole cell sheet or may be much more focal in nature. It may be seen predominantly, if not exclusively, at the edge of the sheet rather than in the middle. The speed of development of the CPE may vary from as short as 18 hours to as long as 4 weeks. Taking all of these factors into account, plus the clinical details relevant to a particular specimen, a trained virologist will be able to make a definitive diagnosis of which virus is present in the culture through

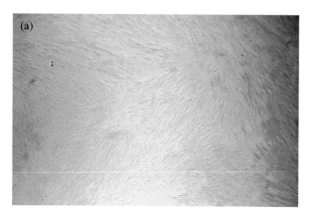

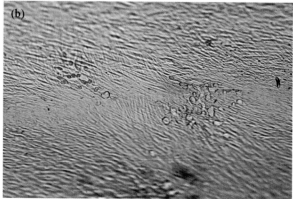

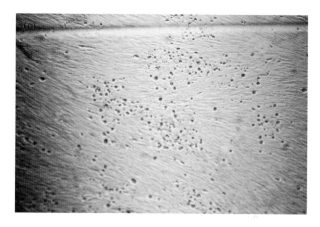

Figure 19.1 Cytopathic effects. (a) A normal cell sheet of fibroblasts. The cells have grown to confluence and are spindle-shaped. (b) Some of the cells are rounded up and swollen. This appearance in discrete foci separated by normal-looking cells is typical of the cytopathic effect induced by cytomegalovirus. (c) Several cells all over the cell sheet have rounded up to give a 'flick-drop' appearance. This is the characteristic appearance of a rhinovirus-induced CPE

light microscopy observation of the CPE alone. Thus, a CPE originating from a vesicle swab consisting of ballooning cells appearing after 24 hours of culture and thereafter spreading rapidly to destroy the whole cell sheet is highly likely to be due to herpes simplex virus. In contrast, a vesicle swab causing a CPE to appear only after 10 days in culture, in only two or three foci of swollen cells in the centre of the sheet, which spread slowly over the next several days, is likely to be due to varicella-zoster virus. Illustrations of CPEs characteristic to specific viruses are shown in Figure 19.1.

Passaging of viruses

Virus replication within a cell sheet is not the only cause of a visible CPE. Material inoculated onto the sheet may be cytotoxic, a problem especially frequent with faecal samples, or contamination with other microorganisms may occur, despite all the precautions taken. If there is any doubt as to the origins of a CPE, a simple way to distinguish between a virus as opposed to a toxic effect is to attempt to passage the putative virus. The cells remaining in the cell sheet are scraped into the culture

supernatant, and a few drops of the resultant material inoculated into a fresh cell culture tube. If there was indeed a virus in the original culture, then not only will the CPE reappear within the new tube, but the speed of development should be much enhanced, as the amount, or titre, of virus will have increased significantly following viral growth in the first culture. However, if the original CPE arose due to some toxic component of the specimen, then this will have been diluted in the second tube, and the subsequent CPE should develop more slowly and less extensively, if at all.

Passaging of viruses is useful for two other reasons. First, some viruses may not produce a visible CPE when first grown in culture, even though replication is indeed taking place. However, on repeated passaging in the same cell substrate, a CPE may become apparent following adaptation of the virus to growth in that particular cell type. The process of passaging viruses from apparently normal-looking cells is known as *blind passage*, presumably because at that stage, the virologist is unable to see evidence of the presence of virus. The identification of rubella virus growing in rabbit kidney (RK13) cells may require several such blind passages. Second, passaging of viruses is a good method of increasing the amount of virus available for further studies, such as neutralization assays (see below).

Confirmation of virus isolation

In most instances the type of virus in a cell culture can be determined with reasonable certainty by observation of the characteristics of the CPE present in the cell sheet, as outlined above. However, there are instances where confirmation of virus identity may be required, e.g. if the CPE is atypical, does not passage well or is absent or, alternatively, when more information about the particular strain of virus is required. This can be achieved by the use of electron microscopy, antigen detection or neutralization assays.

The process of cell culture acts as a means of increasing viral titre to a sufficient level to allow visualization by electron microscopy (EM). Thus, provided that there is access to an EM, most problems associated with atypical or unusual CPEs can be resolved rapidly by appropriate EM examination of the cells or culture supernatant. Viruses need to be at a concentration of $\geq 10^6$ particles/ml to use this technique successfully.

Cells infected with a particular virus will express antigens derived from that virus. These antigens can be detected by staining with antibodies. Thus, the specific identity of a virus growing in cell culture may be determined by staining the cells with a panel of appropriate monoclonal antibodies, suitably labelled with an immunofluorescent tag. Cells can either be scraped off and sucked out of the cell culture tubes, and then dried onto a multispot Teflon-coated glass slide, or, if it is known in advance that antigen detection will be necessary, the cells can be grown on a flat surface, such as a coverslip, within the cell culture tube, which can then subsequently be retrieved, fixed and stained. Antigen detection will allow distinction between, say, influenza A and B viruses, or parainfluenza 1, 2, 3 or 4 viruses, which all produce a similar positive haemadsorption test (see below).

Neutralization assays are used most commonly to distinguish between the various enteroviruses that grow in culture, or for serotyping adenoviruses. In principle, virus isolated in culture is distributed into a series of tubes, and to each tube a different antiserum is added (e.g. anti-polio-1, anti-polio-2, anti-polio-3 to tubes 1, 2 and 3 respectively). Following incubation of virus plus antiserum for 1 hour, the mixtures are added to individual cell culture tubes, and the appearance of CPE monitored over the next few days. The occurrence of a typical CPE in tubes 1 and 3, combined with the absence of a CPE in tube 2, would indicate that the original virus was poliovirus type 2.

Adaptations of cell culture

Virus isolation by cell culture is usually much slower than bacterial isolation on inanimate media. The fastest growing virus, herpes simplex virus, may produce a CPE after 18 hours, but most viruses require several days (or even weeks) to do so. This is a considerable disadvantage! Thus, various modifications of cell culture have been introduced, with the aim of speeding up the process. Two such modifications that have been widely adopted by diagnostic laboratories are those of haemadsorption and the detection of early antigen fluorescent foci.

Some viruses (e.g. the influenza and parainfluenza viruses, mumps virus) possess a haemagglutinin (i.e. a protein that binds red blood cells). Infected cells will express this molecule on their surfaces. Thus, if red blood cells are added to a cell culture tube in which such a virus is replicating, they will become adherent to the cell sheet, a phenomenon known as *haemadsorption* (see Figure 19.2a). Haemadsorption is demonstrable (by gently rotating the culture tube) for some days before a CPE has become evident. The exact nature of the haemadsorbing virus can be determined by staining with monoclonal antibodies, as described above (antigen detection).

The *detection of early antigen fluorescent foci* (DEAFF test) was developed specifically to accelerate the detection of cytomegalovirus (CMV) in cell culture. In essence, DEAFF is an adaptation of antigen detection, where the antigens to be detected are selected as those that appear early (within 24–48 hours) in the replication cycle of the virus (hence 'early antigens'). Thus, clinical material is inoculated onto a cell sheet grown on a coverslip or other flat surface (a type of culture known as a 'shell vial'). There is a centrifugation step ($2500 \times g$ for 1 hour) which greatly increases the infectivity of the cell sheet by virus. After 24 hours, the sheet is washed and then stained with a fluorescein-labelled monoclonal antibody directed against a CMV early antigen. The coverslip is then examined under UV light. A positive result is indicated by the presence of fluorescent nuclei in isolated cells (i.e. foci), which appear morphologically normal (see Figure 19.2b). This technique has been extended to other slow-growing viruses, e.g. adenoviruses can be detected long before any CPE is evident by staining with antibodies against early adenovirus antigens.

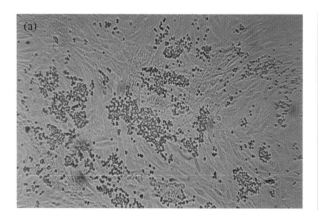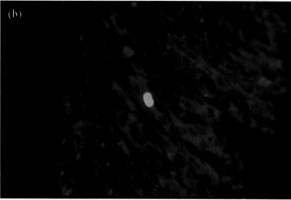

Figure 19.2. Adaptations of cell culture. (a) Haemadsorption. The cell sheet (primary monkey kidney) is normal ie no visible cytopathic effect has yet developed. However, many cells within the sheet are expressing a virally-encoded haemagglutinin on their surface, as the red cells, here seen as small dots overlying the cell sheet, have become attached to the sheet. (b) The DEAFF test. The cell sheet is stained with a fluorescently labelled anti-CMV monoclonal antibody. A single nucleus is seen shining bright apple-green under UV light, indicating the presence of CMV in this cell. All the cells (seen here counterstained with Evan's blue dye) are morphologically normal

Conclusions

Isolation of viruses in cell culture remains an important technique for the diagnosis of virus infections. In theory, a single virus particle within a clinical specimen can be grown in cell culture, and thereby expanded by many orders of magnitude, allowing accurate detection and characterization. The high degrees of sensitivity and specificity inherent in virus isolation are the 'gold standards' against which new techniques should be measured. The methodology is appropriate for a wide range of both clinical specimens and different viruses (Table 19.2). On rare occasions, its use results in the identification of unexpected or even previously unidentified viruses—HIV and the human herpesviruses 6 and 7 were first discovered in cell culture, and the latest virus to be identified in this way is the SARS coronavirus. It is a 'catch-all' technique, well suited to identification of the 'unknown' in clinical specimens.

The two major drawbacks to this approach are that not all viruses can be grown in culture and that some viruses are rather slow-growing. The development of new types of cell culture able to support an ever-widening array of viruses may overcome some of the former problem, whilst there are various adaptations of cell culture that can speed up the process of virus identification.

Table 19.2 Potential viral isolates from clinical material

Clinical specimen	Viruses that may be isolated in routine cell culture
Vesicle fluid or swab	Herpes simplex virus (HSV); varicella zoster virus
Nasopharyngeal aspirate (NPA) and/or throat swab	Respiratory syncytial virus; influenza A and B viruses; parainfluenza viruses 1–4; adenoviruses; rhinoviruses; enteroviruses; HSV; cytomegalovirus (CMV)
Faeces	Enteroviruses; adenoviruses
Cerebrospinal fluid	Enteroviruses; mumps virus
Urine	CMV; mumps virus
Conjunctival swab	HSV; adenoviruses
Blood (buffy coat)	CMV

Further reading

Lennette EH, Schmidt NJ (eds). *Diagnostic Procedures for Viral Rickettsial and Chlamydial Infections*, 7th edu. 1996: American Public Health Association, Washington, DC.

Cann AJ (ed.). *Virus Culture: A Practical Approach.* 1999: Oxford University Press, Oxford.

20

Serological tests in virology

Goura Kudesia

Introduction

Antibodies are produced by the immune system in response to various insults to the body, including infections, and serology is the science of measurement of these antibodies in the serum. Conventionally the term 'serology' also includes the study of serum for antigen and, by extension of the definition, any test involving an antigen–antibody reaction is defined as a serological test. Serological tests take advantage of the fact that most viral and many bacterial, fungal and parasitic infections elicit good antibody responses. These tests have been used for the diagnosis of viral diseases or other diseases where the organisms are not easily isolated, such as *Toxoplasma* and syphilis. In virus infections such as hepatitis B, where there is a prolonged viraemic phase, similar techniques can be used to detect viral antigen. This chapter, although mostly confined to virus serology, will also consider other serological tests currently used in serology laboratories for the diagnosis of infectious diseases and will deal with the principles, techniques, interpretation and future of these tests.

Principles

The class of antibody produced and the functional properties can both be exploited to measure the immune response after infection. The antibody classes most useful for measurement are IgM and IgG. The measurement of both secretory and serum IgA antibody may also be useful but is technically more demanding and therefore not used routinely in diagnostic laboratories. The initial antibody to be produced after primary infection is of the IgM class and generally becomes detectable 1–2 days after the onset of symptoms, remaining detectable for 6–12 weeks. Specific IgG antibody begins to rise at 1–2 weeks and remains detectable for many years, if not for the rest of the lifespan, after the infection. Virus-specific IgG antibody alone is therefore associated with past infection and in most cases denotes immunity to future infection. On the other hand, as the virus-specific IgM antibody is generally undetectable after 3 months, its presence indicates a recent infection. Figure 20.1 shows a graphic representation of the IgM and IgG response after primary infection. The measurement of virus-specific IgG and IgM antibody in a single serum sample can therefore aid in the diagnosis and help distinguish recent from past virus infection. Many techniques, such as enzyme-linked immunoassay (ELISA or EIA), immunofluorescent assay (IFA) and radioimmunoassay (RIA) have been developed to measure specific IgG and IgM. These assays are normally used for a 'qualitative' result, i.e. a positive or negative test result, and are not quantitative. They have similar principles whereby the antibody reaction with antigen is detected by addition of a second antibody directed against human immunoglobulin. The anti-immunglobulin is labelled with fluorescein (IFA), enzyme (ELISA) or radioisotope (RIA). These techniques can also be used for antigen detection.

Antibody produced in response to an infection may also differ in its functional property, i.e. it may be complement fixing, haemagglutinating or neutralizing. The antigens present on the virus determine the functional properties of the antibody produced in response, so only those viruses (e.g. rubella, measles or influenza) that posses haemagglutinin will elicit haemagglutinating antibodies. The knowledge of the antigenic structure of

The Science of Laboratory Diagnosis, Second Edition   Edited by David Burnett and John Crocker

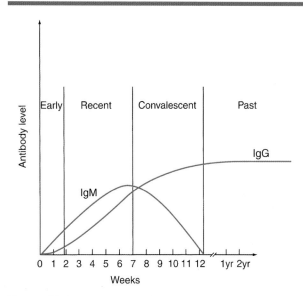

Figure 20.1 IgM and IgG response in early, recent, convalescent and past infection

viruses can be utilized for devising suitable serological tests, such as complement fixation (CF), haemagglutination (HA) or haemagglutination inhibition (HAI) tests. These tests detect both the IgG and IgM classes of antibody at the same time and are able to quantitate the serological response. Serial dilutions of the serum can be made to determine the titre of the antibody present. Paired acute and convalescent serum samples are required to make a diagnosis of recent infection, a four-fold or greater rise in antibody level being diagnostic.

Techniques

Serological techniques can be divided on the basis of the complexity of the test. The simplest are those in which the presence of antibody is shown by a simple interaction with antigen (precipitation or agglutination tests). Next are those that involve indicator systems to detect the antibody–antigen reaction (neutralization or complement fixation). The most complex tests involve the use of a second labelled antibody system, such as enzyme-linked immunosorbent assay (ELISA) or IFA.

Precipitation

Ouchterlony's double diffusion (DD) method can be used to detect either antibody or antigen. In the first case a known antigen is used and in the second case an antibody of known specificity is used. The antibody and antigen

diffuse towards each other in agarose gel and a line of white precipitation indicates a positive reaction. Counter-immunoelectrophorescence (CIE) specifically directs the movement of antigen and antibody towards each other in an electric field and hence is more rapid than DD. CIE was the method originally used in the detection of hepatitis B surface antigen. These methods have mostly been replaced by much more sensitive techniques, although some laboratories still use them for fungal antibody tests.

Haemagglutination and haemagglutination inhibition (HA and HAI)

The haemagglutinin possessed by certain viruses such as influenza, rubella and measles viruses has the property of agglutinating red blood cells (RBC) of selected species. HA tests are most commonly used with influenza viruses. Influenza A and B agglutinate human group O, guinea-pig and fowl RBCs at 4°C and 20°C, whereas influenza C agglutinates only fowl RBCs. HA tests are therefore useful in the detection and titration of viral antigen. HAI utilizes the presence of haemagglutinin on the virus to detect antibody. The test is based on the principle that specific antibody combines with the haemagglutinin and inhibits HA. Serial dilutions of patient's serum are allowed to react with a specified amount of haemagglutinin and appropriate indicator RBCs are then added. If specific antibody is present, it will block the haemagglutinin and a positive reaction is therefore shown by the absence of haemagglutination. Where specific antibody is absent, the viral haemagglutinin is free to agglutinate the indicator RBCs (negative reaction). In the past HAI tests were used extensively to establish immune status and to diagnose recent rubella virus infections. However, the HAI is complicated by the fact that the serum needs prior treatment to remove non-specific inhibitors and has therefore been replaced by more sensitive and specific techniques for the diagnosis of rubella. However, HAI is still used by reference laboratories for the identification and typing of influenza viruses. HA techniques can also be used for viruses that do not possess haemagglutinin. This is achieved by coupling the viral antigen to the surface of RBCs by a coupling agent such as tannic acid. When mixed with serum containing specific antibody, the RBCs are agglutinated because of the viral antigen bound to their surface (indirect or passive HA). Indirect HA has been used for the detection of antibody to toxoplasma. However, because of the instability of RBCs, inert carrier particles such as latex, gelatin and carbon particles are now being used.

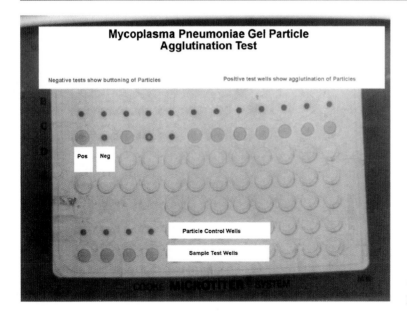

Figure 20.2 Mycoplasma pneumoniae gel particle agglutination assay

Particle agglutination tests

There are many tests based on particle agglutination. These tests are done on either a glass or cardboard slide or in microtitre wells. The following is not an exhaustive list but an example of some of the commonest tests in current use.

Latex agglutination (LA)

Polystyrene latex microparticles are sensitized or coated with viral antigen agglutinate when mixed with patient serum containing specific antibody. The antigen-coated latex particles are mixed with patient's serum on a glass slide or in a microtitre well. A visible agglutination pattern appears if specific antibody is present. These tests are in wide use in virus laboratories because of their speed, simplicity and ease of use. Currently good LA tests are available for rubella, toxoplasma and cytomegalovirus. LA tests are used for screening of both a single serum sample to establish immunity and paired sera to diagnose a recent infection.

Gelatin particle agglutination test (GPAT)

Gelatin particles are coated with antigen and serial dilutions of a patient's serum are tested in microtitre wells. The antibody titre is determined by the highest dilution of serum that agglutinates the antigen-coated particles. Non-specific agglutination may occur, therefore un-

coated gelatin particles are always included as control (Figure 20.2).

VDRL

VDRL is a serological test for screening for syphilis infection. A modification of the test uses antigen containing microparticulate carbon to screen for reagin antibody. The use of carbon particles enhances the visual reading of the test result on a white background.

Complement fixation (CF)

Patient serum, after inactivation at 56°C for 30 minutes to destroy indigenous complement, is added to a known amount of viral antigen and rabbit complement. If antibody–antigen reaction has occurred, then the complement is activated or 'fixed' or bound. An antigen and antibody detector system, in the form of sheep RBCs sensitized with rabbit antibody to sheep RBCs (haemolysin), is then added. If complement has been 'fixed' by the first antigen–antibody reaction, the sheep RBCs are not lysed, indicating a positive reaction and presence of specific antibody in the serum. A negative reaction is indicated by haemolysis of sensitized sheep RBCs by complement. The CF test is a quantitative test. The serum is diluted serially and the level of antibody is expressed as a reciprocal of the highest dilution of the serum giving rise to haemolysis of 50% of the sensitized RBCs. A four-fold rise in titre or seroconversion between

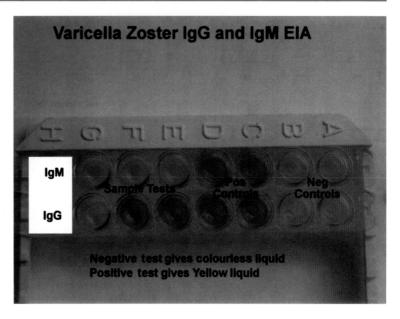

Figure 20.3 Varicella zoster IgG and IgM EIA

an acute and a convalescent sample is diagnostic. This technique requires considerable expertise and is labour-intensive but the serum can be tested against multiple antigens on a single occasion using the same indicator system. CF tests are done only in specialist virology laboratories and are still the tests of choice for the serological diagnosis of respiratory viral and atypical bacterial infections.

Neutralization

The interaction of specific antibody with virus neutralizes infectivity and prevents infection of a susceptible living host system by that virus. A major disadvantage of these tests is that a living host system, in the form of either a cell culture or living animals, is required, and hence many of these tests have been replaced by other techniques. Neutralization tests are still used to detect poliovirus antibody and certain toxins, such as that of *Clostridium difficile*.

Enzyme-linked immunosorbent assays (ELISA)

This is the most popular serological test in current use. There are many variations in methodology but all involve the attachment of antigen to a solid phase which is generally a polystyrene or polyvinyl plate or bead. Patient's serum is added and, after an appropriate length of time to allow the antibody to bind to the antigen on the solid phase, non-specifically bound mate-

rial and excess serum is removed by washing. An anti-human immunoglobulin labelled by conjugation with an enzyme (conjugate) is then added. The conjugate binds to the antibody in the antigen–antibody complex. Excess conjugate is then washed off and presence of the bound labelled anti-human immunoglobulin is detected by the addition of a suitable substrate for the labelling enzyme. If appropriate reactions have occurred, then the substrate is converted to a light-absorbing product and appears coloured. In the absence of antibody, no colour is produced (Figure 20.3). The intensity of the colour is directly related to the amount of antibody bound to the antigen. The colour change can be measured by the naked eye or read by a spectrophotometer to give the exact strength of reaction. The enzyme-substrate systems in common use are horseradish peroxidase (HRP) O-phenylene diamine (OPD), and alkaline phosphatase and p-nitrophenyl phosphatase. To adapt the test for detection of antigen, the solid phase is coated with antibody specific to the antigen to be detected. A second labelled antibody is then added to detect any antibody–antigen complex on the surface of the solid phase. Depending on the sequence of reaction, ELISAs are divided into direct, indirect, capture or competitive assays. Figure 20.4 explains some of the differences between these assays. The assays are specific for IgM or IgG, depending upon whether anti-human IgM or IgG immunoglobulin is used as the second antibody. For a detailed review, the reader is referred to Booth, 1983 (see Further Reading).

ELISA is a very sensitive technique because a small quantity of enzyme can process a large amount

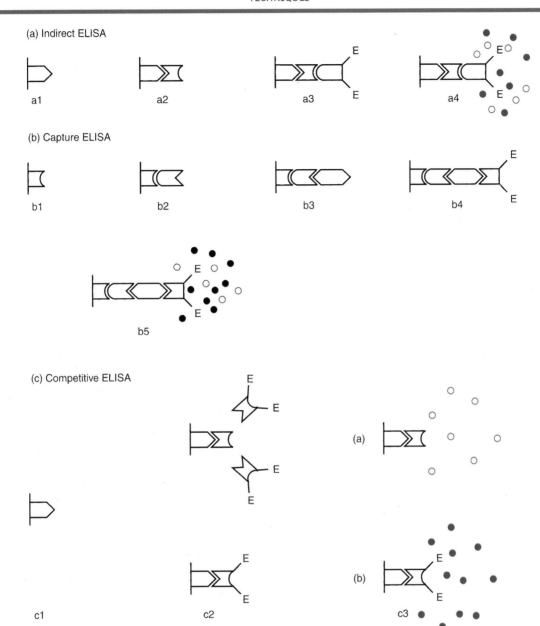

Figure 20.4 Different ELISA formats

(a) Indirect ELISA:
1. Coat solid phase with viral antigen.
2. Incubate with patient's serum. Specific antibody present attaches to antigen bound to solid phase.
3. Add enzyme labelled anti-IgG or -IgM.
4. Add substrate; colour change if reaction is positive.

(b) Capture ELISA:
1. Coat solid phase with anti-IgG or IgM.
2. Incubate with patient's serum. All IgG or IgM present is captured onto solid phase.
3. Add antigen; this will bind to any captured specific antibody.

4. Add enzyme-labelled antiviral IgG.
5. Add substrate; colour change if reaction is positive.

(c) Competitive ELISA:
1. Coat solid phase with antigen.
2. Add patient's serum and enzyme-labelled specific antibody. Specific antibody competes with the conjugate for attachment to solid phase.
3. Add substrate. Positive reaction is shown by no colour in (a), as conjugate has been blocked by specific antibody. Negative reaction is shown by colour in (b), as enzyme-labelled antibody has not been blocked.

of substrate. False negative IgM results may occur in the presence of high levels of specific IgG, which compete for the antigen on the solid phase. This can be avoided by removing the IgG prior to testing of the sample. Non-specific reactions in the IgM assay may also occur because of the presence of rheumatoid factor (RF). RF factor of the IgM class binds to new antigens exposed due to configurational changes on the Fc region of the specific IgG molecule when it binds to the antigen on the solid phase. IgM RF cannot be distinguished from virus-specific IgM, but RF can be removed by absorption with aggregated IgG prior to testing for IgM. Capture assays for IgM are preferred, as they are not affected by RF or specific IgG in the patient's serum. ELISAs have the advantage of being objective, can be easily automated and do not require great technical expertise. They are rapid tests and most assays can be completed within 2–3 hours. Most, if not all, microbiological laboratories are equipped to perform ELISAs, which are in extensive use for screening and serological diagnosis of HIV, viral hepatitis, rubella, cytomegalovirus, Epstein–Barr virus, varicella zoster virus, measles, mumps, toxoplasma, *Chlamydia trachomatis*, etc.

Immunofluorescence (IF)

In the indirect IF for detection of antibody, virally infected cells or bacterial antigen are fixed to wells on Teflon-coated glass slides, patient's serum is added and the antigen–antibody reaction is detected by the addition of anti-human immunoglobulin labelled with fluorescein dye (fluorescein isothionate). The reaction is read under a fluorescent light microscope, positive reactions being indicated by typical apple-green fluorescence. Indirect IF tests for the detection of IgM and IgG antibody to cytomegalovirus, Epstein–Barr and varicella zoster viruses have been in use for many years. False positive reactions due to the expression of receptors on infected cells, to which non-virus specific antibody of IgM class may bind, is a problem. IF tests also requires specialist equipment, such as a fluorescence microscope, and are subject to operator bias in reading. Therefore they have mostly been replaced by ELISAs for antibody detection. On the other hand, the availability of good quality monoclonals to a variety of viral antigens has made direct IF the method of choice for the detection of antigen in various tissues and samples. Infected material is fixed on to a glass slide with help of acetone or alcohol and stained with fluorescein-labelled monoclonal antibody directed against the antigen under test. Direct IF is used widely for the rapid diagnosis of respiratory viruses by testing of epithelial cells from nasopharyngeal aspirates for respiratory syncytical virus, influenza A and B viruses, parainfluenza 1, 2 and 3 viruses and adenoviruses.

Radioimmunoassays (RIA)

These have the same principles as ELISAs. RIA tests use a radioisotope label instead of an enzyme label. Because of the short shelf-life of the radiolabel and special radio-activity disposal requirements, they have been replaced by ELISAs.

Western blot (WB) or line immunoassay (LIA)

This provides a highly specific and sensitive tool for detecting and characterizing antibodies to microorganisms by virtue of their binding to antigens that have been affixed to nitrocellulose membranes. For WB, semi-purified viral or bacterial proteins are separated by electrophoresis on a polyacrylamide gel and then electrophoretically transferred to a nitrocellulose membrane. In LIA the viral antigens, produced by recombinant molecular techniques or artificially synthesized (synthetic peptides), are attached directly to the nitrocellulose membrane. The nitrocellulose membrane is incubated with patient's serum to allow antibody to bind to the antigens fixed on the membrane. Enzyme-labelled anti-human immunoglobulin is then added on a principle similar to that of ELISA. Appropriate washing steps are included. On addition of substrate, antigen bands, to which specific antibody is present, become visible.

The technique is unique in that antibody to single viral or bacterial proteins or antigenic epitopes can be detected, hence making the test very specific. They are used extensively as confirmatory tests for HIV and hepatitis C virus and for the diagnosis of Lyme disease.

Antibody avidity tests

Techniques to measure avidity of IgG antibody have been developed to aid in the timing of infection by serology. Antibody of low avidity is produced initially after primary infection, whereas high-avidity antibody is produced after reinfection or recrudescence. Antibody avidity tests are based on the principle that high avidity antibody–antigen complexes require more energy for dissociation or prevention of complex formation. In the test well, low-avidity antibody is either removed by washing with 8 M urea (dissociation) or bonds are prevented from forming by use of the protein denaturing agent guanidine hydrochloride in the serum diluent fluid. Control wells are treated with normal wash and diluent fluid. Solid phase-complexed antibodies are then detected in both test and control wells. If an antibody is of high avidity, then there is no significant difference between the test and control well reading, as these complexes are not easily dissociated or prevented from being formed. Avidity assays have been invaluable in the management of rubella and *Toxoplasma* infections in pregnancy, by helping to establish the timing of infection.

Serology on non-serum samples

IgG and IgM capture ELISAs have been adapted for the testing of urine and saliva samples. As these are non-invasive samples, they are preferred for children and other groups, such as intravenous drug abusers, where it is difficult to obtain blood samples. Serological diagnosis by testing of saliva is now available for measles, mumps and rubella. Large-scale serosurveillance of HIV infection is being done by testing urine and saliva.

Interpretation and use of serological tests

The ability to semi- or fully automate ELISAs has made these tests available to a vast number of laboratories. The older tests were technically demanding and limited to only a few specialist laboratories. The explosion in ELISA technology, along with awareness of the importance of viral infections in many vulnerable groups of patients, has made serology a mainstay of virus diagnosis.

Serology is now firmly established for the diagnosis of infections, especially viral diseases. Newer technology means that many of the routine diagnostic tests can be performed by general microbiology or other non-specialist laboratories.

Diagnosis of acute infections

Serological studies contribute significantly to the diagnosis of infectious diseases. Normally, a serological confirmation requires examination of a serum sample taken immediately after the onset of illness (acute) and a second sample 1–2 weeks later (convalescent). A four-fold rise in antibody or seroconversion from negative to positive antibody status between the acute and conva-

lescent samples indicates acute infection. New technologies for the detection of specific IgM and IgG, however, enable the laboratory to make a diagnosis or rule out a suspected infection on a single serum sample. For this, ELISAs are used extensively by microbiology laboratories. If neither IgM nor IgG is detected, then the patient has not been exposed to the organism or the sample was taken too early. As IgM antibody to most viruses can be detected within 1 week of the onset of symptoms, a sample taken at this time, if negative for viral IgM, is sufficient to rule out recent or current infection. Specific IgM can normally only be detected for 3 months but more sensitive assays may detect IgM for up to 12 months. As IgG will only be present later, a positive IgM reaction, with or without the presence of specific IgG, indicates recent infection. Specific IgG remains positive for life, therefore the presence of IgG alone, with negative IgM, indicates a past infection and in most cases immunity from further infection to that specific organism. It is clear that the test selection and interpretation of the result depends on the clinical condition and date of onset of symptoms, which should therefore always be communicated to the laboratory.

Detection of antibody to verify immunity

Verification of immunity to infections is required in many clinical situations, such as post-vaccination, pre-employment, pregnancy, pre-transplant or in immunosuppressed patients who may come in contact with infections. Tests to detect protective antibody have to be sensitive and require testing for specific IgG. Viral specific IgG ELISA, IFA or total antibody tests, such as the latex agglutination test, are used.

Post-vaccination seroepidemiological surveys to establish seroconversion and immunity after vaccination to measles, mumps, rubella and hepatitis B have formed a vital part of evaluation of the effectiveness of vaccination programmes. Automatable sensitive ELISAs have made mass post-vaccination screening feasible. Antibody to hepatitis B is expressed in international units and this ability to quantitate allows the clinician to decide on the timing of the follow-up boosters.

Immunity to rubella and hepatitis B is a prerequisite for employment for many health care workers. Immunity to other infections, such as varicella zoster virus, measles and mumps, is also desirable, especially for those working with children or immunocompromised patients, both to protect themselves and to prevent spread of infection to susceptible patients. Those who are susceptible to varicella zoster infection and who are exposed to chickenpox should be excluded from work, to avoid exposing susceptible patients to the infection.

During pregnancy, screening to detect protective antibody to rubella is offered to all patients, susceptible patients being vaccinated post-partum. It is recommended that all patients be screened for hepatitis B virus, and hepatitis B immunization is given to babies of infected mothers to prevent vertical transmission of infection. HIV screening for at-risk mothers enables specific drug treatment of the mother during pregnancy and labour to reduce the risk of vertical HIV transmission. Screening for antibody to other organisms, such as varicella zoster, toxoplasma and cytomegalovirus, enables the clinician to advise susceptible patients about how to avoid infection. All of these screens require a simple IgG ELISA or latex agglutination test. However, in case of recent contact with an infection, IgM assays have to be performed in addition to ensure that the IgG detected is from a past and not a current infection.

Transplanted and immunosuppressed patients

These patients are particularly prone to developing cytomegalovirus (CMV) infections. CMV antibody-negative patients who are given an organ from a CMV-positive donor require prophylaxis to prevent development of primary CMV infection. In addition, donor-acquired toxoplasma infection is a serious problem in heart transplant recipients, so all donors and recipients are screened for antibody to toxoplasma, and negative recipients of a heart from toxoplasma antibody-positive donors are given prophylasis. Immunosuppressed patients are also screened for common infections, such as chicken pox, herpes simplex and measles, as they may suffer from severe disease if exposed to them.

Screening for blood, organ and tissue donation

Many organisms, especially blood-borne viruses, can be transmitted via blood and blood products, organ and tissue transplantation. It is essential that blood be screened for these prior to transfusion. In the UK all blood is screened for HIV, hepatitis B, hepatitis C and syphilis. In the case of HIV and hepatitis C virus, the presence of antibody signifies current infection and screening for viral antigen is not necessary. Blood destined for immunosuppressed patients is also screened for CMV. Because of the importance of discarding infected blood, only the most sensitive tests are used.

Donations found to be positive are then subjected to confirmatory tests by specialist reference laboratories. To cope with the volume of screens required, Blood Transfusion Laboratories have automated ELISA systems for the microbiological screening of blood. Organ and tissue donors are subject to similar screening procedures.

Diagnosis of congenital infection

As maternal IgG crosses the placenta into the fetus, the presence of specific viral IgG in neonatal blood does not necessarily indicate infection. The persistence of IgG antibody beyond 6 months of age indicates congenital infection, as maternally derived antibody should have disappeared by then. The presence of specific IgM at or soon after birth indicates congenital or vertical infection, as the IgM class of antibody does not cross the placenta.

Future of serology

Although many infections can be rapidly diagnosed by the detection of virus-specific IgM by the techniques outlined in this chapter, for others, such as respiratory virus infections, only a retrospective diagnosis can be made because a convalescent sample is required to be tested by CFT. Many immunosuppressed patients may not mount a good antibody response, therefore absence of a virus-specific IgM response does not necessarily rule out infection in this patient group.

The advances in nucleic acid amplification techniques (NAAT), especially in real-time polymerase chain reaction (PCR) using automated technology, have enabled laboratories to offer PCR for routine diagnosis of viral infections. PCR-based assays are rapid; real-time PCR can be done in 2–3 hours. Many laboratories now choose to perform PCR assays to diagnose infection. By virtue of detecting viral RNA or DNA, they can pick up infection much earlier than an antibody response (as measured by the serological assays) is mounted. This is of advantage, especially in immunosuppressed patients.

IgM serological assays will, however, continue to be used to diagnose recent infections in those patients who do not present immediately, as IgM can be detected for up to 3 months post-infection and sometimes longer. Serological assays also have a crucial role in establishing evidence of immunity to infection, whether as a result of past infection or for post-vaccination follow-up. They are also an important epidemiological tool in sero-surveillance studies, which establish the prevalence of infection.

In the future, even though rapid and sensitive NAAT as PCR may replace serology for diagnosing current infection with many viruses, serology will continue to play an important role in supporting PCR in the diagnosis of recent infection. More importantly, it will still remain the mainstay in preventative medicine by establishing evidence of immunity post-vaccination, identifying those who are susceptible to infection so that they can be protected and in studying the epidemiology of virus infections.

Further reading

Booth JC. The use of the enzyme-linked immunosorbent assay (ELISA) technique in clinical virology. *Recent Advances in Clinical Virology*, Waterson AP (ed.). 1983: Churchill-Livingstone, Edinburgh, 73–98.

James K. Immunology of infectious diseases. *Clin Microbiol Rev* 1990; **3**(2): 132–152.

Parry JV, Perry KR, Mortimer PP. Sensitive assays for viral antibodies in saliva: an alternative to tests on serum. *Lancet* 1987; **2**: 72–75.

Thomas HIJ. Specific antibody avidity studies in clinical microbiology: past, present and future. *PHLS Microb Dig* 1995; **12**(2): 97–102.

21

Automated tests in virology

Roger P Eglin

Introduction

Diagnostic testing in clinical laboratories has evolved over the past 50 years from manual operation of tests such as examination of blood films and simple chemistry assays using techniques requiring relatively large quantities of blood, serum or plasma. The 1960s saw the development of the multichannel analyser for clinical chemistry and the introduction of electronic counting methods, e.g. Coulter counter. The continued development of such automated testing began to concentrate on improvements in the quality and consistency of results and to reduce both the times taken for assays and the volume of sample required for each assay. Although sophisticated automated systems have been in routine use in other areas of pathology for the past 20 years, microbiology and particularly virology laboratories used traditional testing methods. For virology these were based around cell culture and virus isolation with antibody tests using reagents produced largely in house. Enzyme immunoassays (EIAs) were introduced in the 1970s and their commercial developments have allowed progress to be made towards automation. Impetus was given to the development of such equipment by the requirement of the Blood Transfusion Service (now National Blood Authority) to screen blood donations for a limited but steadily increasing range of blood-borne virus infections. This began with HBs antigen in the 1970s, then followed anti-HIV in 1984, selective anti-CMV in the 1980s and anti-HCV in 1991. The great expansion in the range of commercial EIAs in the 1980s extended the use of standard protocols and encouraged manufacture of automated systems. It is only since the

early 1990s that a range of such equipment has been developed specifically for the diagnostic virology laboratory. A wide range of routine diagnostic assays is now in the repertoire of these automated machines. The assays available are based around the EIA technique. The early systems were developed for the screening tests most frequently requested, i.e. HBs antigen, anti-HBs, rubella IgG and *Chlamydia trachomatis* antigen. After the initial rush to market a variety of automated equipment in the early 1990s, the marketplace has now become more stable. It has become possible to identify different classes of machines and to identify the type of workload that is most appropriate to each of the classes of instrument. Working definitions of the type of automation to be discussed are as follows.

Liquid handling processor (LHP)

An LHP (a) completes the preparation of a microplate containing appropriately diluted samples and test-specific controls using a worksheet to identify the samples and protocols specific to the test required; and (b) completes the separation of serum from a blood clot and so prepares a serum store from blood samples received.

Automated EIA processor

An automated EIA processor (a) completes an EIA with only the supply of samples and reagents specific to that test; and (b) completes an EIA with only the addition of a microplate containing appropriately diluted samples

The Science of Laboratory Diagnosis, Second Edition   Edited by David Burnett and John Crocker

and reagents specific to that test. The equipment may then be subdivided into the following classes:

- *Random access/batch testing.* EIA processors are generally designed for specific tests on specimens which have been accumulated as a batch and are identified by a specific worksheet. Some processors are also able to run tests on single specimens, to allow response to urgent clinical demand. These single tests require control calibrators for the test in addition to the test sample. It may be possible to interrupt the current testing to run the urgent specimen or it may be introduced at a convenient time between batches of other tests. These random access machines require manufacturer-specific test modules or use of controls that are permanently on board to operate the test.

- *Single tube format/microplate format.* Some processors operate by sampling the specimen tube directly and perform all subsequent operations as single tube tests, e.g. VIDAS, E7001. Other processors accept single tube specimens but set up the test using microplates. This plate format may still be manufacturer-specific, or may allow any standard EIA-based microplate to be used.

- *Manufacturer-specific test system/accept any microplate assay.* The manufacturer's processing system is unique and use of the processor dictates that all the tests to be used must also be purchased from that manufacturer, e.g. VIDAS, AXSYM, PRISM. Other processors have been designed to handle any microplate-based EIA and the choice of manufacturer for each test to be used lies with the laboratory and may be decided by the performance characteristics of the test. Some examples of current equipment available in each class are given in Table 21.1.

Table 21.1 Which automated equipment is most appropriate?

Type of machine	Advantages	Disadvantages
Random access—manufacturer-specific tests	Rapid testing of single samples Requires a full set of control samples once/month Does not require full set of controls for each test, uses calibrators Wide range of assays available covering several disciplines Share costs with other users of machine (biochemistry, immunology)	Daily throughput may be small, e.g. 300/day Total laboratory throughput in a normal working day may be > 400 samples Premium paid for same single commercial supplier of both test modules and equipment Limited range of infectious diseases tests may be available If used as a core laboratory facility, can the current test runs really be interrupted?
Batch testing—two or three microplate-based system	May also include sample dispensing May be able to run any microplate-based system	May be manufacturer-specific tests, e.g. AXSYM (chemiluminescence). Is a full range of infectious diseases tests available? May only achieve three batched runs in a normal working day Careful scheduling of test runs may be required
Open access microplate-based system	Uses any EIA-based microtitre plate assay Capable of accepting next test plate at any time	May require separate sample dispensing equipment
Sample dispensing system	Allows flexibility of unlabelled or unlinked sample handling Can be used for other purposes, e.g. sample aliquots for serum store into bottles/microplates, CFT, SRH	Costs may be increased

How automation works in the diagnostic laboratory

In order to discuss this topic, it is necessary to make the following assumptions: firstly, that the laboratory uses a diagnostic software programme for handling its patient database; secondly, that specimens are given unique identity by means of a bar-coding system with labels on the associated request form, primary blood tube and archived serum sample; and thirdly, that the laboratory is using an automated system comprising an LHP and microplate based EIA processor.

Following reception of the specimen and request form in the laboratory, the first two stages in processing often occur simultaneously.

Worksheets

A set of tests is ordered which is appropriate to the clinical details and date of onset stated on the request form. This set of tests is logged on to the computer and leads to the creation of test-specific worksheets, which may then be called off as required according to the daily planning sheet for the automated system.

Serum separation

After centrifuging the primary blood tube, to spin down the blood clot, the serum is separated by the LHP or manually into a storage tube, which is labelled with the same bar-code identification as the primary blood tube.

Preparing the microplates for the assay

If a random access system is in use then the serum storage bottle will be loaded directly onto the system and the required dilutions made by the machine. The LHP should be able to identify sample tubes or primary blood tubes in racks or carousels. It will check that all the samples on the current worksheet are present and then proceed to make appropriate dilutions of the serum into wells, following the specific protocol. The plate will be bar-coded to allow positive identification and selection of the correct protocol by the software. This will then allow the software to order the appropriate reagents for the specific EIA. It should also add the appropriate standards, both those supplied by manufacturers and laboratory in house samples, and calibration samples

as necessary to allow quality control (QC) of the test run. These QC specimens will be dispensed into wells designated in the protocol. The system will flag up any samples for which it has failed to collect liquid.

EIA processor

The plate is identified by bar-code and the software identifies both the correct worksheet and the correct protocol associated with that test run. The machine checks that the requested EIA reagents have been placed correctly in the system and the volumes of these on board reagents are checked by weight. This checking includes the wash buffer, test reagents and ensures that there is sufficient spare volume in the waste bottle. The first step, which is part of the quality control monitoring of the system, is to take a spectrophotometric reading of the plate to check that a specimen has been added to each of the expected wells. A well with a discrepant optical density (OD) reading identifies where no sample is present. The processor starts the EIA and follows the protocol stored in the software. If an open access system is in use, then the processor will recalculate the time slots for the assays already in process and fit in the new plate to start processing as soon as possible. The start time will be displayed together with a warning if the time delay before starting the assay exceeds the default time for the system. Generally EIAs which use incubations at room temperature are avoided because, although the incubation periods are often longer than those with $37°C$ incubations, the first incubation reactions start immediately the diluted sample is dispensed into the wells. Incubations at $37°C$ or $40°C$ allow a fixed start time and this is necessary for the open access machines. The EIA protocol followed by the processor should include monitoring after each step requiring addition of liquid reagents and also monitoring of the wash heads after each operation to ensure that all the wells have been washed correctly. The read-out from each liquid addition monitoring should be displayed as the EIA proceeds and any errors detected flagged up immediately. If an open access machine is in use then each batch of test reagents should be added when requested by the processor.

Data handling

The final optical density (OD) readings, taken on completion of the assay, are transferred automatically to the system software for manipulation by the data reduction package. This package will, depending on the type of assay, either (a) calculate the cut off value from the controls and apply it to the sample OD values, in which case the results will be expressed as positive, negative or equivocal for each specimen, or (b) generate a standard curve from the controls and apply it to the sample readings in which case the results for the samples will be expressed as units/ml.

The software also checks that the manufacturer's calibrators and standards which have been included in the run are in range and flags up any discrepancies. If the calibrators have acceptable values then the stored standard values are applied to the sample ODs for the current test run. After validation of the displayed results by the experienced technician, the results are transferred automatically to the worksheet. This worksheet may be printed for hard copy storage, and contains all the necessary information to track back the details of the assay should any problems be discovered at a later date. These details include for both assay plate and associated reagents, the type, batch number, expiry date of the plate and reagents, date of assay, worksheet requester, assay performer and results validator. From the worksheet the results are electronically transferred to the individual patient records in the laboratory database.

The software will also perform the required internal quality control (System Process Control) checks on the run by: (a) updating the 20 rolling averages for the control samples and flagging any discrepant results; and (b) updating the Shewhart charts (Costongs et al., 1995) with the new control results. It then applies the associated chosen Westgard rules to check that the run is valid and may be released. Any results which are found to be out of range by these criteria will be flagged up for immediate action.

A model for this automated processing and process control, which achieves a very high level of quality assurance can be found in the Microbiology screening performed in the Testing laboratories at NBS Centres. These 10 Centres process a total of approximately 10,000 donations per day on fully automated screening for HBsAg, anti-HCV and anti-HIV. The assay kits used must all have sample addition monitoring, with positive monitoring of every reagent addition as the ideal. The error rate of the process is less than 0.1%. The screening results are released directly into the national IT system by 2 pm on the day after collection, in order to release for issue the components produced from the blood donation. These laboratories are compliant with General Manufacturing Practice and are regularly inspected.

Should the Laboratory Automate?

The above describes the operation of an automated system within the laboratory. Prior to this, the decision must be made to move to an automated system for EIA testing. The preparative work involved in reaching this decision is considerable and includes several analytical steps. It will also involve major changes in work patterns in the laboratory and the staff must be involved in this development project to achieve new ways of working. The next section describes some of the important factors to be considered during this review process.

Analyse the current laboratory business

This includes the range of viruses, types and number of tests undertaken by the laboratory. Review the current turnaround times for results required by the contracted service level agreements. Is there room for improvement to meet clinical demands for more timely results? Is random access testing a realistic option for small numbers of any test which are currently batched to one or two runs a week? If large volumes of some screening assays are identified, are these tests currently EIA-based and if not, can the test be moved successfully to EIA with no loss of quality and perhaps an improvement in sensitivity and specificity (Figure 21.1)? Decide how to

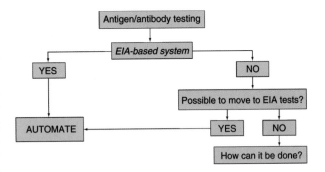

Figure 21.1 Automation flowchart

batch the regular screening tests to one or two runs a day (around 30 tests is usually the minimum number per batch, for economic reasons); is a daily run required; is a same-day result service provided? Define the requirement for one-off urgent or on-call testing and estimate how many could fit into the normal runs without delaying the result unduly (Figure 21.2).

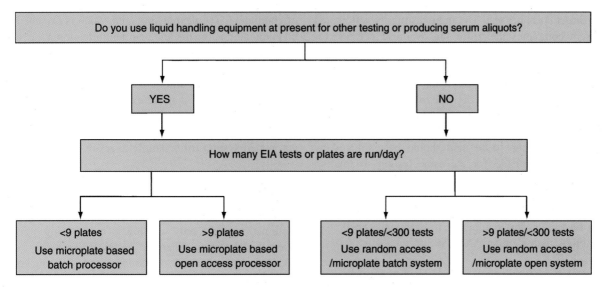

Figure 21.2 Which type of equipment to choose?

Which type of equipment to choose?

A primary laboratory (district general hospital laboratory) undertaking routine screening of a relatively small number of samples can choose a small dedicated machine; make use of the infectious diseases range of tests on the large pathology department analyser; and under- write the cost of equipment by running a screening test on the machine to be used for random access, e.g. antibiotic assays.

A secondary laboratory (teaching hospital laboratory, large referral laboratory) undertaking a wide. range of tests on a large number of samples: requires a large throughput of specimens daily and provides a wide range of tests; consider batch runs, decide how many runs per day are required—most EIAs are completed within three hours. This allows two runs in the normal working day plus one run overnight. For a three-plate system this equates to nine plates/day. Open access systems will complete eight test plates every five hours.

The final choice of equipment requires detailed comparison of their performance, mechanics, quality systems and software and lies beyond the scope of this chapter.

Quality issues

The transfer to an automated system will realise a number of benefits to the laboratory. The system removes subjectivity from all aspects of the procedures used. The runs will be completed reproducibly and follow the protocol exactly on every occasion. Variations in the protocols will only occur when the protocol is amended by the system manager. This standardisation will improve the reproducibility of assays, as judged by the CVs of standards (Westgard *et al.*, 1981). The automated system ensures positive identity of the sample throughout the testing and allows the laboratory to approach the standards already demanded of the NBS laboratories. This security of identity resides with the bar-coding of all specimens and all EIA plates throughout the system. The monitoring of liquid additions and washing stages confirms that all steps of the protocol have been successfully achieved. It allows identification of the point of breakdown in the system in the event of a test run failing the quality control validation. Automated transfer of the worksheet from the laboratory diagnostic software to the automated system software and return of the validated results directly to the patient database removes transcription errors completely. Turnaround times for testing maybe reduced with the results produced in a time frame that is effective in assisting with patient management.

Financial considerations

Changing work practices allows increased numbers of tests per member of staff. This leads to greater income generation, either by fewer staff with the original workload or, if staffing levels do not change, then extra new work can be introduced, driven by customer demands. Increasing the number of tests spreads the staff costs over a large number of specimens and helps to reduce the direct costs per test. The more testing the automated system completes the lower the overhead per test for capital depreciation of the system and annual maintenance charges. The choice between outright purchase rather than leasing or reagent rental must be made and it will depend largely upon the type of equipment required and the financial position of the laboratory at that time. If it is decided to use a manufacturer-specific system then the premium to be paid should be estimated by costing routine EIAs for the same testing. If random access equipment is required, the expected number of samples requiring this urgent treatment should be estimated and a current routine screening test identified that can be run on this equipment to defray the costs, e.g. antibiotic assays on an AXSYM.

Improve the competitive position of the laboratory

Acquisition of an automated system in the laboratory allows for repositioning the role of the laboratory within the pathology department. It should be possible to become the core facility for the provision of EIA-based testing within pathology and cover a large range of testing for virology, bacteriology, immunology and biochemistry. A significant improvement in some turn-around times for results should be achieved. The laboratory is well placed to undertake evaluation work for new test developments and for field trailing tests before they reach the marketplace. The laboratory stores a large range of samples for all routine tests and can offer completely reproducible testing, following protocols that have been set up and trialed by the commercial company.

Other developments in automation

This chapter has discussed the automation of antibody and antigen EIAs for which there is now a wide choice of equipment. The next testing area which is expected to be automated is the nucleic acid amplification assay and specifically the PCR assay. It is already possible to use automated systems which run batches of PCR amplifications and detections automatically. In the next year or two it is anticipated that the extraction of nucleic acids from relatively clean samples, such as serum and plasma will be automated and this will then give a totally automated system from sample to result.

Conclusions

Automation is the only solution to maintaining a cost-effective laboratory. There is downward pressure from all sides on the finances of the laboratory, ranging from cost reductions expected year on year in contracts to the ever-increasing demands for more testing and for an increasing range of new tests. It is essential that old technology is not clung to unnecessarily. New systems are available and re-engineering of the laboratory to make best use of these systems is the way forward. This entails getting the confidence of the staff in making these changes. They need to see the benefits of implementation of new systems and the emergence of completely new areas of work, e.g. viral load, that are continuing to appear at an unprecedented rate. In order to cope with these major changes it will be essential to invest in the staff in terms of retraining and learning new skills.

Further reading

Costongs GM, van Oers RJ, Leerkes B, Janson PC. Evaluation of the DPC IMMULITE random access immunoassayanalyser.. *Eur J Clin Chem and Clin Biochem* 1995; **33**, 887–892.

Westgard JO, Hunt MR, Groth T. A multi-Shewhart chart for quality control in clinical chemistry. *Clin Chem* 1981; **27**(1): 493–501.

22

Molecular techniques in virology

Paul E Klapper

Introduction

Molecular biological techniques pervade virology. Their application in the fields of antiviral drug discovery have aided rational drug design and radically improved the pace of the discovery and application of antiviral compounds; they have aided the development of antiviral vaccines and improved the range of vaccines available for use; and they have revolutionized and continue to revolutionize clinical virology. The application of these procedures has enabled the discovery of many of the newly described human pathogenic viruses (Table 22.1) and dramatically condensed the period of time from initial recognition of a disease-causing agent through to full characterization, development of diagnostic test methods and production of reliable serological tests of infection (e.g. the coronavirus caused severe acute respiratory syndrome (SARS) originating in Guandong Province, People's Republic of China, in November 2002). Not only are molecular diagnostic procedures among the major current methods for diagnosis of virus infection but they also have an increasingly important role in the day-to-day management of patients' antiviral therapy.

Nucleic acid amplification techniques

Nucleic acid amplification techniques (NAATs) form the mainstay of techniques utilized in a modern clinical virology laboratory. The techniques can be classified as 'target', 'probe' or 'signal' amplification procedures. In 'target' NAATs the nucleic acid present in a sample is directly amplified to a level where it may be readily detected. In 'probe' NAATs the action of binding of a specific nucleic acid probe sequence leads to the amplification and subsequent detection of the probe. In 'signal' NAATs the initial binding to a target molecule results in a signal which is itself amplified to a level where the signal can be readily identified. The distinction between the techniques is often blurred because 'target' amplification procedures often include an element of 'signal' and/or 'probe' amplification.

A number of commercially available assays are now available for use under these formats, based upon different principles and with different procedural steps. However, the commercial products are only available for a limited range of viral pathogens and, in consequence, most clinical laboratories will use a combination of commercially available tests and their own 'in-house' (i.e. 'home-brewed', self-manufactured) test procedures, the latter almost exclusively being based upon the polymerase chain reaction (PCR).

Target amplification

Polymerase chain reaction

Due to its versatility and ease of use, the first developed of the NAATs, PCR, is also the most widely employed technique. PCR involves the use of two synthetic oligonucleotide molecules, each of which hybridize to one strand of a double-stranded DNA (dsDNA) target. These oligonucleotide molecules are carefully designed to bind to a specific target region within the nucleic acid of the virus nucleic acid to be amplified. They span a defined

The Science of Laboratory Diagnosis, Second Edition   Edited by David Burnett and John Crocker
© 2005 John Wiley & Sons, Ltd

Table 22.1   A representative list of newly human viral pathogens characterized through the use of molecular biological techniques

Virus	Associated disease	Discovered using
Hepatitis E virus	Infectious hepatitis	Reverse transcription PCR with random primers + animal transmission experiments
Hepatitis C virus	Transfusion-associated hepatitis	Reverse transcription PCR with random primers to produce cDNA library
Sin nombre virus	Hantavirus pulmonary syndrome	Consensus sequence-based PCR
Human herpesvirus 8	Kaposi's sarcoma, Castlemaine's disease	Representational difference analysis
GBV a–c viruses	Transfusion-associated hepatitis	Representational difference analysis
TTV virus	Transfusion-associated hepatitis	Representational difference analysis
Nipah virus	Encephalitis and pneumonia	Reverse transcription PCR with random primers
Metapneumovirus	Respiratory disease	Reverse transcription PCR with random primers
SEN virus	Transfusion-associated hepatitis	Reverse transcription PCR with random primers
SARS—coronavirus	Severe acute respiratory disease	Reverse transcription PCR with random primers

region within that nucleic acid. The hybridization of oligonucleotide to the DNA acts as a primer for a DNA polymerase enzyme (most commonly a heat-stable enzyme originally derived from the thermophilic bacterium, *Thermus aquaticus* and known as Taq polymerase). The enzyme creates a complementary DNA strand by sequentially adding deoxynucleotides. In order to initiate this process, the target dsDNA is heated to a temperature in excess of 90°C. At this temperature the DNA strands dissociate. The reaction mixture is then cooled to a temperature of 50–70°C and the synthetic oligonucleotide primer molecules bind to each of the single strands of DNA. The temperature is then raised slightly to 72–76°C, the optimal temperature for Taq polymerase to effect extension of the complementary DNA strand. By repeating the temperature cycling over 30 or more repetitive cycles, millions of copies of the original target sequence are produced. The rate of temperature change and length of time are controlled by a programmable thermal cycler (Figure 22.1). On completion of

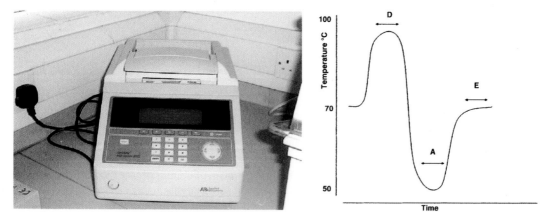

Figure 22.1   Programmable thermocycler. A typical programmable thermocycler, together with an idealized temperature profile of a single PCR cycle. D, denaturation; A, annealing of primers; E, extension of DNA. The programmable instrument automates these extension, heating and cooling cycles of the PCR technique

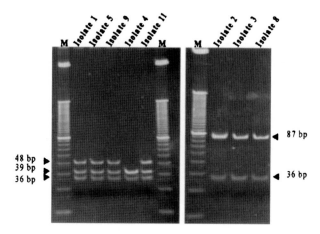

Figure 22.2 PAGE with ethidium bromide staining. An illustration of PCR products separated on 8% polyacrylamide gels. The example shown is of a method for typing adenoviruses by restriction enzyme digestion of PCR products. Ethidium bromide intercalates with double-stranded DNA and is revealed by ultraviolet light transillumination of the gel. M, molecular weight ladder used to calibrate the size of the PCR products

amplification, the reaction mixture is analysed to determine whether specific amplification has occurred. The conventional method has been to electrophorese the reaction mixture in agarose or polyacrylamide gels in the presence of ethidium bromide. Ethidium bromide intercalates with dsDNA and, when exposed to ultraviolet light, will fluoresce to reveal the nucleic acid (Figure 22.2). Southern blotting may be used to confirm the specificity of the test reaction product. In Southern blotting a labelled oligonucleotide designed to bind to the inter-primer region of the nucleic acid reaction product is allowed to hybridize with the electrophoretically separated product and its binding is revealed by detection, using autoradiography. A less laborious hybridization detection method is to denature the amplified DNA and capture the single-stranded DNA onto a solid phase (usually a polystyrene microtitre plate) through the use of avidin or biotin incorporated within one of the oligonucleotide primers. A labelled oligonucleotide is allowed to bind to the captured amplicon DNA and its binding revealed in a reaction involving enzyme-catalysed conversion of a chromogenic substrate.

To detect RNA viruses, an initial reaction to produce a DNA copy (cDNA) of the RNA template is necessary. This is accomplished by the use of reverse transcription, effected by the addition of either a separate reverse transcriptase enzyme or enzymes capable of thermostable reverse transcription and DNA polymerase activity.

A wide variety of modifications of the basic PCR procedure are possible, including nested PCR involving the use of four primer oligonucleotides in two separate reactions. The products of a first round of PCR amplification are re-amplified in a second round of thermal amplification, using a second set of primer oligonucleotides internal to the set utilized in the first round of thermal amplification.

The choice of methodology is dictated by the requirements of desired sensitivity and specificity, coupled with the practical circumstances under which the PCR is performed. A high degree of technical skill, together with dedicated premises and equipment, are required for all PCR procedures, but nested PCR requires additional dedicated premises because of the need to physically separate first- and second-round procedures to prevent carry-over of amplified DNA ('amplicons') from a first round amplification into a second round, leading to false positive test results.

To improve the utility of PCR in the clinical virology laboratory setting, PCRs capable of detecting multiple viral nucleic acid targets have been developed. These 'multiplex' PCR techniques typically incorporate several pairs of primer oligonucleotides within a single reaction. Amplification of any of several target nucleic acids is then possible, using the same thermal cycling conditions and reaction mixture composition.

The large majority of PCR methods in current use provide only qualitative (yes/no) answers. Determination of the amount of virus present in a sample, so-called 'viral quantitation' or 'viral load monitoring', is of increasing importance in assessing the effect of antiviral chemotherapy and in monitoring progression toward disease. For example, monitoring of the blood of bone marrow transplant recipients for cytomegalovirus (CMV) DNA allows pre-emptive therapy with the antiviral drug ganciclovir to prevent the development of CMV disease. Antiviral therapy is usually instituted when a significant rise in blood CMV DNA levels are detected. Serial dilution of a sample in parallel with a standard containing known amounts of viral nucleic acid can provide crude quantitation, but is open to error caused by differential amplification of the two samples, and this renders inter-test comparisons of quantitation difficult. More accurate quantitation is obtained by the competitive co-amplification of an internal control nucleic acid of known concentration, together with the sample nucleic acid of unknown concentration, the internal control molecule being designed to amplify with efficiency equal to the sample target. The method has formed the basis of highly successful commercial assays for hepatitis B and C viruses, human immunodeficiency

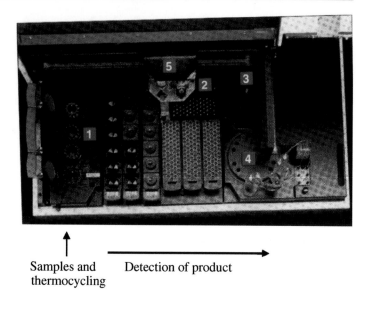

Samples and   Detection of product
thermocycling

Figure 22.3 Internal layout of the Roche Diagnostics Cobas® Amplicor instrument. Thermal cycling and detection of product by an enzyme-linked microparticle-based assay system are automated in this instrument

1 Cyclers 2 x 12 place detection stations   2 Incubator   3 Reader

4 Wash station   5 Automated pipetting unit

virus (HIV) and cytomegalovirus. In the latter system, a high degree of automation of the assay and the detection of product further reduces inter-test variability (Figure 22.3).

Real-time PCR

Kinetic or 'real-time' PCR is a method that is increasingly replacing conventional PCR. This has become possible by the labelling of primers, probes or the amplicon with fluorogenic molecules. As a specific product accumulates, the increased fluorescence emitted from the reaction reveals the accumulation. In contrast to conventional PCR, post-amplification detection of product through manipulation of the reaction mixture is not necessary. The product is detected within a closed sample tube. The possibility of amplicon-derived cross-contamination of tests is thus greatly reduced and, as the accumulation of amplified nucleic acid is detected as it happens, the test is completed much more swiftly. In addition, the range of concentrations over which accurate quantitation of product is possible is much greater than can be achieved in more conventional competitive PCR formats.

Several methods are available to achieve fluorescence detection in real-time PCR. In its most simple guise, compounds such as ethidium bromide or SYBR® green 1 are added to the reaction mixture. These bind to dsDNA and fluoresce when excited by light of an appropriate wavelength. This approach is not ideal, in that the formation of artefactual primer–primer dimers and non-specific amplification of irrelevant non-target DNA can produce false positive fluorescent signals. This problem can be addressed by heating the final product and measuring the temperature of dissociation of products. Primer dimers will dissociate at a lower temperature than that characteristic for the specific PCR product.

The specificity of real-time PCR is greatly improved by the use of labelled oligonucleotide 'probes' labelled with a fluorescent probe. A variety of methods of labelling and detecting the probe are possible. Two of the most popular are the hybrid probe or the 5′ endonuclease (also known as the Taqman®) probe methods. Hybridization probes require two probe oligonucleotides; one is labelled with a 3′ donor fluorophore and the second is labelled with a suitable acceptor fluorophore. The oligonucleotides bind to the target nucleic acid adjacent to one another and, when the fluorophore is

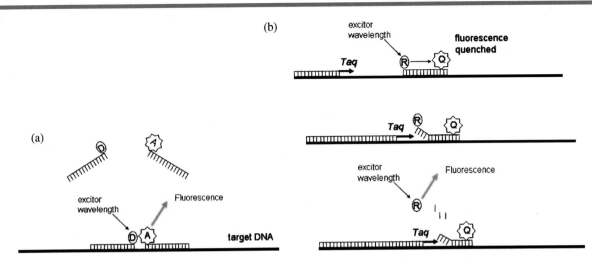

Figure 22.4   Real-time PCR. (a) Hybridization probes. Oligonucleotides bind adjacently to the target DNA; when excited by light of a suitable wavelength, the donor (D) fluorophore transfers energy via FRET to the acceptor fluorophore (A), which emits fluorescent light. (b) Taqman probes. As *Taq* DNA polymerase extends the DNA chain, it encounters the hybridization probe bound to the template DNA. The 5′–3′ endonuclease activity of Taq displaces and degrades the oligonucleotides, releasing the reporter fluorophore (R) from the oligonucleotide, thereby separating it from the quencher fluorophore (Q) and allowing the reporter to fluoresce

activated via light at a suitable wavelength, it fluoresces and, by a process known as fluorescent resonance energy transfer (FRET), transfers energy to the adjacent 5′ acceptor fluorophore, which then emits light at a different wavelength (Figure 22.4). Detection of this emission signals specific binding of the adjacent oligonucleotide probes to their target nucleic acid. An alternative to the use of these dual probes is the use of a single oligonucleotide and the ability of Taq polymerase to act as a 5′–3′ endonuclease. A fluorophore is attached to the 5′ end of a probe oligonucleotide and a second fluorophore is added-usually to the 3′ end of the probe oligonucleotide. Under normal circumstances the excitation of one fluorophore leads to FRET transfer of fluorescence to the other fluorophore. This leads to the emission of light of a different wavelength, which is not usually detected. The fluorescence is said to be quenched. When the oligonucleotide hybridizes with its target nucleic acid, the fluorophores are released by hydrolysis and the fluorescence is no longer quenched (Figure 22.4). Numerous alternatives to these exist, including peptide nucleic acid probes ('Light-up[TM]' probes), hairpin oligonucleotide probes ('molecular beacons') and self-fluorescing amplicons (e.g. 'Sunrise[TM]' primers or 'Scorpion[TM]' primers).

There are now a wide variety of instruments available for use in real-time PCR. One of the most rapid of these instruments is the 'Lightcycler[®]' (Figure 22.5). A plastic seated glass capillary is used as the reaction vessel. The capillary allows very rapid heating and cooling of reactants and also allows direct detection of fluorescence within the reaction vessel. Heating and cooling are achieved using a thermal element and a fan. The capillaries are rotated in front of a blue-emitting laser diode and fluorescence within the capillary is monitored through three photodetection diodes, each with different wavelength filters for activation. The rapid heating and cooling achieved in this system (20°C/second) means that a typical thermal cycle profile of 40 cycles can be completed in 20 minutes.

Automation and PCR

The high level of technical skill required to perform conventional PCR has to some extent been addressed by the increasing availability of commercial test kits. A major stumbling block has been the need for reliable, high-throughput methods for the extraction of nucleic acids. Recent developments in robotics and standardization of reagents have now led to the development of several platforms capable of automating sample preparation and assay set-up. These methods reduce the technical skill required for PCR performance, improve test reproducibility and are conducive to high-throughput testing, helping to introduce NAAT testing to a wider range of clinical laboratories and for a wider range of viral pathogens.

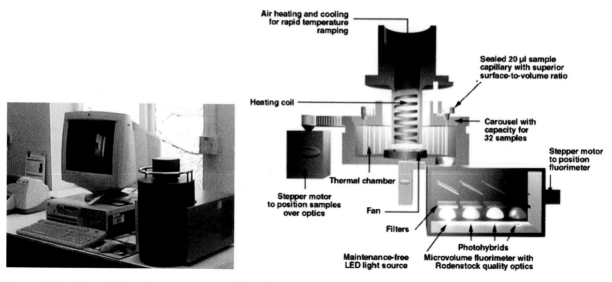

Figure 22.5 The Lightcycler instrument. Schematic drawing of internal layout of instrument. Reproduced from www.lightcycler-online.com, with permission

Transcription mediated amplification

A number of alternative methods for target amplification have been developed. Transcription-mediated amplification (TMA) is an example. Following a proprietary extraction technique to release and stabilize nucleic acid from the virion, the test sample is heated briefly to 95°C to denature the target nucleic acid. In order to amplify nucleic acid, an oligonucleotide to which a promoter sequence for RNA polymerase has been attached binds specifically to the target. If the target nucleic acid is RNA, in an isothermal reaction, a reverse transcriptase enzyme (RT) creates a DNA copy of the RNA template by extension from the 3′ end of the promoter-primer. The RNA in the RNA–DNA duplex is then degraded by the RNAase action of reverse transcriptase. A second oligonucleotide now binds to the cDNA copy and a new strand of DNA is synthesized by RT. The DNA duplex with attached RNA promoter acts as a template for transcription by RNA polymerase. The newly synthesized RNA copies also act as new templates that re-enter the TMA process, producing a new round of replication, leading to an exponential increase in RNA amplicons. Addition of an acridinium ester-labelled DNA probe that binds specifically to the target RNA amplicons allows, after chemical denaturation of unbound probe, detection of the product using chemiluminescence.

Nucleic acid sequence-based amplification

Nucleic acid sequence-based amplification (NASBA) is superficially highly similar to TMA; however, whilst TMA utilizes two enzymes in an isothermal amplification, NASBA uses three. After extraction of nucleic acid using a proprietary silica-based nucleic acid extraction method, an oligonucleotide primer with an attached T7 RNA polymerase promoter is extended by the action of RT, acting in a 3′ to 5′ direction. An RNAase enzyme then degrades the RNA strand and a second primer binds to the cDNA molecule, and RT produces the double-stranded DNA molecule (in recent iterations of the technique, an enzyme combining reverse transcription DNA polymerase and RNAase activity has been used in the same way as in the TMA technique). The T7 polymerase then produces RNA transcripts from the double-stranded DNA, acting as further templates for the NASBA procedure. Detection of amplicons is accomplished by hybridization with an oligonucleotide bound to streptavidin-coated paramagnetic beads and a ruthenium-labelled probe. The paramagnetic beads carrying the hybridized amplicon–probe complex are captured on the surface of an electrode by means of a magnet. Voltage applied to this electrode triggers an electrochemiluminescent reaction. Assays for a wide range of targets have been described and a recent development is the use of 'molecular beacons' in this technology that allows 'real-time' detection and quantitation of HIV RNA.

Strand displacement amplification

Strand displacement amplification (SDA) is a comparative newcomer to the field of nucleic acid amplification but has gained widespread acceptance. The SDA method is based upon the ability of DNA polymerases to initiate DNA synthesis at a single-stranded nick within a double-stranded DNA target molecule. Following extraction and denaturation of the target DNA molecule, a primer oligonucleotide containing a target-specific sequence and a sequence containing a restriction enzyme recognition site (usually BsopI) binds to the single-stranded DNA target molecule. A DNA polymerase enzyme then copies the DNA molecule. However, the dNTPs used for this elongation are modified by α-thiol substitution. When a restriction enzyme is added to the reaction, this attempts to cut the DNA at the BsopI recognition site but can only cut one of the strands of DNA because the newly synthesized strand contains α-thiol substituted dCTP, which the restriction enzyme is unable to cleave. The newly synthesized strand of DNA is thus displaced and the primer–DNA duplex can act as an initiator for a fresh round of DNA polymerase-driven copying. The released copies can serve as an additional template for the reaction. Accumulating product can be detected via chemiluminescence.

Signal amplification

Branched-chain DNA

An example of a 'signal' amplification method for nucleic acid detection and quantitation is found in the commercially available branched-chain DNA (bDNA) assay. Three products to detect and quantify hepatitis B virus DNA, hepatitis C virus RNA and human immunodeficiency RNA are available. The method used for detection of HIV RNA is a sandwich nucleic acid hybridization procedure for the direct quantitation of HIV-1 RNA in human plasma. HIV-1 is first concentrated from plasma by centrifugation. A proprietary nucleic acid extraction procedure is then used to release RNA from virions. The RNA is captured in a microwell by a set of specific, synthetic oligonucleotide capture probes. A set of target probes is then allowed to hybridize to both the viral RNA and the pre-amplifier probes. The capture probes, comprising 17 individual capture extenders, and the target probes, comprising 81 individual target extenders, bind to different regions of the *pol* gene of the viral RNA. The amplifier probe hybridizes to the pre-amplifier, forming a branched DNA (bDNA) complex. Multiple copies of an alkaline phosphatase (AP)-labelled probe are then hybridized to this immobilized complex. Detection is achieved by incubating the complex with a chemiluminescent substrate. Light emission is directly related to the amount of HIV-1 RNA present in each sample, and the results are recorded as relative light units (RLUs) by a luminometer analyser. A standard curve is defined by light emission from standards containing known concentrations of virus. Concentrations of HIV-1 RNA in specimens are determined from this standard curve.

Hybrid capture

A further commercially available signal amplification offers more limited sensitivity than the bDNA method. The hybrid-capture method involves disruption of the sample to release target DNA. The DNA is then combined with specific RNA probes in solution and the DNA–RNA hybrids are captured onto a microtitre plate or reaction tube, using monoclonal antibodies specific for the DNA–RNA hybrids. The captured hybrids are detected using multiple antibodies conjugated to alkaline phosphatase. The bound alkaline phosphatase is detected by a chemiluminescent reaction with a dioextane substrate.

Probe amplification

Ligase chain reaction

Ligase chain reaction (LCR) involves the binding of two complementary oligonucleotide probe sequences to a target DNA (following extraction of nucleic acid from the virion and denaturation of the DNA). A DNA ligase enzyme is used to join the two pairs of complementary probes after they have hybridized to the target molecule. The reaction is heated to separate the DNA strands and the two single-stranded sequences of DNA form templates for further probe binding. The method is somewhat limited by the high background due to blunt-end ligation of probe duplexes, and the hybridization conditions must be highly stringent to reduce non-specific probe binding. Nevertheless, the technique found commercial application in assays for *Chlamydia trachomatis*, *Neisseria gonorrhoea*, mycobacteria and *Borrelia* spp.

Recently, however, the commercial providers of this technology appear to have begun to abandon the procedure in favour of a PCR approach to the detection of microbial targets.

Sequence analysis

Determination of the sequence of the nucleic acid of a virus has important practical application in clinical virology. As the use of cell culture isolation of virus has declined in favour of more rapid methods of virus identification (such as direct detection of viral antigens or detection of viral nucleic acids), there has been a reduction in the amount of epidemiological information concerning circulating virus strains. To address this problem, genomic methods of epidemiological tracing are being introduced. Epidemiological information is of importance in individual patient management; in designing measures to prevent or contain the spread of infection; in contact tracing; and in the design of vaccines and antivirals to prevent or treat infection. In contrast to epidemiological typing schemes based upon either biological properties—such as the ability or absence of ability to haemagglutinate certain types of red cells—or serological typing—based upon the ability of discrete antisera to bind to and neutralize the infectivity of viral infectivity, genomic analysis generally provides more precise biological classification.

In the process of identification of an unknown virus, sequence data, obtained from any region of the viral genome, can be compared with all known viral sequences through the use of powerful sequence alignment programmes (many of which are available within the public domain, e.g. accessible via the Internet), searching international open access nucleic acid databases, such as those maintained at the European Molecular Biological Laboratory or the North American Los Alamos database. With known viruses, discrete databases are available for sequence comparisons. Of course, not all human viruses have yet been sequenced but the number of complete viral sequences increases year on year and for many more viruses partial sequence information is available, meaning that sequence information is becoming the *de facto* method for identification and classification of a novel virus.

Sequence information also has an important role in the management of certain diseases, e.g. the genotype of hepatitis C virus is known to be an important determinant in response to therapy. Patients identified as being chronically infected with hepatitis C virus (persistence of hepatitis C viral RNA in plasma) may be offered a combination of the antiviral drug ribavirin and interferon-α formulated with a polyethylene glycol side-chain (pegylated interferon); however, the response to therapy of an individual has been found to strongly correlate with the genotype of the virus. In consequence, patients entering therapy have the genotype of their virus determined. Those determined as having virus of genotypes 1 or 4 require prolonged antiviral therapy in order to achieve cure of infection.

A very important use of sequencing technology is found in the management of patients infected with HIV. In Europe at least 20% of new cases of HIV infection involve the transmission of virus from a person who has already undergone antiviral drug therapy and has virus resistance to at least some of the antiviral drugs used in the combination therapy of HIV. Determination of the pattern of drug resistance may be crucial to effective therapy. The procedure also has a vital role in selecting an appropriate combination of antiviral compounds in those whose antiviral therapy is failing. There are two main tests for antiretroviral resistance; those that detect genotypic resistance and those that detect phenotypic resistance. Genotypic tests search for alteration in the base sequence of genes of HIV that are known to be associated with the development of drug resistance. For example, a specific mutation, M184V, in the reverse transcriptase gene confers resistance to the nucleoside analogue 3TC. Phenotypic tests measure the concentration of a drug required to inhibit viral replication by 50% or 90% (IC_{50} or IC_{90}, respectively) and require either virus culture or the construction of indicator 'recombinant' viruses.

Phenotypic resistance testing for HIV was (until the late 1990s) based upon plaque reduction assays or peripheral blood monolayer cell (PBMC) culture assays. These had distinct disadvantages. HIV plaque reduction assays required the co-cultivation of virus with HeLa-CD4$^+$ cells and thus could only be used for the minority of clinical isolates that can induce syncytia in cell culture (i.e. viruses that are CXCR4 tropic). PBMC assays are more versatile but require 10–14 days of co-cultivation of the patient's PBMCs with mitogen-stimulated PBMCs from HIV seronegative individuals, together with monitoring of growth via a surrogate marker of infection, such as HIV p24 antigen. A molecular-based approach to such testing is now more commonly utilized. In two commercially available variants of the technique, a reverse transcription PCR is used to amplify the protease, the majority of the RT and a portion of the *gag* genes of HIV-1. In one of these methods the cDNA is incorporated into a *pol*-deleted recombinant virus to create a recombinant HIV-1 isolate by homologous recombination in cell culture. This recombinant is capable of infecting a standard cell line and can be used to measure viral replication in the presence of varying concentrations of antiretroviral drugs by observation of cell death induced by the recombinant virus. In the other method direct, ligation is used to combine the cDNA produced with the pol-deleted HIV-1 vector and tests the recombinant construct during a single round of replication using a luciferase reporter gene assay. Both assays report drug sensitivity in terms of the micromolar concentration of drug required to inhibit HIV-1 replication by 50%. Although phenotypic testing provides a more direct method of measuring resistance, the length of time currently taken to perform testing (up to several weeks) reduces its clinical utility.

Phenotypic changes arise from changes in the genotype, and thus genotypic testing may provide clues about drug resistance before phenotypic tests. Virus extracted from plasma is reverse transcribed and a series of PCRs are performed, designed to allow amplification of regions of the viral protease, reverse transcriptase and/or other regions of the genome (e.g. the HIV-1 gp41 envelope protein gene in those undergoing therapy with HIV fusion inhibitor drugs). Appropriately labelled products are then sequenced (see Figure 22.6). The cDNA sequence is aligned to a 'wild-type' HIV strain and compared with a database, in which point mutations and combinations of point mutations correlated with the development of resistance to individual or multiple combinations of drugs are documented. Proprietary databases are maintained by commercial test suppliers or are available through open access international collaborative databases, such as the Stanford University HIV RT and Protease Database.

In the examination of RNA viruses, such as hepatitis C virus or HIV, RNA extracted from plasma is reverse transcribed and the cDNA amplified by PCR. The sequence may then be examined in several different ways. In the commercially available InnoLipa method for hepatitis C genotyping, denatured cDNA is hybridized with strips of nitrocellulose to which oligonucleotides corresponding with sequences present in the discrete genotypes of hepatitis C virus are bound. One of the oligonucleotide primers used in the PCR reaction is labelled with a biotin molecule. The binding pattern of the cDNA is then revealed by reaction of the immobilized cDNA with an avidin–enzyme complex, followed by a chromogenic substrate; the pattern of bands appearing on the strip reveals the genotype of the virus. Similar commercial resistance assays of HIV-1 reverse transcriptase and protease employ similar methodological principles but here the oligonucleotide probes immobilized on the nitrocellulose are designed to select resistance mutations in the protease or RT genes of HIV-1.

More commonly, however, the cDNA is labelled in a further PCR in the presence of 2′, 3′-dideoxynucleoside triphosphates (ddNTPs). A carefully optimized mixture of deoxynucleotide triphosphates (dNTPs) and ddNTPs are used, together with oligonucleotides in a conventional PCR. The new strand synthesis is randomly terminated by the incorporation of a ddNTP, each of which is labelled with a dye that is specific to the base that it labels. At the end of the sequencing reaction the reaction tube will contain a mixture of partially synthesized DNA copies. Each will have a common 5′ end

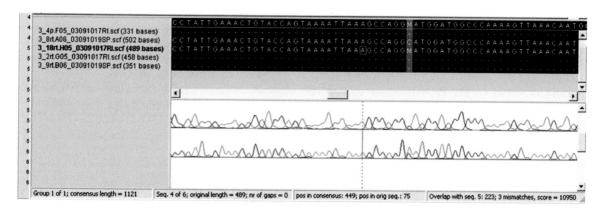

Figure 22.6 Sequencing. An example showing the sequencing of the HIV-1 protease and RT genes. The bases eluting from the capillary sequencer are colour-coded (blue, cytosine; black, guanine; red, thymine; green, adenine), allowing the sequence to be assembled and compared to the sequence of an HIV-1 wild-type strain to determine base changes within the test strain of virus that may be associated with the development of antiviral drug resistance

(defined by the primer oligonucleotide used in the reaction) but will be of differing lengths, varying by 1 base length at the $3'$ end. The mixture is analysed using either polyacrylamide gel electrophoresis (PAGE) and fluorometry or high-throughput automated capillary gel sequencing (Figure 22.6). In the latter method the smallest fragments of labelled DNA have highest mobility and are eluted first from the capillary. Each fragment subsequently eluting from the capillary is one base longer than that preceding it. The separated DNA fragments are revealed by excitation with a laser. Each of the dyes attached to a $2'$ $3'$ terminator base emits light at a different wavelength this allows the individual terminating base to be distinguished. All four colours, and thus bases, can be readily distinguished. The sequence of the fragment is read directly from the capillary eluate.

Alternatives to this procedure include the use of glass slides, silicon wafers or nylon membranes with attached oligonucleotides (DNA microchips). For HIV-1 genotyping, an array was developed to analyse the complete gene sequence of the HIV-1 protease gene and a 1200 base pair region of the RT gene. The chip contained 18 000 probes of 18–22 base pairs, designed to encompass all possible combinations of mutation within this sequence. Every nucleotide in the sequence to be analysed requires at least four oligonucleotide probes in order to determine whether the nucleotide at that position is an A, T, C or a G. To use the array, cDNA resulting from an RT PCR of plasma-derived virus is transcribed to single-stranded RNA and labelled with fluorescent reporter molecules. After hybridization, the chip is scanned using a laser to activate the fluorescent label and the pattern of binding revealed by examination with a confocal microscope. The reporter molecules fluoresce in proportion to the stringency with which the probe binds the nucleic acid. Probes that bind no nucleic acid do not fluoresce, while probes that bind with a single base pair mismatch have up to 35 times less fluorescence than when there is complete matching of sequence. Computer-aided deconvolution of the pattern of binding observed allows the linking of sequences derived from overlapping probes to determine the sequence from the HIV-1 RNA wild-type sequence represented on the chip. The genetic variability of HIV presents an extreme challenge to the use of DNA chips. In comparisons with dideoxynucleotide sequencing, the chip was found to be less reliable in mutation detection and less capable of discerning insertions or deletions of sequence. The chip also performed less well when sequencing non-subtype B strains of HIV-1, which was the subtype on which the chip was designed. Despite this setback, the versatility and high-throughput capabilities

of DNA microchips has led to their continued commercial development, and chips for genotypic analysis of hepatitis B and hepatitis C viruses are approaching commercial release. An interesting approach to wider use of this technology is the description of a long oligonucleotide (70-mer) DNA microarray that has been shown capable of detecting and identifying literally hundreds of different human viruses. Using a random reverse transcription PCR in conjunction with this technology, it was possible to detect multiple viruses in respiratory specimens without the use of PCR, based on sequence-specific or degenerate primers.

Summary

The explosion of applications of molecular biological techniques in virology, and in clinical virology in particular, continues to gather pace. Molecular methods of diagnosis are rapidly replacing conventional methods of diagnosis, such as cell-culture isolation, serology, fluorescence microscopy and electron microscopy. Automation is reducing the technical complexity of testing while improving reproducibility and reliability. Their application has moved clinical virology from a pursuit largely of academic interest to a key science actively involved in the acute stage diagnosis and treatment of patients.

Further reading

Latest data about antiretroviral resistance patterns (genotypic testing) can be found at: Antiviral Drug Resistance Online, www.viral-resistance.com; at Stanford University HIV RT and Protease Database, http://hivdb.stanford.edu/hiv; and the Los Alamos HIV sequence database, http://hiv-web.lanl.gov.

Burd EM. Human papillomaviruses and cervical cancer. *Clin Microbiol Rev* 2003; **16**: 1–17.

Cinque P, Bossacola S, Lundkvist A. Molecular analysis of cerebrospinal fluid in viral diseases of the central nervous system. *J Clin Virol* 2003; **26**: 1–28.

Cockerill FR. Application of rapid-cycle real-time polymerase chain reaction for diagnostic testing in the clinical microbiology laboratory. *Arch Pathol Lab Med* 2003; **127**: 1112–1120.

Ellis JS, Zambon MC. Molecular diagnosis of influenza. *Rev Med Virol* 2002; **12**: 375–389.

Elnifro EM, Cooper RJ, Klapper PE, Bailey AS. PCR and restriction endonuclease analysis for rapid identification of human adenovirus subgenera. *J Clin Microbiol* 2000; **38**: 2055–2061.

Elnifro EM, Ashshi AM, Cooper RJ, Klapper PE. Multiplex PCR: optimization and application in diagnostic virology. *Clin Microbiol Rev* 2000; **13**: 559–570.

Hawkey PM, Bhagani S, Gillespie SH. Severe acute respiratory syndrome (SARS): breath-taking progress. *J Med Microbiol* 2003; **52**: 609–613.

Hill CG. Molecular diagnostic testing for infectious diseases using TMA technology. *Expert Rev Mol Diagn* 2001; **1**: 445–455.

Humar A, Kumar D, Boivin G, Caliendo AM. Cytomegalovirus (CMV) virus load kinetics to predict recurrent disease in solid-organ transplant patients with CMV disease. *J Infect Dis* 2002; **186**: 829–833.

Kellam P. Post-genomic virology: the impact of bioinformatics, microarrays and proteomics on investigating host and pathogen interactions. *Rev Med Virol* 2001; **11**: 313–329.

Kiechle FL, Holland-Stanley CA. Genomics, transcriptomics, proteomics and numbers. *Arch Pathol Lab Med* 2003; **127**: 1089–1097.

Kuiken T, Fouchier RA, Schutten M, Rimmelzwaan GF *et al.* Newly discovered coronavirus as the primary cause of severe acute respiratory syndrome. *Lancet* 2003; **362**: 263–270.

Lednicky JA. Hantaviruses, a short review. *Arch Pathol Lab Med* 2003; **127**: 30–35.

Mackay IM, Arden KE, Nitsche A. Real-time PCR in virology. *Nucleic Acids Res* 2002; **6**: 1292–1305.

Ngui SL, Watkins RL, Heptonstall J, Teo CG. Selective transmission of hepatitis B virus after percutaneous exposure. *J Infect Dis* 2000; **181**: 838–843.

Niesters HGM. Clinical virology in real time. *J Clin Virol* 2002; **25**: S3–S12.

Podzorski RP. HIV-1 genotyping: we can't resist. *Rev Med Microbiol* 2003; **14**: 25–34.

Wang D, Coscoy L, Zylerberg M, Avila PC *et al.* Microarray-based detection and genotyping of viral pathogens. *Proc Natl Acad Sci USA* 2002; **99**: 15687–15692.

23

Virology: other tests

Alex WL Joss

This chapter includes description of techniques not covered in previous sections, in three areas which are outwith the remit of most viral diagnostic laboratories: prion disease, antiviral susceptibility and cell-mediated immunity.

Detection of prion infection

Prions are classed as a separate infectious entity because most research workers believe they lack any nucleic acid and consist solely of proteinaceous infectious particles. They belong in this section for several reasons: they are subviral in size; historically, they were termed 'slow virus infections'; and minority opinion still maintains that they are really viruses, 'nemaviruses'. They cause brain disease, transmissible spongiform encephalopathy (TSE), whereby accumulation of prion protein results in nervous tissue vacuolation and neurodegeneration, manifesting clinically as slowly progressive dementia, ataxia, sleep and eating disorders and leading inevitably to eventual death. Diseases include scrapie in sheep, BSE in cattle and four types of human disease, Gerstmann–Straussler–Schinker disease (GSS), fatal familial insomnia (FFI), Creutzfeldt–Jakob disease (CJD), kuru, plus a fifth if the variant CJD (vCJD) associated with the BSE epidemic is included (Figure 23.1). It is too early to determine whether a second zoonotic infection, by a TSE from deer or elk (chronic wasting disease), should also be included, although three men have died of neurodegenerative disease following wild game feasts in the USA. Before considering the question of diagnosis, it is essential to understand some of the back-ground and theoretical mechanism of the infectious process. Only then can the difficulties inherent in ready diagnosis be appreciated.

The essence of prion disease is the corruption of the α-helical conformation of a normal, essential neuronal membrane protein (PrP^c) to a protease-resistant β-sheet conformation (PrP^{Res}), the deposition of which leads to neurological degeneration (Figure 23.1). The proposition that protein alone (PrP^{Res}) can induce this change is supported by *in vitro* evidence. New evidence suggests that neurodegeneration is triggered by oxidative stress due to alteration of the metal binding affinity of PrP^c. PrP^c is a copper-binding antioxidant anchored to neuronal cell membranes and the protective effect may be lost when PrP^{Res} binds other metals, such as zinc and manganese.

Of the human prion diseases, GSS and FFI arise from various point mutations in the PrP^c gene, which are genetically 'transmitted' within families (Figure 23.1). CJD arises sporadically (sCJD), again with evidence of point mutation, or perhaps also overexpression of the PrP^c gene. The infectious aspect of CJD is its proven iatrogenic transmission, from dural or corneal grafts, neurosurgical instruments or pituitary hormone extracts, and the possibility of accidental infection when handling brain tissue. Kuru, recognized as the consequence of cannibalistic practices in Papua New Guinea, more easily fits the picture of an infectious process. Similarly, artificial cannibalism of ovine or bovine brain leads to BSE infection, and subsequent ingestion of BSE-infected neural tissue may have produced vCJD, which is histologically and epidemiologically distinct from sCJD. Interspecies transmission occurs more readily

The Science of Laboratory Diagnosis, Second Edition   Edited by David Burnett and John Crocker

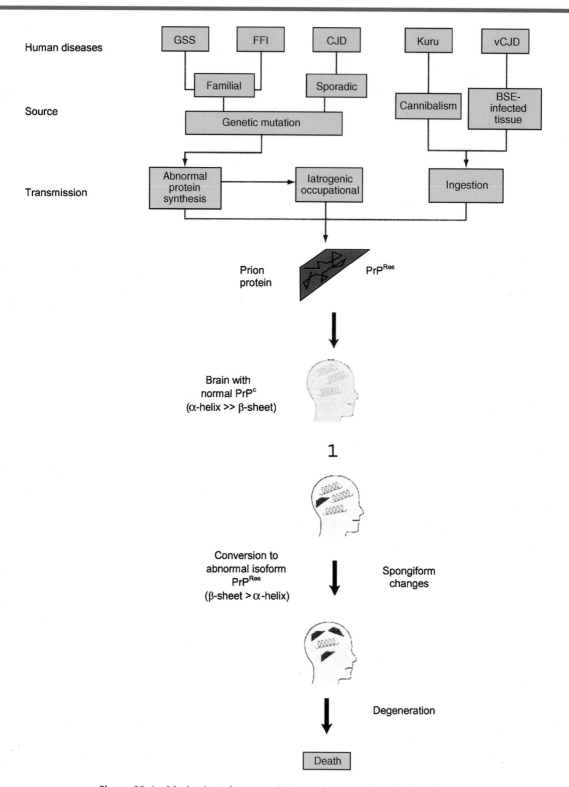

Figure 23.1 Mechanisms for transmission and progression of prion disease

the more closely related the PrP^c of the recipient is to that of the source. Ovine and bovine PrP^c only differ at seven residues, whereas bovine and human PrP^c differ by 30 residues. Nevertheless, all TSEs with the exception of FFI have been transmitted experimentally to a range of species.

Diagnosis

The characteristics that make diagnosis so difficult are the disease site, the close relatedness of the pathogen to its host equivalent, and its apparent lack of nucleic acid. Brain is unlikely to be biopsied when therapy remains unavailable, unless to exclude other treatable diseases, and small samples may be falsely negative. Clinical signs of CJD, such as rapidly progressive dementia, myoclonus, ataxia, visual disturbances or alien-hand syndrome, are not diagnostic, but may be more so in a younger person, as in vCJD. Physiological measurements are generally unhelpful.

Histology

Definitive diagnosis of prion disease requires evidence of PrP^{Res} deposition, in human brain itself, or after transmission to animal brain. Congo red-stained amyloid plaques, loosely packed PrP synaptic deposits, spongiform changes, neurofibrillary tangles and subcortical gliosis are all histological features consistent with the diagnosis. However, all of these features are shared to varying degrees with other neurodegenerative disorders, e.g. amyloid plaques in Alzheimer's disease. They can be specifically related to prion disease using immunohistochemistry.

Prion-specific antibody is not easy to produce but polyclonal rabbit antisera have been raised: against purified amyloid plaque cores from human brain or CJD-infected mouse brain; and against synthetic peptides equivalent to the altered sequences in human prion. Formalin-fixed paraffin-embedded tissue can be tested but, after deparaffinization, pre-treatment with a protein denaturant is essential to enhance immunoreactivity.

Formic acid is the simplest and most effective denaturant, but may be superseded by 'hydrolytic autoclaving' to 121°C for 10 minutes in an appropriate concentration of hydrochloric acid. Prion deposition is then identified by binding specific antibody, which is visualized by reaction with an enzyme-labelled (biotin–streptavidin or peroxidase–antiperoxidase) or fluorescent conjugate. Different prion strains produce varying proportions of the two principal pathologies, amyloid plaques (GSS, Kuru) or punctate synaptic deposits (sCJD), while human vCJD and BSE-infected macaque monkey brains yield abundant florid cortical plaques interspersed with vacuoles in a 'daisy-like' pattern.

Electron microscopy

Tubulofilamentous particles, often over 1 μm long, are diagnostic features seen in impressions of moistened freshly cut brain tissue, touched on to electron microscope grids and negatively stained with phosphotungstic acid. These are distinguishable from the neuro-fibrillary filaments seen in Alzheimer's disease. Electron microscopy diagnosis may fail due to random sampling of uninfected tissue, but it can find positive evidence of infection in animals before other histological changes become apparent.

Culture

Apart from FFI, prion 'infections' can be confirmed by passage in mice or hamsters. Diagnosis is slow, requiring at least 60 days to demonstrate characteristic histology in inoculated brains, and longer than a mouse's lifetime for some slower-growing strains. Transmission success can be low, but BSE crosses the species barrier more easily and may be transmitted orally. Human prions can be expressed in tissue culture (e.g. Chinese hamster ovary cells) but no cytopathic effect is evident. Cell-free *in vitro* culture, if it can be so described, has been developed in which radiolabelled PrP^c was converted to PrP^{Res} in 2 days on exposure to unlabelled scrapie prion. However, the latter had to be purified and added in 50-fold excess, suggesting that the technique requires refinement to have diagnostic applications.

Immunoblotting

Rapid diagnosis, within one day, can be achieved on small brain samples by immunoblotting. Proteinase k-digested tissue, separated on polyacrylamide SDS gels and electrophoretically transferred to nitrocellulose membranes, yields three or four bands of 16–31 kDa molecular weight which react with prion-specific antiserum. Their size and intensity ratios can distinguish vCJD from sCJD. These are not found in Alzheimer's disease and normal PrP^c is fully digested by proteinase K.

Tests in other tissues or body fluids

All methods discussed so far are performed on brain tissue. Diagnosis would be simpler on more accessible material. Monoclonal antibody to PrP^c can be used to diagnose CJD by detecting protease-resistant PrP in samples other than brain. PrP^{Res} has been detected in urine of CJD patients by SDS-polyacrylamide gel electrophoresis (SDS-PAGE) and immunoblotting of proteinase K-digested ultracentrifugation pellets. It can also be detected in formalin-fixed embedded tonsils and lymph nodes, after deparaffinization, formic acid treatment and hydrolytic autoclaving, using biotin–avidin conjugate, but only in vCJD patients.

Tests in cerebrospinal fluid for surrogate markers of neuronal destruction are now part of the accepted repertoire for diagnosis of CJD. The most commonly used is an immunoblotting assay using rabbit polyclonal antibody to detect a 30 kDa highly conserved neuronal protein, 14–3–3. As appearance of this protein in CSF can occur in other neurodegenerative diseases, including some Alzheimer's cases, the test is only 88–95% specific. It is less sensitive for vCJD (50%) than sCJD, but testing in conjunction with a commercial ELISA for tau, an axonal microtubular phosphoprotein, can improve the vCJD sensitivity to 86%.

Non-invasive techniques

Electroencephalography is generally regarded as useful, although not specific. Periodic sharp wave complexes and reactivity to external stimuli or drugs are prominent observations. The current imaging test of choice is diffusion-weighted magnetic resonance imaging (MRI), which yields multifocal cortical and subcortical hyperintensities, a marker which is claimed to be 100% sensitive and specific in sCJD patients.

In conclusion, the nature of prion disease severely limits the usual approaches to diagnosis, and diagnosis is usually slow, invasive and often achieved only at autopsy. However, vCJD has provided urgent impetus for more rapid and less invasive techniques. Testing CSF for 14–3–3 protein is now the current 'gold standard' and developments in MRI have improved the prospects of non-invasive diagnosis.

Antiviral susceptibility tests

Antiviral susceptibility assays are not yet regularly carried out in many routine virology laboratories. Tests take several days or weeks to perform and are therefore only likely to benefit patients who require lengthy therapy for otherwise very severe clinical problems. They are more likely to occur in laboratories dealing with large numbers of immunocompromised patients, perhaps to monitor human immunodeficiency virus (HIV) antiviral resistance, or to identify resistant Herpes group viruses in such patients. In practice, decisions to change antiviral therapy are based often on empirical evidence of resistance, i.e. failure to respond clinically (Figure 23.2). Alternatively, surrogate resistance markers are measured, such as failure of viral antigen or nucleic acid levels in blood to fall in response to therapy. True susceptibility assays are of two categories: phenotypic, which measure the effect of the antiviral on virus growth *in vitro*; and genotypic, which directly detect the presence of mutants that confer resistance.

Phenotypic assays

Phenotypic assays provide definitive proof of antiviral resistance. They measure the antiviral concentration required to inhibit either the overall cytopathic effect (CPE) of virus growth on culture cells or specific stages of viral metabolism, viz. DNA or protein synthesis. Virus has first to be propagated in tissue culture, a step which itself can confound the result by altering the proportion of resistant mutants subsequently tested. Tests are therefore preferably done on low-passage isolates. HIV is often isolated from peripheral blood mononuclear cells (PBMC) by co-culture with a lymphoblastoid cell line, another added complication.

Plaque reduction (PR) assays

When cell monolayers are seeded with diluted virus in conditions which limit virus movement, i.e. under a solid agar or cellulose overlay, or liquid containing antiviral immunoglobulin, each virus plaque forming unit (pfu) produces a discrete CPE plaque. Addition of serially diluted antiviral together with fixed titrated amounts of virus (15–500 pfu) allows measurement of antiviral susceptibility as the concentration that causes 50% plaque reduction (ID_{50}). PR assays only detect resistant strains which constitute more than 20–25% of the isolate. Lower proportions may be detected using a 90% plaque reduction threshold, but ID_{90} measurements are less accurate than ID_{50}.

PR assays use relatively inexpensive routine culture techniques, but disadvantages are the volumes of reagents, media and virus used and the time required to standardize cell, virus and antiviral concentrations and manually count plaques in replicate cultures. Overall test time is at least 2 weeks. The virus:cell ratio must be optimized to avoid generating falsely high or low susceptibility estimates when ratios are, respectively, too low or too high. Preliminary Herpes simplex (HSV) susceptibility results can be obtained in 3 days by pre-screening isolates in parallel with titrating their infectiv-ity, by incubation of serial viral dilutions, with and without acyclovir, at 1.5 times the accepted resistance threshold concentration.

PR assays are the gold standard for detection of HSV, cytomegalovirus (CMV) and Varicella zoster (VZV) resistance. Accepted resistance thresholds have been established: 2 µg/ml for acyclovir, 100 µl/ml for foscar-net, and for ganciclovir a three- to four-fold increase in ID_{50} compared to pretherapy. However, the lengthy

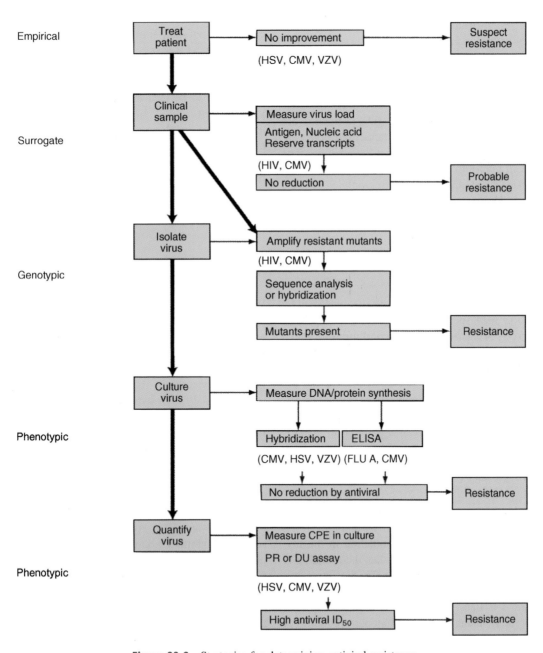

Figure 23.2 Strategies for determining antiviral resistance

procedures involved and low isolation rates, frequently as low as 30%, make HIV PR assays less clinically useful than more rapid genotypic assays.

Dye uptake (DU assays)

The semi-automated technology of a DU assay suits laboratories with a higher throughput. Similar principles apply, testing constant virus concentrations against serial dilutions of antiviral, but the CPE after 2–3 days incubation is measured spectrophotometrically. The amounts of neutral red dye absorbed by surviving viable cells, in 1 hour, then eluted into buffered alcohol, produce optical density readings which are inversely proportional to CPE and virus titres. They can be read objectively and computed automatically to ID_{50} values. Because liquid overlays are used, ID_{50} estimates are higher than in PR assays and resistance thresholds are therefore raised, e.g. from 2 to 3 µg/ml for acyclovir. The technique, in microtitre plates, requires less reagent and will detect resistant strains constituting only 3–9% of a total isolate. However, PR assays more accurately predict clinical failure due to resistance.

DNA synthesis assays

Viral DNA synthesis in culture cells can be quantified by hybridization with specific radiolabelled DNA probes. Antiviral ID_{50} is measured as the concentration which causes 50% reduction in the signal from bound probe. DNA from cells lysed at the end of a defined period of virus growth is transferred either to nylon 'wicks' and quantified using ^{125}I-labelled probes (commercial Hybriwix assay), or to nitrocellulose filters, then hybridized with ^{32}P-labelled probes. These assays are faster than PR assays, producing results in 4–6 days, and have been used to detect resistance in HSV, CMV and VZV strains. Drawbacks are their cost and the short shelf-life of the probes.

Acyclovir resistance in HSV or VZV strains may be confirmed by demonstrating the mechanism of resistance. Most resistant strains show mutation in the thymidine kinase (TK) gene, which makes them unable to phosphorylate and activate acyclovir. TK deficiency can be measured in radiolabel incorporation assays in appropriate cell lines, as a reduced signal on plaque autoradiography, using either ^{125}I-iododeoxycytidine or ^{14}C-thymidine. This correlates well with inability to phosphorylate acyclovir.

Protein synthesis assays

For some viruses, growth can be monitored by the appearance of readily identifiable virus proteins in culture cells. The best example is influenza A haemagglutinin, which can be detected on canine kidney monolayers 18 hours after infection, using monoclonal antibody in an enzyme-linked immunosorbent assay (ELISA). Resistance to amantadine or rimantadine is demonstrated as a failure to reduce ELISA optical density readings, i.e. haemagglutinin synthesis, except at high antiviral concentrations. This assay clearly discriminates resistant from susceptible strains more successfully than PR assays, and is the method of choice for influenza A. With the advent of the licensed anti-neuraminidase agents oseltamivir and zanamivir, antiviral resistence can be measured as diminished inhibition of viral enzyme activity in influenza tissue culture supernates, using a fluorogenic substrate. Viral antigen expression assays are also available for HSV, VZV and CMV, detecting early or late proteins. The degree of inhibition of antigen expression by antivirals can be measured by flow cytometry, which is faster than PR assays and more automated.

Genotypic assays

When point mutations within specific virus genes are known to confer antiviral resistance, they can be directly assayed, in either virus isolates or clinical specimens, usually blood. Mutations are usually identified by polymerase chain reaction (PCR) amplification of relevant DNA sequences in clinical samples, followed by sequence analysis or hybridization with mutation-specific probes. A considerable range of in-house or commercial assays are now available, with sequence analysis probably the most sensitive detection method. The complexity of the methodology and its interpretation requires testing in specialist laboratories, where it is now done routinely for HIV resistance. Susceptibility results are reported on individual antivirals within each of the three main anti-HIV groups: nucleoside reverse transcriptase inhibitors, non-nucleoside reverse transcriptase inhibitors and protease inhibitors. Mutations in CMV phosphotransferase or DNA polymerase genes, and influenza A transmembrane protein gene, have also been linked with antiviral resistance, thus providing targets for genotypic assays. The advantage of this approach is its directness, avoiding the need to isolate, grow and quantify virus. It is not just technically faster;

resistance mutants may be identified in blood before resistant virus is isolated. Disadvantages are the inability to detect resistance when the specific mutation(s) are unknown, or to detect mutations present as a low proportion (e.g. <10–25%) of the total viral population in a sample.

Conclusion

In clinical practice, decisions to change antiviral therapy on empirical or surrogate marker evidence are likely to continue. However, there is still a place for *in vitro* susceptibility testing to confirm resistance. CMV or HIV resistance may display focal heterogenicity, e.g. resistant CMV retinal isolates concurrent with sensitive systemic isolates, which will influence treatment strategy. Recent years have seen rapid innovation in antiviral therapy and screening potentially useful compounds has obviously relied on good susceptibility assays. Introduction of more new antivirals, the assessment of combined therapy and investigation of conflicting data on *in vitro* and *in vivo* resistance should all increase demand for this methodology. With current improved management of HIV infection using multidrug therapy, genotypic HIV antiviral resistance testing has become part of the management repertoire when treatment fails.

Cell-mediated immunity

An effective cellular immune response is important in overcoming viral infection, yet routine laboratory investigations centre almost exclusively on the humoral response. Cellular immunity tests are much less amenable to large throughput than are serological tests. Apart from research studies, these tests are reserved for investigations of deficiency, such as failure to overcome herpes group infections. Typical *in vitro* assays assess two aspects of lymphocyte function, ability to recognize virus (using proliferation assays) and ability to destroy infected cells (using cytotoxicity assays).

Proliferation assays

Patients' fresh peripheral blood lymphocytes (PBL) in culture medium are stimulated to proliferate by external activators, mitogens such as phytohaemagglutinin (PHA) or, more specifically, viral antigens. Several days incubation are required, following which proliferation is measured as the amount of radiolabelled thymidine incorporated into DNA in the last few hours,

quantified by liquid scintillation counting of acid precipitated, washed cells. Tests compare the response of patient T lymphocytes to a particular virus to that of unstimulated (negative) or PHA-stimulated (positive) controls. Assays are done at least in triplicate and, when done on serial dilutions of PBL, estimate the number of circulating T lymphocytes that recognise virus antigen, the responder cell frequency. Individual purified antigens or crude infected cell extracts can be assessed.

Cytotoxicity assays

Cytotoxicity assays can be performed on a variety of different leukocyte populations—antibody-dependent killer cells, non-specific natural killer cells, monocytes—but it is the cytotoxic T lymphocyte (CTL) response that is most relevant in this context. These can be enriched from the PBL fraction by adsorption–elution procedures using monoclonal antibodies or flow cytometry. The test again involves several days' culture, to measure effector activity on virus-containing target cells. Target cells should be histocompatible with patients' CTL and may be fibroblasts, B lymphocytes, macrophages or tumour cells expressing viral antigens, following either infection, transfection or pulses with viral peptides. Activity of CTL is measured by the release of radioactive chromium from labelled target cells over a short period at the end of the incubation. Tests of replicate cultures, usually of serially diluted CTL, measure the number of effector cells killing a specific percentage of a predetermined number of target cells. Data analysis is complex, and a well-controlled test protocol, with appropriate statistical methology, is essential. Active CTL should be detectable in patients with acute, persistent or reactivated viral infection.

Flow cytometry

The measurement of CD4 markers in HIV infection is technically an investigation of cellular immunocompetence. Flow cytometry is routinely used to measure CD4:CD8 ratios in HIV patients to assess progression, or immune recovery following treatment. More recently the method has been used to determine the persistence of cell-mediated immunity following measles or varicella vaccination. Patient lymphocytes are incubated with viral antigen for several days, and subsequent expression of CD25 antigen in the CD4 population indicates persisting immunity. These data have provided reassuring evidence for the efficacy of varicella vaccination in immunocompromised patients.

In summary, proliferation and cytotoxicity assays are time-consuming, use radioactivity, have all the maintenance problems of the most complex in-house methods and require a regular supply of fresh age- and sex-matched control PBL from volunteers. Properly controlled cytotoxicity assays should monitor day-to-day variation in results on cryopreserved high- and low-toxicity control CTL. Normal ranges should be established from a large group of volunteers. Tests are therefore performed in specialist centres, usually for research purposes. Nevertheless, individual patients with severe recurrent HSV, VZV or EBV infections require investigation to reveal the precise dysfunction in cellular immunity, and to suggest and monitor treatment strategies. Flow cytometry is routinely used for immunocompromised patients, but its scope is limited by its expense and requirement for sophisticated equipment and interpretive expertise.

Further reading

Demaerel P, Sciot R, Robberecht W, Dom R *et al*. Accuracy of diffusion-weighted MR imaging in the diagnosis of sporadic Creutzfeldt–Jakob disease. *J Neurol* 2003; **250**: 222–225.

Green AJE, Thompson EJ, Stewart GE *et al*. Use of 14–3–3 and other brain-specific proteins in CSF in the diagnosis of variant Creutzfeldt–Jakob disease. *J Neurol Neurosurg Psychiat* 2001; **70**: 744–748.

Oitani K. Expression of interleukin-2 receptor, CD25, on CD4 lymphocytes in response to *Varicella zoster virus* antigen among patients with malignancies immunised with live attenuated varicella vaccine. *Pediatr Int* 1999; **41**: 32–36.

Safrin S, Elbeik T, Mills J. A rapid screen test for *in vitro* susceptibility of clinical *Herpes simplex virus* isolates. *J Infect Dis* 1994: **169**, 879–882.

Swierkosz EM, Arens MQ. Susceptibility test methods: viruses. In *Manual of Clinical Microbiology*, 8th edn, Murray PR, Baron EJ, Jorgensen JH, Pfaller MA, Yolken RH (eds). 2003: ASM Press, Washington, DC, 1638–1649.

24

Mycology

David W Warnock

Introduction

Among the 50 000–250 000 species of fungi that have been described, fewer than 500 have been identified as human pathogens. With few exceptions, these organisms are found in the environment and human infections are acquired through inhalation, ingestion or traumatic implantation. Mycotic diseases of humans can be divided into three broad groups: superficial, subcutaneous or systemic.

The superficial mycoses are infections limited to the outermost layers of the skin, the nails and hair, and the mucous membranes. The principal infections in this group are dermatophytosis and candidiasis. The aetiological agents of these diseases are dependent on the living host for their survival, but differ from one another in the manner by which this is achieved. The aetiological agents of dermatophytosis (the dermatophytes, *Epidermophyton*, *Microsporum* and *Trichophyton* species) depend on person-to-person spread for their survival, while the aetiological agents of candidiasis, of which *Candida albicans* is the most important, are normal commensals of the gastrointestinal tract. These organisms do not produce disease unless some change in the host lowers its natural defences. In this situation, endogenous infection results in superficial or systemic infection.

The subcutaneous mycoses are infections involving the dermis, subcutaneous tissues and adjacent bone. Among the infections in this group are chromoblastomycosis, mycetoma and sporotrichosis. These diseases are most common in tropical and subtropical regions and are usually acquired as a result of the traumatic implantation of organisms that are found in the environment.

The disease may remain localized at the site of implantation or spread to adjacent soft tissue and bone. More widespread dissemination of the infection, through the blood or lymphatics, is uncommon, and usually only occurs if the host is in some way debilitated or immunocompromised.

The systemic mycoses are infections that usually originate in the respiratory or gastrointestinal tracts, but may spread to many other organs. The organisms that cause these diseases can be divided into two distinct groups: the true pathogens and the opportunists. The first of these groups consists of a small number of organisms, such as *Histoplasma capsulatum*, that are able to invade the tissues of a normal host with no recognizable predisposition. Apart from histoplasmosis, the principal infections caused by members of this group are blastomycosis, coccidioidomycosis and paracoccidioidomycosis. In many instances, these infections are asymptomatic or mild and of short duration. Individuals who recover from these infections often enjoy lasting resistance to reinfection, while those with chronic or residual disease often have a serious underlying illness.

The second group of systemic fungal pathogens, the opportunists, consists of a much larger group of less well-adapted organisms, such as *Aspergillus fumigatus*, that are only able to invade the tissues of a debilitated or immunocompromised host. Apart from aspergillosis, the principal infections caused by members of this group are candidiasis, cryptococcosis and mucormycosis (zygomycosis). With the exception of candidiasis, which is usually acquired from the individual's own endogenous reservoir, most opportunistic fungal infections are acquired from the environment, rather than as a result of person-to-person spread. These infections are

The Science of Laboratory Diagnosis, Second Edition   Edited by David Burnett and John Crocker
© 2005 John Wiley & Sons, Ltd

associated with high mortality rates, but estimates of their incidence are thought to be quite conservative in comparison with their true magnitude, because many cases go undiagnosed or unreported.

As with other microbial infections, the diagnosis of fungal infections depends upon a combination of clinical observation and laboratory investigation. Superficial and subcutaneous infections often produce characteristic lesions that suggest the diagnosis, but laboratory tests are essential where this is not the case, either because the clinical signs mimic those of other conditions or because the appearance of lesions has been altered by previous treatment. In most situations where systemic fungal infection is entertained as a diagnosis, the clinical presentation is non-specific and can be caused by a wide range of infections, underlying illnesses or complications of treatment.

The successful laboratory diagnosis of fungal infections depends in major part on the collection of adequate specimens for investigation. It is also dependent on the selection of appropriate microbiological, serological and histopathological test procedures. These differ from one disease to another, and depend on the site of infection as well as the presenting symptoms and clinical signs. Interpretation of the results of laboratory investigations can sometimes be made with confidence, but at times the findings can be unhelpful or even misleading. It is in these situations that close liaison between the clinician and the laboratory is particularly important.

Laboratory methods for the diagnosis of fungal infections remain based on three broad approaches: the microscopical detection of the aetiological agent in clinical material; its isolation and identification in culture; and the detection of a serological response to the pathogen or some other marker of its presence, such as a fungal cell constituent or metabolic product. New diagnostic procedures, based on the detection of fungal DNA in clinical material, are currently being developed, but have not yet had a significant impact in clinical laboratories. In the sections that follow, the value and limitations of current diagnostic procedures for fungal infections are reviewed.

Microscopic examination

The direct microscopic examination of clinical material is often helpful in the laboratory diagnosis of fungal infections. Various methods can be used: unstained wet preparations can be examined by light-field, dark-field or phase-contrast illumination, or dried smears can be stained and examined. In some instances, direct

microscopic examination will permit a tentative or definitive diagnosis to be made, long before growth is apparent in culture. In other instances, observation of fungal elements in a clinical specimen is more significant than isolating the fungus in culture, particularly if the organism is a common contaminant.

Although fungal cells are larger than bacterial cells, these organisms are often present in much smaller numbers in clinical specimens. For this reason it is often essential to increase the concentration of fungal elements in a specimen before it is examined. Fluids and secretions should be centrifuged and the deposit retained for mycological investigation. Other specimens, such as sputum, must be digested before centrifugation.

There are several methods of preparing specimens for direct microscopic examination. Gram-stained smears are often used to detect fungal cells in fluids and secretions (Figure 24.1). India ink is useful for negative

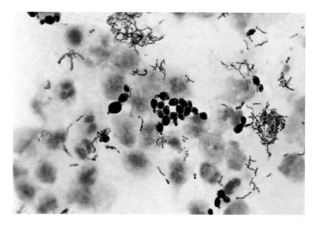

Figure 24.1 Gram-stained smear of peritoneal drain fluid, showing clusters of budding yeast cells and numerous much smaller bacterial cells

staining of cerebrospinal fluid (CSF) sediment to reveal encapsulated *Cryptococcus neoformans* cells. Both Giemsa stain and Wright's stain can be used to detect *Histoplasma capsulatum* cells in bone marrow preparations or blood smears. The Papanicolaou stain can be used on sputum or other respiratory tract samples to detect fungal elements.

Skin scrapings and other dermatological specimens should be examined after digestion with 10–20% potassium hydroxide solution, which clears the specimen without damaging the fungal cells. These samples can be examined without stain, as a wet preparation (Figure 24.2). The addition of chemical brighteners, such as calcofluor white, is helpful in revealing fungal elements

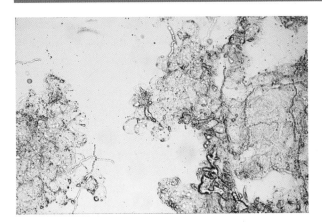

Figure 24.2 Unstained potassium hydroxide preparation of skin, demonstrating the presence of branching dermatophyte hyphae, some of which are fragmenting in arthrospores

in wet preparations of these and other clinical materials, such as sputum, when examined under a fluorescence microscope. The fungal elements appear brightly staining against a dark background.

In certain situations, direct microscopic examination of fluids or other clinical material can establish the diagnosis of a subcutaneous or systemic fungal infection. Instances include the detection of encapsulated *Cryptococcus neoformans* cells in CSF, or *Histoplasma capsulatum* cells in peripheral blood smears. More often, however, only a tentative diagnosis of deep fungal infection can be made on the basis of microscopic examination. Nevertheless, this can help to determine whether an organism recovered later in culture is a contaminant or a pathogen, and can assist in the selection of the most appropriate culture conditions to recover organisms visualized on direct smear.

Histopathological examination of tissue sections is one of the most reliable methods of establishing the diagnosis of subcutaneous and systemic fungal infections. However, the ease with which a fungal pathogen can be recognized in tissue is dependent not only on its abundance, but also on the distinctiveness of its appearance. Many fungi stain poorly with haematoxylin and eosin and this method alone may be insufficient to reveal fungal elements in tissue. There are a number of special stains for detecting and highlighting fungal organisms, including methenamine–silver (Grocott or Gomori) and periodic acid–Schiff. Mucicarmine can be used to stain the capsule of *Cryptococcus neoformans*.

These staining methods, although useful at revealing the presence of fungal elements in tissue, seldom permit the precise fungal genus involved to be identified. For instance, the detection of non-pigmented branching,

septate hyphae is typical of *Aspergillus* infection, but it is also characteristic of a large number of less common organisms, including species of *Fusarium* and *Scedosporium*. Likewise, the detection of small, budding fungal cells seldom permits a specific diagnosis. Tissue-form cells of *Histoplasma capsulatum* and *Blastomyces dermatitidis*, for instance, can appear similar, and may be confused with non-encapsulated *Cryptococcus neoformans* cells.

To overcome this problem, a number of methods have been developed for the specific identification of fungal organisms in tissue. Immunoperoxidase and immunofluorescent staining reagents, both monoclonal and polyclonal, are available for some fungi, and can facilitate the identification of atypical fungal elements and the detection of small numbers of organisms. Currently under investigation are a number of techniques that involve specific binding of DNA probes to the nucleic acid of the fungal agent, either directly on the slide (*in situ* hybridization) or in a test tube.

Culture

Isolation in culture will permit most pathogenic fungi to be identified. Most of these organisms are not fastidious in their nutritional requirements and will grow on the media used for bacterial isolation from clinical specimens. However, growth on these media can be slow and development of the spores and other structures used in fungal identification can be poor. For these reasons, most laboratories use a specific medium, such as Sabouraud's dextrose agar, to isolate fungi (Figure 24.3). Many clinical

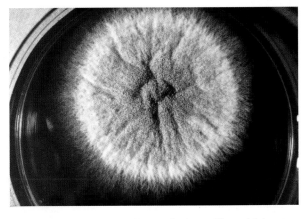

Figure 24.3 Typical culture of *Aspergillus nidulans* on Sabouraud's dextrose agar. Note the powdery appearance of the colonial surface, due to the presence of enormous numbers of spores

specimens submitted for fungal culture are contaminated with bacteria and it is essential to add antibacterial antibiotics to fungal culture media. If dermatophytes or dimorphic fungi are being isolated, cycloheximide (actidione) should be added to the medium as well, to prevent overgrowth by faster-growing fungi.

The optimum growth temperature for most pathogenic fungi is around 30°C. Material from patients with a suspected superficial infection should be incubated at 25–30°C, because most dermatophytes will not grow at higher temperatures. Material from subcutaneous or deep sites should be incubated at two temperatures, 25–30°C and 37°C. This is because a number of important pathogens, including *Histoplasma capsulatum*, *Blastomyces dermatitidis* and *Sporothrix schenckii*, are dimorphic and the change in their growth form, depending on the incubation conditions, is useful in identification. At 25–30°C these organisms develop as moulds on Sabouraud's dextrose agar, but at higher temperatures on an enriched medium (such as brain–heart infusion agar), these organisms grow as budding yeasts.

Some pathogenic fungi grow slowly and cultures should be retained for at least 2 weeks, and in some case up to 4 weeks, before being discarded as negative. However, many common pathogenic fungi, such as *Aspergillus* and *Candida* species, will produce identifiable colonies within 1–3 days. Cultures should be examined at frequent intervals (at least three times weekly) and appropriate sub-cultures made, particularly from blood-enriched media, on which fungi often fail to sporulate.

It is important to recognize that growth of an organism in culture does not necessarily establish its role as a pathogen. Only if the organism is identified as an unequivocal pathogen, such as *Trichophyton rubrum* or *Histoplasma capsulatum*, can the diagnosis can be firmly established. If, however, an opportunistic organism such as *Aspergillus fumigatus* or *Candida albicans* is recovered, its isolation may have no clinical relevance unless there is additional evidence of its involvement in a pathogenic process. In this situation, culture results should be compared with those of microscopic examination. Isolation of opportunistic fungal pathogens from sterile sites, such as blood or CSF, often provides reliable evidence of significant infection, but their isolation from material such as pus, sputum or urine must be interpreted with caution. Attention should be given to the amount of fungus isolated and further investigations undertaken.

Many unfamiliar moulds have been reported as occasional causes of lethal systemic infection in immunocompromised patients. No isolate should be dismissed as a contaminant without careful consideration of the clinical condition of the patient, the site of isolation, the method of specimen collection, the amount of organisms recovered, and the likelihood of contamination.

Although culture often permits the definitive diagnosis of a fungal infection, it also has some limitations. Chief amongst these is failure to recover the organism. This may be due to inadequate specimen collection or delayed transport of specimens. Incorrect isolation procedures or inadequate periods of incubation are other important factors.

Identification

Once isolated in culture, moulds and dermatophytes (filamentous fungi) are identified on the basis of their macroscopic (colonial) and microscopic morphologic characteristics. Macroscopic characteristics, such as colonial form, surface colour and pigmentation, are often helpful in identification, but it is essential to examine slide preparations of the culture under a microscope. If well prepared, these will often give sufficient information on the form and arrangement of the spores and spore-bearing structures for identification of the fungus to be accomplished (Figure 24.4). Because

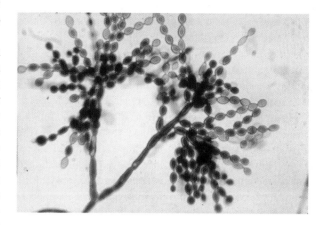

Figure 24.4 Lactophenol cotton blue stain of *Cladophialophora carrionii*, showing the characteristic long branching chains of spores by which this organism is identified

identification is usually dependent on visualization of the particular structures an organism produces when it is sporulating, identification is usually dependent on the ability of the organism to sporulate. Moulds often grow best on rich media, such as Sabouraud's dextrose agar, but overproduction of mycelium often results in loss of sporulation. If a mould isolate fails to produce spores after 2 weeks, it should be subcultured to a less-rich medium to encourage sporulation. The use of DNA-based identification methods may in future eliminate this requirement.

Yeasts (unicellular, budding fungi) are usually identified on the basis of their morphological and biochemical characteristics. Useful morphological characteristics include the colour of the colonies, the size and shape of the cells, the presence of a capsule around the cells, and the production of hyphae or pseudohyphae. Useful biochemical tests include the assimilation and fermentation of sugars, and the assimilation of nitrate and urea. Most yeasts associated with human infections can be identified using one of the numerous commercial identification systems, such as API 20C AUX (bioMerieux-Vitek Inc., Hazelwood, MO), that are based on the differential assimilation of various carbon compounds. However, it is important to remember that morphological examination of Dalmau plate cultures on cornmeal agar is essential to avoid confusion between organisms with identical biochemical profiles. A number of simple rapid tests have been devised for the presumptive identification of some of the most important human pathogens. Foremost among these is the serum germ tube test for *Candida albicans*, which can be performed in less than 3 hours, and the urease test for *Cryptococcus neoformans*. In recent years a number of rapid commercial tests have been developed. These include the RapID Yeast Plus system (Innovative Diagnostic Systems, Norcross, GA) that contains conventional and chromogenic substrates and requires 4 hours to perform. Most of these rapid test systems are more accurate in the identification of the common rather than unusual yeast pathogens.

In the past, dimorphic fungi such as *Blastomyces dermatitidis* and *Histoplasma capsulatum* were identified by observing the conversion of mycelial growth at 25°C to yeast-like growth at 37°C. However, development of DNA probe-based tests (Accuprobe, GenProbe Inc., San Diego, CA) has enabled these pathogens to be identified using only a small amount of mycelial material.

Serological tests

Serological testing often provides the most rapid means of diagnosing a systemic fungal infection. Most tests are based on the detection of antibodies to specific fungal pathogens, although tests for fungal antigens are now becoming more widely available. At their best, individual serological tests can be diagnostic, e.g. tests for antigenaemia in cryptococcosis and histoplasmosis. In general, however, the results of serological testing are seldom more than suggestive or supportive of a fungal diagnosis. These tests must be interpreted with caution and considered alongside the results of other clinical and laboratory investigations.

Tests for antibodies have proved useful in diagnosing infections, such as histoplasmosis and coccidioidomycosis, in immunocompetent persons. In these individuals, the interval between exposure and the development of symptoms (2–6 weeks) is usually sufficient for a humoral response to develop. Tests for *Histoplasma capsulatum* and *Coccidioides immitis* antibodies are most helpful when paired serum specimens (acute and convalescent) are obtained, so that it can be determined whether titres are rising or falling. Tests for antibodies also have an established diagnostic use in the different forms of *Aspergillus* infection that occur in immunocompetent individuals. In contrast, these tests are seldom helpful in diagnosing invasive aspergillosis in immunocompromised persons, many of whom are incapable of mounting a detectable humoral response to infection. Tests for *Candida* antibodies have been extensively evaluated but remain of limited usefulness in the diagnosis of invasive forms of candidiasis. These tests are complicated by false-positive results in patients with mucosal colonization or superficial infection, and by false negative results in immunocompromised individuals.

Testing for fungal antigens in serum, CSF and/or urine is an established procedure for the diagnosis of cryptococcosis and histoplasmosis, and similar tests are currently being evaluated for aspergillosis and candidiasis. The LPA test for *Cryptococcus neoformans* capsular polysaccharide antigen is sensitive and specific, giving positive results with serum and CSF specimens from well over 90% of infected patients. High or rising titres indicate progression of infection, while falling titres indicate regression of disease and response to treatment. Antigen detection in urine has proved a useful method for the rapid diagnosis of histoplasmosis in patients presenting with acute disease, as well as in those with disseminated infection. In acute disease, antigen can be detected in urine within the first month after exposure before antibodies appear. Several test formats have been developed, including RIA and ELISA.

Antigen detection tests have also been extensively evaluated for the rapid diagnosis of invasive forms of aspergillosis in immunocompromised individuals. Two tests have been marketed to detect circulating galactomannan, a major cell wall component of *Aspergillus* species. Both utilize the same monoclonal, in either an

LPA or sandwich ELISA format. The latter test (Platelia Aspergillus, Sanofi Diagnostics Pasteur, Paris, France) is more sensitive than the former (Pastorex Aspergillus, Sanofi Diagnostics Pasteur) and can detect galactomannan in serum at an earlier stage of infection.

New directions in diagnosis

New approaches to the diagnosis of invasive fungal infections include the detection of fungal genomic sequences in clinical specimens. Most of the diagnostic methods that have been devised have been based on the use of conventional PCR formats, but many modified approaches have also been evaluated, including multiplex PCR and nested PCR methods. Several regions within the fungal genome have been evaluated as potential targets for detection, but much effort has focused on the ribosomal DNA (rDNA) gene complex. This section of the genome includes the relatively conserved regions of the 18S, 5.8S and 28S genes and the more variable intervening transcribed spacer (ITS) regions. The latest developments in fungal molecular diagnostics involve the use of real-time PCR methods, in which thermocycling is combined with fluorescence monitoring of the amplified product during its generation. These techniques permit quantification of the amounts of fungal nucleic acid that are present in clinical specimens, thus allowing the microbial load to be measured.

Despite recent progress, the goal of developing simple, rapid and cost-effective clinical tests for the molecular diagnosis of acute life-threatening fungal infections remains elusive. Although numerous research laboratories now offer 'in-house' procedures for molecular detection of fungal infection from tissue specimens or from body fluids, the sensitivity, specificity and predictive value of these tests have not always been thoroughly investigated. It is to be hoped that, in the future, the relevance of serial monitoring of fungal antigens and fungal-specific nucleic acid sequences in blood and other biological fluids will be demonstrated, and that reliable tests will become available to a much broader group of clinical laboratories.

Further reading

Campbell CK, Johnson EM, Philpot CM, Warnock DW. *Identification of Pathogenic Fungi*. 1996 Public Health Laboratory Service, London.

Chen SC, Halliday CL, Meyer W. A review of nucleic acid-based diagnostic tests for systemic mycoses with an emphasis on polymerase chain reaction-based assays. *Med Mycol* 2003; **40**: 333–357.

Richardson MD, Warnock DW. *Fungal Infection: Diagnosis and Management*, 3rd edn. 2003: Blackwell, Oxford.

Yeo SF, Wong B. Current status of nonculture methods for diagnosis of invasive fungal infections. *Clin Microbiol Rev* 2002 **15**: 465–484.

25

Parasitology

Robert WA Girdwood

Introduction

In the context of this book, diagnostic parasitology can be defined as the demonstration of evidence of the presence of protozoan or metazoan organisms which live in or on human beings or other animals (the hosts). The evidence may be direct or indirect. Direct evidence is usually achieved by the examination of samples from the putative host, such as faeces, urine, blood and other tissues, for a stage of the parasite or a portion of the parasite. Indirect evidence can be obtained by demonstrating characteristic inflammatory responses, parasite products or specific antibodies in the putative host. The direct demonstration of a parasite stage in a host sample, e.g. a helminth ovum in a sample of faeces, is usually incontrovertible evidence of infection but the possibility of specimen contamination must always be considered. Conversely, a failure to demonstrate ova in a faecal sample does not necessarily exclude a diagnosis, as it takes time for parasites to mature in their hosts and produce the looked-for stage, or the parasite stage may be scanty or intermittently present in the samples examined. Indirect evidence of infection, such as demonstration of antibodies, must also be treated with caution, especially because of the possibility of cross-reactions with other parasites. It is for these reasons that a detailed knowledge of parasite life cycles, modes of transmission and times taken for the various stages to be completed are prerequisites for a soundly based diagnostic approach. This knowledge is required to decide what samples to examine and what tests are most appropriate in relation to the possible time of exposure to infection and the disease manifestations, if present.

The cornerstone of most diagnostic parasitology is based on morphology and morphometrics. Thus, although in microbiological terms the transmissive stages (i.e. ova, cysts, oocysts or larvae) tend to be relatively large—in the order of tens to hundreds of microns (μm) — the conventional transmitted light microscope remains the most important diagnostic tool. Similarly, although most adult worms and most arthropod parasites (or vectors) are macroscopic, microscopy is usually required to detect the often subtle morphological features necessary for species identification. In this latter instance, a low-magnification stereomicroscope is most useful.

Microscopy

The conventional transmitted light microscope, providing total magnifications of $\times 100$, $\times 400$ and $\times 1000$, is the parasitologist's basic instrument. Because an accurate measurement of the size of protozoan cysts, oocysts and helminth ova is so important, an accurately calibrated eyepiece graticule is essential. Transmitted light microscopy requires that the specimen to be examined is sufficiently transparent to allow light to pass through it and provide adequate definition of morphology. This means that the samples have to be thin, in the order of microns, and when relatively opaque have to be rendered more transparent by clearing agents. When the parasites themselves have a refractive index similar to that of the sample containing them, they require to be differentially stained so that the stain(s) used are taken up preferentially by the parasites. Less frequently, the surrounding

The Science of Laboratory Diagnosis, Second Edition   Edited by David Burnett and John Crocker
© 2005 John Wiley & Sons, Ltd

tissues or medium can be stained and the contained parasites remain unstained: this is negative staining. An alternative approach is to use different illumination systems such as dark-ground, phase-contrast or differential interference contrast (Nomarski) microscopy.

Wet mounts

In parasitology the most frequently examined sample is the wet mount, where a few drops of the specimen or a suspension of the specimen are placed on a microscope slide, covered with a coverslip and examined at total magnifications of ×100 and ×400. The specific details of the preparation of the specimen will depend on the number of parasites likely to be present in the sample relative to the presence of contaminating or obscuring material. Thus, while direct examination of unconcentrated drops of blood or urine or saline suspensions of faeces may be useful, concentration of the sample is usually necessary because the parasite is present in small numbers relative to the volume of the specimen requiring to be examined. Transparent fluids, such as urine, can be scrutinized by centrifugation and examination of a wet mount of the resuspended deposit or by filtration and similar examination of the residue. Faecal material presents a more complex problem in that scanty parasites may be present in a mass of opaque and obscuring debris. Techniques of selective concentration are employed, in which parasite ova, cysts and oocysts are concentrated and separated from the faecal debris, or vice versa (Figure 25.1). Such techniques use flotation and/or centrifugation, in which the differences between the densities of the parasite stages and the contaminating debris are exploited by using various suspending media

of different specific gravities. Depending on the technique used, the 'cleaned' concentrated sample to be examined microscopically will be taken from the centrifuged deposit, the interface between suspending media of differing specific gravities or the surface meniscus from flotation. Examples of such techniques include Ridley's formol-ether differential flotation/centrifugation, sucrose gradient concentration and zinc sulphate flotation. The same principles are used for the detection of parasite cysts, oocysts and ova in environmental samples, such as water, soil, sludge and sewage. In such samples the parasites are often even more scanty and further concentration techniques, such as anti-parasite antibodies attached to magnetized particles, are being used.

Parasites in the bloodstream are present at low concentration and, again, techniques that involve concentration of the parasites and allow the examination of larger volumes of blood are employed. Thus, detection of microfilariae which, although relatively large (200–300 μm), tend to be very scanty, invokes these techniques by either: (a) filtration of a large volume of anticoagulated blood through a membrane filter, which retains the microfilariae and allows the smaller cellular components of blood to pass through, with subsequent staining, clearing and microscopy of the filter; or (b) lysis of the erythrocytes in a large volume of blood (about 5 ml) and the sedimentation of any contained microfilariae, which are examined in a wet mount of the resuspended deposit.

Films and smears

Films and smears are used widely to detect parasites in samples of blood, bone marrow and faeces. Blood samples for the detection of protozoan parasites, such as malaria and trypanosomes, are usually examined as Romanowsky-stained thin or thick films (Figure 25.2). Thin blood films, one cell thick, are fixed prior to staining and, because of this, retain the morphology of the erythrocytes and, in the case of malaria, the contained intracellular parasites. With thick films the erythrocytes are lysed prior to staining and fixation, thus the final preparation reveals only leukocytes, platelets and parasites. The advantage of the thick film is that more material can be examined, but the disadvantages are that important morphological changes in the erythrocytes produced by the malaria parasite cannot be detected, and parasites can be confused with platelets and vice versa. Bone marrow smears stained with a Romanowsky stain are used to detect intracellular *Leishmania* spp.

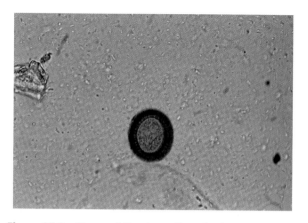

Figure 25.1 Ovum of *Taenia* sp. Formal-ether concentrated faecal suspension (×400).

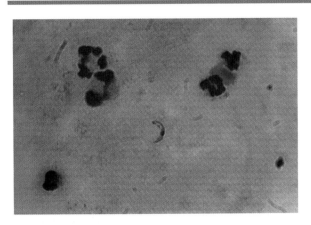

Figure 25.2 Trypomastigotes of *Trypanosoma rhodesiense*. Romanowsky stained thin blood film (×400)

Fixed and stained smears are required for the detection of protozoan trophozoites in faeces. Such techniques are necessary because trophozoites rupture in unfixed material and visualization of the fine details of nuclear structure and intracytoplasmic inclusions is required for the species identification of amoebae. Iron haematoxylin, trichrome and Giemsa stains are widely used for these purposes. In addition, stained faecal smears are used to detect *Cryptosporidium* spp. oocysts and microsporidial spores.

Less frequently, stained impression smears from tissue biopsy or necropsy material are employed to diagnose *Leishmania* spp. infections.

Histopathology

Conventional tissue sections can provide diagnostic information for the parasitologist, either by revealing characteristic tissue responses to the infection or by demonstration of the parasite (protozoan) or sections of the parasite (metazoan). Here again, micrometry is important and, in the context of examining histological sections of worms and their ova, due cognizance must be given to shrinkage due to fixation and alterations to dimensions if sections are other than truly cross-sectional or sagittal. Special stains are frequently employed to accentuate certain components of the parasite sections but description of their use is beyond the scope of this chapter.

Fluorescence

The ability of materials to become luminous when viewed with ultraviolet light is utilized in diagnostic parasitology in three ways: autofluorescence, fluorochrome staining and fluorochrome labelling. Autofluorescence refers to the intrinsic property of the organism or a component of the organism to fluoresce, and is exemplified by the blue appearance of *Cyclospora* spp. oocysts when viewed in unstained wet mounts under ultraviolet light. Fluorochrome staining refers to the direct staining of the organism or a component of the organism with the fluorochrome. The apple-green fluorescence produced by *Cryptosporidium* spp. oocysts when stained with auramine phenol is an example of this method. Fluorochrome labelling usually involves immunological methods, in which parasite-specific antibodies (polyclonal or monoclonal) are conjugated to a fluorochrome, such as fluorescein isothiocyanate, and used to enhance the detectability of parasites in clinical material. The success of this technique depends largely on the specificity of the antibody used to bind the fluorescent label to the parasite. Examples of useful assays include the detection of structurally damaged *Giardia duodenalis* cysts in faecal samples and the detection of *Entamoeba histolytica* trophozoites in tissue sections or abscesses. Indirect methods, which use fluorescence microscopy and the specific parasite as a fixed substrate to detect antibodies in serum, are described briefly in the serology section below. The incorporation or exclusion of fluorochromes is being advocated increasingly as a surrogate method of determining viability, and therefore potential infectivity, of cysts or oocysts isolated from environmental samples. Thus, the exclusion of propidium iodide and the inclusion of 4,6-diamidino-2-phenylindole (DAPI) by *Cryptosporidium* spp. oocysts is currently under evaluation.

Electron microscopy

With the exception of microsporidial infections, electron microscopy has little place in diagnostic parasitology. Although alternative diagnostic procedures are being developed, transmission electron microscopy of faeces, intestinal biopsies and other tissues is the definitive, if somewhat inconvenient, technique for diagnosing infections with these organisms, primarily because they are small (1–2 μm), intracellular and stain poorly.

Culture

A very basic form of culture is employed for the diagnosis and speciation of nematode larvae, such as hookworms and *Strongyloides* spp. While *Strongyloides* larvae are voided in the faeces of the host and ova are not usually present, the converse is true of the hookworms *Ancylostoma duodenale* and *Necator americanus*, where ova only are voided in fresh faeces. As the ova of the latter two are morphologically indistinguishable, speciation can only be effected by creating conditions in which ova hatch and develop into distinguishable third-stage larvae. In addition, the motility of the larvae of all three species is utilized to facilitate collection. This is particularly useful in the diagnosis of strongyloidiasis, where larvae present in faeces may be scanty and do not concentrate well when conventional techniques such as formol-ether are used. The conditions that pertain in the natural transmission of these parasites are recreated in the Harada–Muri (or similar) technique. Here, faecal material is smeared on filter paper strips, the lower ends of which are suspended in a well of distilled water contained in sealed test-tubes and incubated at 28°C for about 10 days. Under these conditions, the hatched hookworm larvae and the *Strongyloides* larvae migrate down the filter paper to be collected in the water. The larvae are then speciated by detecting morphological differences. It should be noted that no replication of parasites occurs in this 'culture' technique.

In vitro culture of clinical material for diagnostic purposes is used relatively infrequently in parasitology compared with the other microbial disciplines. This is because protozoans and metazoans have more complex metabolic requirements which, in the majority of cases, cannot be met in current *in vitro* culture systems. Nevertheless, true replicative cultural methods have a limited role in diagnostic parasitology, where alternative methods are used but have other limitations. Thus, Robinson's culture system for the isolation of *Entamoeba histolytica* as a diagnostic technique is fairly cumbersome and insensitive but it does offer the advantage, when successful, of yielding trophozoites for isoenzyme analysis. Zymodeme determination of isolates can distinguish between pathogenic and non-pathogenic strains. Similarly, *in vitro* culture of biopsy material is used widely in the diagnosis of both cutaneous and visceral leishmaniasis, frequently as an adjunct to direct microscopy of a suitably stained portion of the same material. The advantage of microscopy is that it is quick and, if positive, diagnostic, but this is offset by the frequent paucity of parasites. Culture is relatively slow—days to weeks—but has the advantage, when positive, of yielding viable organisms that can be speciated by molecular, serological or enzyme analyses and, in addition, can be used for drug susceptibility testing. It must be emphasized again that negative culture results do not exclude the diagnosis.

Increasingly, with the sophistication of *in vitro* culture techniques, parasites are propagated in axenic culture so that the parasites, fractions prepared from them or their metabolic products can be harvested, purified and characterized for use in immunological diagnostic procedures. Two basic examples of the use of cultural methods for immunodiagnostic purposes are: first, *in vitro* culture of *Entamoeba histolytica* trophozoites, which are harvested, attached to microscope slides and used as antigen in the indirect fluorescent antibody test for amoebiasis; second, the maintenance of hatched second-stage *Toxocara canis* larvae *in vitro* and the harvesting, concentration and standardization of the excretory/secretory products they produce for use as antigens in an ELISA test for the detection of circulating *Toxocara* antibodies.

Animal infection

The inoculation or feeding of clinical material into susceptible species of laboratory-maintained experimental animals was once the mainstay of all disciplines of diagnostic microbiology. A diagnosis was established by the sacrifice of the animals after an appropriate incubation period and the demonstration of the organism, or the characteristic pathology produced by it, in the organs or tissues by conventional microscopic and histological techniques. Increasingly, alternative diagnostic methods are being used, but animals are still required, either for the maintenance of parasites for use as antigens when there are no *in vitro* culture techniques available, or for the production of anti-parasite antibodies used in diagnostic tests. It seems likely that in the former instance the use of construct antigens or the development of tissue culture techniques will reduce further this requirement, e.g. continuous cell culture for the production of *T. gondii* has replaced animal culture.

Xenodiagnosis

This unusual method falls somewhere between culture and animal inoculation and utilizes a natural vector or intermediate host in the parasite's life cycle to concentrate the parasite and thus make it more readily detectable. The classic example of xenodiagnosis uses one of the insect vectors of *Trypanosoma cruzi* to facilitate the diagnosis of Chagas' disease (South American trypanosomiasis). Laboratory-reared (parasite-free) nymphal stages of the reduviid bugs are allowed to feed on the patient and are sacrificed some 4 weeks later. The contents of the hindgut are expressed, stained and examined microscopically for trypomastigotes. This almost unique example of xenodiagnosis acknowledges that parasites are extremely scanty in the peripheral blood of the host and the reduviid bugs are extremely efficient vectors.

Serology

Serodiagnosis is generally less reliable than the more direct microscopic methods because of the problems of cross-reactivity (poor specificity), low sensitivity and, frequently, the inability to distinguish between past and current infections. Of the three major groups of serological assays, i.e. detection of antibody, detection of antigen and the detection of immune complexes, it is the first category which is most widely used in diagnosis. Such serological techniques are usually employed when material for direct examination for the presence of the parasite is not available. Thus, generally, serological tests for the diagnosis of intestinal parasites would not normally be recommended, because specific diagnosis by the demonstration of ova or cysts in the usually readily available faeces would be the method of choice. Conversely, in tissue-invasive parasitic diseases, such as echinococcosis, toxoplasmosis or toxocarosis, the demonstration of circulating antibodies may be more productive than tissue biopsy examination. The interpretation of serological results in relation to the stage of the disease produced by the parasite (acute or chronic) can be improved by determining the immunoglobulin class and isotype involved in the antibody response. Greater sensitivity and specificity of the test can, in some instances, be achieved by immunoblotting. Similarly, better characterization of antigen preparations, e.g. using monoclonal antibodies, can achieve the same goal. Because antibodies can persist for years following infection and following successful treatment, the detection of parasite antigen in clinical material is, in theory, more attractive because the presence of antigen must indicate current or very recent infection. Examples of the value of this approach are (a) the use of the ELISA technique to detect filarial antigen in the serum, urine and hydrocoele fluid of patients with *Wuchereria bancrofti* infections (where in the chronic stages microfilariae are difficult to demonstrate in the peripheral blood) and (b) in the serum and urine of patients with *Onchocerca volvulus* infections. A potential additional advantage of antigen detection is that quantification of circulating or excreted antigen may correlate with worm burden and, by extrapolation, symptomatology and transmissibility.

The detection of immune complexes is not yet sufficiently specific for diagnostic purposes, but dissociation of these complexes to detect the antigen and/or antibody components is a more promising approach.

Molecular methods

The use of DNA probes and the PCR technique has proliferated throughout all fields of microbiology in the last 20 years. While this is true in parasitological research, where such techniques now predominate, in the fields of diagnostic parasitology the role of molecular methods remains limited at present. The main advantage of nucleic acid-based detection methods is their sensitivity. Thus, in diagnosis it is only when the parasite burden is low that these techniques can improve on the more conventional approaches. South American trypanosomiasis is a good example, where in the chronic stage of the disease parasitaemias are so low as to be beyond the limit of detection by conventional microscopic methods (see Xenodiagnosis, above). Also in this disease, because of its endemicity, serodiagnosis not only lacks specificity but cannot distinguish between infection past or present and current disease status. Specifically, a conserved mini-repeat sequence of kinetoplast DNA minicirclets used as a probe, followed by PCR amplification, has proved more sensitive and specific than microscopy, xenodiagnosis or serology. Molecular methods can also be valuable diagnostically where more conventional approaches are jeopardized by changes in the host. A prime example is the problem of diagnosing toxoplamosis in the immunocompromised host. *Toxoplasma gondii* has a worldwide distribution, with a high incidence of subclinical infection. Diagnosis of infections past or present is usually made by assaying the various classes of specific antibody. In the immunocompromised host, latent infection can progress to potentially fatal disease and, because of the immune deficiency, serodiagnosis is unhelpful. PCR assays targeting the B1 gene or the P30 gene have been applied to amniotic fluid and thereby the diagnosis of foetal infection can be made without foetoscopy.

Antigen production, by either hybridization or recombinant DNA technology, is providing potentially useful specific and sensitive diagnostic reagents, and the use of molecular techniques to detect parasite-bearing vectors is a further example of the exciting promise of molecular research. However, enthusiasm for the potential of such techniques must be tempered by awareness of the disadvantages of relative expense and the problems of false positive results due to contamination of samples.

Table 25.1 Some advantages and disadvantages of the major approaches used in diagnostic parasitology

Method	Advantages	Disadvantages
Microscopy	Fast (for individual specimen) Direct visualization of parasite Positive result usually definitive	Requires skilled microscopist Requires relatively numerous parasites, i.e. negative result does not exclude diagnosis Slow for mass screening
In vitro culture	Detects only viable parasites Provides isolates for further characterization, sensitivity testing and antigen preparation	Slow Only available for limited number of species/strains Negative culture does not exclude diagnosis
Animal infection	As above	As above Expensive
Serology	Simple Fast Can be used for mass screening	Lack of standard reagents (antigens) Difficult to differentiate between past and present infection False positive results due to cross-reactivity
Xenodiagnosis	Simple Cheap Specific	Low sensitivity Very limited application Slow ?Unpleasant
Molecular methods	Fast Sensitive Can detect live and dead parasites Direct detection of parasite	Expensive Detects live and dead parasites False negatives from PCR inhibitors False positives from contamination

The main diagnostic procedures with some of their advantages and disadvantages are summarized in Table 25.1.

Further reading

Basic Laboratory Methods in Medical Parasitology. 1991: World Health Organization, Geneva.

Cook GC (ed.) *Manson's Tropical Diseases.* 1996: WB Saunders, London.

Fleck SL, Moody AH. *Diagnostic Techniques in Medical Parasitology.* 1988: Wright, London.

Gillespie SH, Hawkey PM (eds). *Medical Parasitology—A Practical Approach.* 1995: Oxford University Press, Oxford.

Kettle DS (ed.). *Medical and Veterinary Entomology.* 1995: CAB International, Wallingford.

SECTION 5

HAEMATOLOGY

26

Blood cell and bone marrow morphology

Supratik Basu

Peripheral blood morphology

Cell morphology is an essential part of any haematological investigation, and is best assessed by examining a well-spread, well-stained film. A blood film may be made from non-anticoagulated (native) blood, obtained from either a vein or a capillary, or EDTA anti-coagulated blood. A well-made film is evenly spread and has a tongue-shaped edge. Once made, the film should be rapidly air-dried and then fixed in absolute methanol for 10–20 minutes.

Staining

All films once fixed should be stained as soon as possible. Blood and bone marrow films are stained by Romanowsky dyes consisting of a mixture of methylene blue and eosin. Methylene blue stained acidic components, e.g. nuclei and cytoplasmic RNA blue, while eosin stains basic components, such as haemoglobin, red. A popular Romanowsky stain is May–Gruenewald–Giesma stain. In certain situations, such as differentiating various types of leukaemias, special stains are employed (see Table 26.5).

Technique for examination of film

Films should first be examined under a low magnification, in order to get an idea of the quality of preparation, number, distribution and staining of red cells, leukocytes and platelets. A low magnification is also best suited to detect the presence of abnormal precipitates and agglu-

tination. Once a satisfactory low-power examination has been made, a suitable area of the film should be examined in greater detail under higher power or an oil immersion objective.

Red cell morphology

In health, red cells vary little in size and shape. The majority of red cells are round and smooth and have a diameter within a narrow range (mean $\pm 2SD$) of 6.0–8.5 µm with a central pallor. In examination of a film in which the red cells are well spread and do not touch each other, less than 10% of the red cells should be oval in shape. A very small percentage (less than 0.1%) may be contracted or fragmented. In premature and normal infants this proportion may be higher (0.3–5.6%) (for normal peripheral blood morphology, see Figure 26.1).

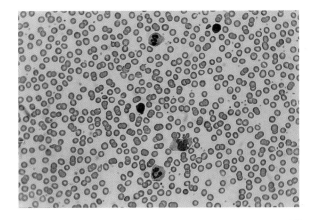

Figure 26.1 Normal peripheral film showing neutrophil, lymphocyte, monocyte

The Science of Laboratory Diagnosis, Second Edition   Edited by David Burnett and John Crocker
© 2005 John Wiley & Sons, Ltd

Table 26.1 RBC abnormalities

Terminology	What it means	Associated conditions
Anisocytosis	Greater variation in size than normal.	Non-specific feature. Pronounced in severe anaemia
Anisochromia	Dual population of cells. Some, but not all, RBC stain palely.	Iron deficiency being treated, or transfused. Combined hematinic deficiency
Acanthocytosis	Small cells with regular, multiple spiky projections.	Post-splenectomy (Hyposplenic), McLeod phenotype, α-β lipoproteinaemia, starvation
Auto-agglutination (Fig. 26.2)	Irregular clumping of red cells.	Cold agglutinin diseases, autoimmune haemolytic aneamia
Basophilic stippling (Fig. 26.3)	Deep blue small inclusions in RBC. Best seen under oil immersion.	Lead poisoning, pyrimidine 5′ nucleotidase deficiency, myelodysplasia, megaloblastic anaemia, unstable haemoglobin disease, thalassaemia
Crenated cells	RBC showing evenly spaced blunt projections.	Artefact, hypothyroid, old age, renal failure
Elliptocytosis	Oval or elliptical cells.	Megaloblastic anaemia, iron deficiency, myelofibrosis, hereditary elliptocytosis/ovalocytosis
Howell Jolly bodies (Fig. 26.4)	Darkly staining, round, dot-like inclusion within cells (nuclear remnant).	Hyposplenism of any cause, megaloblastic anaemia
Hypochromia (Fig. 26.5)	Pale red cells (MCH <27 pg)	Iron deficiency anaemia, thalassamia, sidroblastic anaemia
Macrocytosis (Fig. 26.6)	Large cells (MCV >100 fl)	Megaloblastic anaemia, myelodysplasia, hypothyroid, aplastic anaemia, liver disease
Microcytosis (Fig. 26.5)	Small cells (MCV <75 fl)	See hypochromia
Nucleated RBC (Fig. 26.7)	Presence of red cells with nuclei.	Any severe anaemia, myelofibrosis, severe haemolysis, thalaxssaemia (post-splenectomy), marrow infiltration.
Normal in cord blood, large numbers found in haemolytic disease of newborn
Poikilocytes	Red cells with abnormal shape.	Any anaemia, specially associated with abnormal erythropoiesis, e.g. thalassaemia, myelofibrosis
Polychromasia	Presence of red cells staining bluish grey. These are reticulocytes.	Haemolysis, blood loss, extramedullary erythropoiesis
Rouleaux (Fig. 26.8)	Stacking of RBC in columns.	Some degree is normal, myeloma, macroglobulinaemia, chronic infection, and inflammation
Schistocyte (Fig. 26.9)	Fragmented red cells.	DIC, carcinoma, micro-angiopathic haemolytic anaemia (MAHA)
Sickle cell (Fig. 26.10)	Thin, elongated crescentic, cells.	Sickle cells diseases
Spherocytes (Fig. 26.7)	Small density straining cells with no central pallor.	Hereditary spherocytosis, ABO haemolytic disease of newborn, autoimmune haemolytic anaemia
Spur cell	Cells with irregular, sharp projections.	Liver disease, pyruvate kinase deficiency
Stomatocytes	Cells with slit-like mouth at centre.	Hereditary stomatocytosis, alcoholism, artefact
Target cells (Fig. 26.11)	RBC with central dense staining area and disease, rim of haemoglobin at the periphery, with clear ring in between these two.	Haemoglobinopathies e.g. HbCC, SC liver disease
Tear-drop cells (Fig. 26.12)	Self-explanatory (type of poikilocytosis).	Myelofibrosis, thalassaemia

Abnormalities of RBC morphology

A complete description of all normal variations and abnormalities is not possible in this small chapter. For this a detailed atlas should be consulted. Some common abnormalities affecting the red cells with their associated disorders are listed in Table 26.1.

White cell morphology

Normal peripheral blood leukocytes are classified as polymorphonuclear leukocytes and mononuclear cells. The latter term refers to lymphocytes and monocytes. In a blood film monocytes and neutrophils are concentrated at the edge and at the end of the film. Vital information is obtained by scanning the film for abnormal forms and numbers at a lower magnification. Detailed study of granulation and nuclear and cytoplasmic morphology is then best done under oil immersion or a higher power of magnification.

Normal morphology

The normal white cells are of five types:

- *Neutrophils*: The mature neutrophil measures 12–15 μm in diameter. The cytoplasm is acidophilic with fine granules. The nucleus with clumped chromatin is divided into two to five distinct lobes by filaments which are dense heterochromatin. In females, some neutrophils have a drumstick-shaped nuclear appendage linked to the nucleus by a filament. This represents an inactive X chromosome (Figure 26.1).

- *Eosinophils*: These are slightly larger then neutrophils, being 12–17 μm in diameter. The nucleus is usually bilobed. Eosinophil granules are spherical, larger, coarse and reddish orange in colour (see Figure 26.13).

- *Basophils*: Basophils are similar in size to neutrophils. The nucleus is obscured by purple-black, coarse granules.

- *Lymphocytes*: These are 10–16 μm in diameter. The smaller lymphocytes (10 μm), which predominate, have a scanty cytoplasm and a round nucleus with condensed chromatin. About 10% of the lymphocytes are larger, have more abundant cytoplasm and less condensed nuclear chromatin. Lymphocytes may have a small number of granules containing lysosomal enzymes (azurophilic granules). Occasional larger cells with more abundant cytoplasm have quite prominent azurophilic granules. These are called large granular lymphocytes (for normal lymphocyte morphology, see Figure 26.1).

- *Monocytes*: These are the largest cells, with a diameter of 12–20 μm. The nucleus is irregular and lobulated. Cytoplasm is plentiful with a greyish-blue colour. Fine azurophilic granules can be seen. The cell outline is often irregular and the cytoplasm may also be vacuolated (Figure 26.1). Delay in making films with EDTA blood gives rise to sequestrine changes. This shows as vacuolation of the nucleus and cytoplasm. It first affects the monocytes and then the neutrophils.

Abnormalities of WBC morphology

Some common abnormalities affecting the leukocytes are listed in Table 26.2.

Platelets

Normal platelets measure 1–3 μm in diameter. They contain fine granules which are either dispersed or concentrated in the centre. A rough guess can be made of their number while examining a film. In EDTA anticoagulated blood platelets generally remain separate. In fresh films they are often clumped. A poorly collected specimen can cause a spuriously low platelet count. Some common abnormalities of platelets are listed in Table 26.3.

Examination of bone marrow and bone marrow morphology

The distribution of haemopoietic marrow is age-dependent. In neonates, haemopoietic marrow occupies almost all of the bone marrow cavity. Haematopoiesis occurs in virtually all bones. With age, haemopoietic marrow contracts and is replaced by fatty marrow. In young adults haemopoietic marrow is confined to the skull, spine, ribs, clavicle, sternum, pelvis and proximal portions of the long bones. However, haemopoietic marrow can expand in response to increased demand.

Examination of bone marrow

Bone marrow should be examined for morphology by both aspiration biopsy and a trephine biopsy. Bone marrow aspirations are commonly carried out from the sternum,

Table 26.2 WBC abnormalities

Terminology	What it means	Associated conditions
Atypical lymphocytes (Fig. 26.14)	Large lymphocytes with basophilic cytoplasm. Often wraps around red cells.	Viral infections, drug reactions
Auer rods	Rod-like red inclusion in immature cells (blasts).	Myeloid leukaemias
Blast cells	Immature primitive cells.	Leukaemias
Döhle bodies (Fig. 26.15)	Blue cytoplasmic inclusions in neutrophil cytoplasm.	Infection, inflammation
Hypogranular neutrophils	Neutrophils with abnormal and reduced granulation.	Myelodysplasia
Leucoerythroblastic	Presence of nucleated red cells and early granulocytes in blood.	Marrow infiltration, myelofibrosis, acute haemolysis
Leucocytosis	White cell count more than $11 \times 10^9/1$.	Infection, inflammation, leukaemia
Lymphocytosis	Lymphocyte count $> 4 \times 10^9/1$ in adults.	Chronic lymphatic leukaemia, lymphoma in leukaemic phase
	$>7 \times 10^9/1$ in children.	Pertussis, viral infection
Neutrophilia	Neutrophils $>7.5 \times 10^9/1$.	Infection inflammation, leukaemoid reaction, chronic myeloid leukaemia
Pelger–Huët anomaly	Neutrophils with two unsegmented lobes (bilobed).	Myelodysplasia, myeloid leukaemia, hereditary form
'Shift to left'	Presence of early myeloid cells.	(see Neutrophilia)
'Shift to right'	Neutrophils five or more lobes.	Megaloblastic anaemia
Smear cells	Smudged, degenerating lymphocytes.	Chronic lymphatic leukaemia
Toxic granulation (Fig. 26.16)	Neutrophils with coarse purple granules.	Infection, inflammation
Turk cells/plasmacytic cells	Reactive lymphoplasmacytic cells.	Severe bacterial, viral infection, rarely plasma cell leukaemia

the iliac crest or the medial surface of the tibia in babies up to the age of 18 months. Special aspiration needles are available for this procedure. Aspiration specimens are suitable for fine and detailed cytological examination when spread properly on a slide. Aspiration marrow is also suitable for flow cytometric studies, karyotypic analysis and other molecular studies, and also for bone marrow culture studies.

Trephine biopsies are best and easily done from the iliac crests. Special trephine biopsy needles are available for this purpose. Trephines are essential for a proper histological and cellularity assessment. Cellularity of the

Table 26.3 Platelet abnormalities

Abnormality	What it means	Associated conditions
Large platelets	Platelets of above average size.	Immune thrombocytopenia, 'giant' platelets of Bernard–Soulier syndrome
Platelet clumping	Clumping of platelet in film, giving rise to low platelet count.	Anticoagulant related, poorly collected specimen, partially clotted specimens, small clumps normal in fresh films
Thrombocytopenia	Low platelet count of $<150 \times 10^9/1$.	Immune thrombocytopenia (ITP), marrow aplasia, or infiltration, myelodysplasia, hypersplenism
Thrombocytosis (Fig. 26.17)	High platelet count $>500 \times 10^9/1$.	Infection, inflammation, myeloproliferative states

marrow can, however, also be assessed by examining fragments of the aspirated marrow.

Cellularity decreases steadily with age, with an accelerated decline above the age of 70. Trephine biopsies are always performed when a 'dry tap' or a dilute sample is obtained by aspiration. This often happens when a marrow is fibrotic, hypercellular or abnormally infiltrated with disease. Aspiration and trephine biopsies should be regarded as complementary procedures.

Bone marrow morphology

Once a marrow has been aspirated it should be spread into films as described above. Bone marrow films, after staining, should be scanned under a low-power objective (×10) for overall cellularity, distribution or haemopoietic cells, presence of abnormal clusters of non-haemopoietic cells, megakaryocyte numbers and morphology.

Maturation of erythroid and myeloid components, their relative proportions and abnormal patterns of maturation (e.g. megaloblastic or dysplastic) should then be noted. The normal myeloid to erythroid ratio (M:E ratio) is 2.5:1–8:1. Ideally, a differential count (myelogram) of at least 200 nucleated cells should be done. This is important if abnormal infiltration with leukaemia, myeloma, or lymphoma is suspected. Children have a large number of small lymphocytes; this number decreases with age. In adults about 5–15% of nucleated cells are lymphoid. Other cells to look out for are megakaryocytes, plasma cells, macrophages and mast cells. Both their number and morphology are important. Parasites are often best found in macrophages.

A Prussian blue stain of the marrow should be made for assessing iron stores and distribution. The entire haemopoietic marrow originates from a totipotent haemopoietic stem cell in the marrow. A simple diagrammatic representation is given in Diagram A.

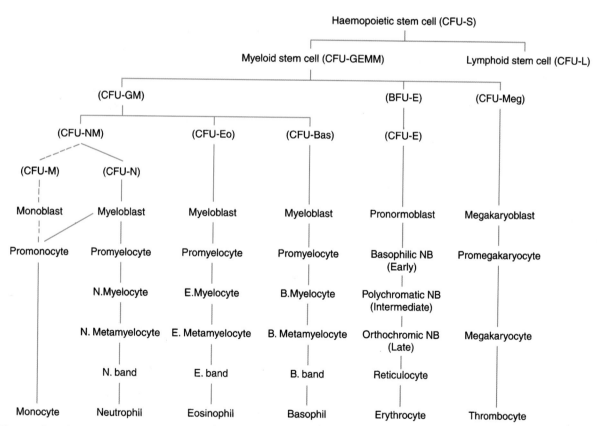

Diagram A Diagramatic representation of haematopoiesis. CFU-S, colony forming unit—spleen; CFU-GEMM, colony forming unit-granulocyte, erythroid, macrophage, megakaryocyte; LSC (CFU-L), lymphoid stem cell (colony forming unit—lymphoid); CFU-GM, colony forming unit—granulocyte; BFU-E burst forming unit—erythroid; CFU-Meg, colony forming unit—megakaryocyte; CFU-NM colony forming unit—neutrophil, monocytes; CFU-Eo, colony forming unit—eosinophil; CFU-Bas, colony forming unit—basophil; CFU-E, colony forming unit—erythroid; CFU-M, colony forming unit—monocytes/macrophage; CFU-N, colony forming unit—neutrophil; N, neutrophilic; E, eosinophilic; B, basophilic; NB, normoblast

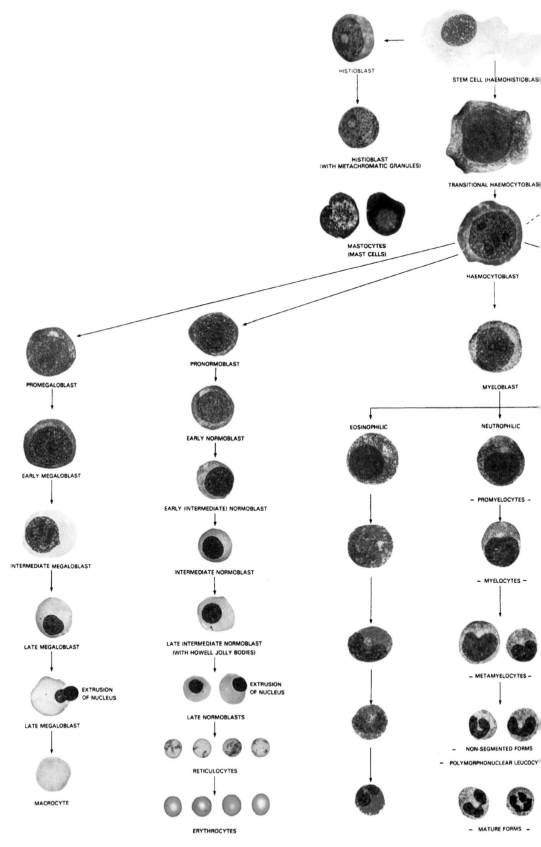

Diagram B   Maturation chart. Reproduced with permission from Churchill Livingstone, 'Atlas of Haematology'

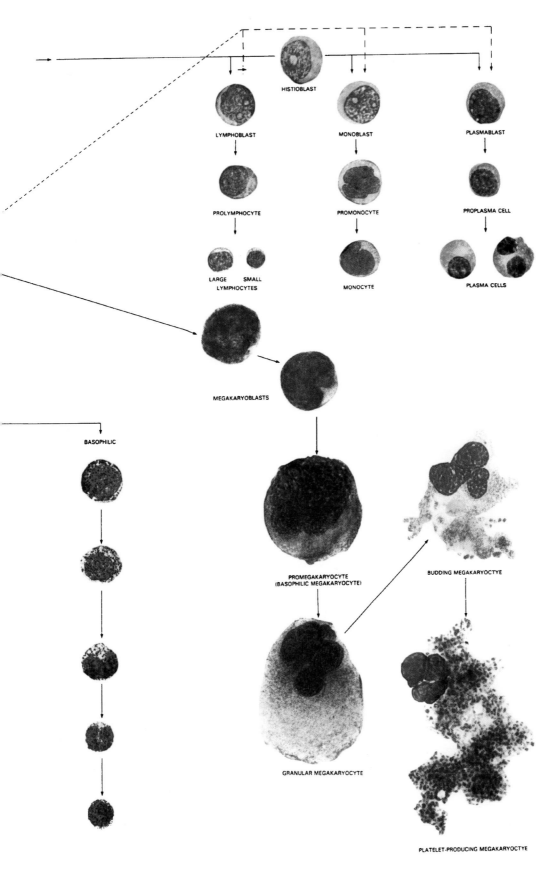

HISTIOBLAST

LYMPHOBLAST

MONOBLAST

PLASMABLAST

PROLYMPHOCYTE

PROMONOCYTE

PROPLASMA CELL

LARGE SMALL
LYMPHOCYTES

MONOCYTE

PLASMA CELLS

MEGAKARYOBLASTS

BASOPHILIC

PROMEGAKARYOCYTE
(BASOPHILIC MEGAKARYOCYTE)

BUDDING MEGAKARYOCTYE

GRANULAR MEGAKARYOCYTE

PLATELET-PRODUCING MEGAKARYOCTYE

A. McDonald, J. Paul and B. Cruickshank. 5th edition, 1989

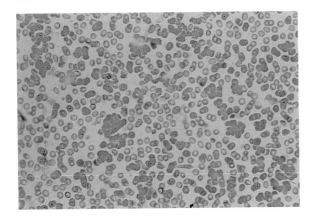

Figure 26.2   Auto-agglutination of red cells

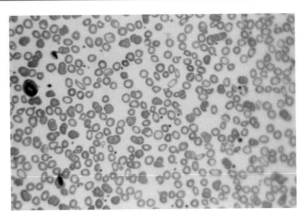

Figure 26.5   Hypochromic, macrocytic red cells

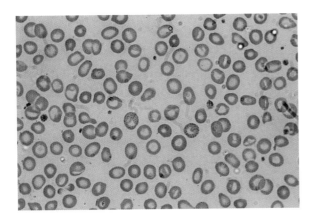

Figure 26.3   Basophilic stippling of red cells

Normal erythropoiesis

The earliest recognizable erythroid precursor, the pro-normoblast, develops progressively and differentiates into a normal erythrocyte. In this process it acquires a rising haemoglobin content and gradually loses it cytoplasmic basophilia, as well as its nucleus. This entire process is arbitrarily divided into three stages: early normoblast, intermediate normoblast and late normoblast.

Late normoblasts do not divide but lose their nucleus by extrusion and give rise to a marrow reticulocyte. These spend up to 2 days in the marrow before entering the peripheral blood, where they make up less than 1% of the red cell population. Reticulocytes have a characteristic bluish-grey staining property and are best demonstrated and counted using a supravital stain. Mature red cells survive about 120 days before destruction in the reticulo-endothelial system. Normal erythropoiesis and haematopoiesis are illustrated in Diagram B.

Some common disorders mainly affecting erythropoiesis

Megaloblastic anaemia

This arises from a deficiency of either vitamin B_{12} or folic acid. Principally due to defective formation of thymidylate, DNA synthesis in the S phase of the cell cycle is slowed down. Nuclear division is thus retarded, and nuclear cytoplasmic synchronization in development is affected. Apart from erythroblasts, most proliferating cells are affected, including the gut mucosa, granulocytes and platelet precursors. The megaloblastic marrow

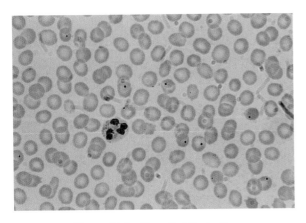

Figure 26.4   Howell–Jolly bodies

is hypercellular. Erythropoiesis is left-shifted with increase in cell size and opening up of the nuclear chromatin network system. Premature haemoglobinization with loss of nuclear cytoplasmic developmental synchronization is common (megaloblastic features). Parallel changes in granulocyte precursors include the presence of giant myelocytes or metamyelocytes and multi-lobated neutrophils (right shift). Megakaryocytes also show nuclear hypersegmentation. Peripheral blood shows the presence of macrocytes and right-shifted neutrophils (Figures 26.6 and 26.18).

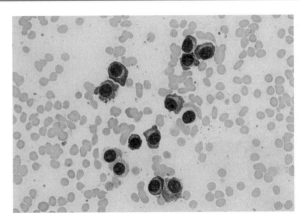

Figure 26.8 Rouleaux with abnormal plasma cells in myeloma

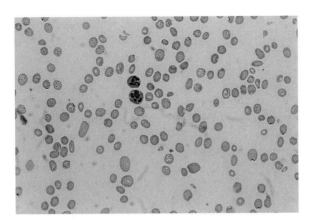

Figure 26.6 Macrocytic and hypersegmented neutrophils

Haemolytic anaemias

Haemolytic anaemias (excessive destruction of red cells) of any cause show compensatory marrow erythroid hyperplasia. The M:E ratio is reduced, with normoblastic hyperplasia and obliteration of fat spaces. Apart from

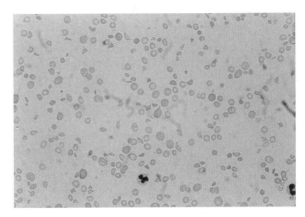

Figure 26.9 fragmented RBC in microangiopathic haemolytic anaemia (MAHA)

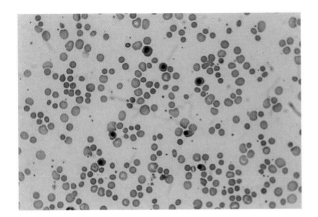

Figure 26.7 Spherocytes with nucleated RBC in autoimmune haemolytic anaemia (AIHA)

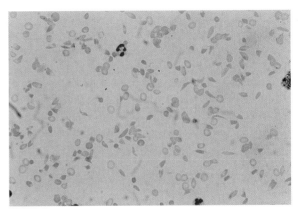

Figure 26.10 Sickle cell disease

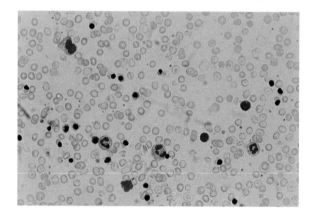

Figure 26.11   Thalassaemia with nucleated red cells

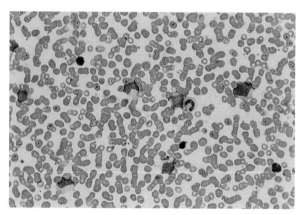

Figure 26.14   Atypical lymphocytes in infectious mononu-
cleosis

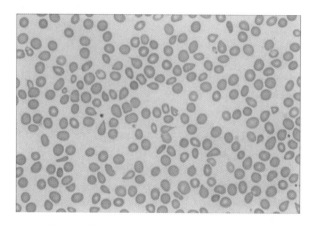

Figure 26.12   Tear-drop cells in myelofibrosis

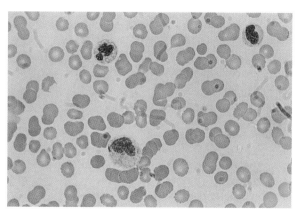

Figure 26.15   Döble body in neutrophil

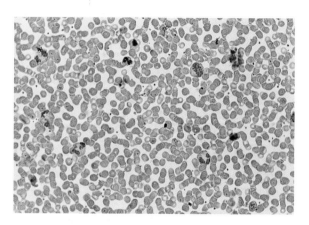

Figure 26.13   Eosinophils

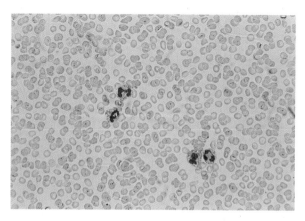

Figure 26.16   Toxic granulation in neutrophils

this common shared feature, further helpful diagnostic clues are best obtained from peripheral red cell morphology, and appropriate supplementary laboratory investigations for haemolysis.

Aplastic and hypoplastic states

These disorders commonly present with anaemia, leukopenia and thrombocytopenia, e.g. pancytopenia. The causes can be variable but are often idiopathic. Pancytopenia in some cases can become progressively severe. The anaemia is often normochromic and normocytic with undetectable reticulocytes in peripheral blood. The marrow is poorly cellular with a predominance of fatty spaces. A relatively higher proportion of lymphocytes and plasma cells can be found. Marrow aspirate is acellular and a definitive diagnosis is best made by trephine biopsy. Hypoplasia can affect one lineage only, as in pure red cell aplasia when the red cells lineage is predominantly altered.

Myelodysplastic syndromes

This is a group of morphologically heterogeneous conditions which are consequent on an acquired myeloid stem cell disorder, leading to abnormal proliferation and disorderly maturation of one or more lineages of haemopoietic cells. It is characterized by ineffective haematopoiesis, which causes peripheral blood cytopenia and a propensity for leukaemic transformation. The FAB (French, American and British) classification subdivides myelodysplasia syndromes into several subgroups.

Morphologically, the marrow shows dysplastic features affecting all three lineages. Erythroid dysplasia is evidenced by ragged haemoglobinization, abnormal and irregular nuclear morphology, and cytoplastic bridging. In a subgroup known as *sideroblastic anaemia* the red cell precursors show the presence of abnormal siderotic granules (Prussian blue stain) arranged in a ring fashion around the nucleus of the erythroblast (see Figure 26.27). Common peripheral red cell changes include anisocytosis, poikilocytosis, macrocytosis and, quite often, the presence of hypochromia or a dimorphic blood picture. Corresponding changes in white cell series include neutropenia and the presence of *hypogranular* neutrophils in the peripheral blood, with pseudo-Pelger changes. Similar abnormalities can also be detected in granulocyte precursors in marrow.

Polycythaemia

Primary proliferative polycythaemia (PRV or PPP) is clinically characterized by high haemoglobin, high haematocrit, high red cell count and mass. The white cell and platelet counts are often elevated and splenomegaly is common. The bone marrow shows obliteration of fat spaces with triliniage hyperplasia. Chromosomal changes can also occur. The transition to the myelofibrotic state can occur in up to 15–20% of cases. When this happens the trephine shows increased reticulin and marrow fibrosis. 'Tear drop' poikilocytes and leukoerythroblastic features appear in the peripheral blood. Terminal transformation to acute myeloid leukaemia or a myelodysplastic state can also occur.

Secondary polycythaemia is a condition which affects the red cell series only without showing leukocytosis or thrombocytosis. This happens mostly in chronic cardiovascular or pulmonary diseases, causing decreased oxygen saturation which, in turn, causes compensatory polycythaemia. Morphologically, erythroid hyperplasia predominates without a parallel increase in other lineages.

Anaemia of blood loss and iron deficiency

Chronic blood loss can cause iron deficiency anaemia. The peripheral red cells show hypochromia and microcytosis with pencil cells. Erythropoiesis in the marrow is hyperplastic. The erythroblasts are often small and poorly haemoglobinized with irregular and ragged outline (micronormoblasts).

The Prussian blue stain fails to show any storage iron. A condition called anaemia of chronic disease (resulting from inflammation or chronic infection) can give a similar blood picture. In these conditions the marrow shows an increase in storage iron. Intra-erythroid iron stores are, however, reduced.

Erythroleukaemia

This is a form of acute myeloid leukaemia in which the erythroid lineage is predominantly affected. The erythroid precursors are usually markedly abnormal with bizarre nuclear lobulation. Erythropoiesis can also be megaloblastic or sideroblastic. Prominent red cell abnormality may be found in the peripheral blood, including many circulating nucleated red cells.

Leukoerythroblastic anaemia (including idiopathic myelofibrosis)

This condition is characterized by the presence of 'teardrop' poikilocytes, nucleated red cells and early granulocytes in the peripheral blood. This picture can arise when the marrow is infiltrated with metastatic tumour or foreign tissue, or when the marrow is fibrosed. Prominent marrow fibrosis can be the primary manifestation of a myeloproliferative state. This is called primary idiopathic myelofibrosis. The marrow shows an increase in reticulin and extensive fibrosis. Bone marrow aspirate is difficult or unhelpful in this condition. A trephine biopsy should always be performed and is diagnostic.

Normal myelopoiesis and megakaryopoiesis

The earliest recognizable cells of the granulocyte series is a myeloblast, which gives rise to a sequence of promyelocytes, myelocytes, metamyelocytes, stab cells and mature neutrophils (Diagram B). From the promyelocyte onwards, specific granules (neutrophilic, eosinophilic, basophilic) become increasingly conspicuous in the cytoplasm and differentiate the common neutrophil granulocytes from the less common eosinophilic and basophilic precursors. Monocytes and their precursors, monoblasts and promonocytes are only present in small numbers in normal marrow. In abnormal states, notably leukaemia, they can become very conspicuous.

Megakaryocytes are easily recognized in the marrow by their large size and nuclear lobulation. With maturation the cytoplasm fragments and gives rise to platelets. Megakaryocytes are smaller and can be very similar to myeloblasts in appearance.

Common disorders predominantly affecting myelopoiesis and megakaryopoiesis

Acute myeloid leukaemia

In acute myeloid leukaemia the bone marrow is infiltrated with primitive myeloblasts numbering more than 30% of the total myeloid cell lines. Myeloblasts are often present in the peripheral blood as well. The myeloblasts are primitive cells showing an open nuclear chromatin pattern and a nucleolus.

Cytoplasmic granulation and Auer rods may or may not be present (Figures 26.19 and 26.20). Morphologically, acute myeloid leukaemia has been subdivided into various subtypes by the FAB group, depending on the degree of differentiation and the nature of predominant

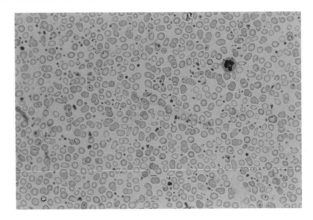

Figure 26.17 Raised platelet count in essential thrombocythaemia with some large forms

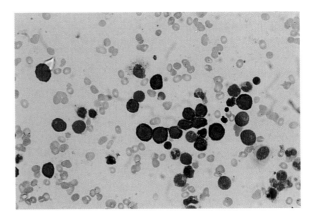

Figure 26.18 Megaloblastic bone marrow

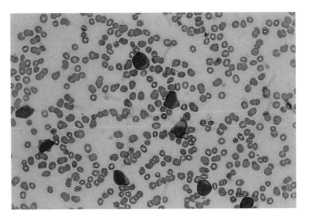

Figure 26.19 Acute myeloid leukaemia

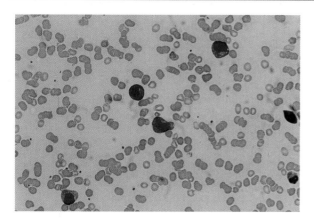

Figure 26.20 Acute promyelocytic leukaemia

cells in the marrow. Sometimes primitive myeloblasts and monoblasts are difficult to differentiate by Romanowsky stains, and may not be easily distinguished from lymphoblasts. Special cytochemical stains are sometimes used in this situation (Tables 26.4 and 26.5). Recently, cytochemistry has been superseded by immunophenotyping (see Chapter 32).

Acute myeloid leukaemia is a malignant disease. Chromosomal changes are readily demonstrated in 50% of cases. Clinically the patient often presents with anaemia, low platelet count, bleeding and infection. Circulating blasts are commonly found in peripheral blood. Bone marrow testing is mandatory and diagnostic.

Chronic myeloid leukaemia

This is a stem cell disorder which is characterized by a high leukocyte count and the presence of granulocyte precursors, notably myelocytes and metamyelocytes, along with numerous circulating neutrophils. The marrow shows hypercellularity with granulocytic hyperplasia, frequent eosinophilia or basophilia (Figure 26.21). Megakaryocytic hyperplasia with a raised platelet count is also common. The distinctive chromosomal abnormality is the presence of the Ph chromosome (Philadelphia chromosome). This is a reciprocal translocation between parts of the long arm of chromosome 22 and the long arm of chromosome 9, t(9:22) (q34:q11). This results in the transfer of the *abl* oncogene from 9q to a site on 22q, known as the breakpoint cluster region (BCR). Transformation to acute leukaemia (AML or ALL-like state) occurs after a variable length of time. This is the so-called blast crisis, the median interval being about 3–4 years.

Reactive changes in granulocytes and monocytes

In infective and inflammatory states the WBC count increases above 11×10^9/l.

Neutrophils show a shift to the left with toxic granulation. Some circulating myelocytes and occasional myeloblasts may also be seen. Marrow shows a myeloid

Table 26.4 French-American-British (FAB) classification of acute myelocytic leukaemias

	Category	Morphologic criteria (bone marrow)
M1	Myeloblastic without maturation	$\geq$90% of myeloid-line cells are blasts.
M2	Myeloblastic with maturation	30–89% of myeloid-line cells are blasts, >10% are promyelocytes to PMN (often dysplastic), <20% are monocytes.
M3	Promyelocytic	Hypergranular promyelocytes with heavy to dust-like granules, often Auer rods; nucleus often bilobed; microgranular variant may occur.
M4	Myelomonocytic	30–80% of myeloid-line cells are myeloblasts plus maturing neutrophils; >20% of myeloid-line cells are monocytic lineage. In addition, >5000/μ/l monocytic cells in peripheral blood.
M4	With eosinophilia	As above, with $\geq$5% abnormal eosinophils that may have unsegmented nucleus and both eosinophilic and large basophilic granules.
M5	Monoblastic, monocytic	>80% of myeloid-line cells are monoblasts, promonocytes, or monocytes; in M5a, 80% of myeloid-line cells are monoblasts; in M5b, <80% are monoblasts, and remainder are promonocytes and monocytes.
M6	Erythroleukemia	$\geq$50% of bone marrow cells are erythroid precursors; $\geq$30% of non-erythroid myeloid-line cells are blasts.
M7	Megakaryocytic	Blasts in marrow or blood are identified as megakaryocytic lineage; if marrow inaspirable, biopsy shows large numbers of blasts, frequently with increased numbers of megakaryocytes and reticulin.

PMN: polymorphonuclear leukocytes

Table 26.5 Special stains and assays used in classifying acute leumaemias

Leukaemia	Peroxidase or Sudan black B	Esterases Specific[a]	Esterases Nonspecific[b]	PAS[c]
		Stain		
AML-M1	+	+	—	—
AML-M2	+ to +++	+	—	—
AML-M3	+++	+++	—	—
AML-M4	++ to +++	+ to +++	+ to +++	—
AML-M5	+	—	+++	—
AML-M6	—	—	—	+++
AML-M7	—	0 to ++	0 to + +(punctate)[d]	++ (punctate)
ALL	—	—	—	+++
Normal neutrophils	+++	+++	—	+++
Normal monocytes	+	—	+++	+++
Normal lymphocytes	—	—	—	±

[a]α-naphthol AS-D chloroacetate.
[b]α-naphthyl acetate esterase and α-naphthyl butyrate esterase.
[c]Periodic acid—Schiff.
[d]Megakaryoblasts negative for α-naphthyl butyrate esterase.

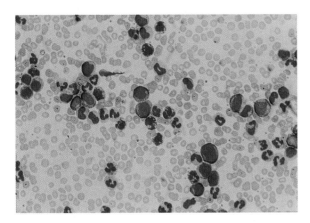

Figure 26.21 Chronic myeloid leukaemia

hyperplasia with predominance of promyelocytes and myelocytes.

The overall picture can, in severe cases, resemble a leukaemic process and is sometimes called a 'leukaemoid reaction'. The clinical background of the patient, immunophenotyping, chromosomal study and clonality studies may be needed to separate this condition from leukaemia.

Myelodysplastic states

This heterogeneous group of disorders has been mentioned earlier (see p. 257). Severe myelodysplastic states, particularly those involving trilineage dysplasia, can progressively show an increasing proportion of blasts in the marrow and, ultimately, transform to acute myeloid leukaemia. A special subcategory, known as chronic myelomonocytic leukaemia (CMML), shows features of both dysplasia and a myeloproliferative condition. This is characterized by the presence of peripheral blood monocytosis of $> 1 \times 10^9$/l. The monocytes are often abnormal in morphology. Associated dysplastic features are also present in the red cells and other white cells.

Megakaryocytes and platelet disorders

Thrombocytopenia

A low platelet count of $< 150 \times 10^9$/l can be due to increased peripheral consumption (immune or nonimmune) or decreased marrow production of platelets, i.e. marrow aplasia or infiltration. In idiopathic thrombocytopenic purpura (IT), anti-platelet antibodies cause an increased reticuloendothelial destruction of platelets. In ITP or other consumptive states, the bone marrow shows a normal to increased number of megakaryocytes. Platelet production disorders are best diagnosed by bone test. Here the megakaryocytes may be absent, diminished, or show dysplastic morphology. The bone marrow aspirate also shows the presence of an abnormal infiltration.

Thrombocytosis

A persistently raised platelet count of over $1000 \times 10^9/l$ occurs in essential thrombocythaemia (ET), which is a myeloproliferative disease predominantly involving the megakaryocyte lineage. The presence of large platelets or even megakaryocyte fragments is also characteristic of this disorder. Marrow aspiration can be difficult, as it may clot readily before spreading. Bone marrow trephine shows hypercellularity with a conspicuous increase in the count of megakaryocytes, which are often atypical in morphology. An associated increase in reticulin or fibrosis of the marrow is also common.

Reactive thrombocystosis (due to infection or inflammation) can sometimes cause a similar picture and can, at times, be difficult to differentiate from essential thrombocythaemia by morphology alone (see Figure 26.17)

Lymphocytes, plasma cells and their disorders

Morphological variation in both lymphocytes and plasma cells cover a much wider range than among granulocytes. In infections, particularly viral infections, lymphocytes show activated or immunoblastic features, with cytoplasmic basophilia and the appearance of nucleoli. Children often have relative lymphocytosis, which diminishes with age. Plasma cells typically have more abundant basophilic cytoplasm, with an eccentric nucleus showing clumped chromatin ('clock-face' appearance). Cytoplasmic inclusion of immunglobulins can sometimes be seen.

Common disorders affecting lymphocyte and plasma cell lineage

Acute lymphoblastic leukaemia (ALL)

This is a monoclonal neoplastic disease arising from lymphoblastic precursors of lymphocytes. It accounts for about 85% of all acute leukaemias below the age of 16. Abnormal lymphoblasts are often present in peripheral blood associated with anaemia and a low platelet count.

The bone marrow shows abnormal infiltration with lymphoblasts that have a higher nuclear cytoplasmic ratio than a typical myeloblast. The FAB group have classified acute lymphoblastic leukaemia into three morphological subtypes (see Table 26.6). A pure morphological distinction between a lymphoblast and an undifferentiated myeloblast can be difficult in some cases. Flow cytometry and special stains are very helpful in this situation (see Table 26.5 and Figure 26.22).

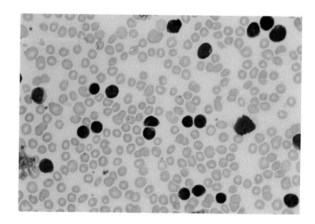

Figure 26.22   Acute lymphocytic leukaemia

Table 26.6   FAB classification of acute lymphocytic leukaemia

Cytology	L1	L2	L3
Cell size	Small	Large	Large, homogeneous
Nuclear chromatin	Homogeneous	Variable	Finely strippled
Nuclear shape	Regular	Irregular	Oval to round
Nucleoli	Rare	Present	1–3
Cytoplasm	Scanty	Moderate	Moderate, vacuolated
Cytoplasmic basophilia	Moderate	Variable	Intense
Incidence in children	85%	13%	2%
Incidence in adults	35%	63%	2%
Immunologic markers	Early B or thymic T	Early B or thymic T	Differentiated B (SIg positive), Burkitt type leukaemia/lymphoma

Chronic lymphocytic leukaemia (CLL)

The disease is uncommon before middle age and its incidence increases with age. Typically it presents with peripheral lymphocytosis, lymphadenopathy and hepatosplenomegaly. The peripheral blood and bone marrow show the presence of many monomorphic small mature-looking lymphocytes. Smear cells are characteristically found in this disorder. CLL cells have also a distinctive immunophenotypic profile (Figure 26.23).

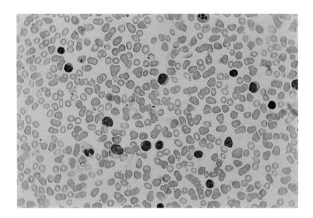

Figure 26.23   Chronic lymphocytic leukaemia

Myelomas

This is a disease characterized by clonal, neoplastic growth of plasma cells. Patients present with paraprotein, hypercalcaemia, lytic bone lesions, anaemia and renal failure. Bone marrow, which is diagnostic, shows the presence of abnormal plasma cells in a large proportion (>30%) (see Figure 26.8).

Lymphomas

Lymphomas are a complex, heterogeneous group of clonal neoplastic diseases, predominantly arising from lymph nodes but which can also involve peripheral blood or bone marrow. Lymphoma is a disease with many subtypes. The neoplastic cells can be small and can look similar to small lymphocytes (low-grade lymphoma). On the other hand, some lymphoma cells have very immature, large, blast-like morphology (high-grade lymphoma). Hodgkin's disease (HD), classified as a type of lymphoma, is characterized by the presence of Reed–Sternberg cells.

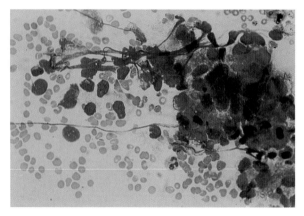

Figure 26.24   Metastatic carcinoma cells

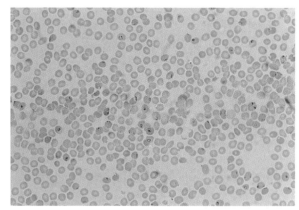

Figure 26.25   Malaria parasites in blood

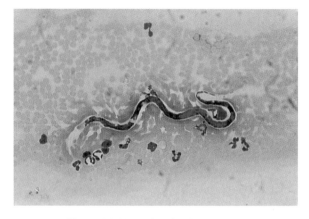

Figure 26.26   Microfilariae in blood

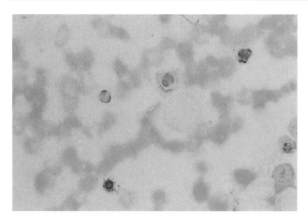

Figure 26.27   Sideroblasts

Non-haemopoietic cells and parasites in blood and marrow

A bone marrow aspirate and trephine is a useful test to detect metastatic carcinoma cells, especially in the presence of a leukoerythroblastic blood picture (Figure 26.24). Malaria parasites are best detected in peripheral blood film. Uncommonly, microfilariae can also be found (Figures 26.25 and 26.26). Expertise and confidence in cell morphology come with practice. For a more exhaustive review on this subject, see Hayhoe and Flemans 1992.

Further reading

Bennet JM, Catovsky D, Daniel MT *et al.* Proposal for classification of myelodysplastic syndrome. *Br J Haematol* 1982; **51**: 189.

Bennet JM, Cartovsky D, Daniel MT *et al.* Proposal for classification of acute leukaemia. *Br J Haematol* 1976; **33**: 451.

Hayhoe FGJ, Flemans RJ. *A Colour Atlas of Haematological Cytology*, 3rd edn. 1992: Wolfe, London.

Holtbrand AV, Pettit JE. *Clinical Haematology*, 2nd edn. 1994: Sandoz Atlas, London.

27

Principles of automated blood cell counters

Graham Martin

Introduction

The full blood count (FBC) has come a long way from just being a measurement of haemoglobin and the cellular components in the peripheral blood. The development and adaptation of different technologies has yielded a huge variety of different cellular parameters, some very useful and some that have yet to prove their worth. In parallel with the measuring technology, automated instruments have been developed that can sample very small amounts of blood using closed-tube sampling and have very high sample throughputs.

The many measurements provided by automated and semi-automated instruments are mostly modifications of the original manual techniques but there are several exciting applications of new technologies. These instruments are precise and accurate, and measurements are reproducible. There are several instrument manufacturers employing similar technologies and measuring systems, measuring the same parameter in slightly different ways. There are advantages and disadvantages for all systems and it could be argued that one set of problems may be exchanged for another.

In this chapter I propose to review the different technologies and their principles of operation. The main parameters are:

1. Haemoglobin (Hb) measurement.

2. Red cell (RBC) measurement.

3. Reticulocyte and nucleated RBC measurement.

4. White cell (WBC) measurement.

5. Platelet measurement.

Hb measurement

Measurement of Hb (Figure 27.1) is based upon the linear relationship between the amount of light absorbed at a particular absorbtion band and the concentration of the absorbtion entity in the sample (Beer's Law) (Skoog DA, West DM, 1965).

Most automated counters employ a cyanmethaemoglobin method reading absorbance at wavelengths of 525 or 540 nm. Sysmex systems use sodium lauryl sulphate, with the advantage of no cyanide in the waste from the analyser.

Red cell measurements

Red cells can be counted by aperture impedance, light-scattering techniques – using Laser LED or tungsten or a combination of the two technologies.

Aperture impedance

This was patented in 1956 by Wallace Coulter and is known as the Coulter principle (Figure 27.2). It has been used to count RBCs, WBCs, and platelets. An electrical current flow is established through an aperture of known dimensions. When a cell or particle passes through the aperture, the cell or particle impedes the current flow and causes a voltage surge. The voltage, first rising above and then falling below a certain threshold, indicates that a cell or particle has passed through the sensing zone. Cells and particles are counted by monitoring the number of voltage pulses that occur during a specified measurement interval. The volume of the cell can be

The Science of Laboratory Diagnosis, Second Edition   Edited by David Burnett and John Crocker
© 2005 John Wiley & Sons, Ltd

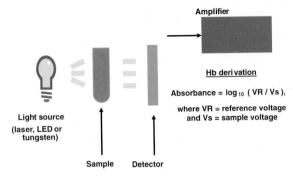

Figure 27.1 Hb measurement

determined by measuring the magnitude of the pulse generated. Thresholds or electronic gates are set, allowing the analyser to discriminate RBC pulses from smaller platelet pulses, debris and electrical noise.

Coincidence

Inaccuracy may be introduced by coincidence. If two or more cells enter the aperture sensing zone, the resistance change either creates a single high pulse or a double-peaked pulse. Statistical corrections are applied in the analyser software to correct this. To avoid recirculation of cells around the aperture, causing false measurements of numbers and volume, cells are usually injected into the aperture chamber in the centre of a sheath fluid

stream or, once counted, are removed from the sensing zone by a sweep fluid.

Light-scattering techniques

Light scatter estimates the relative size of the cell based on forward scatter, which is more a measurement of cross-sectional diameter. The amount of light scattered is proportional to the surface area and hence the volume of the cell. Lasers have superior optical properties compared to tungsten light sources and detectors can be placed to collect forward, narrow- and wide-angle scattered light (Figure 27.3). Laser light is used to measure both volume and cellular Hb concentration on Bayer instruments. The amount of light scattered at low angle (2–3°) is dependent on the RBC size and the amount scattered at high angle (5–15°) is related to the refractive index of the cell.

Depending on the way they are projected to the laser, non-spherical cells such as platelets and RBCs can give very different signals to the detectors. Bayer has overcome this problem by a technique known as iso-volumetric sphering. Sodium dodecyl sulphate and gluteraldehyde in the red cell reagent causes sphering and partial fixation of the red cells and platelets, eliminating erroneous results. This has allowed accurate measurement of the % hypochromic cells? and has proved to be a useful parameter for optimizing erythropoetin and iron therapy (Richardson *et al.*, 2001).

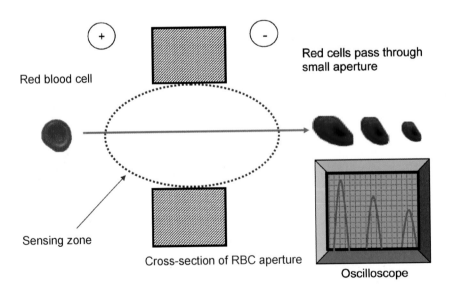

Figure 27.2 The Coulter principle

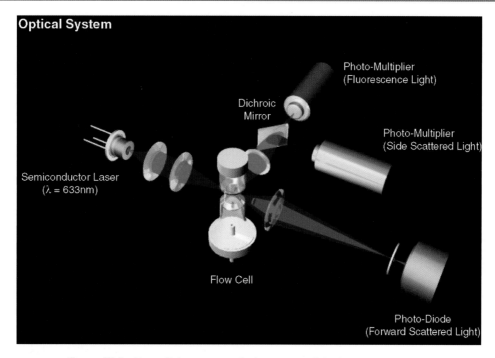

Figure 27.3   Laser light scatter optical system used by Sysmex instruments

Reticulocyte and nucleated RBC measurement

Reticulocyte counting

All cell counter manufacturers provide reticulocyte analysis on their instruments. Some systems measure reticulocyte and related parameters using fluorescent dyes for RNA with laser light (references from ALM in H p90 Takubo *et al.*, 1989; Tichelli *et al.*, 1990; Davis *et al.*, 1996; Kim *et al.*, 2003). Other systems use supravital basic dyes causing precipitation and staining of reticular substance, which is then measured by light absorbance and scattering (references from ALM in Hp90 Buttarello *et al.*, 1995, 1996, 1997; Van den Bossche J *et al.*, 2001; Rudenski, 1997; Wysocka J, Turowski D. 2000).

Summary of current analyser methods

It is also possible to measure reticulocyte maturity, due to the fact that immature reticulocytes have a greater proportion of RNA and therefore stain deeper or give a greater fluorescence. Monochromatic light scatter measuring volume plotted against absorbtion is used on the Advia to provide a reticulocyte maturation index and reticulocyte Hb content.

Table 27.1   Reticulocyte counting techniques

Company	Analyser	Method	RNA stain
Abbott	Cell-Dyn 4000 + Sapphire	Fluorescence	CD4K530
ABX	ABX Pentra 120	Fluorescence	Thiazole orange
Bayer	ADVIA 120 + 2120	Light scatter and absorbtion	Oxazine 750 on sphered cells
Beckman Coulter	GEN-S + LH750	Light scatter	New methylene blue on sphered cells
Sysmex	XE 2100	Fluorescence	Auramine O

Nucleated RBCs

Instrument manufacturers have adopted differing approaches to differentiate nucleated RBCs. Nuclei are counted using combinations of light scatter and impedance after the RBC cytoplasm has been stripped (Beckman Coulter). The counting is done in the WBC channel and the total WBC corrected for the presence of NuRBC. In Sysmex analysers, NuRBC counts are determined via flow cytometry and laser light. The sample is aspirated and mixed with a RNA/DNA stain. NucRBC are counted using side fluorescence, giving RNA/DNA information and forward scatter, a measure of cell size.

In all analysers the NucRBC count is expressed as NucRBC/100 WBC, from the formula:

$$NucRBC\% = \frac{NucRBC \times 100}{NucRBC + WBC}$$

White cell measurements

White cells can be counted and differentiated into a wide number of categories by a variety of technologies. There are advantages and disadvantages to all. The development of sheath flow-based counting systems, enabling the passage of single cells through the sensing zone, has led to multi-parameter analysis on the same cell by combining the signals from several sensors. Depending

Table 27.2 Current analyser technologies

Company	Analyser	Technology
Abbott	Cell-Dyn 3500	Forward light scatter Narrow angle light scatter Orthogonal light scatter Polarized light scatter
	Cell-Dyn 4000 + Sapphire	All the above, plus nucleated RBC count following binding to fluorescent dye
ABX	Pentra 60	Cytochemistry Focused flow impedance Light absorbance Flow cytometry
	Pentra 120 Retic	Cytochemistry Focused flow cytometry impedance and absorbance Light absorbtion following staining of eosinophils Impedance following preferential stripping of cytoplasm from basophils at low pH Argon-ion laser
Bayer	Advia 60	Cytochemistry Focused flow impedance Light absorbance Flow cytometry
	ADVIA 120, 2120, H1, H2 and H3	Light scattering following peroxidase reaction Light absorbance following peroxidase reaction Light scattering following stripping of cytoplasm from cells other than basophils by a lytic agent at low pH
Beckman Coulter	A^{c}T 5diff	Impedance measurement following differential lysis Impedance measurements and absorbance cytochemistry
	GEN-S + LH750	Impedance with low-frequency electromagnetic current Conductivity with low-frequency electromagnetic current Laser light scattering
Sysmex	SE 9000	Impedance with low-frequency electromagnetic current Impedance with radio-frequency electromagnetic current Impedance with low-frequency electromagnetic current at low and high pH
	XE 2100	Impedance with low-frequency electromagnetic current Impedance with radio-frequency electromagnetic current Forward light scatter Sideways light scatter Fluorescence intensity following reaction with fluorescent dye

upon the manufacturer, the sensing zone can be either optical, conductance, impedance or a combination of all, and the sensors can be placed to look at forward light scatter, side scatter, narrow- or wide-angle scatter, polarized light scatter or fluorescence. The technologies each current instrument uses are summarized in Table 27.2.

Aperture impedance

By first partially stripping the cytoplasm from white cells, aperture impedance (Figure 27.4), as previously

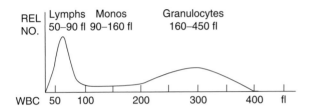

Figure 27.4 A 256 channel histogram display of the WBC cell population between 35 and 450 fl using aperture impedance data only. Reproduced by permission of Beckman Coulter

described, will give a measurement of the size of the nucleus and cytoplasmic granularity. By using this method alone it is possible to quantify lymphocytes, monocytes and granulocytes.

Aperture impedance and light scatter

Beckman Coulter instruments achieve a five-population differential by making three simultaneous measurements on each cell: volume (v), using standard aperture impedance; conductivity (c), using high-frequency electromagnetic waves; determining cell complexity and light scatter (s), measuring cell surface characteristics and the lobularity of each cell (VCS 3-D cluster analysis: Figure 27.5).

Adaptable cluster analysis algorithms have largely displaced the earlier use of fixed discriminators as boundaries between cell populations. The development of 'diagnostic assist' systems is seen as a further improvement in the laboratory's ability to interpret electronic differential findings.

Both three- and five-part differential systems are equipped with flagging algorithms, alerting the user to possible morphological or other abnormalities, requiring review of the data or some other form of intervention, such as morphology review.

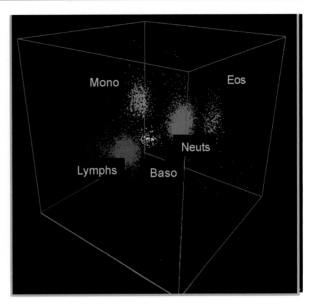

Figure 27.5 VCS three-dimensional cluster analysis. Reproduced by permission of Beckman Coulter

Flow cytometry and light scatter

WBC and differential counts in the Sysmex XE instruments are determined using a flow cytometry method combined with a semiconductor laser. Cell information is obtained using forward light scatter to determine cell volume, lateral light scatter to evaluate cell internal structure and lateral fluorescent light to give DNA/ RNA information. By aspirating the blood sample into six separate channels with different reagents, a complex cluster analysis can be applied to separate all normal and abnormal cell variants. Competitive learning algorithms allows optimal adaptation to biological differences between samples, including very abnormal cells.

The polymethine dye combines with nucleic acids (nuclear DNA and RNA in cytoplasmic organelles) The Sysmex XE has the capacity to count reticulocytes, recognize RNA-containing platelets, recognize and count nucleated RBCs and recognize cells with the characteristics of haemopoietic progenitor cells (HPC), which can be used to predict an increase in CD34[+] cells.

Cytochemistry and light scatter

The Bayer series of instruments derive a differential from two channels. The peroxidase channel uses a cytochemical reaction in which the peroxidase of neutrophils, eosinophils and monocytes act on a substrate, 4-chloro-1-naphthol, to produce a black reaction product.

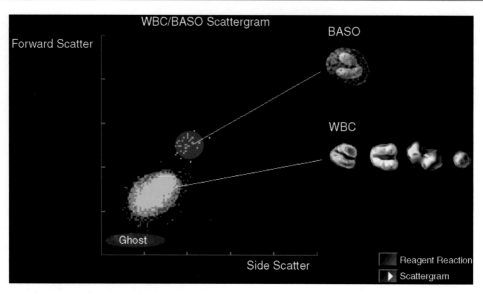

Figure 27.6   Forward scatter plotted against side scatter. Reproduced by permission of Sysmex UK Ltd

Light scatter, which is proportional to cell size, is plotted against light absorbance, which is proportional to the intensity of the peroxidase reaction. Neutrophils, eosinophils, monocytes and lymphocytes fall into four clusters, separated by electronic thresholds. Because basophils fall into the lymphocyte region, they are separated from the other cells in a separate channel on the basis of their resistance to acidic cytoplasmic stripping. Basophils are sized larger than other cells by forward scatter. This channel is also used to detect blasts. Forward scatter is plotted against high-angle light scatter to measure nuclear density and lobulation (Figure 27.6).

Platelet counting

Ever since they were first identified in the mid nineteenth century and referred to as 'the blood dust', platelets have presented a challenge in terms of the accuracy of counting techniques. Modern therapies require accuracy, not only in the critical clinical range, but also the ability to differentiate small red cells and large platelets. Platelets can be counted and sized using impedance, light scatter, a combination of the two and flow cytometry using fluorescence (Figure 27.7).

Impedance

Beckman Coulter instruments utilize impedance to obtain a platelet count, which is derived from the number of cells under the curve (Figure 27.8). By using curve-fitting software, the accuracy of this count is improved when platelets larger than 20 femtolitres (fl) are present. The platelet count beyond the 35 fl limit is extended up to 70 fl.

Optical platelet counting

The Advia range of instruments from Bayer combine high-angle (5–15°) and low-angle (2–3°) scatter signals for each cell. These are transformed into volume plotted on a vertical axis and refractive index values plotted on the horizontal axis to give a platelet scatter cytogram (Figure 27.9). The curved lines represent a grid of varying refractive index along which the platelets fall. By also plotting the refactive index against platelet volume range, macroplatelets and red cells can be separated.

Combination of impedance and optical counting

The Sysmex XE range of instruments use an impedance channel as the default count and a fluorescent channel on instances of abnormality. Platelet measurements are made using forward scatter to determine size, side scatter looking at the internal structure and fluorescence measuring RNA/DNA stained.

Immuno-platelet counts

As well as optical and impedance counting, the Cell-Dyn 4000 and Sapphire are able to count platelets by measur-

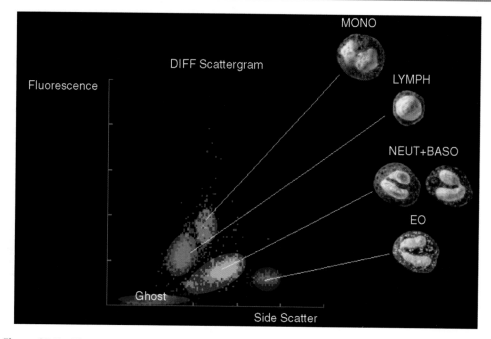

Figure 27.7 Fluorescence plotted against side scatter. Reproduced by permission of Sysmex UK Ltd

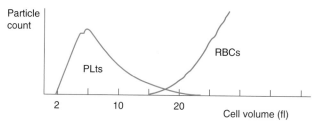

Figure 27.8 Coulter plot showing cell size distribution of platelets (PLTs) and red blood cells (RBCs)

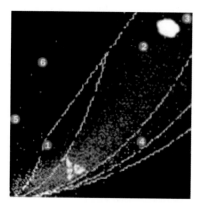

Figure 27.9 Platelet scatter cytogram. 1, platelets; 2, large platelets; 3, RBCs; 4, RBC fragments; 5, debris; 6, RBC ghosts. Reproduced by permission of Bayer plc

ing green fluorescence from CD61. A monoclonal antibody, present in one of the reagents, binds to the CD61 antigen found on all normal platelets. Fluorescein isothiocyanate (FITC) is the dye used that fluoresces when excited at 488 nm. This technique is useful in the presence of large numbers of RBC or WBC fragments.

Further reading

Buttarello M, Bulian P, Pra MD, Barbera P, Rizzotti P. Reticulocyte quantification by Coulter MAXM VCS (volume, conductivity, light scatter) technology. *Clin Chem.* 1996; **42**(12): 1930–1937.

Buttarello M, Bulian P, Temporin V, Rizzotti P. Sysmex SE-9000 hematology analyzer: performance evaluation on leukocyte differential counts using an NCCLS H20-A protocol. National Committee for Clinical Laboratory Standards. *Am J Clin Pathol.* 1997; **108**(6): 674–686.

Buttarello M, Bulian P, Venudo A, Rizzotti P. Laboratory evaluation of the Miles H.3 automated retriculocyte counter. A comparative study with manual reference method and Sysmex R-1000. *Arch Pathol Lab Med* 1995; **119**(12): 1141–1148.

Davis BH. Diagnostic utility of red cell flow cytometric analysis. *Clin Lab Med* 2001; **21**(4): 829–840.

Kim YR, van't Oever R, Landayan M, Bearden J. Automated red blood cell differential analysis on a multi-angle light scatter/fluorescence hematology analyzer. *Cytometry*, 2003; **56B**(1): 43–54.

Richardson D, Bartlett C, Will EJ. Optimizing erythropoietin therapy in hemodialysis patients. *Am J Kidney Dis* 2001; **38**(1): 109–117.

Skoog DA, West DM. *Analytical Chemistry*. 1965: Holt, Reinhart and Winston, New York, pp. 451–455.

Takubo T, Kitano K, Ikemoto T, Kikuchi T, Shimizu A. Ring eosinophils in patients with lowered eosinophil peroxidase activity. Article in Japanese. *Rinsho Byori* 1993; **41**(4): 468–470.

Tichelli A, Gratwohl A, Driessen A, Mathys S, Pfefferkorn E, Regenass A, Schumacher P, Stebler C, Wernli M, Nissen C, et al. Evaluation of the Sysmex R-1000. An automated reticulocyte analyzer. *Am J Clin Pathol* 1990; **93**(1): 70–78.

Van den Bossche J, Devreese K, Malfait R, Van de Vyvere M, De Schouwer P. Comparison of the reticulocyte mode of the Abx Pentra 120 Retic, Coulter General-S, Sysmex SE 9500, Abbott CD 4000 and Bayer Advia 120 haematology analysers in a simultaneous evaluation. *Clin Lab Haematol* 2001; **23**(6): 355–360.

Wysocka J, Turowski D. New reticulocyte indices and their utility in hematologic diagnosis (Article in Polish). *Pol Merkuriusz Lek* 2000; **8**(49): 498–502.

28

Methods for the identification of the haemoglobinopathies

Nick Jackson and **Anne Sermon**

Introduction

The haemoglobinopathies and thalassaemias are the most common inherited genetic disorders. The molecular defects are located in the globin genes and affect the synthesis of haemoglobin (Hb) in the developing erythrocyte. They manifest clinically as haemolytic anaemia and inheritance is usually autosomal recessive or co-dominant. The mutations that produce a haemoglobinopathy are diverse; the study and characterization of the human haemoglobin gene can be used as an example to demonstrate most of the known types of genetic mutation. The clinically significant defects are found in the α and β genes (found on chromosomes 16 and 11, respectively), but mutations can be identified in any of the globin-producing genes. The resulting abnormalities give rise both to qualitative and quantitative abnormalities of Hb synthesis. Haemoglobinopathies result from the production of a structurally abnormal variant Hb; the thalassaemias arise from a reduction in the rate of synthesis of one or more of the types of globin chains.

Point mutations leading to amino acid substitutions or abnormal termination of gene transcription account for the majority of the globin gene defects and are typical of haemoglobinopathies and β-thalassaemia. Gene deletion is the usual cause of α- and $\delta\beta$-thalassaemia. There are currently over 1000 identified globin gene variants, which can be divided broadly into the following groups: (a) clinically silent (the majority); (b) thalassaemic

haemoglobins; (c) unstable haemoglobins; (d) haemoglobins with altered oxygen affinity; (e) miscellaneous atypical effects, e.g. sickle haemoglobin (HbS).

HbS is the most common clinically significant variant Hb and in the homozygous state (HbSS) or in combination with HbC or β-thalassaemia trait produces severe health problems. Tissue ischaemia secondary to acute sickling results in painful and potentially fatal crises. HbS is commonest in populations originating from: sub-Saharan Africa, but is also found in people from India, Saudi Arabia and the Mediterranean Basin. The thalassaemias are found in populations from all tropical areas of the world and the Mediterranean. Screening is generally aimed at those ethnic populations at risk of carrying these genes, but with increasing ethnic mixing screening may have to become universal in order not to miss any cases or carriers.

Screening techniques

Current screening methodology allows rapid detection and accurate identification of the clinically significant haemoglobin disorders, as well as their heterozygous states. These techniques can also be applied reliably in the screening of neonates to detect unexpected disease, as well as carrier states. It is possible to assess genetic risk through the identification of carriers and offer prenatal diagnosis of the fetus. Policies are established in most laboratories for the screening for adults and

The Science of Laboratory Diagnosis, Second Edition   Edited by David Burnett and John Crocker
© 2005 John Wiley & Sons, Ltd

neonates. Techniques for prenatal diagnosis of fetuses are based on DNA analysis and are normally carried out in national centres.

In order to interpret fully the results of Hb analysis in an individual, the following information should be available: age, sex, ethnic origin, clinical status (e.g. pregnant or not) and full blood count (FBC). For those with red cell microcytosis (MCV < 80 fl), a reliable measure of iron status is required (e.g. serum ferritin) to exclude iron deficiency. Samples from patients targeted for screening should then channel through a flexible protocol of laboratory investigations, which may include high-performance liquid chromatography (HPLC) or electrophoresis, sickle solubility and measurement of HbA$_2$ and HbF levels. Diagnosis of the majority of the common carrier and disease states, i.e. α- and β-thalassaemia, HbS, HbC, HbD and HbE, can usually be achieved by assessment of these test results.

Laboratories handling small numbers of samples may use Hb electrophoresis and Hb A$_2$ estimation by microcolumn as their primary screening tools. However, with increasingly wide screening policies, most laboratories are now screening samples by HPLC. Hb electrophoresis and other techniques are used to confirm the identity of variant haemoglobins found on HPLC. The sickle solubility test is mainly used for the exclusion of sickle cell disorders before emergency surgery in populations at risk.

Laboratory diagnosis of haemoglobinopathies and thalassaemias

Full blood count, blood film and ferritin

In the majority of the structural haemoglobinopathy carrier states the FBC shows no abnormality, although the film may show certain features (e.g. target cells in HbC and HbE traits). Basophilic stippling is found in β-thalassaemia trait and irregularly contracted cells in α-thalassaemia trait. The red cell indices are important indicators in the assessment for thalassaemia trait, which is characterized by microcytosis and a normal or near-normal Hb. A mean cell volume (MCV) of < 80 fl or a mean cell Hb (MCH) of < 27 pg are indicative of possible thalassaemia, especially when the RBC count is normal or raised ($> 5 \times 10^{12}$/l) and serum ferritin is normal (> 30 μg/l). However, these delineators may vary slightly from one laboratory to another, according to the

method of automated measurement and the normal ranges assigned by the laboratory. The FBC from patients who are symptomatic (e.g. β-thalassaemia major, HbSS) may show the features of anaemia to variable degrees and more severe morphological abnormalities of the red cells. Polycythaemia may be found in cases of haemoglobins with increased oxygen affinity.

Detection, identification and quantitation of haemglobinopathies

The principles of detection, identification and quantitation of haemoglobins are based on the physical separation of haemoglobins in solution, according to their charge. The amino acid substitutions in most variants introduce a change in overall surface charge which is integral to their detection. A limitation of these techniques, therefore, is that Hb variants cannot be distinguished from HbA if they have the same surface charge. For correct interpretation of all these tests, it is important to ensure that the sample is not taken within three months after a blood transfusion.

Detection and identification

Electrophoresis

Basic screening methodology relies on the migration of a charged molecule (Hb) in an electric field towards a cathode or anode. The strength and polarity of the charge is determined by the pH of the buffered environment. The rate of migration is governed by the pore size of the supporting medium and the magnitude of the charge on the molecule.

Cellulose acetate is a commonly used medium, being inexpensive and having an indefinite shelf-life; agar is a widely used alternative. The pH for preliminary screening is alkaline, fixed at pH 8.4–8.9 with Tris–EDTA borate or Tris-barbitone buffers. At this pH most haemoglobins are negatively charged and will migrate from the cathode towards the anode. Many variants separate from HbA under these conditions, enabling visible detection, which can be made more obvious by staining with a protein-specific dye, e.g., Ponceau S or Amido black. The pattern of migration, marked by reference controls, can then be compared to a variant map to give probable identification. Fixed pH techniques are relatively insensitive to the discrete separation of groups of variants with similar charges. At pH 8.4, two groups of common variants—HbS, HbD and HbG; and HbC, HbE and HbO Arab—co-migrate. This makes distinction between the variants in each group impossible without further investigation. A differential change in charge in the haemoglobins can be induced by changing the buffer to acid (e.g. to pH 6.3, usually in citrate agar), which alters the rate and characteristic pattern of migration. The relative mobilities of the variant Hb at acid and alkaline pH are cross-referenced on variant maps and this usually allows its confident identification, e.g. at pH 6.3, HbC will become distinct from HbE and HbO Arab, and HbS will separate from HbD and HbG. The identity of some variants will remain unresolved, and may be established with further analysis by different techniques, e.g. iso-electric focusing (IEF) or HPLC. Some rare cases may require definition of the exact mutation at the molecular level.

Sickle solubility

The sickle solubility test is a simple, rapid screen for the presence of HbS. A positive screen does not distinguish between homozygotes and heterozygotes and should have a sensitivity down to approximately 20% HbS concentration. This test is most useful where a rapid screen is required, e.g. prior to general anaesthetic in a patient from an 'at-risk' ethnic group whose haemoglobinopathy status is unknown.

The detection of HbS is based on its relative insolubility when deoxygenated and the subsequent deformation of the RBC membrane into the classic sickle shape. In the test tube, deoxygenation is induced by sodium dithionite with trace saponin added. If HbS is present, then the deoxy form polymerizes to form the classic tactoid crystals. A positive test retains an opaque appearance (due to sickled RBCs in suspension), whereas the deoxyhaemoglobin in negative samples gives a clear haemoglobin solution. There are six other rare variants which also have sickling properties, so this screen is not unique for HbS, but rather for 'sickling' haemoglobins. The identity should always be confirmed by electrophoresis. Conversely, a variant band which migrates in the position of HbS should always be confirmed with a sickle solubility test.

This screen is insensitive to very low levels of HbS, such as those found in newborns, and therefore is not useful as part of a neonatal screen. However, it can be used to detect the HbS gene in individuals where electrophoresis is not available as a first-line investigation, e.g. Third World countries.

Isoelectric focusing (IEF)

Isoelectric focusing is a highly sensitive and much more sophisticated form of electrophoresis and is based on the separation of haemoglobins according to their isoelectric point. Low molecular weight carrier ampholytes with a range of isoelectric points are incorporated into polyacrylamide gel or agar to create a pH gradient. For the purposes of Hb separation, a pH range of 5.5–8.5 is used. As the haemoglobins migrate through the gradient, they become neutral at their isoelectric point (pI) and stop migrating, i.e. they become focused at their pI. Since the pI is specific to the surface charge on a molecule, even haemoglobins with a very small differential charge will separate discretely. On precast gels, the haemoglobins focus reproducibly in the same place, thereby offering much greater certainty of identification on a single separation (Figure 28.1). Due to the increased sensitivity of IEF, even variants that are present in very small concentrations can be resolved, e.g. Constant Spring, A_2 variants, H, Bart's. This technique is therefore also suited to the cord blood screening of neonates.

Quantitation

Quantitation of Hb fractions is mainly of use in the distinction of α- and β-thalassaemia traits in people with RBC microcytosis and normal iron status. It is also of value in: (a) the further characterization of some variants, e.g. α-chain variants, HbE; (b) the diagnosis of compound haemoglobinopathy syndromes; (c) the diagnosis of hereditary persistence of fetal Hb (HPFH) disorders; and (d) the monitoring of transfusion regimens in sickle cell disorders. Estimation of Hb fractions can be achieved by a variety of techniques, including separation of the variant by electrophoresis, followed by elution, microcolumn chromatography, HPLC, radial immunodiffusion and ELISA.

Microcolumn chromatography

Microcolumn chromatography is principally used for determining the percentage of HbA_2 for the detection

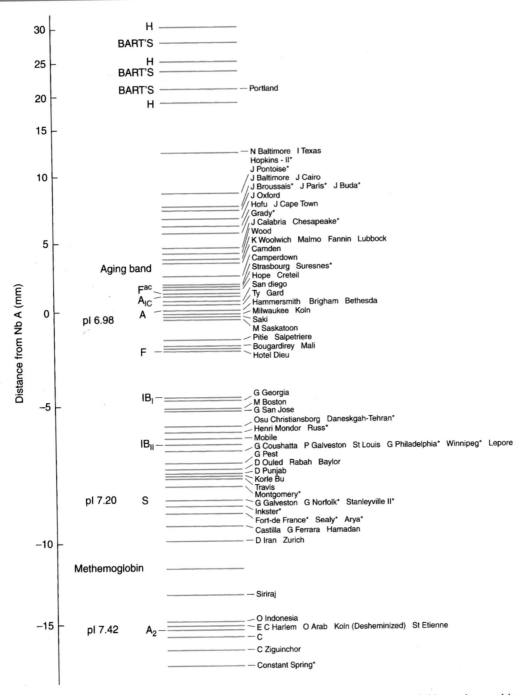

Figure 28.1 Diagrammatic representation of thin layer isoelectric focusing of normal haemoglobins and several haemoglobin structural variants. IB$_1$ and IB$_2$ are ferrous–ferric hybrids of Hb A. [Courtesy of Dr Yves Beuzard.]

of β-thalassaemia trait, but may also be modified for the quantitation of major fractions, e.g. HbS. The principle of separation is dependent on adsorption and binding of charged Hb molecules onto a resin with a polar side-chain. On the addition of a developer buffer to the column, the bound protein is displaced by stronger charged buffer ions, hence the term 'ion exchange chromatography'. Displaced haemoglobins are subsequently washed from the resin in the eluate. Estimation of the percentage concentration of the fraction is then measured against a diluted total by optical densitometry. DEAE (diethylaminoethyl) cellulose is an anion exchange resin, which is paired with a glycine–KCN or Tris–HCl buffer, pH 8.3.

The normal range for HbA$_2$ is 1.8–3.5%, with raised levels (up to about 7.5%) indicating β-thalassaemia trait. Borderline levels (3.3–3.7% need careful interpretation, and possibly DNA analysis, to confirm normality or a mild (β^+) thalassaemia. In α-thalassaemia trait, the HbA$_2$ level may be normal or low. Reduced HbA$_2$ levels are also found in severe iron deficiency, HbH disease and δ-thalassaemia.

Measurement of HbF

HbF comprises $< 1\%$ in normal adults and is mildly raised in approximately half of β-thalassaemia carriers. HPFH and $\delta\beta$-thalassaemia both give rise to significantly raised HbF levels and are distinguished by normal, as opposed to reduced, MCV and MCH, respectively. The Kleihauer test may also be useful, as some types of HPFH are 'pancellular' (with an even distribution of HbF in the RBCs), whereas others are 'heterocellular' (with an heterogeneous distribution of HbF in the RBCs). In $\delta\beta$-thalassaemia, the distribution is typically heterocellular. However, it may be necessary to perform DNA analysis to be sure of this distinction, especially if α-thalassaemia is a possible coexistent condition causing a low MCV.

A widely used method for HbF assay was first introduced by Betke and is based on the selective denaturation of other haemoglobins by alkali, leaving intact HbF, which is resistant. A dilute lysate solution is subject to a fixed incubation of 2 minutes with NaOH, which oxidizes all other fractions. The resulting methaemoglobins are precipitated with a saturated salt solution, which also neutralizes the oxidation. HbF, which remains in solution, can be separated from the precipitate by filtration or preferably by high-speed centrifugation. The proportion of the HbF fraction is determined by optical densitometry against a total Hb dilution.

An HbF level of $< 1\%$ constitutes the adult normal range; 1–5% is found in up to 50% of β-thalassaemia carriers; 5–20% is characteristic of the $\delta\beta$-thalassaemia trait and some HPFH cases; 20–45% is characteristic of pancellular African-type HPFH. In some homozygous cases, HbF can represent $> 90\%$ of total Hb.

High-performance liquid chromatography (HPLC)

HPLC combines detection, identification and quantitation of haemoglobins in a single technique and is eminently suited to screening large numbers of samples quickly, accurately and cheaply. The principle of separation remains the same as that of microcolumn chromatography, although the resin has a polyaspartate side-chain, i.e. is a cation exchanger and the fluid phase is a Cl$^-$ ion. The analysis is automated with an autosampler injection onto the column and a pump that exerts a constant pressure of elution buffer onto the top of the lysate. This controls and regulates the elution time. The sensitivity of the separation is vastly increased through the use of two buffers, which differ in ion concentration and/or pH. Hb fractions are sequentially eluted from the column by the creation of an elution gradient, achieved by mixing the two fluid phases. This enables the separation of previously unresolved variants, i.e. D from G, and E from O. The optical density of the eluates is measured directly as they pass from the column and plotted continuously to create a chromatogram (Figure 28.2). Identification is achieved by comparison of the retention times to those of known variants. Both major and minor components can be quantitated accurately by integrating the area under each peak;

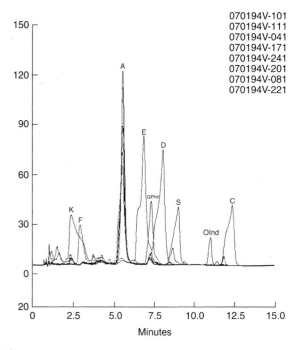

Figure 28.2 HPLC chromatogram overlay plot of the common Hb variants

α- and β-thalassaemias are distinguished readily, as the HbA$_2$ level is calculated automatically. It is recommended that the identity of a variant Hb that is detected by HPLC is confirmed by a second technique (e.g. electrophoresis or sickle solubility).

Detection of RBC inclusion bodies

The redox reaction of supravital stains can be used to stain red cell inclusion bodies, formed from Hb derivatives. This property is useful in the further characterization of Hb disorders.

HbH is a tetramer formed from the excess β chains (β_4) in α-thalassaemia and is detectable by electrophoresis or HPLC when present in significant quantities (i.e. in HbH disease). Intracellular HbH is soluble but very unstable and is precipitated by incubation with brilliant cresyl blue. The precipitate attaches to the RBC membrane to give a typical 'golf ball' appearance to the RBCs, with multiple stained bodies. HbH inclusions are present in 1–2 cells/1000 in α-thalassaemia trait but can be difficult to detect microscopically. They are much more numerous and obvious in HbH disease.

Heinz bodies (see unstable haemoglobins) are not visible on a standard Romanowsky-stained film, but are detectable as large, round and usually single intracellular precipitates following incubation with methyl violet. Their presence is usually detected only in acute haemolysis and may not be obvious if splenic function is intact or if the stain is performed on very fresh blood.

Detection of unstable haemoglobins

Molecular instability of Hb may arise from amino acid substitution in the haem binding groups, the $\alpha\beta$ contact areas or in the interior of the haem pocket. These defects confer weakness in the haem–globin contacts and in the overall tetrameric or helical structures. This leads to a reduced tolerance to physiological stress, with a tendency to the irreversible oxidation of haem iron and intracellular precipitation of Hb in the form of Heinz bodies. There are over 180 known unstable haemoglobins, some of which lead to congenital Heinz body haemolytic anaemias, the severity of which varies depending on the nature and position of the molecular defect.

Electrophoresis may not be particularly helpful in the diagnosis of unstable Hb disease, since the majority of these mutations show no change in the net charge of the molecule. Instability is detected using two denaturation screens based on either exposure to a solvent or precipitation by heat. The samples should be fresh and a cord blood may be used as a positive control (HbF has a relative intolerance to heat and hydrophobic stress compared to normal adult Hb).

The heat instability test

This screen subjects haemoglobin to incubation at 50°C, which exerts further stress on already weakened internal van der Waals' bonds, causing the sub-units to dissociate more readily than normal.

Isopropanol stability test

Incubation with isopropanol induces hydrophobic stress. Isopropanol is more polar than water and weakens the hydrophobic bonds, allowing water to enter the haem pocket and facilitating the oxidation of haem iron.

In both screens, normal haemoglobin remains in solution, whilst unstable variants are detected by variable flocculation and precipitation.

Molecular analysis

The standard screening techniques described above are adequate for the detection and characterization of the common mutations, but are limited in the identification of rare variants and the specific definition of the thalassaemia defects. The identification of the precise molecular lesion is essential for the purposes of genetic counselling, prenatal diagnosis and, sometimes, for clinical management. This is achieved by analysis of genomic DNA extracted and amplified from peripheral blood leukocytes, or from chorionic villus samples (CVS) for prenatal diagnosis. Recent rapid progress has been made in the development of diagnostic techniques for DNA analysis. A detailed description of these and their applications are beyond the scope of this chapter. However, a brief outline is given on use of the polymerase chain reaction (PCR) in haemoglobinopathy diagnosis.

Polymerase chain reaction

PCR is primarily applied to the detection of point mutations, deletions and DNA polymorphisms. This technique amplifies a region of the DNA of interest, simply and rapidly, and is particularly appropriate to prenatal diagnosis, since it requires only a very small sample which can be obtained by CVS at about 12 weeks gestation.

The principle of PCR involves the synthesis of DNA using synthetic primers (short single-stranded DNA sequences), which flank the DNA region of interest, and a thermostable DNA polymerase (Taq polymerase). The enzymatic amplification of large quantities of DNA permits direct visualization of stained DNA fragments in an agarose gel. A single base substitution can be identified by the change in DNA fragment sizes following digestion of the PCR product with restriction enzymes that recognize specific DNA sequences, followed by 'Southern blotting'. However, this is time-consuming and involves radioisotopes.

New techniques have been developed, based on PCR, that allow testing for specific mutations without the use of restriction enzymes or radioisotopes if the precise molecular defect being sought is known beforehand, thus allowing results to be available within 24 hours. One such technique is the 'amplification refractory mutation system' (ARMS), using allele-specific primers. In this technique two different primers are used, one complementary to the normal allele and the other to the mutant allele, i.e. they differ at the site of mutation only. The primers yield a PCR product if the primer and the DNA sequences are complementary. Thus, the normal and mutant primers will amplify the normal and mutant alleles, respectively. Using this technique, the patient's DNA can be tested for a specific gene mutation, e.g. HbS. Primers have been synthesized for β_A, β_S, β_C, β_E and most of the common β-thalassaemia genotypes. In β-thalassaemia, a limited number of defects have been found to be prevalent in each ethnic group. Thus, the ethnic origin of the patient will determine a particular set of primers to be used first in analysis, with a high probability of positive identification in the first screen.

GAP-PCR is a technique whereby large 'gaps' (deletions) in DNA are detected, and is useful in the diagnosis of the common forms of α^+ and α^0 thalassaemias, which are mostly deletional in origin. It is also used in the molecular diagnosis of Hb Lepore, $\delta\beta$-thalassaemia and deletional forms of HPFH. Multiplex PCR is a useful technique for the simultaneous demonstration/exclusion of a number of different mutations (e.g. all known α^+ and α^0 thalassaemias) in a single test.

The PCR-based techniques mentioned above are used when screening for specific mutations or deletions. However, if the molecular defect remains undetermined, the putative mutation may be identified by directly sequencing the gene.

Acknowledgements

Thanks to Jaspal Kaeda FIBMS PhD (Leukaemia Unit, Imperial School of Medicine, Hammersmith Hospital, London) for help with the PCR section, and to Yvonne Elliott CSI FIBMS (Walsgrave Hospital, Coventry) for critical review of the manuscript.

Further reading

Bain BJ. *Haemoglobinopathy Diagnosis*. 2001: Blackwell Science, Oxford.

Huisman THJ, Carver MFH, Efremov GD. *A Syllabus of Human Hemoglobin Variants*. 1996: Sickle Cell Anemia Foundation, Augusta, GA.

International Committee for Standardization in Haematology (ICSH). Recommendations for neonatal screening for haemoglobinopathies. Clin Lab Haematol 1988; **10**: 335–345.

Thalassaemia Working Party of the British Committee for Standards in Haematology, General Haematology Task Force. Guidelines for the investigation of α- and β-thalassaemia traits. *J Clin Pathol* 1994; **47**: 289–295.

Vulliamy T, Kaeda J. Molecular techniques. In *Dacie and Lewis Practical Haematology*, 9th edn, Lewis SM, Bain BJ, Bates I (eds) 2001: Churchill Livingstone, London, 493–526.

Wild BJ, Stephen AD. The use of automated HPLC to detect and quantitate haemoglobins. *Clin Lab Haematol* 1997; **19**: 171–176.

Working Party of the General Haematology Task Force of the British Committee for Standards in Haematology. The laboratory diagnosis of haemoglobinopathies. *Br J Haematol* 1998; **101**: 783–792.

Working Party of the General Haematology Task Force of the British Committee for Standards in Haematology. Guidelines for the fetal diagnosis of globin gene disorders. *J Clin Pathol 1994;* **47**: 199–204.

29

Special von Willebrand factor investigations

Mohammad S Enayat

Introduction

von Willebrand disease (VWD) was first described by Erik von Willebrand in 1926 in several members of a large family from Åland archipelago in Finland. In 1953, an association between decreased factor VIII (FVIII) procoagulant activity and VWD was identified, leading to some confusion concerning the nature of the protein responsible for haemophilia A and VWD. But it was not until the late 1970s that a better understanding of the immunological and molecular structures of FVIII and VWF led to gene mapping and cDNA cloning of FVIII in 1986 and VWF in 1989.

VWD is the commonest of the congenital bleeding disorders, with a heterogeneous phenotype. It results from quantitative (types 1 and 3) or qualitative (type 2 variants) defects of VWF in plasma and/or platelets. This large multimeric glycoprotein ($10–20 \times 10^6$ kDa) has two major roles in haemostasis; acting as carrier and proteolytic protector of FVIII, and acting as the mediator of platelet adhesion to the subendothelium after vessel injury. VWF is synthesized in the endothelial cells and megakaryocytes by a $\sim$9 kb mRNA transcription resulting from the 180 kb *VWF* gene on the telomeric end of chromosome 12 at 12p13.2 → pter (Figure 29.1). Localization studies using a cDNA probe from the mid-portion of VWF has identified not only the authentic gene on this chromosome, but also a pseudogene sequence on chromosome 22 at 22q11–23. This pseudogene is 21–29 kb long, with DNA corresponding to both exons and introns of the region encoding exons 23–34 of the *VWF* gene and with only 3.1% divergence in sequence.

VWF gene has 52 exons, spanning approximately 178 kb, encoding a translation product of 2813 amino acid (aa) precursor (Prepro-VWF) with large internal repetition of homologous domains. The propeptide (763 aa) and the mature subunit (2050aa) of VWF is composed of repeating domains in the following order: D1–D2–D′–D3–A1–A2–A3–D4–B1–B2–B3–C1–C2–CK. Before secretion, VWF undergoes an extensive post-translational processing, including D1–D2 propeptide cleavage, followed by glycosylation with 12 *N*-linked and 10 *O*-linked oligosaccharides and multimerization. Some of the *N*-linked oligosaceharides of VWF have the unusual property of bearing ABO blood group determinants. Several functional domains (see Figure 29.1) have been identified in the VWF molecule and most of the mutations responsible for various types of VWD have been mapped to these regions.

Results from phenotypic and genotypic tests form the basis of the diagnosis and classification of different types of VWD. However, as more details have emerged from these types of tests, more precise diagnosis and complex classification have regularly been put forward. A revised classification of VWD was published in 1994, but it has already been modified and, as more mutations responsible for each type of VWD are identified, a newer classification based on functional defects and mutations is proposed. In the 2003 XIX Congress of the International Society on Thrombosis and Haemostasis in Birmingham, UK, several presentations emphasized the need for a new classification of VWD, based on molecular diagnosis and improved multimeric analysis of VWF. With so many unclassifiable patients with type 1

The Science of Laboratory Diagnosis, Second Edition   Edited by David Burnett and John Crocker
© 2005 John Wiley & Sons, Ltd

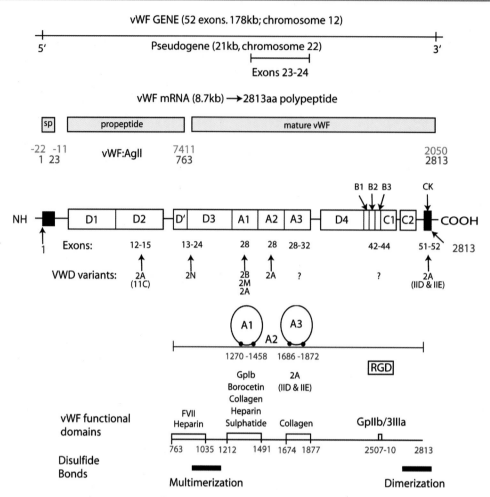

Figure 29.1   Schematic representation of human VWF gene and protein. From top to bottom: structural features of VWF gene, pseudogene and cDNA; locations and old and new numbering of the signal peptide (SP), prepro-peptide and mature VWF. Prepro VWF contains 2813 (2050 old numbering) amino acids, of which 1–22 (-22-1 old numbering) are the signal peptide, 23–763 are the propeptide and 764–2813 are the mature subunit. The lettered boxes denote regions of internally repeated homologous domains; the approximate locations of the cluster of mutations responsible for different types of VWD; A1 and A3 disulphide loops and the positions of the functional domains; positions of disulphide bonds responsible for dimerization and multimerization VWF. Platelet glycoprotein IIb-IIIa ($^\alpha IIb^\beta 3$) binds to the Arg–Gly–Asp (RGD) sequence indicated in the C1 domain

VWD group, it has now been suggested that such an improved multimeric method would help in future classification of these patients.

In this chapter three special phenotypic tests that are now used for diagnosis and classification of VWD are described. They are multimetic analysis of VWF:Ag, used for differential diagnosis of all types of variant VWD; ristocetin-induced platelet aggregation, which is essential for diagnosis of type 2B VWD; and finally VWF/ FVIII binding assay for diagnosis of type N 'Normandy' VWD. Although it is not long since the *VWF* gene was identified, molecular tests have now been extensively

introduced and a brief methodology and some of the approaches for mutation detection are also described.

Phenotypic tests

Multimeric analysis of VWF

In 1981 a non-reducing SDS–gel electrophoresis for high resolution of VWF:Ag multimers was reported by Ruggeri and Zimmerman. This original method has since been modified and improved by others, but the principle of the method has remained the same. The modifications include variations to the actual method, the type of the media in which the protein is separated, semi-automation, and different types of antibodies and methods of visualization of the multimer bands. All of these methods are used for identification of qualitative abnormalities VWF:Ag, such as those seen in variant or type 2 VWD, where there is loss of high and/or intermediate molecular weight multimers. For comprehensive multimer analysis of VWF:Ag used in diagnosis and classification of type 2 VWD, both plasma and platelet VWF:Ag should be examined in a range of 1.0–2.2% agarose gel concentrations. The method described here is Enayat and Hill's (1983) modification of the original Ruggeri and Zimmerman (1981) method. This is a SDS–agarose gel electrophoresis using a discontinuous buffer technique. The multimer band visualization is by autoradiography, using a ^{125}I-labelled mono- or polyclonal anti-VWF antibody. Other non-radioactive methods for band visualization are also possible after transfer of the multimer bands from agarose gels onto different types of fillers.

Gel preparation

A sandwich set made of a piece of gel bond film (Flowgen), covering one glass plate and separated from a second glass plate by a 1 mm thick U-shaped plastic spacer, is used for preparing the gels. The running gel (Agarose Type VII LGT; Sigma) is poured in between the glass plates and, after it has set, the top glass plate is removed and a 3 cm strip from the top of the gel is cut away and is replaced with stacking gel made up of 0.8% agarose (SeaKem HGT (P) Agarose, Flowgen Instruments Ltd). The sample wells are cut out in the stacking gel. Samples to be tested are incubated for 30 minutes at 56°C in a buffer containing bromophenol blue dye, to monitor molecular migration, and sodium dodecyl sulphate (SDS) for complete dispersion of VWF molecules and providing a negative charge to all the multimers.

Electrophoretic conditions

Each electrophoresis instrument has to be optimized for this method but, in general, electrophoresis is initially carried out rapidly at 2 mA/cm for the samples to move out of the wells into the stacking gel. The empty wells are filled with molten stacking gel and electrophoresis is carried out at lower rate of 1.0 mA/Cm overnight. When electrophoresis is completed, the gels are fixed in iso-propanol solution, pressed dry and washed in 10% rabbit serum solution. Autoradiography is performed by incubating the gels in ^{125}I-labelled anti-human VWF antibody (DAKO Ltd) overnight. After a thorough wash to elute out unreacted antibody, the gels are dried and autoradiograph plates are produced using X-ray films and kept at −70°C for 2–5 days prior to development.

Interpretation of the results

Autoradiography is an extremely sensitive method and, by varying the amount of exposure, different autoradiographs with different intensities can be obtained from the same gel. The normal VWF:Ag pattern in plasma shows the full range of multimer bands of von Willebrand Factor. These are made up of high, intermediate and low molecular weight multimers (Figure 29.2). Each multimer band is composed of a triplet band, the main central and two faint but equally stained satellite bands (a and b). The best spread of VWF:Ag multimers is seen in medium resolution (1.3–1.5%) agarose gel, loss of high molecular weight multimers is best investigated in low resolution (1.0–1.3%) agarose gels (Figure 29.2A) and the triplet band abnormalities in high resolution (1.8–2.2%) agarose gels (Figure 29.2B). Therefore, for a full multimeric analysis two or three different gel concentrations should be used. This is not an easy technique and each run can vary from another and need individual optimization of electrophoretic conditions. Densitometric analysis of each multimer pattern can also help in quantification of the amount of multimer gain or loss in some type 2A VWD patients (Figure 29.2C).

Normal platelet VWF:Ag multimer bands are different to those seen from plasma. Much larger multimers are present in platelets than in plasma and the multimeric organisation is also different (Figure 29.3). Smaller multimer bands appear to be made up of a doublet and the central bands migrate less than the corresponding multimers in plasma. Information from platelet multimer analysis can help in deciding on the type of treatment of some type 2A VWD patients and corresponds to the type of mutation present in these patients.

Ristocetin-induced platelet aggregation assay (RIPA)

One of the major functions of VWF glycoprotein is to promote platelet adhesion to the subendothelium at the site of vascular injury, through interaction with GPIb in the platelet membrane GPIb–IX receptor complex. This

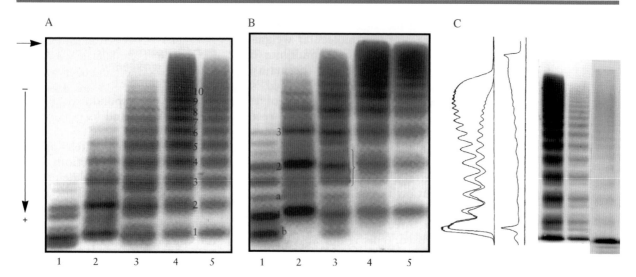

Figure 29.2 Autoradiographs of different patterns seen in plasma VWF:Ag multimers from type 2A (lane 1), 2D (lane 2), 2B (lane 3), normal (lane 4) and type 1 VWD (lane 5) electrophoresed in 1.2% (A) and 1.8% (B) agarose gels. The triplet for band 2 is marked by a bracket and the satellite bands a and b can best be seen in band 1 of the plasma from type 2A VWD (lane 1). Arrow at the top of the gel points to the line between the stacking and separating gels. Direction of electrophoresis is from top to the bottom. (C) A 1.0% gel showing the presence of ultra-high molecular weight multimers, as seen in type 2 Vincenza (1) and some unclassified type 2 VWD patients (2). The next panel illustrates the densitometric scan of one of the two abnormal gels and the area for the ultra-high molecular weight multimers

functional domain mapped to the A1 domain of VWF plays an important role in primary haemostasis. Defects in this domain results in increase in the affinity of VWF for platelet GPIb. However, this does not cause thrombosis but, paradoxically, causes bleeding. This rare phenotype of variant type 2 VWD is referred to as type 2B, and its characteristic functional abnormality is detected by the ristocetin-induced platelet aggregation assay (RIPA). The antibiotic ristocetin induces binding of VWF to platelet GPIb in platelet-rich plasma (PRP) and the degree of platelet agglutination with different concentrations of ristocetin forms the basis of this assay. Aside from this abnormality, 2B VWD is also characterized by selective absence of the high molecular weight multimers (HMWMs) in plasma, which is identified by multimeric analysis of VWF:Ag. In fact, patients with type 2B VWD can synthesize a full range of VWF multimers, as shown by normal multimeric VWF:AG multimer patterns in platelets and endothelial cells, but the HMWMs, are cleared from the circulation because of the increased affinity of the abnormal VWF for the platelet GPIb receptor.

RIPA methodology described here is a modification of the original work described in 1977. Ristocetin (Paesel-Lore) is reconstituted in Trisbuffered saline, pH 7.4, and five different solutions, giving the final concentrations 0.50, 0.1, 0.125 and 0.15 mg/ml, are prepared for use in the assay. PRP is prepared by centrifuging the test and control blood samples at 800 rpm for 10 minutes. The platelet count in the supernatant (PRP) is adjusted to about $250 \times 109/l$. 200 µl of the patient's blood or normal control (blank) is added to cuvettes containing a magnetic stir bar and placed in the 37°C heating blocks of Bio/Data 4 channel platelet aggregometre for 2 minutes. Each cuvette is then inserted in one of the channels of the aggregometre and aggregation is started. 20 µl of ristocetin (starting with the weakest sample) is added to each of the specimens. Aggregation is allowed to occur for a minimum of 3 minutes. A trace of pattern of aggregation that is proportional to the light transmitted is printed out and a typical one is given in Figure 29.4. Samples from type 2B VWD require less ristocetin to achieve a comparable aggregation pattern than normal samples.

VWF/FVIII binding assay

VWF and FVIII are closely associated and in plasma they form a non-covalent molecular complex. The integrity of the FVIII binding domain on the VWF molecule is an important factor for the formation of this and the stability and transport of the VWF/FVIII complex in plasma. In an investigation of several cases of VWD, it

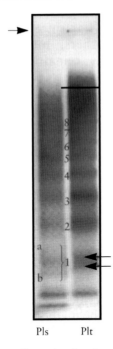

Pls   Plt

Figure 29.3 Autoradiograph showing different multimer patterns seen in normal plasma (Pls) and platelet (Plt) VWF:Ag, electrophoresed on 1.4% agarose. Arrow at the top of the gel points to the sample application wells. Two small arrows at the bottom point to the doublet band pattern best seen in 1.4% agarose. Note the presence of very high molecular weight multimers in the platelet sample

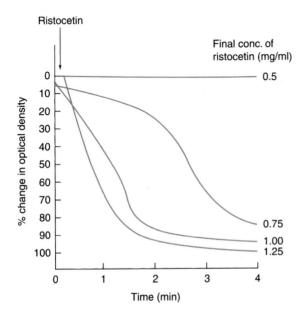

Figure 29.4 A typical trace of the pattern of aggregation for plasma from a normal individual with platelets in the presence of different final concentrations of ristocetin

was noticed that VWF has a defective binding capacity to FVIII, causing reduction in the level of this factor, leading to a condition similar to mild haemophilia A. This condition was initially referred to as 'pseudohae-mophilia' but later it was recognized as a VWF abnorm-ality and renamed 'Normandy' (after the area where the first defined patient came from) or type 2N VWD. The VWF:Ag multimers in this variant VWD are normal, as the mutational defects present in these patients do not affect the mechanism of VWF multimerization. Recently, specific mutations within VWF and responsi-ble for this condition have been mapped to the D' and D3 domains and most of the mutations are grouped in exons 18–24, between Arg 19 and Cys297.

The method described here for determining the bind-ing of FVIII to VWF is the Nesbitt et al. (1996) modification of the original reported method. A suitable concentration of an anti-VWF monoclonal antibody, MAS 533p (Sera Lab), is bound to microtitre plates (Immulon 4, Dynatech Laboratories) overnight at 4°C. The plates are washed twice in 50 mM Tris, 100 mM NaCl, pH 8.0 (TBS), containing 0.1% BSA. Serial dilutions of patient's plasma containing 1 U/dl, 0.5 U/dl, 0.25 U/dl and 0.125 U/dl of VWF:Ag are added in TBS containing 3% BSA and incubated again overnight at 4°C. The plates are washed as before and endogenous FVIII in the samples is removed by incubating with 0.35 M $CaCl_2$ for 1 h at room temperature. Recombinant FVIII (Bioclate, Baxter) at 0.05 U/ml diluted in TBS/1% BSA with 10 mM $CaCL_2$ and 0.002% Tween 20 is added and incubated for 2 h at 37°C. After washing the FVIII bound to VWF is determined using the Coamatic FVIII Chromogenic kit (Quadratech) and detected at 405 nm.

The results are plotted as VWF:Ag dilution (%) against absorbance at 405 nm for FVIII binding. In the example given here (Figure 29.5), the samples used are from a normal control, a homozygous and two hetero-zygous (P1 and P2) type 2N VWD patients with the Thr28Met mutation as positive controls. For determina-tion of any abnormal result, a range of normal control samples should be used.

Genotypic tests for mutation identification

Screening for mutations

The mutations associated with all types of VWD have been identified since late 1980. However, because of the large size and complexity of the VWF gene and the presence of the pseudogene on chromosome 22, with exclusion of large deletions, generally there had been less information about molecular defects in type 1 and

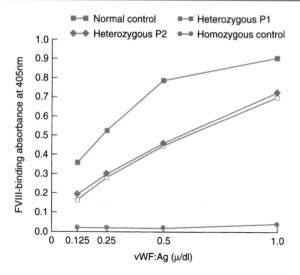

Figure 29.5 Binding of FVIII to VWF in normal control, two heterozygous patients, P1 and P2, with the Thr28Met mutation and a homozygous control with the same mutation

type 3 than in type 2 VWD. Search for the mutations responsible for 2A, 2B, 2N and 2M sub-types have been more successful and these result from the clues provided by the phenotype studies. A protease-sensitive region within the A2 domain, near the Try842 to Met843 cleavage site, was reported to induce the structural changes similar to those seen in 2A VWD, and this domain has been targeted for mutation detection in 2A VWD. In 2B VWD, where there is an increased affinity for platelet GpIb, the mutation detection studies have been directed to the A1 domain of VWF, which contains the functional binding domain for GpIb. Indeed, almost all of the mutations responsible for these two subtypes of VWD have been found in exon 28, which maps to the A1 and A2 domains of VWF. Similarly, exons 18–24 have been targeted for mutation detection in type 2N VWD. A database of point mutations, insertions and deletions identified in VWD, together with a large numbers of polymorphisms found in VWF, was published in 1993. However, since this list is continuously increasing as more information becomes available, a new VWF on-line mutation and polymorphism database was created and maintained by a consortium of VWD investigators on the Internet. This site has now been changed and a new one created on behalf of the ISTH VWF Scientific and Standardization Committee, maintained by Sheffield University, UK. This website (http://www.sheffield.ac.uk/VWF) contains up-to-date information on the latest reported mutations and polymorphisms in the *VWF* gene. Although most of these reported mutations have been confirmed by functional studies, where the

recombinant VWF is expressed in a cell-line culture in which the mutation have been introduced by site-directed mutagenesis, others have yet to be expressed. In some of the reported mutations the entire *VWF* gene has not been investigated to exclude the possibility of changes elsewhere.

In types 1 and 3 VWD, where the mutations could be found anywhere in the entire length of the *VWF* gene, a pre-screening by chemical mismatch cleavage detection (CMCD), conformational sensitive gel electrophoresis (CSGE) or denaturing gradient gel electrophoresis (DGGE) have been reported. For mutation screening by CMCD, the whole of the *VWF* gene is amplified in seven segments from cDNA, obtained by reverse transcription of the 'illegitimate' mRNA found in peripheral lymphocytes by means of polymerase chain reaction (RT-PCR). These segments can then be screened by CMCD for mutation. DGGE is as sensitive as CMCD, but requires synthesis of special primers and use of the electrophoresis gel technique. CSGE methodology is a simple and non-radioactive detection method; however, it does involves amplifications and analysis of up to 60 segments for *VWF* gene investigation.

Mutation detection and authentication

DNA sequencing

Screening methods such as CSGE and CMCD only identify the position and sometimes the type of a molecular change in a small area of the gene, and where mutations could be found. The actual nature of the mutation, however, could only be determined by direct DNA sequencing. The older methods of preparation of single-stranded DNA PCR products needed for sequencing (using appropriate biotinylated primers and streptavidin-coated magnetic beads, or by asymmetric PCR) have now been replaced by cycle sequencing. This method relies on the synthesis of a new strand of DNA from a small amount of original double-stranded template in a cycle sequencing process, using a special thermostable Taq enzyme and fluorescently labelled dideoxy-dNTPs. With the introduction of automated genetic analysers with 16–96 capillary electrophoresis systems, it is now possible to perform hundreds of sequencings per day.

Following detection of a mutation, it can be authenticated by site-directed mutagenesis and its expression in a cell-line culture or by one of the following methods:

1. *Restriction endonuclease analysis.* A single base pair substitution can create or destroy a restriction

endonuclease enzyme site. For confirmation of such a change, restriction products of relevant PCR products with one of the hundreds of suitable restriction enzymes can be analysed by electrophoresis on agarose or acrylamide gel and the restricted DNA bands can be visualized by ethidium bromide staining. In type 2NVWD almost all of the reported mutations can be detected in this way.

2. *Allele-specific oligonucleotide (ASO) hybridization.* In mutations where no restriction enzyme is available to detect the change, ASO-H or dot-blot analysis can be used. Here a short oligonucleotide (about 15 bp) with wild-type and mutant sequences are synthesized. Purified PCR products of the relevant exon are denatured in NaOH. Normal and patient's PCR products from the appropriate exon are applied to Hybond N^+ nylon strips (Amersham International), manually or using one of the commercially available apparatus. The nylon filter strips are then hybridized with the two different types of oligonucleotides labelled with ^{32}P-ATP, using DNA polymerase I Klenow fragment (Pharmacia). After hybridizations, the filter strips are washed three times in differing concentrations of SSC with SDS for 10–20 minutes at an optimal temperature empirically determined for each ASO probe. Using autoradiography, it is possible to visualize positive (annealed) and negative (not annealed) samples.

At the present time, at least 40 missense mutations, four small deletions and one insertion are listed in the database to cause type 2A VWD. A rare dominant form of type 2A VWD (formally type IID) was found to have a missense mutation in the carboxyl-terminal CK domain. A series of missense mutations responsible for type 2B VWD have now been identified and they are all grouped in the 2A domain of VWF, which contains the functional binding domain for GPIb. With few exceptions, these are all confined to a short peptide (amino acids 540–578). The most frequent mutations are R1306W, R1308W, V1316M and R1341Q, which account for about 90% of type 2B VWDs. Fifteen missense mutations, in the D' and D3 domains associated with exons 18–24, currently appear in the database for type 2N VWD, the majority being the R854Q missense mutation.

As mutations for types 1 and 3 could be present in any part of the *VWF* gene's 52 exons, mutation detection in these types of VWD was slow and only a handfull with large deletions had been reported by the early 1990s. However, with the introduction and relative ease of direct DNA sequencing, a large number of mutations have now been reported for type 3 VWD, mostly in homozygous form in patients from families with consanguineous marriages. As the result of a multicenter European (MCMDM-1VWD) study and a Canadian study into the diagnosis and management of type 1 VWD, many more mutations have now been identified. These results indicate that heterozygous missense mutations in mature VWF are an important cause of type 1 VWD and that several other types of mutations can result in reduced VWF expression levels and contribute to this type of VWD phenotype.

Further reading

Budde U, Drewake E, Mainnusch K, Schneppenheim R. Laboratory diagnosis of congenital von Willebrand Disease. *Semin Thromb Hemost* 2002; **28**: 173–190.

Enayat MS. Multimeric analysis of von Willebrand Factor. *Methods Mol Med* 1999; **31**: 187–200.

Evan Sadler J, Matsushita T, Dong Z *et al.* Molecular mechanism and classification of von Willebrand disease. *Thromb Haemost* 1995; **74**: 161–166.

Ginsburg D. Molecular genetics of von Willebrand disease. *Thromb Haemost* 1999; **82**: 585–591.

Goodeve AC. Laboratory methods for the genetic diagnosis of bleeding disorders. *Clin Lab Haematol* 1998; **20**: 3–19.

Goodeve AC. Laboratory methods for the genetic diagnosis of bleeding disorders. *Clin Lab Haematol* 1998; **20**: 3–19.

Jenkins PV. Screening for candidate mutation causing von Willebrand's Disease. *Methods Mol Med* 1999; **31**: 169–177.

Keeney S, Cumming AM. The molecular biology of von Willebrand disease. *Clin Lab Haemotol* 2001; **23**: 290–230.

Nesbitt IM, Goodeve AC, Guillatt AM *et al.* Characterisation of type 2N von Willebrand disease using phenotype and molecular techniques. *Thromb Haemost* 1996; **75**: 959–964.

Ribba AS, Lavergne JM, Bahnak BR *et al.* Duplication of a methionine within the GPIb binding domain of von Willebrand factor detected by denaturing gel electrophoresis in a patient with type IIB von Willebrand disease. *Blood* 1991; **78**: 1738–1743.

Ruggeri ZM, Ware J. The structure and function of von Willebrand factor. *Thromb Haemost* 1992; **67**: 594–599.

Ruggeri ZM, Zimmerman TS. The complex multimeric composition of factor VIII/von Willebrand factor. *Blood* 1981; **57**: 1140–1143.

Sadler JE, Mannucci PM, Berntorp E *et al.* Impact, diagnosis and treatment of von Willebrand disease. *Thromb Haemost* 2000; **84**: 160–174.

Schneppenheim R, Budde U, Ruggeri ZM. A molecular approach to the classification of von Willebrand disease. *Best Pract Res Clin Haematol* 2001; **14**: 281–298.

30

Platelet investigations

Steven Walton and Peter E Rose

Introduction

Platelets are small fragments of megakaryocyte cytoplasm with a mean diameter of 1–2 μm and a mean volume of 5–8 fl, having an average lifespan in the peripheral circulation of 1–10 days. Their function is to maintain the integrity of the vessel wall and to initiate haemostasis upon damage to the vasculature. Their functionality can be divided into three main areas: adhesion to the vascular endothelium; aggregation to each other; and release of chemicals into the plasma. This chapter will describe the principle behind the techniques used to investigate each of those areas.

In clinical situations, loss of this functionality is expressed by patients showing increased bruising, petechial rashes or prolonged bleeding following minor traumas, such as venepuncture or dental treatment. Patients who present with these problems should have a screen of platelet function, together with quantitation of the platelet count.

Structure and function

Platelet function is closely related to the platelet structure. The platelet external membrane is a highly functional organelle, containing different glycoproteins that transect the standard bilipid cellular membrane. Several of these glycoproteins are capable of activating various biochemical pathways within the platelet to induce any of the functions required in a normal platelet response. Abnormal platelet function has been shown to result from a lack of expression of one or more of these glycoproteins (see Table 30.1 and Figure 30.1). Abnormal platelet adhesion is seen in Bernard–Soulier syndrome, in which the platelet membrane glycoprotein Ib has been shown to be deficient. This glycoprotein has a specific binding capacity for the plasma protein von Willebrand's factor, which coats subendothelial matrix upon exposure to plasma, thus adhering platelets to the site of vascular injury via the glycoprotein Ib. Deficiency of complex glycoprotein IIb/IIIa causes an abnormality in the platelets' ability to aggregate (see Figure 30.1). This condition is known as Glanzman's thrombasthaenia. These and other glycoproteins act as a physiological receptor for various low and high molecular weight platelet agonists. Once one or more of these glycoprotein receptors have become activated, there is a signal transduction into the internal organelles of the platelet. This is commonly via activation of the enzyme phospholipase C, which is exposed on the internal ends of the glycoproteins upon activation by their respective ligands.

Within the platelet cytoplasm are many of the internal structures found in other secretory cells; however, the platelet does not have a great capacity for the synthesis of proteins. The platelet contains very little rough endoplasmic reticulum and Golgi apparatus (see Figure 30.2). It does contain extensive smooth endoplasmic reticulum, which is often referred to as 'the dense tubular system'. The cytoplasm also contains many α-granules and dense granules. These granules contain a wide variety of chemicals which are involved in the inflammatory response and, more importantly, in accelerating the process of localized haemostasis. The α-granules contain coagulation factors such as factors V, VII and fibrinogen, along with growth factors to aid

The Science of Laboratory Diagnosis, Second Edition   Edited by David Burnett and John Crocker

Table 30.1 Factors involved in a normal platelet response

Glycoprotein	Ligands	Platelet function
GP IIb-IIIa	Vitronectin von Willebrand factor Fibrinectin Fibrinogen	Aggregation and adhesion at high shear rates
GP Ia-Iia	Vitronectin von Willebrand factor Fibrinectin Fibrinogen	Adhesion
GMP 140 (PADGEM)	Various glycoproteins and glycolipids	Platelet to leukocyte interaction

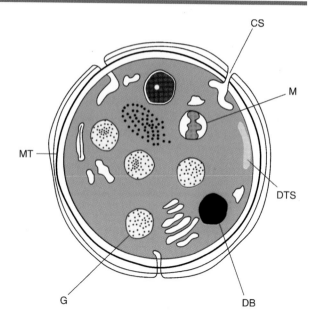

Figure 30.2 Schematic representation of platelet structure. The diagram illustrates the main internal structures of a discoid platelet. (CS) is the surface connected canalicular system. (M) is the platelet mitochondria. (DTS) is the dense tubular system. (DB) is a dense body. (G) represents one of the platelet granules. (MT) represents the circumferential band of microtubules

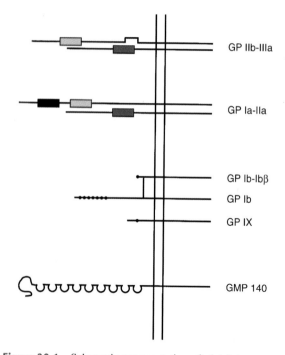

Figure 30.1 Schematic representation of platelet receptors

vascular repair, notably platelet-derived growth factor (PDGF) and endothelial growth factor (EGF). Another substance stored in the α-granules is platelet factor IV and this is one of the main factors assayed to assess the platelet release response.

The dense granules contain a large proportion of the platelet's available nucleotides, mainly adenine and guanine diphosphate and triphosphate, along with cal-

cium and magnesium ions and 5-hydroxytryptamine (5-HT). ADP is a major accelerant for platelet aggregation, whilst ATP has an inhibitory effect on ADP and is therefore a part of the control mechanism to localize the thrombus formation. 5-HT is another powerful platelet aggregator, the platelet membrane containing numerous receptors for 5-HT. These receptors are members of the superfamily of G proteins, a coupled neurotransmitter and hormone receptor, found both on nerve cells and in the gut endothelium in large numbers.

Platelet counting

It is important to obtain an accurate platelet count before proceeding to tests of platelet function. Platelet numbers can be approximated by microscopy of a Romanowski-stained blood film. Platelet morphology for size and granularity is helpful in disorders associated with large platelets, such as Bernard–Soulier syndrome.

Automated blood count machines capable of counting platelets are routine laboratory equipment (see Chapter 27). Greater accuracy than manual techniques enables counts to be measured as low as $5 \times 10^9/1$ and in excess of $1000 \times 10^9/1$.

Platelet antibodies

Reduced platelet counts result either from a failure of marrow production (e.g. following cytotoxic chemotherapy) or from increased platelet consumption. The production of antibody to a platelet's membrane component or to a substance carried on the membrane of the platelet may result in increased sequestration in the spleen. The presence of the platelet membrane-activated immunoglobulin is therefore an important investigation. The presence of platelet-directed plasma immunoglobulins does not correlate with clinical severity of autoimmune thrombocytopenia, while the concentration of platelet-bound immunoglobulin is a better marker of disease activity.

The demonstration of platelet-bound immunoglobulin is more difficult than red cell association immunoglobulin. Due to low platelet numbers and the difficulty in visualizing platelets, the method of choice is to use a flow cytometer and combine the antihuman globulin reagent with a fluorescent dye. A platelet-rich plasma is prepared by slow centrifugation. This plasma is then centrifuged hard in the presence of a buffer containing EDTA or some other platelet inhibitor to form a platelet button, which is then washed several times to remove any trapped plasma containing human globulins. Finally, the platelets are resuspended in 5% bovine albumin. An aliquot of the platelets is then mixed with an antihuman globulin with either fluorescein isothiocyanate or another fluorochrome detectable by the flow cytometer. After incubation in the dark, platelets are given a final wash in PBS EDTA buffer and resuspended in a sufficient quantity of buffer to allow easy flow through the flow cytometer. The patient's platelets without fluorescent dye tagged to them are used as a negative control. A positive reaction occurs when the fluorescent index is higher in the platelets tagged with the fluorochrome than in those platelets without the dye.

Bleeding time

One of the simplest platelet function tests is a bleeding time. An incision is made into the skin on the forearm, using a bleeding device, and the time taken for the bleeding to stop is measured. In order to improve reproducibility of the method, the technique is performed by making a dual incision, using a spring-loaded lancet of standard area. The spring is of a standard tension to give reproducible depth to the cut, while a sphygmomanometer cuff is inflated to a standard pressure of 40 mmHg. The time for bleeding to cease is measured by a stop-watch and detection is by mopping the excess blood from the arm with clean filter paper. Any major platelet defect will give a prolonged time, as will disorders of von Willebrand protein.

Platelet adhesion

Physiologically, the first stage of platelet activation is the adhesion of platelets to the subendothelial matrix. The measurement of platelet adhesion is difficult and is seldom performed in routine laboratories. Several methods are reported that can be used to give a crude estimation of platelet adhesive function. The simplest is to take a citrated blood sample without venous occlusion and perform a platelet count on the sample. An aliquot of the sample is then passed at constant pressure over a tube containing standardized glass beads and a second platelet count performed on the emerging sample. The percentage of platelet adhesion can be calculated. A modification to this standard technique, using a subcellular matrix such as collagen, may give a better physiological picture. Problems with reproducibility of results have restricted use of this method to research laboratories, including pharmaceutical companies evaluating the efficacy of drugs modifying platelet adhesion or activation. A more complex method involves a system to simulate normal venous pressure and requires the production of a loop of inert plastic with an area of subendothelial matrix. Blood is then passed into the system at normal physiological shear rates.

Investigations of platelet aggregation

A measurement of platelet aggregation is probably the most commonly used technique in the investigation of platelet disorders. Aggregation studies are based on a photometric technique. Aggregation is recorded as the change in the absorbance of a mixture of platelet-rich plasma as aggregates form. The larger the clumps, the heavier they are, and as they fall out of the light path a higher transmission of the light is detected. There are several commonly used agonists, including ADP, adrenalin, collagen and the antibiotic ristocetin. Ristocetin is an unusual agonist in that it has no direct effect on platelets but modifies part of the factor VIII complex known as von Willebrand factor. When modified, this protein changes from a globular to a linear structure. The linear structure then binds to several platelets and gives pseudoaggregation. An abnormal response to ristocetin is seen in patients with quantitative and qualitative changes in von Willebrand protein.

Platelet function analyser PFA-100

The PFA 100 device (Dade) is increasingly used in routine laboratories to measure the collagen/epinephrine-induced closure time. The device measures platelet plug formation on a collagen-coated capillary under shear stress. Citrated venous blood is drawn through a capillary tube to contact a membrane coated with epinephrine, resulting in platelet activation. Blood is then aspirated through a precision aperture in the membrane, while platelets start to adhere to the circumference until a stable plug forms to occlude the aperture. The closure time is therefore the time taken for blood to stop passing through the aperture and is a measure of *ex vivo* platelet plug formation. This methodology now represents the first line of platelet investigation for many laboratories.

Investigations into platelet release

Techniques studying platelet release can be divided into two, those that use radioisotopes and those that use the production of light using the enzyme luciferinase. Isotopic techniques can be performed in two ways. Platelets can be incubated with a radioisotope that can be incorporated into the molecule under investigation, such as ^{14}C-labelled 5-hydroxytryptamine (5-HT) to look for release of 5-HT. In these methods, platelet-rich plasma is incubated for a time period with a relevant radioactive compound. The platelets are then separated from the plasma and excess radioisotope removed. To do this, the platelets are spun through an albumin density gradient, leaving the platelet pellet at the bottom with the radioactive plasma on the top. The platelet pellet is then resuspended in a buffer, washed again and counted. After platelet aggregation with a potent agonist, the platelet-poor plasma is also counted and the amount of radioactivity in the platelet-poor plasma expressed as a percentage of the activity in a full platelet sample.

A second technique using radioisotopes is to perform a radioimmune assay (RIA). With this methodology the compound under investigation is mixed with a portion of the same compound labelled with a radioactive tracer. To this mixture is added a specific andibody to the compound under investigation. After incubation, antibody-bound compound is separated from unbound, usually by the addition of activated charcoal followed by centrifugation. It is possible to count the radioactivity in either the pellet or the free supernatant. Because the antibody binds radiolabelled and non-radiolabelled samples in equal quantity, the proportion of radioactivity bound by the antibody is inversely proportional to the amount of compound in the plasma under investigation. The method is quantified by using known concentrations of control plasmas to construct a graph and then readings for samples are measured from the graph.

Chemiluminescence is another technique used in investigation of platelet release reaction. This is based on the same chemical reaction that takes place in the firefly, where ATP and luciferinase reacts on luciferin to produce photons of light. The reaction is dependent upon the amount of ATP being produced. In the platelet reaction, luciferinase and luciferin are added to a reaction vial along with platelet release compounds. The amount of ATP in the reaction vial determines the amount of light produced. A higher production of light results from a higher release of ATP from the platelets.

Flow cytometry

Flow cytometry is increasingly used to investigate platelet function against specific antigens expressed on platelets. The methodology of flow cytometry is discussed in Chapter 32. For platelet investigations there are two main proteins that can be identified; those required for the binding of the platelet to the cell wall and those required for aggregating platelets to each other. Glycoprotein Ib is a surface antigen that is required for binding platelets to the subendothelial matrix via von Willebrand's factor. Glycoprotein IIb/IIIa is one of the main components required for the platelet aggregation reaction. A deficit of platelet function can therefore be identified using monoclonal antibodies raised against either of these proteins.

To investigate abnormalities in platelet membrane-bound glycoproteins, a platelet-rich plasma is prepared by slow centrifugation. The plasma is then diluted in either platelet-poor plasma or albumin to give a platelet count of approximately $1 \times 10^9/1$. An aliquot of this is then mixed with a fluorescently-tagged monoclonal antibody specific to the glycoprotein. After incubation, the whole amount is again diluted to give about 0.5 ml. The sample is then analysed by a flow cytometer. For positivity, the fluorescence index must be higher than a control sample of the same patient's platelets without the fluorochrome present. Platelets are the smallest cellular constituent of blood and it is not necessary to lyse the red cells or to remove any debris from the sample, as it is simple to gate around the platelets under investigation.

There is increasing interest in the role of platelets in thrombotic disorders. This has led to the investigation of platelets to identify activated populations of platelets during thrombotic episodes, e.g. after prosthetic heart valve replacements. Two major markers of activation have been identified. One is due to changes to the conformational shape of membrane glycoproteins, notably IIb/IIIa. This change exposes sites to the external environment which, in the resting platelet, are hidden within coils on the molecules. Many antibodies have been produced to these activation epitopes. These activation antigens are only demonstrable on platelets that have been activated with weak thrombin solutions and are negative on untreated platelets. A second type of activation protein is identified when parts of the α-granules are expressed on the surface membrane of platelets. This happens when granules have gone through the secretory process and the membrane of the granules has become incorporated into the platelet external membrane. The name for these has been given as platelet activation-derived granular to external membrane (PAD-GEM). Using antibodies to these markers, either singly or in combination, and using a flow cytometer with the technique discussed above, it is possible to determine the proportion of activated platelets.

Thromboelastogram

A more physiological and global approach to platelet function is measured using a thromboelastogram. The thromboelastogram measures temperature-adapted coagulation, fibrinolytic factors and platelet function by monitoring the clot's physical properties and its ability to perform mechanical work throughout its development and degradation. $CaCl_2$ is added to citrated venous blood in a temperature-regulated (37°C) disposable cup which oscillates at an angle of 4° 45′. A disposable pin is placed into the sample immediately after recalcification. The torque of the rotating cup is transmitted to the immersed pin after fibrin platelet bonding has linked cup and pin together. The magnitude of the pin motion depends on the strength of bonding, with strong clots moving the pin directly in phase with the cup motion. As the clot retracts or dissolves, the bonds are broken and the transfer of the cup motion is diminished. Information is provided on the time to fibrin strand formation, the kinetics of clot formation and clot dissolution. This approach is increasingly used in the intensive care setting to monitor coagulation status.

Further reading

Ahn YS *et al.* Activated platelet aggregates in thrombotic thrombocytopenic purpura: decrease with plasma infusions and normalisation in remission. *Br J Haematol* 1996; **95**: 408–415.

Chand IF, Keiffer NA, Phillips BR. Platelet membrane glycoproteins. In *Haemostasis and Thrombosis*; 3rd edn. 1994: Lippincott, London.

Dacie JV, Lewis SM (eds). Basic haematological techniques. In *Practical Haematology*, 7th edn. 1991: Churchill Livingstone, London.

Rosenfield CS, Nicholls G, Bodensteiner DC. Flow cytometric measurement of antiplatelet antibodies. *Am J Clin Pathol* 1987; **87**: 518–522.

White JG. Platelet ultrastructure. *Haemostasis and Thrombosis*, 2nd edn. 1987: Churchill Livingstone, London.

31

A hospital transfusion service

Steven Walton and Peter E Rose

A hospital blood transfusion service undertakes three major serological investigations: (a) to identify a patient's blood group; (b) to detect and identify irregular antibodies, including those inducing haemolytic anaemia; (c) to provide compatible blood components to patients.

Blood group identification

The laboratory methods applied to transfusion serology are rapidly changing to accommodate an increasing need to simplify and automate many aspects of the service. The principles of serology, however, remain the same. There are over 100 recognized antigens on the red cell membrane, the presence of which can be identified by agglutination of red cells on exposure to the corresponding antibody or antiserum. Most blood group antigens are naturally occurring and exposure of the antigen may stimulate a primary antibody response in a person lacking the antigen. The resultant alloantibody is specific for that antigen, and further exposure to the antigen may stimulate a rapid and prolonged antibody response, with the potential to induce significant transfusion reaction. Rapid intravascular haemolysis may follow the binding of the antibody (usually IgM) to the antigen and complement activation. This results in ABO incompatibility when anti-A or anti-B, naturally present in the recipient's serum is exposed to the appropriate antigen. Usually an individual produces naturally occurring antibodies against the AB antigens that are absent from his/her own red cells, due to stimulation from the same antigen found on other biological substances, such as pollen or bacteria. An individual blood group can therefore be determined directly by adding specific antisera to the test red cells and indirectly by addition of red cells of known antigen specificity to the test sera. To determine a patient's blood group requires the characterization of red cell antigens. For routine blood grouping, this requires identifying A, B and D antigens. People expressing the A antigen on the cells do not produce anti-A but can produce anti-B. People expressing B antigen do not normally produce anti-B but can produce anti-A, whilst group O do not express either A or B antigen. Historically, antigen identification was performed using purified antibodies from previously typed patients. Nowadays, most typing antibodies are chemically modified monoclonal antibodies. For ease of use, commercial antibodies have a specific coloured dye added to anti-A and anti-B antibodies. An indirect method of checking a patient's blood group is to react a patient's serum, which contains the antibodies, with cells of known ABO specificity, which gives a reverse or back group. Thus, a group A patient's serum will react with B cells, group B patients will react with A cells, and group O patients will react with both A and B cells. The rare patients who possess both A and B antigens react with neither cell. A further check and part of the investigation for irregular antibodies is to put the patient's serum with group O cells, which should not react, irrespective of the patient's blood group.

It is important to include appropriate negative controls, such as the patient's own cells or O cells. The control cells are necessary to identify reactions due to cold antibodies in the sample other than anti-A and anti-B.

The Science of Laboratory Diagnosis, Second Edition Edited by David Burnett and John Crocker
© 2005 John Wiley & Sons, Ltd

Table 31.1 Expected results for common blood groups

Group	Anti-A	Anti-B	Anti-AB	A Cells	B Cells	O Cells	Anti-D1	Anti-D2
A Rh$^+$	+	−	+	−	+	−	+	+
A Rh$^-$	+	−	+	−	+	−	−	−
B Rh$^+$	−	+	+	+	−	−	+	+
B Rh$^-$	−	+	+	+	−	−	−	−
AB Rh$^+$	+	+	+	−	−	−	+	+
AB Rh$^-$	+	+	+	−	−	−	−	−
O Rh$^+$	−	−	−	+	+	−	+	+
O Rh$^-$	−	−	−	+	+	−	−	−

The rhesus system

The rhesus (Rh) system is the second most important blood group system to be identified. Unlike the ABO system, antibodies are not present naturally in the absence of the antigen; however, antibodies can be readily formed following exposure of rhesus-positive (Rh$^+$) cells in a rhesus-negative (Rh$^-$) recipient. The antibodies formed are usually IgG, and can cross the placental barrier, resulting in second or subsequent pregnancies in which the mother is Rh$^-$ and the fetus Rh$^+$ developing haemolytic diease of the newborn (HDN). It is therefore important that every effort be made to avoid sensitization of Rh$^-$ females of child-bearing age to the D antigen. Rhesus grouping should be performed in duplicate, using an IgM monoclonal anti-D. Positive and negative controls must be included in each batch of tests and the results read microscopically after centrifugation of tubes for 1 minute at a low speed. In the UK, national guidelines recommend the use of two different anti-D reagents. The D antigen is a complex antigen made up of many different subantigens (epitopes). Monoclonal antibodies are highly specific and may react to single epitopes; therefore, if the particular epitope to which the reagent reacts is missing there will be a false negative result.

Using these eight reagents (anti-A, anti-B, anti-AB, anti-D, anti-D2, A cells, B cells and O cells), it is possible to identify the common blood groups (see Table 31.1).

Methods for blood grouping

There are many methods using these basic reagents to group patients, which can broadly be divided into five categories: (a) methods based on individual tubes with no enhancement, requiring approximately 1 hour of incubation at an optimum temperature of 16°C; (b) methods in individual tubes with enhancement (rapid groups), usually requiring centrifugation and only performed in cell typing; (c) methods using microtitre plates; (d) methods using a solid-phase matrix; (e) automated methods based on continuous flow principles. The method chosen depends on the volume of work to be undertaken and its urgency. Rapid methods usually only check the patient's antigens without a back-check.

Visualization of results varies depending on the method employed. For tube and microtitre methods, it is dependent upon agglutination of the red cells, which can be interpreted either micro- or macroscopically. Microtitre and rapid group methodologies tend to use macroscopic visualization, while non-enhanced methods tend to be read microscopically.

Microtitre methods

Microtitre methodologies allow multiple groups to be performed easily in batches. A standard microplate consists of 96 wells in a solid plastic block, aligned in 12 rows of eight. Using eight reagents for a full group, 12 patients' bloods can be grouped on a single plate. Visualization of all the groups on the plate can be rapid, using backlight to see positive and negative results. There are systems available using computers and micro-robotics to automate or semi-automate microtitre grouping systems. These systems incorporate microplate readers, which can be programmed to identify blood groups by the reactivity pattern of the microtitre plate.

Gel systems

Gel-phase systems rely on trapping the reacted cells in a solid or semi-solid matrix, with negative results falling

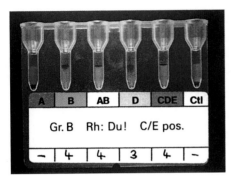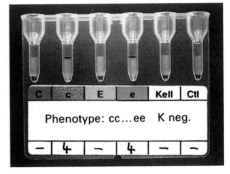

Figure 31.1 ABO grouping of gel system. Showing a group B Rh⁺ sample. Reproduced by permission of DiaMed-GB Ltd

through the gel. This occurs by having the monoclonal antibodies mentioned above chemically bonded to the matrix. Thus, cells containing the corresponding antigen are stuck (trapped in the matrix) when they are pulled through the gel by centrifugation (Figure 31.1). This method is particularly useful for grouping patients at high risk from blood-borne microorganisms, such as hepatitis or HIV. The high cost of manufacturing gels incorporating specific antibodies needs to be considered when implementing this methodology into routine laboratory practice.

Automated systems

Automated methods using equipment that can use positive sample identification are required in laboratories with high workloads. The benefit from using automated equipment is a reduction in sample handling time, while patients benefit from the removal of clerical errors, as results can be reported directly from reading with no transcription. The large capital outlay required makes automated systems too expensive for laboratories with a low workload. Most laboratories will use two techniques, a rapid system for urgent analysis and a routine batch system for the bulk of the workload. Rapid grouping is performed to identify the patient's blood group in an emergency when blood is required for cross-matching, thus allowing a group-compatible blood to be selected with little delay.

Antibody screening

Screening patient's sera for the presence of any irregular antibodies has now become a routine part of every hospital blood bank. It is now rare to undertake a blood group identification without antibody screening

at the same time, with the possible exception of neonatal samples, where antibody production has not commenced and sample size is small.

For many patients undergoing elective and emergency surgical procedures, blood grouping and antibody screening is all that is recommended. This policy has dramatically reduced blood wastage, with cross-matched blood reserved for procedures with a greater than 30% likelihood of requiring cells. For patients in whom a clinically significant antibody is identified in the screening test procedure, a full cross-match is necessary.

There are a number of physiochemical properties displayed by different antibodies that are important in their identification. First, different blood group antibodies can be distinguished from each other on the basis that some antibodies agglutinate red cells better at low temperatures (cold antibodies), while others are active at 37°C. Cold antibodies are often IgM antibodies and may not be detectable or clinically significant at higher temperatures. Some naturally occurring antibodies, such as anti-A and anti-B, will still react at 37°C; however, the titre will be much higher at 0–4°C. Warm antibodies are usually IgG and agglutinate red cells more quickly at 37°C. Historically, antibodies have also been classified as complete or incomplete, depending on whether they agglutinate red cells suspended in normal saline. Incomplete antibodies do not agglutinate red cells under such circumstances, and this has led to the search for other techniques to enhance the sensitivity. Red cells suspended in 20–30% bovine albumin can help to identify many incomplete antibodies. Other methods employing polybrene or enzyme-treated cells have been routinely used. Enzymes such as trypsin, papain, bromelain or ficin have been used to remove neuraminic acid from the red cell surfaces and reduce the negative charge, causing the incomplete antibody to agglutinate the enzyme-treated cells. Saline tests at room temperature, albumin and enzyme methods have been superseded by the

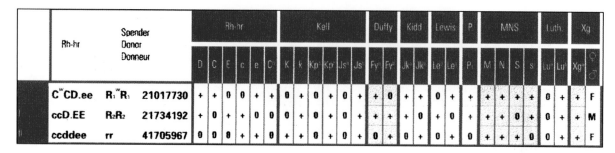

Rh-hr	Spender Donor Donneur		Rh-hr						Kell						Duffy		Kidd		Lewis		P	MNS				Luth.		Xg	
			D	C	E	c	e	Cʷ	K	k	Kpᵃ	Kpᵇ	Jsᵃ	Jsᵇ	Fyᵃ	Fyᵇ	Jkᵃ	Jkᵇ	Leᵃ	Leᵇ	P₁	M	N	S	s	Luᵃ	Luᵇ	Xgᵃ	♀♂
CʷCD.ee	R₁ʷR₁	21017730	+	+	0	0	+	+	0	+	0	+	0	+	+	0	+	+	0	+	+	+	+	+	+	0	+	+	F
ccD.EE	R₂R₂	21734192	+	0	+	+	0	0	0	+	0	+	0	+	+	+	+	0	+	0	+	+	+	0	+	0	+	+	M
ccddee	rr	41705967	0	0	0	+	+	0	+	+	0	+	0	+	0	+	0	+	0	+	0	+	+	+	0	0	+	+	F

Figure 31.2 Example of antibody screening cells. Reproduced by permission of DiaMed-GB Ltd

indirect antiglobin test (IAT). The latter test is superior in identifying clinically significant antibodies and does not have the disadvantage of identifying irrelevant antibodies, which can result in a serious delay in the laboratory, as further assessment and identification of the antibody is necessary.

Antibody screening is undertaken by reacting red cells containing the majority of common blood group antigens with the patient's serum. It is usual to have a set of three cell samples, and the antigens known on each cell sample are given on an information sheet (Figure 31.2).

The antibody screen can be performed using any of the techniques found in the laboratory, but commonly the indirect antiglobulin test is used as the initial screen. This is because the IAT test is the most sensitive test for most antibodies. Using the new gel systems, it is being proposed that a negative IAT-based antibody screen and selection of ABO Rh-compatible blood are sufficient to issue blood for a patient, and that cross-matching is no longer necessary. In the majority of cases this is true, but there is a risk that incompatible blood might be issued to a patient with antibodies to a rare antigen.

The indirect antiglobulin test

The IAT using red cells suspended in low-ionic strength saline (LISS) is the recommended method for antibody screening. In normal saline the ionized groups on both antigen and antibody are partially neutralized by oppositely charged ions in the solution. The minimum incubation time for normal ionic strength techniques is 45 minutes and is no longer recommended.

If LISS is used as the medium, antigen and antibody reactions are more rapid. LISS is a solution of sodium glycine containing 0.03 M sodium chloride. Rarely, LISS-dependent autoantibodies may be detected, and in these circumstances normal ionic strength techniques may be helpful.

The screening cells used in antibody detection should have homozygous expression of appropriate antigens (Rh, Cc, Ee, Jkᵃ, Jkᵇ, Fyᵃ, Fyᵇ, Ss). It is expected that 99.9% of antibodies would be detected, with only antibodies to red cells of very low frequency not detected. Following incubation of test serum with screening red cells, the cells are washed to remove any unbound antibody. Any contamination by free globulin will neutralize the antiglobin component in the antiglobulin reagent, and must be avoided.

Monospecific anti-IgG may be used instead of a polyspecific antiglobulin reagent containing anti-complement sera, using the LISS IAT method. This avoids the undesirable susceptibility to interface from low thermal amplitude and LISS-dependent antibodies that are complement binding. When an irregular antibody is identified, further investigation to identify the specificity of the antibody is necessary.

Antibody identification

If a positive result is obtained in any of the antibody screening cells it is essential to identify the antibody specificity. This requires reacting the sera with a larger panel of typed cells. Commonly, commercial panels contain 11 cell types and are supplied with an antigram of the corresponding antigens (Figure 31.3). Antibody identification is produced by matching the antibody reactive pattern with the pattern of the antigens. If blood is required for transfusion, only units negative for the corresponding antigen should be selected. As with the antibody screen, any method can be used but it is best to start with the same technique as gave the positive reaction in the antibody screen. Frequently this is the IAT. Inconclusive, results from this panel can frequently be clarified by repeating the panel using an enzyme-enhanced technique. If identification is still inconclusive, a different panel of cells should be used.

	Rh-hr	Spender Donor Donneur		Rh-hr						Kell						Duffy		Kidd		Lewis		P	MNS				Luth		Xg		Spez. Antigene special types antigènes part.
				D	C	E	c	e	C^w	K	k	Kp^a	Kp^b	Js^a	Js^b	Fy^a	Fy^b	Jk^a	Jk^b	Le^a	Le^b	P_1	M	N	S	s	Lu^a	Lu^b	Xg^a	♀ ♂	
1	$C^wCD.ee$	$R_1^wR_1$	403/37728	+	+	0	0	+	+	0	+	0	+	0	+	+	+	+	+	0	0	+	+	0	0	+	+	+	0	M	
2	CCD.ee	R_1R_1	504/38187	+	+	0	0	+	0	+	+	0	+	0	+	0	+	+	+	0	+	v.w. +	+	0	+	0	0	+	+	M	
3	ccD.EE	R_2R_2	43/37566	+	0	+	+	0	0	0	+	0	+	0	+	+	+	0	+	0	+	+	+	0	+	+	+	+	nt	M	Co^b+, Co^a-
4	Ccddee	r′r	38016	0	+	0	+	+	0	0	+	0	+	0	+	+	+	0	+	0	0	+	+	+	+	+	+	+	0		Co^b+
5	ccddEe	r″r	36849	0	0	+	+	+	0	0	+	0	+	0	+	+	+	+	0	0	+	+	+	+	0	+	0	+	+		
6	ccddee	rr	112727	0	0	0	+	+	0	+	+	0	+	0	+	+	0	0	+	0	+	0	0	+	0	+	0	+	+	M	Co^b+
7	ccddee	rr	95/36818	0	0	0	+	+	0	0	+	0	+	0	+	+	+	+	0	+	0	w +	+	+	0	+	0	+	+	M	Bg^a+
8	ccD.ee	R_{0r}	818/38098	+	0	0	+	+	0	0	+	0	+	0	+	+	+	0	+	0	+	0	+	+	+	+	0	+	0	M	
9	ccD.EE	R_2R_2	71034080	+	0	+	+	0	0	+	+	0	+	0	+	0	+	+	0	0	+	0	+	+	0	+	0	+	+	M	Co^b+
10	ccddee	rr	01776470	0	0	0	+	+	0	0	+	0	+	0	+	+	0	0	+	0	+	+	+	0	+	0	0	+	0	M	
11	CCD.ee	R_1R_1	2573669	+	+	0	0	+	0	0	+	+	+	0	+	0	+	+	0	+	0	+	+	0	+	0	0	+	+		

Figure 31.3 Example of an antigram showing a wide range of antigens. Reproduced by permission of DiaMed-GB Ltd

Inconclusive results may require a fresh sample to be taken to ensure the antibody is real and not a sample contaminant. If the identity of the antibody remains unknown, it may be necessary to refer the sample to the reference centre, where a larger donor panel will be available to aid identification.

Cross-matching

Cross-matching is the procedure performed to ensure that potential donor blood is compatible with the recipient. Once the patient's ABO Rh group and a negative antibody screen has been obtained, cross-matching the blood should be straightforward. Donor units should, where possible, be selected from the same ABO and Rh group. The type of red cell product will need to be considered, e.g. whole blood, concentrated red cells, cells with added supplement, leukocyte-poor or -depleted. This will depend on the condition requiring transfusion and on the age of the recipient. Furthermore, it is necessary to ensure that women aged under 50 years are given Kell-negative red cells. This is because antibodies produced to the Kell antigen are able to cross the placenta. Women stimulated to produce anti-Kell by transfusion, who become pregnant, may have an infant develop a haemolytic anaemia in utero.

Once the correct product has been selected, the cross-match procedure is relatively straightforward, as cells from the donor bag are washed and reacted with the recipient's serum. The choice of technique is the same as for antibody screening, but must include an indirect antiglobulin method. Any units that give a positive reaction should not be transfused. Rarely there are instances where it is impossible to obtain compatible units, e.g. in patients with strong autoantibodies in the serum. In these patients, an auto-cross-match (recipient's cells against recipient's serum) should be performed. Units that exhibit no greater strength of reactivity than in the auto-autologous cross-match can be issued.

All autoantibodies should be further investigated to identify the specificity and thermal range of the antibody. This may require elution techniques.

Elution methods

It is possible to remove antibodies bound to red cell antigens without altering their antigenic specificity, by a process that is termed elution. There are three main elution processes; temperature, low pH and organic solvents.

Temperature

The most commonly used temperature elution system is to heat washed red cells to 56°C for 5 minutes. After centrifugation, the supernatant contains the antibodies. Freezing washed cells suspended in albumin elicits the same haemolysed supernatant which, after centrifugation, is ready for investigation. Both these methods are quick and easy to undertake in any laboratory.

Low pH

If washed red cells are suspended in buffers with a pH below 3.5, IgG antibodies may be recovered from the cell membranes without lysis. Although low pH is the recommended elution technique, a pH above 10 appears to give better results for IgM antibodies.

Organic solvents

Although results of eluates using ether or xylene are very good for IgG antibodies, the hazards to workers from exposure to these solvents restricts their use to laboratories with extraction hoods. Once an eluate has been prepared, the eluate is substituted for serum in an antibody identification method.

Transfusion practice

Current hospital transfusion practice should include systems to minimize the use of blood products where possible. Potential viral transmission of hepatitis B, hepatitis C, HIV and CMV in blood products, together with a potential risk of variant CJD, have resulted in a number of measures to improve the safety of blood products. These include improved systems for donor selection, routine viral screening, the use of inactivated plasma products and leukocyte depletion of red cell products. Measures to minimize the use of transfusion products include the use of maximal blood ordering schedules, the development of autologous transfusion practice and participation in the Serious Hazards of Transfusion (SHOT) reporting system. The latter is a UK voluntary reporting system for serious adverse events following transfusion. Acute adverse events of transfusion include haemolytic transfusion reactions, infusion of bacteria-contaminated blood products, transfusion-related acute lung injury, fluid overload, severe allergic reactions or anaphylaxis and post-transfusion purpura. Potential longer-term complications result from viral infection (see above), chronic graft vs. host disease in the severely immunosuppressed, and iron overload. In every case the risks of transfusion do need to be balanced against the risks of not receiving blood products. Patients should, therefore, be properly informed of transfusion risks and have access to appropriate information.

Further reading

Guidelines for Pretransfusion Compatibility Procedures in Blood Transfusion Laboratories. *Transfusion Med* 1996; **6**: 273–283.

Issitt PD. *Applied Blood Group Serology*, 3rd edn. 1985: Montgomery Scientific; Miami, FL.

Knight RC, DeSilva M. New technologies for red cell serology. *Blood Rev* 1996; **10**: 101–110.

Mollison PL, Engelfriet CP, Contreras M. *Blood Transfusion in Clinical Medicine*, 9th edn. 1993: Blackwell Scientific, Oxford.

32

Flow cytometry and molecular biology in haematology

Ian Chant

Introduction

The diagnostic utility of flow cytometry and molecular biology continues to expand into diverse areas of clinical haematology. The combination of an immunobiological and molecular approach to diagnosis and subsequent patient monitoring has proved to be more useful in regard to haematological neoplasms than in any other area of cancer biology.

In flow cytometry, the development of new benchtop analysers and commercially available monoclonal antibody combinations permits a multiparametric approach to diagnosis. This allows an accurate definition of the immunophenotype of specific cells. The accumulation of immunophenotypic data has proved to be important, not only from a diagnostic point of view but also in terms of prognostic evaluation. In several haematological neoplasms, the expression or absence of certain antigens has been shown to have prognostic significance. In addition, flow cytometry is now used in treatment monitoring, particularly in terms of the detection of minimal residual disease.

Similarly, molecular biology continues to expand as a vital tool in both diagnosis and disease monitoring. The most important molecular technologies in diagnostic haematology are fluorescence *in situ* hybridization (FISH) and polymerase chain reaction (PCR) methodologies. Molecular approaches are vital in the demonstration of specific genetic lesions that are seen in the haematological neoplasms. In addition, the demonstra-

tion of clonality in the lymphoproliferative disorders is achieved by molecular techniques.

The importance of a combined immunophenotypic and molecular approach to leukaemia and lymphoma diagnosis is demonstrated by the recent publication of the World Health Organization (WHO) classification of haematopoietic and lymphoid neoplasms. This system links previous classifications with new data generated from flow cytometry and molecular biology, incorporating these into a system with clinical relevance. This is exemplified by the development of treatment modalities that target specific genetic abnormalities.

In other areas of haematology, flow cytometry and molecular biology continue to evolve as vital diagnostic and clinical tools. The genetic basis of the haemaoglobinopathies continues to be elucidated, while molecular techniques are increasingly important in the diagnosis of coagulopathies.

This chapter will outline the major applications of these two technologies in the haematology laboratory and illustrate how the combination of immunobiological and molecular information has had a profound impact on diagnosis and our understanding of the biology of haematological disorders.

Flow cytometry and immunophenotyping

The most important application of flow cytometry in the diagnostic haematology laboratory is the identification

The Science of Laboratory Diagnosis, Second Edition   Edited by David Burnett and John Crocker

of cell lineage in leukaemias and lymphomas. The expression of cell surface antigens that are lineage- and differentiation-dependent permits the use of fluorochrome-labelled monoclonal antibodies specific to these antigens. The monoclonal antibodies that recognize specific epitopes of antigens are identified by cluster of designation (CD) number. At the time of writing, appximately 250 CD numbers have been assigned and a number of these are particularly important in immunophenotyping haematopoietic cells.

The approach to leukaemia and lymphoma diagnosis is the utilization of a panel of monoclonal antibodies that will identify the specific lineage of a cell population and provide a specific immunophenotype for a putative population of malignant cells. Together with morphological and molecular information, this flow cytometric data is an essential tool in the classification of the malignant cell.

Immunophenotyping of the acute leukaemias

The aim of immunophenotyping a newly diagnosed leukaemia is primarily to discriminate between lymphoid and myeloid malignancies. This can be achieved using a relatively small panel of monoclonal antibodies, which detect lineage-specific antigens expressed on immature myeloid or lymphoid cells, discriminating acute myeloid leukaemias (AMLs) from the lymphoblastic leukaemias (ALLs). The first-line acute panel should also differentiate B cell or T cell lineage in ALL and allow further definition of subtype, e.g. monocytic and megakaryocytic markers in AML. Table 32.1 shows a typical first-line antibody panel for acute leukaemia diagnosis. This initial panel includes B lineage (CD10, CD19, CD20, CD22), T lineage (CD2, CD3, CD7) and myeloid-associated (CD13, CD33, CD117) markers, plus others that offer information on the degree of cellular differentiation (TdT, CD34).

Acute myeloid leukaemias

The most useful myeloid-specific markers used to discriminate myeloid cells from those of lymphoid origin are CD13, CD33 and CD117. Expression of lymphoid antigens will be absent on AML cells, with the exception of CD7 and Tdt, which may be positive in a small number of cases.

Acute myeloid leukaemias are traditionally classified by the French–American–British (FAB) system on morphological and cytochemical grounds (Table 32.2). In

Table 32.1 A first-line panel of antibodies used to determine lineage and differentiation in acute leukaemias

Lymphoid lineage	CD3	Pan-T (also cytoplasmic CD3)
	CD7	Pan-T
	CD19	Pan-B
	CD10	Pre-B
	CD79α	Pan-B (cytoplasmic expression)
Myeloid lineage	CD13	Granulocytes, monocytes
	CD33	Myeloid progenitor, monocytes
	CD14	Monocytes
	CD64	Monocytes
	CD15	Granulocytes, monocytes
	CD117	Myeloid progenitor
	MPO	Myeloperoxidase
Non-lineage restricted	HLA-DR	Progenitor cell
	CD34	Progenitor cell
	Tdt	(Nuclear expression)

Table 32.2 Classification of acute myeloid leukaemias by the French–American–British (FAB) system

AML M0	AML with no maturation
AML M1	AML with minimal maturation
AML M2	AML with maturation
AML M3	Acute promyelocytic leukaemia
AML M4	Acute monocytic leukaemia
AML M5a	Acute monoblastic without differentiation
AML M5b	Acute monoblastic with differentiation
AML M6	Acute erythroleukaemia
AML M7	Megakaryocytic leukaemia

AML, although there are no specific markers that distinguish the AML M1-M5 subtypes, immunophenotyping correlates reasonably well with the FAB subtype, some markers being preferentially expressed within certain groups. These include the monocytic markers CD14 and CD64 in the M4 and M5 categories, whilst the rarer AML M6 and M7 subtypes can be characterized by their expression of red cell- and platelet-specific antigens, respectively. AML M0 cells lack differentiation and express myeloid antigens plus CD34, the haemopoietic stem cell marker, whilst in AML M1 there is usually expression of myeloid antigens only. Table 32.3 lists the general immunophenotypes seen in AML in relation to their FAB classification.

Table 32.3 Typical immunophenotypes in AML with correlation to the FAB classification

CD	Antibodies	M1, M2	M3	M4, M5	M6	M7
Myeloid lineage						
CD11b	Mo1, Leu15	±	±	++	−	−
CD13	MY7, Leu-M7	++	++	++	++	+
CD14	MY4, Mo2, Leu-M3	±	−	++	++	−
CD15	Leu-M1	++	++	++	++	−
CD33	MY9, Leu-M9	++	++	++	++	+
T lineage						
CD2	T11, Leu-5b	±	±	±		
CD3	T3, Leu-4	−	−	−	−	−
CD5	T1, Leu-1	−	−	−	−	−
CD7	3A1, Leu-9	+−	±	±	±	+
B lineage						
CD10	CALLA, J5	−	−	−	−	−
CD19	B4, Leu-12	±	−	±	−	−
CD20	B1, Leu-16	−	−	−	−	−
Erythroid lineage						
Glycophorin A	D2.10	−	−	−	++	−
CD71	T9	−	−	−	++	−
Megakaryocyte lineage						
CD41	gpIIb/IIIa	−	−	−	−	++
CD42	gpIb	−	−	−	−	++
CD61	gp/IIIa	−	−	−	−	++
Stem cell						
CD34	MY10, HPCA-1	+	−	±	+	+
CD38	Leu-17	+	+	+	+	+
Non-lineage-dependent						
HLA-DR	Ia, I3	++	−	++	++	±

The recent WHO classification of AML places emphasis on morphological, immunophenotypic and molecular features, As such, AML is classified according to specific recurrent genetic abnormalities, and these are often associated with specific immunophenotypic profiles. In cases of AML, where such genetic abnormalities are not evident, these are described according to their degree of differentiation and/or differentiation along monocytic, megakaryocytic or erythroid lineages. As such, the immunophenotype is essential in characterization of the leukaemic cells in the same way as its utilization in the FAB system.

Acute lymphoblastic leukaemias (ALLs)

Acute leukaemias of lymphoid origin are routinely classified according to their B cell or T cell origin. T cell ALL cells express one or more of the T cell antigens (CD2, CD3, CD7) and Tdt. The CD3 antigen is expressed in the cytoplasm early in T cell maturation and is the most useful marker for T-ALL. One of the first surface antigens in T cell development is CD7 and this is generally present on all T-ALL cells.

The B cell lymphoblastic leukaemias can be classified into three groups, relating to their degree of maturation, which is associated with generally characteristic phenotype. Null cell ALL, an immature leukaemia, has cells that express B cell markers (CD19, CD22) plus TdT and CD34. Common ALL is distinguished by the presence of CD10 expression, along with the B cell antigens and TdT. B-ALL cells express all the usual B cell antigens but are distinguished by the absence of TdT and CD10.

Chronic lymphoproliferative disorders

Flow cytometry is an essential tool in the diagnosis of chronic or mature lymphoproliferative disorders. Immunophenotyping is designed to demonstrate the B or T cell nature of the malignant cell, to demonstrate potential clonality of κ or λ surface light chain expression on B cells. The approach is generally to use a first-line panel of antibodies specific to a number of B and T cell antigens, which will identify clonality or abnormal antigen expression. A second-line panel can then be applied selectively according to these results, plus any pertinent morphological or clinical indications. Table 32.4 illustrates typical first- and second-line panels.

B cell malignancies represent the majority of mature lyphoproliferative disorders and these are generally associated with particular patterns of B cell antigen

Table 32.4 A first-line panel for the investigation of a lymphocytosis to establish B and T cell lineage

	Antibody	Lineage
T lineage	CD2	T cells, NK cells
	CD3	Pan-T
	CD4	T helper
	CD8	T suppressor
	CD7	Pan-T
B lineage	CD19	Pan-B
	CD20	Pan-B
	CD22	Mature B
	CD23	Immature B, CLL
	CD103	Hairy cell
	λ SIg	
	κ SIg	

expression. In addition to the presence or absence of certain antigens, the interpretation of immunophenotypic data needs to look at the intensity of antigen expression, demonstrated by flow cytometry as fluorescence intensity. For example, in chronic lymphocytic leukaemia (CLL), the mature B cells co-express CD5 (an antigen normally present on B cells) plus CD23. Characteristically in CLL, the B cell antigens CD19 and CD20 are downregulated, as is surface light chain expression. By contrast, B lineage lymphoma cells demonstrate strong reactivity with CD19, CD20 and κ or λ surface light chains. In cases where a diagnosis of hairy cell leukaemia is suspected on morphological or clinical grounds, antibodies to CD11c, CD25 and CD103 will be added, whilst in potential cases of possible lymphoplasmacytic or plasma cell proliferation, CD38 and CD138 will be included.

The T cell lymphoproliferative disorders show an overlap of CD antigen expression and the malignant cells often show antigen loss or abnormal expression of T cell markers. Certain markers are characteristic, such as strong expression of CD25 in adult T cell leukaemia (ATLL), strong reactivity with CD7 in adult T cell prolymphocytic leukaemia, and CD56 expression in large granular lymphocyte (LGL) leukaemia.

In the B and T cell disorders, diagnosis is therefore based not only on the immunophenotypic pattern revealed by the antibody panels, but also with reference to the levels of antigen expression, as revealed by the intensity of fluorescence during flow cytometric analysis. This is illustrated by Table 32.5, which shows the

Table 32.5 Immunophenotypic patterns in the T and B cell lymphoproliferative disorders. B cell lymphoproliferative disorders

B-cell lymphoproliferative disorders	CD5	CD10	CD19	CD20	CD23	CD25	FMC7	κ or λ
CLL	+	−	+	+ (w)	+	−	−	+ (w)
PLL	−	−	+	+ (s)	−	+	+	+ (s)
NHL (diffuse)	−	−	+	+ (s)	−	−	±	+ (s)
Mantle cell lymphoma	+	−	+	+ (s)	−	−	−	+ (s)
Follicular lymphoma	−	+	+	+	±	−	−	+ (s)
Hairy cell leukaemia	−	−	+	+ (s)	−	+	+	+ (vs)

T-cell lymphoproliferative disorders	CD2	CD3	CD4	CD5	CD8	CD16	CD25	CD56
T-PLL	+	+	+	+	−	−	−	−
L-GL	+	+	−	−	±	+	−	−
Sezary cell	+	+	+	+	−	−	−	−

(w), weak reactivity; (s), strong reactivity; (vs), very strong reactivity. CLL, chronic lymphocytic leukaemia; PLL, prolymphocytic leukaemia; NHL, Non-Hodgkin's lymphoma. L-GL, large granular lymphocytic leukaemia.

main immunophenotypic patterns seen in these disorders.

Assessment of platelet function by flow cytometry

Platelet dysfunction is seen in a variety of systemic disorders, including renal disease, hepatic failure, connective tissue disorders, myeloproliferative and myelodysplastic disorders, malignancy and cardiovascular disease. The availability of monoclonal antibodies that recognize specific antigens on both resting and activated platelets provides a means for assessing platelet function. These include antibodies to P-Selectin (CD62P), an adhesion molecule, which is translocated to the platelet surface upon activation. Antibodies to this molecule only bind to degranulated platelets. Antibodies are also available to GPIIb/IIIa (CD41/CD61), an epitope that appears when the platelet is activated. It results from a conformational change that leads to the binding of fibrinogen to the platelet surface and subsequently to platelet aggregation.

At present, flow cytometric analysis of platelet function has not replaced standard clinical tests of platelet function, such as the bleeding time and platelet aggregometry. This is partly due to cost and operator expertise, although flow cytometry does offer several advantages: whole-blood analysis is possible, thereby minimizing platelet activation, and extremely small volumes of blood are required (20 μl), making neonatal studies possible. The platelets of patients with profound thrombocytopenia can also be analysed accurately.

Molecular biology in haematology

The greatest impact of molecular biology techniques in haematology has been in the identification of genetic abnormalities associated with leukaemias and lymphomas. The identification of the chromosomal translocation that gives rise to the Philadelphia chromosome, a hallmark of chronic myeloid leukaemia, was the first human cancer for which a genetic basis was established. Indeed, we understand more about the molecular pathogenesis of haematological malignancies than for any other group of human cancers. Table 32.6 illustrates some of the genetic abnormalities that are associated with selected haematological neoplasms.

The main tools of molecular biology used to demonstrate such genetic aberrations are *in situ* hybridization, especially FISH and PCR. Both techniques are highly sensitive and more rapid than conventional cytogenetic analysis, and DNA or RNA can be extracted from blood, bone marrow or a variety of body fluids for molecular analysis. These two techniques have been used to identify both chromosomal abnormalities and abnormal genes or mRNA, e.g. oncogene expression. These include translocation-induced gene rearrangements involving oncogene activation, plus normal gene rearrangements involving immunoglobulin heavy and light chain genes, which are used to demonstrate clonality in

Table 32.6 Some of the frequent cytogenetic and molecular features seen in haematological neoplasms which are useful in diagnosis and as targets for disease monitoring

Disease	Karyotype	Abnormal gene	Use in diagnosis
CML	t(9;22)(q34;q11)	*BCR-ABL*	CML diagnosis
AML	t(8;21)(q22;q22)	*AML 1-ETO*	AML with maturation
	t(15;17)(q22;q21)	*PML-RARA*	Acute promyelocytic
	inv(16)(p13;q22)	*CBFβ-MYH11*	Myelomonocytic
ALL	t(12;21)(p13;q22)	*TEL-AML1*	Precursor B-ALL
	t(4;11)(q21;q23)	*MLL-AF4*	Often neonatal presentation
	t(8;14)(q24;q32)	*MYC* dysregulated	Burkitt type ALL
	t(1;14)(p32;q11)	*TAL1* dysregulated	T-ALL
	t(7;9)(q34;q32)	*TAL2* dysregulated	T-ALL
Lymphomas	t(14;18)(q32;q21)	*bcl-2* dysregulated	Follicular centre lymphoma
	t(11;14)(q13;q32)	*bcl-1* dysregulated	Mantle cell lymphoma

CML chronic myeloid leukaemia.
AML acute myeloid leukaemia.
ALL acute lymphoblastic leukaemia.

lymphoid neoplasms. The examples outlined below illustrate how FISH and PCR are used to identify these genetic rearrangements in haematological malignancies.

FISH to demonstrate the Philadelphia chromosome in CML

The Philadelphia chromosome results from a reciprocal translocation, t(9;22) (q34;q11), causing gene rearrangement involving a cellular oncogene, *c-abl*, and the *BCR* gene (Figure 32.1). This rearrangement is seen in 95% of

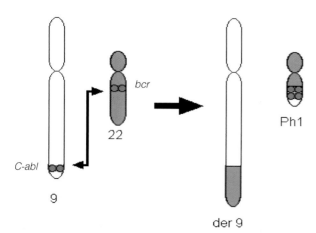

Figure 32.1 Reciprocal translocation between chromosomes 9 and 22 results in a longer chromosome 9 (der 9) and the Philadelphia chromosome Ph1, containing the fused *bcr–abl* gene

chronic myeloid leukaemia (CML) patients, producing a *BCR–ABL* fusion gene, which codes for a protein with increased tyrosine kinase activity. Increased activation of growth regulatory proteins by *bcr-abl* increase the rate of mitosis and protects cells from apoptosis.

FISH can be used to visualize the *ABL* and *BCR* genes via nucleic probes complementary to DNA sequences in the two genes (Figure 32.2). Using a biotin-labelled probe for *BCR*, the *BCR* gene can then be detected with avidin-FITC, which binds to the biotin-labelled probe and can be visualized as green dots by fluorescence microscopy. A probe for the *ABL* gene can be labelled with digoxygenin and detected with anti-digoxygenin rhodamine, which will fluoresce as red dots. The presence of the fused *BCR-ABL* gene on the Philadelphia chromosome is therefore demonstrated by the combined red and green dots.

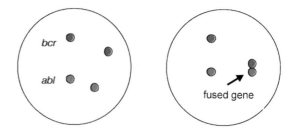

Normal interphase nucleus   Interphase nucleus of leukaemic cell with the Philadelphia chromosome.

Figure 32.2 Visualization of the *bcr* and *abl* genes using FISH to demonstrate the fused *bcr–abl* gene on the Philadelphia chromosome

A large number of labelled probes are commercially available which target the frequently-seen genetic abnormalities seen in leukaemias and lymphomas, and this will possibly permit the transfer of FISH methodologies into the routine diagnostic laboratory.

Demonstration of clonality by gene rearrangement studies

The diagnosis of the lymphoproliferative disorders has been based on immunophenotypic methods to demonstrate clonality and cell lineage. In the B cell malignancies, κ or λ light chain restriction can often be assessed, but for the T cell malignancies clonality is less easily determined. The use of molecular biology techniques to detect clonality in T or B cells has therefore been an important diagnostic development.

B cell clonality analysis by PCR

During B cell development there is rearrangement of the immunoglobulin heavy chain (IgH), involving V (variable), D (diversity) and J (joining) regions, which are brought together to form a functional unit. In a normal B cell population, each cell uses a different combination of V, D and J segments, plus there is the insertion of random numbers of base pairs at the V–D and D–J junctions (Figure 32.3).

The PCR method utilizes two primers, one that corresponds to a consensus sequence found in the majority of V segments, and the other a consensus sequence common to most J segments. When the DNA

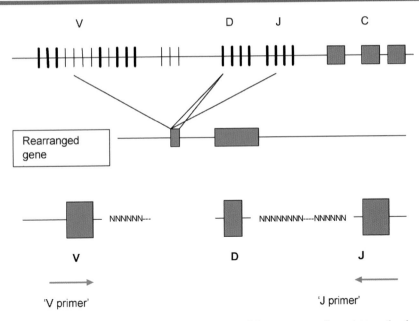

Figure 32.3 During B cell development, one each of several V, D and J segments are brought together by gene rearrangement. Using V and J primers, PCR analysis of immunoglobulin gene DNA produces a variety of PCR products in normal B cells. In a B cell lymphoproliferative disorder, clonality is demonstrated by a single PCR product

is amplified, the length of the PCR product will be determined by the number of random nucleotides inserted during VDJ joining. In a normal population of B cells, each PCR product will have a slightly different size, so that when the PCR products are separated by electrophoresis, a smear will be seen on the gel. In the case of a neoplastic population of B cells, all will have the same VDJ rearrangement, thereby producing a single-sized PCR product, which is visualized by the appearance of a discrete band on electrophoresis.

B cell clonality analysis by PCR has several advantages. It can be performed on peripheral blood, bone marrow, fresh or frozen tissue and paraffin-embedded samples. Very small samples of DNA are required and, as with *in situ* hybridization, results are available much more quickly than with conventional cytogenetic analysis.

T cell receptor gene rearrangement studies

The receptor for the antigen on most mature T cells (TCR) comprises two polypeptides, α and β, which are linked and associated with the CD3 molecule. A smaller population of T cells have a different heterodimer, composed of two different polypeptides designated γ and δ, which have a degree of homology with the α and

β chains, respectively. Normal T cell development involves rearrangement of these chains to give a heterogenous population of T cell receptor genes.

Clonality of T cells is commonly assessed by PCR, using the TCRγ locus. This is the most appropriate single chain to examine, since immature T cell expansions may not have undergone $\alpha\beta$ recombination, while the δ gene is deleted during a gene recombination. Generally, three sets of consensus primers for the TCRγ chain are used and the amplified products are separated by electrophoresis. A polyclonal T cell population results in a smear of PCR products, whereas a monoclonal population of malignant T cells will be demonstrated by just one or two distinct bands visible on the electrophoretic gel.

Detection of minimal residual disease

Minimal residual disease (MDR) is defined as those malignant cells that survive following initial remission-induction chemotherapy. The detection of a potentially very small population of malignant cells, e.g. in a bone marrow that is morphologically in remission, may have important prognostic and therapeutic implications. Both flow cytometry and molecular biology techniques have been used to monitor MDR.

One of the main problems with flow cytometry has been the identification of a tumour-specific immunophenotype. However, some haemopoietic antigens are found on malignant cells in combinations not present in normal blood or bone marrow, e.g. in most cases of T cell acute lymphoblastic leukaemia (T-ALL), the malignant cells express nuclear TdT as well as CD3, CD5 and CD1. This pattern is not normally seen in T cells outside the thymus and can be used to demonstrate T-ALL cells in blood or bone marrow. Other immunophenotypic combinations have been used in MRD analysis for B cell ALL and acute myeloid leukaemia (AML), with varying degrees of success. A major problem with immunological techniques will always be limitations on sensitivity, and flow cytometry is capable of detecting one target cell in 10^4–10^5 background cells. Most studies of residual disease therefore utilize the extreme sensitivity of PCR to identify known genetic abnormalities present in the target malignancy. For example, detection of BCR–ABL fusion genes has been used extensively in the follow-up of patients with CML, including following bone marrow transplants. In lymphoproliferative disorders, unique clonal rearrangements can be used as targets for PCR-based analyses with nucleic acid probes specific to a particular patient's malignant cells. Such approaches are labour-intensive, but as more information becomes available they will play a role in assessing prognosis and eligibility for specific treatment modalities.

Diagnosis of haemoglobinopathies

Molecular biology has had profound benefits in relation to the identification of specific common mutations giving rise to abnormal globin chain synthesis. PCR has been primarily applied to the detection of point mutations, deletions and DNA polymorphisms, to provide a rapid screening test that has been particularly important in prenatal diagnosis. The choice of a specific technique depends upon the degree to which the disease has been defined at the genetic level. For example, in sickle cell disease the affected gene is known at the level of the DNA sequence, and several approaches can be taken to amplify and analyse a patient's DNA profile with PCR. Knowledge of the specific point mutation has allowed the development of fluorescence amplification techniques for rapid screening. These methods utilize oligonucleotide primers for the normal and mutant DNA sequences, labelled differentially with red and green fluorescent markers. By pairing each with an unlabelled second primer, the PCR products can be analysed for differential red and green fluorescence in a fluorimeter, providing a rapid screening technique.

With diseases such as the thalassaemias, the genes are cloned and sequenced but genetic mutations are heterogenous. The approach to inheritance studies is therefore based on linkage studies, using restriction fragment length polymorphisms (RFLP). These are DNA mutations, generally in non-coding sequences of DNA, which are inherited in association with a gene and can therefore become useful markers for detection of a mutant gene in prenatal diagnosis.

Genetic abnormalities in the coagulopathies

As for the haemoglobinopathies, an increasing number of disease-specific mutations have been identified that lead to abnormalities associated with blood coagulation. The demonstration of point mutations in genes encoding coagulation factors is used for diagnostic and familial screening studies.

A widely used test is the PCR-based detection of the factor V Leiden mutation. It is estimated that 2–6% of the normal population carry this mutation, and homozygosity of the alleles is reported to carry an 80-fold increased risk of thrombosis. Detection of the mutation utilizes sequence-specific primers, one a sense primer, which is complementary to both normal factor V and FV Leiden, and a second antisense primer complementary to either the normal FV allele or the FV Leiden allele. The nature of the FV genotype can then be determined by analysis of the amplification products, since either the normal or FV Leiden-specific primer will produce an amplified product.

Summary

Flow cytometry and molecular biology have jointly played a vital role in the diagnosis of leukaemias and lymphomas. The recognition of abnormal immunophenotypic and genetic markers that are associated with particular haematological disorders have led to a re-analysis of the classification system for haematological malignancies. The recently published World Health Organization (WHO) classification system takes more account of these developments and attempts to utilize immunological and genetic features along with morphological observations. This produces a classification system that has more clinical value in terms of prognosis and treatment modalities.

Future breakthroughs in the treatment of these disorders will come from modalities that may target specific immunological or genetic features of the disease. It is clear that even within distinct disease entities, the exact prognostic outlook for a particular patient depends on a variety of factors, involving the expression of many genes, some as yet unidentified. An exciting development involves the technique of DNA microarrays, which permit the quantification of thousands of genes. Distinct genes are represented by cDNA fragments on a solid substrate, thousands of which can be accommodated on a single glass slide. Labelled cDNA or RNA probes are prepared from the patient's cells and hybridized to the microarray. The amount of probe hybridizing to the microarray element is proportional to the expression of mRNA from the corresponding gene in the patient's cell.

This extremely powerful, broad picture of gene expression will certainly, in the future, provide us with an increasing knowledge of the factors involved in the malignant process and hopefully lead to improvements in treatment of the haematological neoplasms.

Further reading

Jennings CD, Foon KA. Recent advances in flow cytometry: application to the diagnosis of hematologic malignancy. *Blood* 1997; **90**: 2863–2892.

Provan D, Gribben J (eds). *Molecular Haematology.* 2000: Blackwell Science, Oxford.

Stamatoyannopoulos G (ed.). *The Molecular Basis of Blood Diseases.* 2001: W.B. Saunders, Philadelphia, PA.

33

Haematinic investigations

Frank Wells

Anaemia may be caused by loss of blood, destruction of red cells or by a failure in red cell production. Failure to produce cells is most frequently caused by the separate or combined deficiencies of the 'haematinics'—iron, vitamin B_{12} and folate. Vitamin B_{12} is more properly known by its chemical name, cobalamin, and that nomenclature is used here.

The starting point for the laboratory investigation of anaemia is the blood count. Macrocytosis and pancytopenia are characteristic findings in the megaloblastic anaemias caused by cobalamin and folate deficiency, whilst microcytosis and hypochromia characterize deficiency of iron. Microscopic examination of blood and marrow yields characteristic findings but in the case of megaloblastic anaemia cannot differentiate folate and cobalamin deficiency. The measurement of the vitamins and iron in blood is of significant value, but results require careful interpretation, based on possible interactions between folate and cobalamin, other coexisting pathologies, effects of binding proteins and the possible presence of mild deficiency states. In the case of iron, a functional deficiency may occur in the presence of adequate iron stores. All these factors are briefly discussed, together with methods for clarifying the cause of the identified deficiencies and the investigation of iron excess.

Cobalamin (vitamin B_{12}) and folate

Cobalamin and folate are essential to a number of single carbon transfers, and in the present context the most important of these relate to DNA synthesis. A simplified view of the metabolic pathways involving the two vitamins is shown in Figure 33.1. The active form of folate is tetrahydrofolate (THF) and this carries and utilizes the single carbon unit in different oxidation states as 5-methyl THF ($>N–CH_3$), 5,10-methylene THF ($>N–CH_2–N<$) or 10-formyl THF ($>N–CHO$). A single carbon insertion (from formate via 10-formyl THF) is required twice in the synthesis of purines, and methylene THF is utilized in the conversion of uridine to thymidine in pyrimidine synthesis. 5-methyl THF and cobalamin are together required for the methylation of homocysteine to methionine. Much of the methionine is further converted to S-adenosylmethionine, a universal donor of methyl groups required in a wide range of methylation reactions involving DNA, RNA, hormones, neurotransmitters, membrane lipids and myelin basic protein. Failure of this last function results in the subacute degeneration of the cord associated with severe cobalamin deficiency. Cobalamin is also an essential cofactor for the mutase that converts methylmalonic acid to succinic acid.

Both cobalamin and folate exist in protein-bound forms in blood. The main binding protein for cobalamin is transcobalamin II. In chronic myelogenous leukaemia, transcobalamin III, which is produced in large quantities by granulocytes, can cause spuriously high measured concentrations of serum cobalamin.

Analysis of cobalamin and folate in blood

Methods of laboratory analysis are often strongly affected by the need to analyse large numbers of specimens.

The Science of Laboratory Diagnosis, Second Edition   Edited by David Burnett and John Crocker
© 2005 John Wiley & Sons, Ltd

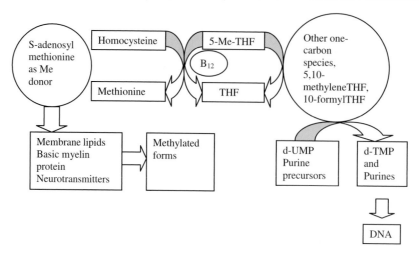

Figure 33.1 Metabolic transformations involving cobalamin (vitamin B_{12}) and folate. Reproduced by permission from Klee (2000)

This militates against procedures that require manual intervention or steps that cannot be readily incorporated into a continuous automated process. Early methods for analysis of both vitamins depended on the growth of organisms having an absolute requirement for one of the vitamins. For cobalamin this was *Euglena gracilis* or *Lactobacillus leichmannii* and for folate a chloramphenicol-resistant *Lactobacillus casei*. Growth was measured by increase in turbidity of the culture medium with all other required nutrients in excess. Although these assays still have value as a measure of biologically active vitamin, they have been replaced in routine practice by competitive protein binding assays.

Competitive protein-binding assays

The principle of these assays can be summarized in respect of cobalamin and is represented schematically in Figure 33.2. A protein that binds cobalamin strongly and specifically is added to a mixture of natural cobalamin (the specimen) and a labelled form of cobalamin. The binding protein is present in a concentration significantly less than that of the vitamin and its labelled analogue. The natural and labelled forms of the vitamin compete for the restricted number of binding sites on the protein during a period of equilibriation. At equilibrium the ratio of natural to labelled cobalamin bound to the specific protein will be approximately the same as the ratio of natural to labelled cobalamin in the original solution. The bound cobalamin is then separated from the solution

and the amount of labelled cobalamin attached to the binding protein is measured. The label may be a fluorescent species or an enzyme, and sensitive measurement techniques, such as chemiluminescence, may be employed.

Comparison of the result with a standard curve permits quantification of the amount of natural cobalamin in the original sample and allows for the fact that the binding constant for natural and labelled cobalamin may not be exactly the same, and that non-specific binding may also occur with other serum proteins. The details of this process vary with different analysers, but the principle is common to most. When the concentration of cobalamin in the specimen is very high, the amount of labelled cobalamin bound to the binding protein approaches zero, and when the concentration of cobalamin in the specimen is zero, the binding of labelled cobalamin reaches a maximum.

The first competitive protein binding assays utilized radioisotopes for labelling cobalamin, but the hazards involved and difficulties in automating such techniques caused their use to decline.

Assay of cobalamin

The vitamin is separated from the natural binding protein, transcobalamin II, by sodium hydroxide (pH 12.9). Potassium cyanide converts the vitamin to its cyanocobalamin form. Earlier methods used a lower pH but involved boiling the mixture to release the cobalamin from its natural binding proteins. Hog intrinsic

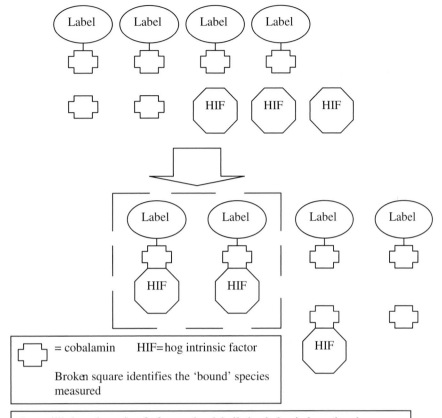

Figure 33.2 Schematic of principle of competitive protein binding assay

factor (HIF) is added as the specific protein binder. In one particular form of the assay, free cobalamin from the specimen competes with cobalamin which is 'labelled' by virtue of being bound to a solid support (a plastic bead). These constituents are incubated with an HIF antibody conjugated to alkaline phosphatase (ALP–HIFAb). The ALP–HIFAb is only immobilized to those beads which have HIF attached. The beads are washed free of all excess reagents and the amount of bound HIF determined by means of the attached alkaline phosphatase enzyme. If there is very little cobalamin in the specimen, much of the HIF will be attached to the cobalamin on the beads, and conversely if the cobalamin concentration in the specimen is high, there will be little HIF, and thus little alkaline phosphatase attached to the bead. Although the sequence of events differs slightly, the principle of this process can be seen to be identical to that of the schematic in Figure 33.2.

Assay of folate

Folate may be measured in serum or in red cells. Red cell folate is potentially the more meaningful measurement, as it represents a time-averaged view of folate availability during the period over which the circulating red cells were formed, whereas serum folate is very dependent on recent dietary intake. The principle of folate assays is very similar to that of cobalamin, described above, although the details will vary considerably with different analytical systems. The specific binding protein used in the competitive assay is β-lactoglobulin (a binder of folate in milk).

Dissociation of folate from binding proteins is again achieved by alkalinization with sodium hydroxide. If folate is measured in serum and in whole blood, the two results can be used, together with the haematocrit, to determine red cell folate. The method is more imprecise than measurement of serum folate because of the additive nature of analytical error. In general, the coefficient of variation of an analysis involving three measurements is given by:

$$CV_t = \sqrt{(CV_1^2 + CV_2^2 + CV_3^2)}$$

where CV_t is the overall coefficient of variation of the analysis and CV_1, CV_2 and CV_3 are the coefficients of variation of the individual analyses involved, in this case serum folate, whole blood folate and haematocrit. The more complex matrix of the whole blood haemolysate may also cause interference. For these reasons, laboratories may choose to measure either serum folate, because the analysis is less imprecise, or red cell folate, because the result is more meaningful, or both.

The interpretation of the assay is hindered by the fact that, like cobalamin, folate has poor precision at the low end of the range, and also folate reference ranges are sometimes inappropriate, particularly in populations with supplemented folate intake. Different analytical methods for folate show differing bias, and laboratories should determine local reference ranges.

Alternative measures of cobalamin and folate status

Although assays of these vitamins in blood give valuable information, a number of factors can cause misleading results. Cobalamin can be falsely increased by myeloproliferative disorders, and falsely decreased by folate deficiency, pregnancy, binding protein deficiencies and myelomatosis. Deficiency of cobalamin alone can reduce intracellular folate concentrations, and this may result in a normal serum folate associated with low red cell folate and low serum cobalamin. There is also evidence that clinically significant sequelae can follow from mild vitamin deficiency with serum concentrations in the low normal range.

Figure 33.1 showed the role of cobalamin *and* folate in conversion of homocysteine (HC) to methionine. Cobalamin alone is also involved in the important conversion of methylmalonic acid to succinic acid. Deficiency of either vitamin thus results in increased serum concentrations of homocysteine, and isolated cobalamin deficiency results in increased serum levels and excretion of methylmalonic acid (MMA). Measurement of these two substances, plasma HC and urine or plasma MMA, can thus confirm deficiency of the vitamins, and comparison of the two can differentiate single and combined deficiencies and may, in general, improve the specificity of diagnostic testing, particularly in cases with borderline low cobalamin or folate. There is evidence that elevated concentrations of these two metabolites can detect clinically significant vitamin deficiency before this is clearly evident from measurement of the vitamins themselves and before there is evidence of macrocytosis. At present the analytical difficulties in measurement of MMA and HC have prevented their widespread use, but together they hold the prospect of a functional assessment of cobalamin and folate status, which may be helpful in a wide variety of situations but particularly in the elderly, in whom marginal cobalamin deficiency is thought to be relatively common.

Investigation of the cause of folate and cobalamin deficiency

Folate deficiency is usually caused by malabsorption or inadequate dietary intake (or a combination of one of these with increased requirement, as in pregnancy). Supplementation is straightforward, and in some countries foods are routinely fortified with added folate, but care is necessary because administration of folate to a cobalamin-deficient patient can cause subacute combined degeneration of the cord. An important cause of cobalamin deficiency is pernicious anaemia (PA), in which the gastric parietal cells are no longer able to produce intrinsic factor which is essential for ileal cobalamin absorption. Preliminary investigation may involve assessment of gastric parietal cell antibodies and intrinsic factor antibodies. The former are positive in 90% of cases of PA, but have poor specificity for the condition, being present in 3–10% of normal subjects. Intrinsic factor antibodies are quite specific for PA, but their sensitivity is low. There are two types of intrinsic factor antibody, that which blocks binding of IF to cobalamin and that which blocks the uptake of the IF–cobalamin complex by the terminal ileum. The former antibody is the one routinely measured and it is present in 50% of cases of PA. In the past, the Schilling test (measuring absorption of radioactive cobalamin in the presence and absence of added intrinsic factor) was used to determine the ability to absorb administered cobalamin and to identify whether this was due to intrinsic factor deficiency (as in PA) or some other cause, such as ileal disease. Prior saturation with unlabelled cobalamin, administered by intramuscular injection, ensures that all the labelled cobalamin absorbed is excreted. The Schilling test is used less now than in the past because of the problems involved in the use of radioisotopes, and the general inconvenience of the test.

Approximately 80% of cases of PA have increased serum gastrin as a result of the associated achlorhydria

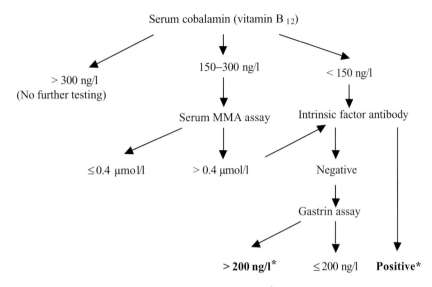

Figure 33.3 An investigative procedure for pernicious anaemia. *Indicates consistent with pernicious anaemia

due to failure of parietal cells to produce hydrochloric acid, thus serum gastrin can have value in the investigation of PA. Interestingly, the absence of gastric acid is significant in its own right, as failure to release dietary cobalamin (and folate) from natural binding proteins in the diet may impair absorption. A normal Schilling test (measuring absorption of free cobalamin) may thus occur in a patient who malabsorbs protein-bound cobalamin from natural foods.

A laboratory cascade for investigation of pernicious anaemia is shown in Figure 33.3. This avoids the use of the Schilling test but involves measurements not routinely available in a number of laboratories, certainly in the UK. Methylmalonic acid is seldom available, and gastrin, although available, is little used in this context. Because oral supplementation of cobalamin is ineffective in the treatment of PA, a precise diagnosis is important.

Iron

Iron is an important element, involved not only in haemoglobin synthesis but in many haem- and non-haem-containing metalloporoteins involved in the utilization of molecular oxygen. The most obvious effect of its deficiency is iron-deficient anaemia, but there may be more subtle changes resulting from its involvement in other metabolic processes. The existence of iron in two principal oxidation states, Fe(II) and Fe(III), and the

resultant ease with which it can partake in one electron transfers, result in it being a potential source of oxygen free radicals, which have important use in defence of the host against bacteria but which, if not confined to their appropriate location, are highly damaging to host tissues. The absorption and transport of iron is thus tightly controlled to avoid the presence of free iron, and conditions of iron overload have serious clinical consequences.

Laboratory measures of iron deficiency and overload

Apart from haemoglobin itself, the laboratory measures of iron status most frequently used are serum iron and iron-binding capacity, serum ferritin, red cell zinc protoporphyrin and, more recently, serum transferrin receptor (TfR) concentration.

Serum iron and iron-binding capacity

Serum iron is the most obvious measure of iron status, but its concentration is affected by a number of factors, including the concentration of its binding protein, transferrin. Some measure of transferrin is thus essential in the interpretation of serum iron concentration, either by direct measurement of the protein, or by assessing chemically the iron-binding capacity of the serum, which is equivalent to the transferrin concentration.

Ferritin

Ferritin is made up of 24 protein subunits around a core, which can contain up to 4500 atoms of iron and comprises the major storage form of available iron found in most body tissues. In denatured form, ferritin forms haemosiderin. The concentration of ferritin in plasma is directly related to the level of iron stores, with each μg/l of serum ferritin being equivalent to about 8 mg of storage iron. It is also, however, an acute phase protein, the concentration of which rises in response to infection, inflammation and malignancy, and this may result in 'normal' levels of serum ferritin in an iron-deficient patient with inflammatory disease.

Zinc protoporphyrin (ZPP)

In the synthesis of haemoglobin, the ferrochetalase enzyme inserts iron (II) into the protoporphyrin ring system to give haem. In the absence of adequate iron, zinc is inserted (again enzymatically) and the zinc protoporphyrin remains in the red cell during its entire life. The concentration of ZPP is thus increased when iron is unavailable in the marrow, due either to simple iron deficiency or to a functional iron deficiency in the presence of adequate iron stores. This latter situation pertains in the anaemia of chronic disease. Measurement of ZPP thus has the merit of identifying decreased availability of iron in the marrow, but does not always give direct information on iron stores. Increased ZPP also reflects longstanding problems in haem synthesis (of the order of red cell lifespan) and may be normal in iron deficiency of rapid onset caused by gastrointestinal blood loss, for example. Although it is seldom an interpretive problem, ZPP is also raised in lead toxicity.

Serum transferrin receptor (TfR)

The nucleated red cells in the bone marrow carry the vast majority of transferrin receptors, although they occur in other cells in numbers reflecting the cells' iron requirements. These receptors, situated in the cell membrane, internalize transferrin, which, after releasing its iron, is returned to the extracellular fluid. The transferrin receptor consists of two identical protein subunits of molecular mass 95 kDa. The synthesis of TfR is controlled by iron supply, decreasing when the cell is iron replete. The TfR is present in plasma, bound to transferrin, and its concentration in plasma or serum reflects the number of cellular transferrin receptors and, so long as iron stores are adequate, this reflects the number of developing red

cells in the marrow. Iron deficiency causes an increase in serum TfR in parallel with the rise in cellular receptors. Increased serum TfR may thus reflect decreased iron availability, or increased erythropoeisis, or both.

Investigation of suspected iron deficiency

The blood count is the first line of investigation. More specific haematological indices, such as the percentage of hypochromic cells, are viewed by many authors as one of the best measures of iron deficiency.

Measurement of serum ferritin

The analysis of serum ferritin utilizes a two-site or immunometric assay. In contrast to the competitive protein binding described for cobalamin and folate, the anti-ferritin antibodies used to capture ferritin are greatly in excess of normal concentrations of ferritin. Effectively all the ferritin in the serum specimen is captured by anti-ferritin antibodies on a solid support (bead or well). A second anti-ferritin antibody, which attaches to a different epitope on the ferritin molecule, is then added, also in excess. This second antibody forms a sandwich, with ferritin in the middle. The second antibody carries a label; originally this was a radioisotope, but now it is commonly an enzyme or fluorescent species. After washing to remove all the reagents not bound to the bead or well, substrate is added that reacts chemically with the labelled antibody to give a measurable signal, which is compared to that produced by a series of standards. Because the method relies on an excess of both antibodies, there is a possibility that exceptionally high concentrations of ferritin may saturate the antibodies and give spuriously low values (the 'high-dose hook' effect). There are means of assay design which minimize this risk, but if in doubt the serum specimen is analysed in dilution, and if the 'hook' effect is present, the diluted specimen will give a higher apparent value for the serum ferritin. The immunometric assay is shown schematically in Figure 33.4.

Measurement of zinc protoporphyrin

Some confusion exists regarding the relationship of ZPP and free protoporphyrin, mainly because earlier methods of measurement of ZPP involved acid extraction, which removed the zinc to give free protoporphyrin. Except in rare porphyrias, free protoporphyrin comprises 5% or

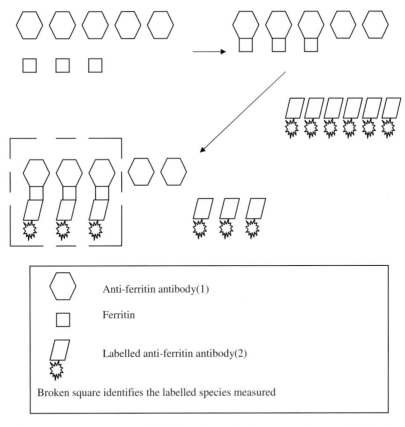

Figure 33.4 Schematic of principle of two-site immunometric assay for ferritin

less of the total non-haem porphyrin in red cells, the vast majority existing as ZPP.

Zinc protoporphyrin absorbs light of wavelength around 425 nm (the Soret band) and fluoresces, emitting light at a wavelength of 595 nm. The commonest method of measuring zinc protoporphyrin involves the technique of front face fluorimetry. A drop of whole blood is pretreated with a reagent that converts haemoglobin to cyanhaemoglobin and eliminates the interfering effect of variable oxyhaemoglobin content. The diluted blood is placed on a glass slide and a beam of incident light (415 nm) is directed onto the lower side of the glass slide. The layer of red cells on the flat glass surface absorbs the incident light, and the ZPP fluoresces, light at 595 nm being emitted in all directions. That light emitted downwards, back through the glass slide, suffers minimal reabsorption by haemoglobin and is detected by a photomultiplier tube. The concentration of ZPP is expressed as μmol ZPP/mole haem. Interference occurs from haemolysis, high serum bilirubin or riboflavin concentrations. Washing the red cells removes these interferences, but is time consuming.

Measurement of serum transferrin receptor

Measurement of serum TfR is by a two-site immunometric assay, similar in principle to that for serum ferritin. The analysis is usually an enzyme-linked immunosorbent assay (ELISA). Unfortunately, differences in procedures used to purify membrane-bound transferrin receptors for use as standards in the assay result in reference ranges which vary with the particular assay system, although the qualitative differences between patient groups are similar, irrespective of assay formulation. The reference range is largely unaffected by age and sex (unlike, for example, ferritin), although information in infants and children is sparse. Iron deficiency results in a three- to four-fold increase of serum TfR concentration compared to normals.

Measurement of serum iron and iron-binding capacity

Iron in serum is in the Fe(III) form and bound to transferrin. At a pH less than 4.5 and in the presence of ascorbic acid as a reducing agent, the trivalent iron is released from transferrin and reduced to Fe(II). It is then forms a complex with a chromophore, e.g. ferene [3-(2-pyridyl)-5,6-bis-2-(5-furyl sulphonic acid)-1,2,4-triazine] or alternatively ferrozine. The absorbance of the iron-ferene complex at 700 nm is measured. This method is homogeneous (involves no protein precipitation), the reaction mixture containing detergent to maintain protein in solution, and thiourea to minimize interference by copper.

Iron binding capacity may be measured by adding excess Fe(III) solution to totally saturate transferrin and leave some free iron. After reduction by ascorbic acid, the free iron is measured as the ferene complex at pH 8.6, at which pH the transferrin-bound iron remains unavailable. The solution is then acidified and the iron assay repeated. The increase in iron due to acidification is the iron-binding capacity of the serum, which is equivalent to the transferrin-bound iron.

Alternatively, transferrin can be measured directly by immunological methods. These involve the formation of antigen–antibody complexes in solution between transferrin and anti-transferrin antibodies. The concentration of these complexes is measured by their ability to scatter light. Either the decrease in transmitted light is measured in a spectrophotometer (turbidimetry) or the actual scattered light is assessed by detectors at 90° to the path of transmitted light (nephelometry). Standardization of the transferrin assay presents some problems, and there is little to chose between the transferrin assay and the iron-binding capacity as methods of measuring transferrin concentration.

The place of laboratory tests in the investigation of iron deficiency

In uncomplicated cases, no further laboratory investigation may be necessary when a microcytic, hypochromic anaemia is identified and treatment with oral iron is successful, although recurrence of anaemia in the presence of normal dietary iron intake will require explanation. Possible malabsorption or occult blood loss may require endoscopy or other modes of investigation.

An important diagnostic problem occurs in the differentiation of iron deficiency anaemia (IDA) and the anaemia of chronic disease. The anaemia of chronic disease may present with a normocytic, normochromic or a microcytic, hypochromic picture and may occur in the presence or absence of adequate iron stores. It may

be defined as a hypoproliferative anaemia occurring in association with infection, inflammation or neoplastic disease. It is characterized by low values for serum iron, serum transferrin and percentage transferrin saturation, increased serum ferritin, increased reticuloendothelial iron stores, increased ZPP, moderately increased TfR and reduced iron absorption. A moderate shortening of red cell lifespan occurs. The precise mechanism of the process is still not completely clear and disordered iron metabolism is not the only element, as iron delivery to the erythroid marrow remains possible and erythropoietin therapy can correct the condition, whereas it cannot correct iron deficiency. The effect of inflammatory cytokines appears central. The anaemia of chronic disease can be differentiated from iron deficiency anaemia by examination of the marrow, with the presence of stainable iron in the reticuloendothelial cells excluding IDA as a cause of anaemia, but this test is not suitable for widespread use.

Serum iron has serious shortcomings as a test of iron deficiency. It shows significant diurnal variation and is affected by recent food intake as well, resulting in high intraindividual variability. In the anaemia of chronic disease, serum iron is depressed irrespective of iron stores and, although use of transferrin saturation partially overcomes this (as transferrin or IBC is depressed in the same situation), its predictive value is not high. Oestrogenization (in pregnancy, oral contraceptive or oestrogen replacement therapy) can confuse the situation by increasing serum transferrin (and IBC).

Serum ferritin in an otherwise healthy person is a good index of body iron stores, but inflammation and liver disease cause increases in serum ferritin irrespective of iron status, which impairs its diagnostic value. Although a serum ferritin of less than 20 µg/l is consistent with IDA and a ferritin in excess of 100 µg/l makes IDA unlikely, even in the presence of inflammatory disease, this leaves a large group of patients with intermediate ferritin values in whom the diagnosis may be uncertain.

Zinc protoporphyrin, unlike serum ferritin, is unaffected by liver disease, and not directly affected by the acute phase reaction. The fact that it is positive in lead toxicity is seldom a problem. In rheumatoid disease it correlates with the percentage of hypochromic cells, but is frequently raised when the latter is normal and in renal failure it is raised non-specifically when percentage hypochromic cells is normal. It is a test of functional deficiency, in that it is increased when iron is unavailable at the time of erythropoesis, and this is true of the anaemia of chronic disease. Although it is said to be unaffected by thalassaemia trait, there is evidence that 50% of patients with this condition do have a raised ZPP. Thus, a raised ZPP is not diagnostic of iron deficiency, but it does give information on functional availability of iron to the developing red cell, except possibly in thalassaemia trait.

Serum transferrin receptor is related well to iron stores in healthy people and is increased in iron deficiency or when increased erythropoeisis occurs. This latter situation includes ineffective erythropoeisis. In chronic disease, concentrations are increased even in the presence of adequate iron stores, possibly related to the occurrence of ineffective erythropoeisis. However, a relationship to iron stores still remains. The ratio of serum TfR to serum ferritin has been shown to be an excellent measure of iron stores in the healthy, and a better indicator of iron deficiency in the anaemia of chronic disease than serum ferritin alone. Serum TfR may be particularly helpful in pregnancy. Pregnancy may cause anaemia through haemodilution, is often associated with a lowered ferritin, even in the presence of adequate iron stores, and an increase in IBC caused by oestrogens may suggest iron deficiency. Serum TfR appears, from preliminary evidence, to be relatively unaffected by pregnancy, allowing its use in the assessment of iron deficiency.

Although its manual nature makes it inappropriate in some laboratories, ZPP is a cheap and good first-line test for iron deficiency, measurable on the initial full blood count sample. Ferritin is a good second-line test, if its deficiencies are recognized. Serum transferrin receptor may assume a greater role when it is more readily available on major analysers and its role more clearly defined, but there is probably little to be gained at present by adding measurement of serum TfR to the existing range of tests available in laboratories. It is important, when new laboratory tests are introduced, that investigative protocols are reassessed, to avoid ever broader panels of tests being used without due discrimination.

The investigation of iron overload

Acquired iron overload may occur in association with chronic haemolytic anaemias, parenteral iron overload, or chronic liver disease, but the origin is usually clear from the patient's history and the investigation and management of this condition is not described here.

Genetic susceptibility to haemochromatosis is common in the general population (1 in 100–300), although the incidence of symptomatic disease is probably one-twentieth of the incidence of genetic mutation. It is an important condition to exclude in anyone with unexplained elevation of liver enzymes, because it is potentially fatal but readily treatable, and discovery of index cases allows investigation of close relatives to establish future risk. The first abnormality to develop is an increase in transferrin saturation, and values greater than 55% in females or 60% in males suggest iron accumulation. The effect of food and diurnal variation is best avoided by use of an early morning fasting specimen. Serum ferritin is increased at a later stage in iron accumulation, when liver iron has become elevated. Values in excess of 500 µg/l are suspicious of iron overload but other conditions involving inflammation must be ruled out, and transferrin saturation is a superior test in this respect also, as inflammatory disease causes a decreased saturation and thus less diagnostic uncertainty.

If genetic haemochromatosis is suggested by these preliminary investigations, HFE mutation analysis should be performed, using a polymerase chain reaction (PCR). The commonest form of inherited iron overload (approximately 90% of cases) is associated with mutations in the HFE gene, in particular the C282Y mutation, in which a cysteine (C) at position 282 is replaced by a tyrosine residue (Y). The other mutation is H63D, in which histidine (H) at position 63 is replaced by aspartic acid (D). Homozygosity for the C282Y mutation is associated with iron overload, and up to 10% of men and 5% of women with the phenotype HH/YY go on to develop symptomatic iron overload. The situation with compound heterozygotes (e.g. HD/CY) is less clear and, similarly, homozygotes for the H63D mutation (DD/CC) are less seriously affected.

Assessment of liver iron is not a necessary part of the diagnostic process, but may be used to assess severity of disease in selected patients. Treatment is by regular venesection until borderline iron deficiency is achieved.

Summary

The investigation of haematinic deficiencies always starts with the full blood count. Measurement of serum cobalamin and serum and/or red cell folate can assist in identifying the specific deficiency, although an understanding of the limitations of the tests is necessary and other tests, some not readily available at present, may become more important, particularly in the investigation of marginal deficiency. There are several measures of adequacy of iron stores with ferritin, despite its imperfections, remaining the best readily accessible test, although zinc protoporphyrin has a role, and in the future serum transferrin receptor may be the test of choice. Although serum iron, iron-binding capacity and transferrin saturation are of less value in the assessment of iron deficiency, they are the most sensitive tests for iron overload, and the presence of genetic haemochromatosis can be unequivocally demonstrated by assessing HFE gene mutation by PCR. Investigation of iron overload may be stimulated by unexplained abnormalities of liver function tests.

As always with laboratory tests, interpretation must be in the context of a full clinical assessment of the patient and with an evidence-based knowledge of the strengths and deficiencies of individual laboratory tests.

Further reading

Scott J M. Folate and vitamin B_{12}. *Proc Nutrit Soc* 1999; **58**: 441–448.

Klee G G. Cobalamin and folate evaluation: measurement of methylmalonic acid and homocysteine vs. vitamin B_{12} and folate. *Clin Chem* 2000; **46**(8B): 1277–1283.

Spivak J L. Iron and the anemia of chronic disease. *Oncology* 2002; **16**(9) suppl: 25–33.

Worwood M. Serum transferrin receptor assays and their application. *Ann Clin Biochem* 2002; **39**: 221–230.

Braun J. Erythrocyte zinc protoporphyrin. *Kidney Int* 1999; **55**: S57–S60.

Dooley J S. Diagnosis and management of genetic haemochromatosis. *Best Pract Res Clin Haematol* 2002; **15**: 277–293.

34

Laboratory investigation of haemolysis

Paul Revell

Introduction

In normal life, red cells are recycled every 120 days. The haemolytic disorders are those in which there is accelerated red cell destruction, accompanied by a compensatory increase in red cell production. If the marrow cannot 'keep up' with the increased demand for new cells, anaemia will result. The accelerated destruction is usually because the red cell is abnormal. The associated abnormalities detectable in the laboratory are shown in Figure 34.1 and summarised in Table 34.1. Some of these are illustrated in Figure 34.2.

Clinical features

What happens to the patient is often rather non-specific and dependent on the *speed of onset* as much as the particular disease causing the haemolysis. The main clinical features seen in haemolytic anaemias are summarised in Table 34.2.

In very rapid onset conditions (e.g. incompatible blood transfusion) there will be prostration, fever and backache with haemoglobinuria and malaise, rather than the features in Table 34.2. The more chronic conditions often reach a 'steady state' with destruction and production in balance, although usually some test results remain abnormal. This steady state can be punctuated by exacerbations of illness or 'crises'. There are four main types of crisis:

1. A *haemolytic crisis* is the result of an increase in the accelerated haemolysis, often brought on by an intercurrent illness, such as a viral infection. This causes an increase in jaundice and anaemia and a pouring out of reticulocytes (and sometimes nucleated red cells) from the marrow. This is one facet of a 'sickle crisis'.

2. An *aplastic crisis* is where the marrow stops working for a while, for example in parvovirus infection. In most people this has little effect but in a haemolytic condition, the patient can quickly become very anaemic and ill, since for most of the time they rely on a very active marrow to 'keep up'.

3. A *sequestration crisis* occurs in some conditions, like sickle cell disease in children, when the spleen suddenly enlarges and engulfs the cells. The patient is either very ill or dead on arrival at hospital: fortunately this is rare.

4. A *megaloblastic crisis* is caused by the marrow running out of folate (usually) from the excessive production of red cells required to 'keep up,' and a frank megaloblastic anaemia results. 'Megaloblastic' refers to a characteristic bone marrow appearance, where the nucleated red cells look abnormal because the maturation of the nucleus and cytoplasm are out of step with each other.

General management of the patient

When the patient first presents, the diagnostic priorities are to establish that haemolysis is occurring (Figures and Tables 34.1 and 34.2) and to try to ascertain whether the

The Science of Laboratory Diagnosis, Second Edition   Edited by David Burnett and John Crocker

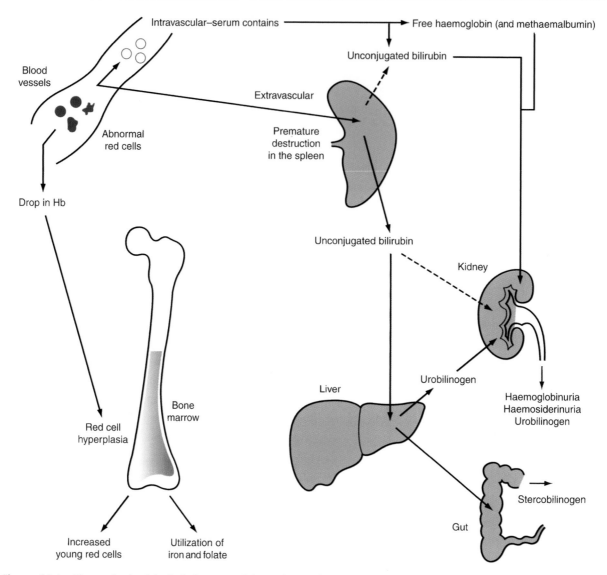

Figure 34.1 The pathophysiological features of haemolysis. If destruction occurs within the blood vessels, then free haemoglobin is liberated, which will appear in the urine (see also Fig. 34.2). If the destruction is extravascular (spleen; sometimes liver) then this will be avoided but excessive unconjugated bilirubin will be liberated. This may result in the patient appearing jaundiced (yellow; pale yellow if also anaemic, first seen in the whites of the eyes) and the secondary product, urobilinogen, will be detected in the urine on testing (it does not discolour the urine). Increased production results in a shift of red cells to younger forms, which creates polychromasia, a blue tinge, on the peripheral blood film, reflected in an increased reticulocyte count. Nucleated red cells, usually only seen in the marrow, can also be seen in the blood in active haemolysis

process is slow or fast, intra- or extravascular. Tests to find the cause of the haemolysis then follow logically. Patients will generally need their vitamin B$_{12}$ and folate levels checked and then be started on treatment doses of folic acid by mouth. Transfusion will be necessary in extreme clinical states. If the cause is found, then specific treatment will be started, such as corticosteroids

by mouth for immune haemolysis. Complications may need treatment, such as the removal of symptomatic pigment gallstones in hereditary spherocytosis. Removal of the spleen (splenectomy, to reduce destruction) will have to be considered in some cases.

Extra medical input is needed in times of stress (pregnancy, surgery, etc.) and support and education of

Table 34.1 Laboratory abnormalities in haemolysis

These are not all found in every patient. The relative severity of each may depend on the stage in the illness that has been reached. Reduced red cell lifespan is rarely measured directly, but see Fig. 34.5 for an example.
In general:

- Low haemoglobin if decompensated
- Increased reticulocyte count
- Increased (unconjugated) bilirubin
- Urobilinogen in urine
- Reduced red cell lifespan
- Abnormal red cells (depending on cause)

And if there is intravascular haemolysis:
- Haemoglobinaemia
- Methaemalbuminaemia
- Haemoglobinuria
- Haemosiderinuria
- Low serum haptoglobin

Table 34.2 Clinical features of haemolysis

The clinical information provided by doctors can assist in the selection of primary as well as secondary investigations in suspected haemolysis.

- History of previous episodes
- Association of episodes with: infections
- Anaemia   drugs
- Jaundice   cold
- Pigment gallstones   foods
- Leg ulcers
- Growth retardation
- Family history of anaemia/jaundice
- Enlarged spleen
- Skeletal abnormalities

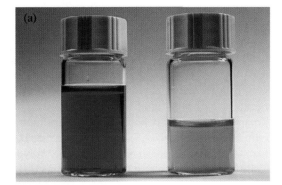

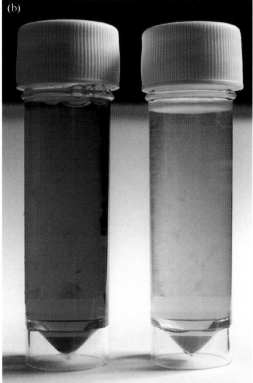

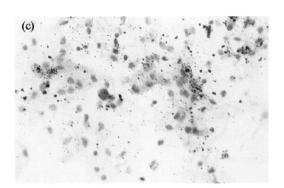

Figure 34.2 Some laboratory findings in intravascular haemolysis. (a) Haemoglobin is released into the serum, producing a 'muddy-brown' appearance. A normal serum is shown for comparison. (b) Some of this appears directly in the urine, causing a similar discolouration. This should not be confused with the much commoner occurrence of haematuria, where whole red cells appear in the urine. In haemoglobinuria, therefore, the stick test for blood will be positive but no red cells will be seen on microscopy of urine. (c) Some haemoglobin is taken up by kidney cells, which are shed into the urine (red counterstain) and show up as small haemosiderin granules (blue). See also Table 34.7

the patient and family are always needed in chronic conditions. Genetic counselling and family studies may be appropriate in certain cases.

Haemolytic disorders

There are hundreds of different conditions and many have had large tomes written about them! Table 34.3 gives a general outline of the broad groups and the common or important examples. A brief word about each of these is provided to illustrate where they fit into this general scheme; previous chapters give greater detail about some of the individual conditions. There is also a reading list at the end of the chapter.

Sickle cell anaemias and other haemoglobin variants

The red cell contains haemoglobin made from abnormal globin chains. Haemoglobin A (HbA) is normal. HbF is a variant but would be normal in the fetus. The abnormal haemoglobin S arises from a genetic defect that causes an amino acid substitution in the haemoglobin β chain. In these conditions the red cell contains particular haemoglobins with respect to the genes held. For example, in homozygous sickle disease with two S genes, the red cell will contain mostly HbS and a little HbF but no HbA. In the trait (one S gene) they will contain 45% HbS and the rest HbA. It is worth bearing in mind that

these are the percentages in every cell—in contrast, a homozygous sickle patient who has been transfused normal blood (HbA only) may also have 45% HbS and the rest HbA, but each cell will be *either* all HbS *or* all HbA.

Sickle cell anaemia (SS)

The deoxygenated form of the abnormal Hb is less soluble than normal HbA (in phosphate buffer this forms the basis of the screening test for HbS). HbS causes deformed red cells (sickle cells) due to 'tactoid' formation, and these cells are destroyed in the spleen and peripherally. The patients run a low haemoglobin (5–10 g/dl) and often have raised neutrophil and platelet counts. Sickle and 'boat shaped' cells are visible on the blood film. Diagnosis is by Hb electrophoresis on agarose gel at acid or alkaline pH. Laboratories handling large number of samples may use high performance liquid chromatography (HPLC). The low Hb is sufficient to impair development in some children. Thrombotic phenomena occur due to sickling, which can cause pain, classically in the limbs, and also affect the chest, abdomen and brain. Infarction (localized destruction due to lack of oxygen) of the spleen causes hyposplenism with Howell–Jolly bodies in red cells on the blood film. Good medical care has a significant impact on the quality of life and mortality of patients with the condition.

In *sickle cell trait* (AS) sickling does not occur (as there is less HbS in each cell) except under very hypoxic conditions (e.g. unpressurized aircraft, general anaesthesia). There is little to see on the film.

Table 34.3 The haemolytic disorders

This way of dividing up the conditions enables a limited amount of clinical information to guide subsequent testing.

INHERITED ——— Defect of haemoglobin synthesis, e.g. sickle cell disease or thalassaemia
——— Membrane abnormality, e.g. hereditary spherocytosis
——— Enzyme deficiency, e.g. G6PD or PK deficiency

ACQUIRED ——— IMMUNE ——— Autoimmune, e.g. warm AIHA or cold (CHAD)
——— Haemolytic disease of the newborn
——— Transfusion incompatibility

——— NON-IMMUNE ——— Physico-mechanical, e.g. heart valves
——— Microangiopathies
——— Paroxysmal nocturnal haemoglobinuria

HbC Disease (CC)

This produces mild haemolysis and an enlarged spleen but extra problems arise in dehydration and pregnancy. The trait (AC) is of no significance to the individual except in genetic terms.

HbSC disease (S/C)

This produces mild haemolysis but patients can have sickling problems, especially in pregnancy. Some are troubled by retinopathy (infarctions at the back of the eye) and bony destruction (e.g. of the head of the femur).

Sickle/thal disease (S/Thal)

The severity depends upon the amount of normal Hb produced, which in turn depends on the precise thalassaemia gene. If none, then the disease is every bit as severe as the homozygous SS form.

Thalassaemias

In these conditions, there is abnormal production of globin chains (rather than production of abnormal types of chain). This ranges from β_0-thalassaemia (no β chain) to the mild α-thalassaemias, where there is a slight reduction in α chain synthesis and no clinical problems to speak of. Heterozygotes do not run into trouble but often have blood film abnormalities. Homozygous β_0-thalassaemia is a serious disorder requiring a lifetime of transfusions and is sometimes complicated by hypersplenism (the overactive spleen destroys all the blood cells). Target cells are characteristically seen on the film. The lack of production is of more importance than haemolysis of abnormal cells. Hyperplasia of the marrow leads to the characteristic childhood bony deformities. Children fail to thrive and die without transfusion. Survivors of transfusion suffer the effects of iron overload. If chelation, using an oral chelating drug or desferrioxamine as a nightly subcutaneous infusion to increase iron excretion fails, then endocrine gland (pituitary, gonadal, pancreatic), liver and cardiac infiltration and damage occurs, with fatal result, often before the age of 25. Haemoglobin H disease is a form of α-thalassaemia (*not* an abnormal Hb variant called H!) Here the absence of some α chains causes the excess β chains to form tetramers (β_4), which condense as inclusion bodies (H bodies, seen on cresyl blue staining).

Hereditary spherocytosis

Hereditary spherocytosis is 'autosomal dominant', i.e. with one gene, a person inherits the condition and generally found in Caucasians. There is an abnormality of the red cell membrane contractile proteins which leads to reduced deformability. The abnormal cells are sequestered in the spleen and destroyed prematurely. Anaemia is usually mild and spherocytes are seen on the blood film (but they are easily missed!). The diagnosis is made by an increased 'osmotic fragility' (Figure 34.3) and can be confirmed by electrophoretic analysis of the red cell membrane components using SDS polyacrylamide gels.

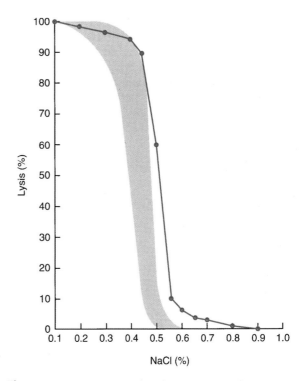

Figure 34.3 The osmotic fragility test. Aliquots of well-mixed oxygenated blood are added to a series of buffered saline concentrations, usually in the range 0.2–1.2% NaCl. The dilutions are incubated at room temperature for 30 minutes before the tubes are centrifuged and the amount of haemolysis in the supernatant read photometrically. Spherocytes are abnormally sensitive to hypotonic solutions and lyse in higher concentrations than normal red cells. An inconclusive osmotic fragility test can be repeated by incubating the blood sample for 24 hours at 37°C prior to testing. This modification is much more sensitive in detecting mild spherocytosis than the original method. The graph for normal red cells will generally appear in the grey area. A representative graph for a patient with hereditary spherocytosis is shown. Some laboratories use a variation—the acidified glycerol lysis time test

G6PD (Glucose 6-phosphate dehydrogenase) deficiency

The red cell has a reduced reductive energy from a lack of the first enzyme in the pentose phosphate shunt pathway of glucose metabolism. It is often a sex-linked recessive condition: the disease is expressed in males with one affected gene on the X chromosome but females need two affected genes. Females with one affected will show variable expression, depending on which X chromosome is inactivated in which cells, according to the Lyon hypothesis. It is mostly seen in black and Mediterranean populations and affects 3% of the world's people. G6PD activity is present in reticulocytes but it falls off rapidly and prematurely in these individuals. Red cell integrity is therefore reduced on exposure to oxidant chemicals and drugs (e.g. sulphonamide antibiotics). Heinz bodies are seen on specially prepared blood films. Diagnosis is by assay of G6PD but only in the steady state (not when there is an excessive number of reticulocytes such as after haemolytic crises). Some episodes are caused by foods (classically, by fava beans—'favism') as well as drugs.

Screening for 6GPD deficiency

Within the pentose phosphate pathway NADP is reduced by G6PD to NADPH. This product fluoresces under ultraviolet light. This forms the basis of the fluorescent spot test. Whole blood is mixed with:

- Glucose 6-phosphate.

- NADP.

- Lysing agent (usually saponin).

- Buffer.

It is then incubated for 5–10 minutes before being spotted onto filter paper, dried and examined under long wave UV light. Normal samples will fluoresce brightly, deficient samples will not fluoresce, or only poorly. Any abnormal screening test must be confirmed by a G6PD assay; here the production of NADPH by G6PD is measured spectrometrically, with a change in optical density over time.

Pyruvate kinase deficiency

Pyruvate kinase deficiency is an 'autosomal recessive' condition (with both genes abnormal a person inherits the condition) and another enzyme problem—the commonest of the rarer non-G6PD diseases. The cells become deformed and vulnerable. The blood film shows poikilocytes (abnormally shaped red cells) and these are haemolysed spontaneously without a drug stimulus. Transfusions may be needed.

Screening for pyruvate kinase deficiency

Pyruvate kinase is the catalyst for the reaction:

$$ADP + phosphoenolpyruvate \rightarrow ATP + pyruvate$$

The product of this reaction, pyruvate, then proceeds into the following reaction which is catalysed by lactate dehydrogenase (LDH):

$$Pyruvate + NADH \rightarrow lactate + NAD$$

NADH will fluoresce under long-wave UV light, whereas NAD will not. Therefore when whole blood is incubated with ADP, phosphoenolpyruvate and NADH, in normal samples NADH is oxidized to NAD, with a consequential loss of fluorescence. Deficient samples will fluoresce brightly. An abnormal PK screening test must be confirmed by a full assay of the enzyme where the oxidation of NADH to NAD is measured by a change in absorbance photometrically over time.

Immune haemolyses

Various conditions (such as those listed in Table 34.4) result in antibody-coated red cells, which have a shortened lifespan. Immune haemolysis is divided in the laboratory into 'warm' and 'cold' types, depending on the thermal range of activity (and agglutination) in the laboratory, classically 37°C in warm and 4°C in cold, although there is sometimes a little overlap. As well as a broad screening direct Coombs (anti-globulin) test, which will be positive (DCT, Figure 34.4), reagents giving a more specific profile (IgG, complement) can be used in warm immune haemolysis. It is usual in suspected cold immune haemolysis to keep the specimen of blood warm until the serum is separated, then test against adult (containing I antigen) and umbilical cord (i antigen-bearing) cells. The DCT is usually only positive with the complement reagent and the blood film shows agglutination, unless made warm. The distinction between warm and cold conditions is important for treatment. In the warm immune haemolyses, steroids and other immunosuppressive treatments aimed at switching off production

Table 34.4 Causes of immune haemolysis

There are many different conditions that can give rise to antibody-coated red cells. The broad groups are shown. The division into 'cold' and 'warm' conditions helps in treatment decisions.

'Cold' —————— Lymphoproliferative disorders, e.g. low-grade non-Hodgkin's lymphoma

Infections, e.g. *Mycoplasma pneumoniae*

Cold haemagglutinin disease (CHAD)

'Warm' —————— Lymphoproliferative disorders, e.g. chronic lymphocytic leukaemia

Connective tissue diseases, e.g. systemic lupus erythematosus

Drugs, e.g. α-methyldopa, used for high blood pressure

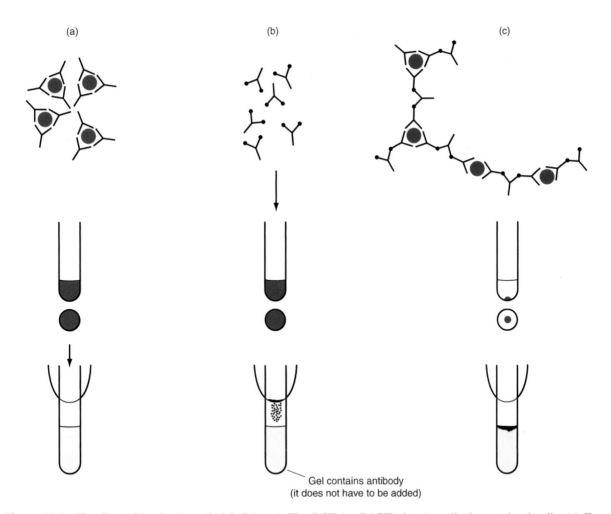

(a)   (b)   (c)

Gel contains antibody
(it does not have to be added)

Figure 34.4 The direct Coombs (or anti-globulin) test. The DCT (or DAGT) detects antibody-coated red cells. (a) To a suspension of the patient's red cells (already coated with antibody) is added (b) broad spectrum anti-globulin (e.g. rabbit anti-human). (c) Agglutination occurs. The result is shown in a traditional tube method (upper) or gel technology (lower)

of, or interfering with, the effect of antibody production are often useful. Splenectomy often works. In cold immune haemolyses, however, cytotoxic chemotherapy (sometimes) and keeping the patient warm (nearly always) help, but not steroids or splenectomy. Transfusion is generally avoided in immune haemolysis, as the autoagglutination interferes with cross-matching. The clinical state of the patient occasionally demands transfusion and he/she should certainly not be allowed to succumb through lack of red cells, in which case the 'least incompatible' blood is issued.

Haemolytic disease of the newborn (HDN)

Rhesus-positive cells from the Rh^+ foetus pass into the circulation of an Rh^- mother, e.g. in haemorrhage during pregnancy or threatened miscarriage. This causes the mother to produce anti-D (anti-rhesus) antibodies which later on in the same or subsequent pregnancies, will pass to the foetus and coat red cells, causing haemolysis if the baby is Rh^+. ABO group incompatibilities can cause similar problems but of a lesser severity. High unconjugated bilirubin levels after birth (due to haemolysis) will cross the blood–brain barrier and cause 'kernicterus', with brain damage. Treatment, which may include exchange transfusion, will prevent this. Spherocytes may be seen on the blood film and the DCT will be positive. In severe cases the baby will be hydropic (anaemia/jaundice/swollen up with oedema). At times of potential feto–maternal haemorrhage, the production of antibody by the mother may be prevented by the passive administration of anti-D by intramuscular injection to mop up Rh^+ cells, which will prevent her producing her own response. The prophylactic use of anti-D in this way is one of the success stories of modern scientific medicine, so affected infants are now rare. They may be treated by intrauterine transfusion (a tricky manoeuvre!) or early induction of labour, with exchange transfusion of the newborn.

Incompatible transfusion

Incompatible transfusion creates an immune-mediated haemolysis. In ABO incompatibility (a very rare occurrence, it is hoped) the donor cells are destroyed intravascularly because of the patient's naturally occurring anti-A or anti-B antibodies (or both). The patient can become ill very rapidly, as previously described, and will develop haemoglobinuria. If the transfusion is not stopped or the patient is under anaesthesia, the condition can be fatal. Incompatibility reactions due to other antigens will usually provoke extravascular haemolysis with anaemia and jaundice. Recovery is usual but there will be cross-matching problems thereafter, on account of the allo-antibodies to red cell antigens.

Non-immune mechanisms

These can result in abnormal red cells (which therefore have a shortened lifespan). Physicomechanical trauma to normal red cells, such as passing through a leaking mechanical heart valve, can lead to fragmentation and either intravascular lysis or early recycling by the spleen.

Paroxysmal noctural haemoglobinuria (PNH) is a rare acquired haematological disease. The patient typically suffers intravascular complement-mediated haemolysis, resulting in haemoglobinuria, iron deficiency, aplastic crises and a predisposition to venous thrombosis. This is a stem cell disorder which produces cells deficient in complement regulatory proteins, resulting in an increased sensitivity of the red cell membrane to lysis by complement. Traditionally the diagnosis was made using a variety of tests. The most sensitive are the acidified serum test (Hams' test) and the sucrose lysis test. These tests have now largely being replaced by the introduction of flow cytometry for the detection of surface molecules CD 55 (decay-accelerating factor-DAF) and CD 59 [homozygous restriction factor-HRF/C8-binding protein (C8bp)]. These antigens are reduced or absent in PNH and flow cytometry is the most sensitive and specific tool available for diagnosis at present. The abnormality can be detected on white as well as red cells in this condition.

Microangiopathies

The microangiopathies cause red cell shearing on fibrin strands in small vessels and are associated with a characteristic blood picture, which contains lots of fragments, some helmet cells and a few microspherocytes. Thrombocytopenia and markers of haemolysis (anaemia, raised reticulocytes and bilirubin) are usually present. There are a number of causes of microangiopathy, which are summarised in Table 34.5. The diagnostic pointers that distinguish between them are shown in Table 34.6. The diagnosis is well worth making because all of these conditions are serious and can kill otherwise young, fit patients, but are often treatable. The correct distinction between them is important because certain blood products are potentially dangerous in some but not in others, and steroids are helpful in some but not in the rest.

Table 34.5 Causes of microangiopathy

These three broad groups contain all the likely causes:

- Disseminated intravascular coagulation (DIC) (in obstetric problems, septicaemia, cancer, etc.)
- Systemic lupus erythematosus (SLE) and other renal and connective tissue disorders
- Thrombotic thrombocytopenic purpura (TTP) and haemolytic uraemic syndrome (HUS)

Table 34.6 Laboratory diagnosis of microangiopathic conditions

The coagulation screen, renal biochemistry and clinical information will usually distinguish the cause.

Cause	Hb/Plats	Clotting	Renal failure	Clinical context
DIC	Low	Abnormal	+	++
SLE	Low	N	+	++++
TTP	Low	N	−	−
HUS	Low	N	+++	+++

Table 34.7 Laboratory investigation of intravascular haemolysis

During haemolysis, haemoglobin is released into the plasma. This binds rapidly to the plasma proteins haptoglobin and haemopexin before being cleared from the circulation by the liver. If haemolysis is severe haptoglobin and haemopexin concentrations are rapidly depleted and haemoglobinuria/aemia and methaemalbuminaemia become detectable.

- Methaemalbumin, with its 'muddy-brown' appearance that can be measured photometrically, has a characteristic absorbtion peak of 624 nm
- Serum haptoglobin and haemopexin levels can be measured in a number of ways, including gel filtration and electrophoretic, photometric and immunological methods. The commonest in use today are the immunological methods, utilizing anti-haptoglobin or anti-haemopexin, allowing demonstration by radial immunodiffusion or Laurell rocket techniques
- Urinary haemosiderin demonstration is by the Perl's Prussion blue iron stain method. A specimen of urine is centrifuged and the deposit spread onto a glass slide, dried in air before being fixed in methanol. Ferric iron present in the deposit reacts with acidified potassium ferrocyanide to produce ferric ferrocyanide, which appears as blue-stained granules on microscopy.

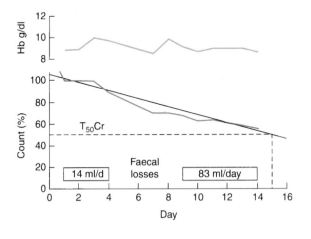

Figure 34.5 Red cell labelling. Mrs ID, aged 76, was suffering recurrent attacks of anaemia associated with palpitations, shortness of breath and exhaustion. She was known to have complex valvular heart disease, including an aortic valve replacement, which had murmurs on listening to the heart, which might indicate leakage. She was on warfarin and was known to have red cell allo-antibodies, making cross-matching difficult. An iron deficiency picture indicated loss of red cells but, with little fragmentation on the blood film, reduced haptoglobin but no haemosiderinuria, it was unclear whether the intravascular destruction was significant. She had no bowel symptoms and full examination of the gastrointestinal tract revealed no anatomical causes of blood loss. The patient's red cells were therefore labelled with ^{51}Cr and re-injected (day 0). Samples of blood were taken daily for isotopic activity and stools collected for activity as shown. Day 1 is taken as 100% to allow for irrelevant early losses. It can be seen that the chromium half-life (T_{50}Cr) is reduced at 15 days (normal 25–33 days), although she maintained her Hb during the study. This modest reduction was accounted for by the considerable loss noted from the gastrointestinal tract shown by the stool isotope counts. The loss is clearly variable and was assumed to be coming from an angiodysplasia in the large bowel (these are not demonstrable anatomically). She needed several elective and emergency transfusions during the first year but none thereafter. It appeared that blood loss had ceased. The heart valve did not need replacing

Additional evidence of intravascular haemolysis can be obtained from the investigations shown in Table 34.7.

Endpiece

There will always be some cases that remain difficult to elucidate and direct measurement by isotope labelling of red cells may be needed (Figure 34.5). There will, finally, be some patients who are clearly haemolysing but in whom no cause can be found. Most of these will have an as-yet undefined disorder of red cell anatomy or physiology.

Further reading

Dacie JV. *The Haemolytic Anaemias*, 3rd edn, vols 1–5. 1988–1999: Churchill Livingstone, Edinburgh.

Greer JP *et al. Wintrobe's Clinical Hematology*, 11th edn. 2004: Lippincott Williams & Wilkins, Philadelphia, PA.

Hall R, Malia RG. *Medical Laboratory Haematology*, 2nd edn. 1991: Butterworth-Heinemann, Oxford.

Lewis SM, Bain BJ, Bates I, Dacie and Lewis'. *Practical Haematology*, 9th edn. 2001: Churchill Livingstone, London.

35

Laboratory investigation of haemostasis

Peter E Rose and **Catherine Caveen**

Introduction

Blood flow within the vascular compartment is dependent upon the balance between procoagulant and anticoagulant activity. Under normal circumstances anticoagulant activity is dominant; however, with damage to endothelial cells lining blood vessels, subendothelium may be exposed, with local clot formation initiated. Initial platelet aggregation forms a platelet plug, while local coagulation produces a firm fibrin clot. Subsequently, a system of clot digestion (fibrinolysis) prevents clot extension and restores patency.

Laboratory investigation is routinely used to assess patients with increased thrombotic or haemorrhagic risk. In many acute medical conditions the normal balance of haemostasis is disturbed and requires correction. Furthermore, monitoring of therapeutic agents to promote anticoagulant activity or agents to restore normal haemostasis form part of routine investigations undertaken in the haematology laboratory. *In vivo* clotting requires both calcium and phospholipid surfaces as an integral component for clot formation. Coagulation factors circulate as inactive precursors, which under appropriate stimuli are converted to active enzymes and co-factors, with generation of thrombin and subsequent conversion of fibrinogen to fibrin. The initial steps in activation of coagulation involve tissue factor, expressed on non-vascular cell membrane surfaces, acting as a co-factor for the activation of factor VII to VIIa, with subsequent activation of factors X and IX and eventual thrombin generation. There are, however, numerous haemostatic interactions between coagulation factors, enabling different factors to act as both anticoagulant and procoagulant factors in different circumstances.

Traditionally, *in vitro* coagulation tests have been conveniently separated into activation of an intrinsic or extrinsic pathway. Non-physiological intrinsic pathway activation results, upon contact to a foreign surface, of factor XII, high molecular weight kininogen and subsequent activation of clotting factors through factors XI, IX, X and prothrombin. *In vivo*, however, small amounts of thrombin generation following activation of the extrinsic pathway will result in an amplification of haemostasis via activation of factor XI (see Figure 35.1).

Prothrombin time

The prothrombin time is used as a measure of extrinsic pathway activity, in which thromboplastin (tissue factor) and calcium are added to plasma and the time taken to clot formation is measured (see Figure 35.2).

A prolonged prothrombin time may be due to:

- Oral anticoagulants.

- Deficiency of factor I, II, V, VII or X, which may be inherited or acquired, e.g. in liver disease or disseminated intravascular coagulation.

- High levels of heparin.

- Inhibitors to specific coagulation factors, including the lupus inhibitor. Further investigation of a prolonged prothrombin time may involve correction studies or assays of clotting factors.

The Science of Laboratory Diagnosis, Second Edition   Edited by David Burnett and John Crocker
© 2005 John Wiley & Sons, Ltd

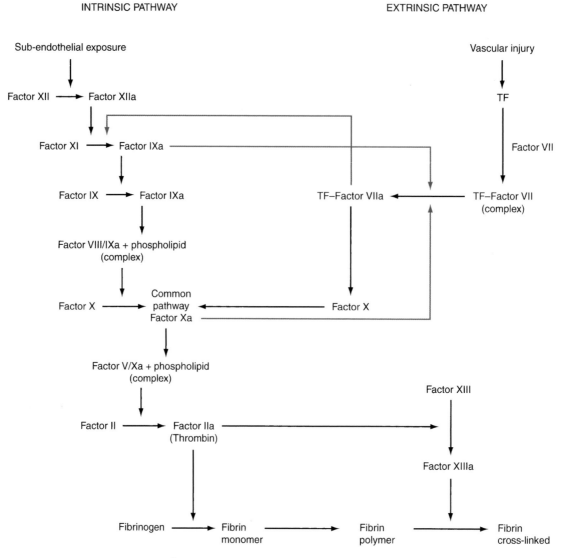

Figure 35.1   The coagulation cascade pathway

A prolonged prothrombin time may be corrected in the presence of normal plasma. The pattern of correction may identify the factor, or factors, that are deficient. Several reagents have been traditionally used in correction studies (see Table 35.1). These tests, however, have been largely replaced by assays of individual clotting factors.

Oral anticoagulant control

The international normalized ratio (INR) is the recommended method for reporting prothrombin time results for anticoagulant control. The INR system has been developed to compensate for the major source of discrepancy in prothrombin time assays, viz. variability in response of different thromboplastin reagents to changes in the vitamin K-dependent clotting factors induced by warfarin. With increasing numbers of patients requiring oral anticoagulant therapy (1 in 80 people in the UK) and the need for regular monitoring of the INR, this represents a major workload. The principle of oral anticoagulation is to provide a level of anticoagulation to prevent thrombotic problems but to avoid bleeding problems from over-anticoagulation. For most venous thrombotic problems, an INR range of 2–3 is satisfactory.

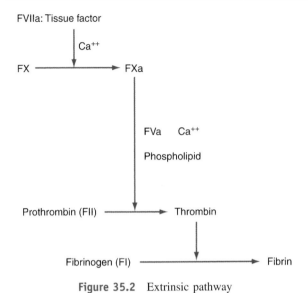

Figure 35.2 Extrinsic pathway

For patients with mechanical heart valves, a higher level of anticoagulation, INR range 2.5–3.5, is needed to prevent valve clot formation (Table 35.2).

The INR is expressed as:

$$INR = \left(\frac{PT}{GMNPT}\right)(ISI)$$

where *ISI* is the International Sensitivity Index of the thromboplastin reagent and *GMNPT* is the geometric mean normal prothrombin time.

Important sources of error remain in INR measurement and may result from problems in measurement of the prothrombin time, *ISI* or *GMNPT*.

Prothrombin errors

Errors with estimation of the prothrombin time can arise from problems with sample collection, the concentration of anticoagulant and the type of collection tube used. Furthermore, differences between manual and automated methods are recognized, with the latter producing shorter prothrombin times. While manufacturers are required to produce an ISI value for each batch of thromboplastin reagent, incorrect calibration of thromboplastin reagents by local laboratory or manufacturers is a problem. For calibration of a thromboplastin, a pool of plasma samples from 20 normal adults and 60 patients on warfarin is recommended. In addition, different international reference preparations from different species may result in ISI differences. The geometric mean normal prothrombin time should be derived from a pool of 20 normal adult plasma samples and the geometric mean calculated from this.

Activated partial thromboplastin time (APTT)

This test measures the intrinsic pathway of coagulation. An activator, such as kaolin, triggers the pathway by activating the contact factors (Figure 35.3). In the presence of calcium ions and phospholipid, this culminates in the generation of thrombin and ultimately fibrin clot formation. The APTT is also used in the monitoring of heparin therapy. A prolonged APTT in a patient with history of a bleeding diathesis would require further investigation, particularly to exclude haemophilia A or B.

Table 35.1 Correction studies of a prolonged prothrombin time

Normal plasma	Aged serum	Absorbed plasma	Oxalated plasma	Factor deficiency	Further tests
+	−	+	+	I	Fibrinogen assay
+	−	−	+	II	Factor assay
+	−	+	−	V	Factor assay
+	+	−	+	VII	Factor assay
+	+	−	+	X	RVV time
−	−	−	−	Inhibitor	Reptilase time
					Protamine neutralization

+ = corrected; − = not corrected; RVV = Russells's viper (the snake *vipera russelli*) venom test.
Normal citrate plasma: this provides all the coagulation factors.
Aged serum: clotted blood is incubated for 24 hours at 37°C; the serum contains factors VII, IX, X, XI and XII.
Absorbed plasma: normal plasma is treated with aluminium hydroxide, which absorbs certain factors; the resultant plasma contains factors I, V, VII, XI and XII.
Oxalated plasma: normal plasma is added to sodium oxalate and incubated for 72 hours at 37°C; contains all factors except V.

Table 35.2 Oral anticoagulants for various clinical conditions

Condition	INR Range	Recommended duration
Venous thromboembolism		
• Postoperative calf vein thrombosis without any risk factors	2–3	6 weeks
• Calf vein thrombosis in non-surgical patients without any risk factors	2–3	3 months
• Calf vein thrombosis in non-surgical patients with risk factors	2–3	Indefinite (while risk factors persist)
• Pulmonary embolus and proximal vein thrombosis	2–3	6 months
• Recurrent DVT and/or PE	2–3	Indefinite
• Recurrent DVT and/or PE while on warfarin (INR range 2–3)	3–4	Indefinite
Atrial fibrillation		
• Atrial fibrillation or other high-risk arrhythmias	2–3	Indefinite
Heart valve prostheses and other cardiac indications		
• Mechanical prosthetic valves	2.5–3.5	Indefinite
• Bioprosthetic heart valves (not aortic)	2–3	3 months
• Cardiomyopathy, mural thrombus or akinetic segment	2–3	Indefinite
Aspirin is first-line therapy for the following conditions; if aspirin is contraindicated, the following INR ranges for warfarin therapy are recommended:		
• TIA/ischaemic stroke	3–4	Indefinite
• Peripheral arterial thrombosis and grafts	3–4	Indefinite
• Coronary artery thrombosis	3–4	Indefinite
• Coronary artery graft thrombosis	3–4	Indefinite
• Coronary angioplasty and coronary stents	3–4	Indefinite

[*]Discontinue warfarin if there is no AF, intracardiac thrombus or history of systemic embolism. Patients not requiring warfarin should be considered for anti-platelet therapy (e.g. aspirin).

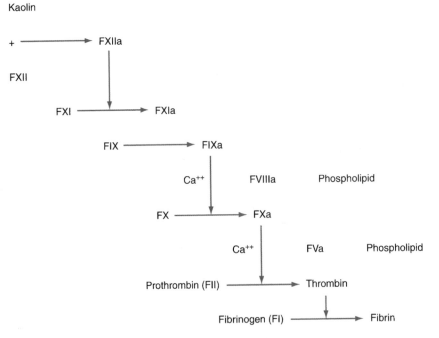

Figure 35.3 Intrinsic pathway

Laboratory investigation of a prolonged APTT

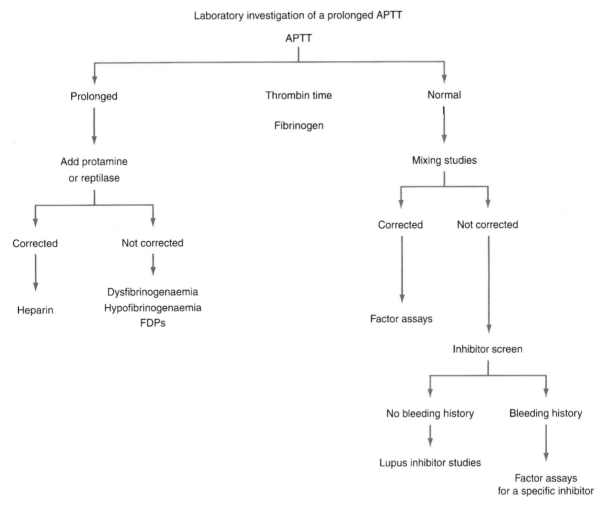

Figure 35.4 Laboratory investigation of a prolonged APTT

A prolonged APTT may be caused by deficiency of factors I, II, V, VIII, IX, X, XI, or XII, which can be inherited or acquired due to liver disease or consumption, as in disseminated intravascular coagulation. Heparin therapy, inhibitors to specific coagulation factors, the presence of lupus anticoagulant or high levels of FDPs (fibrinogen degradation products) may also produce a prolonged APTT. Correction studies may also be used to investigate further the cause of a prolonged APTT. If mixing studies show correction of the APTT, then specific factor assays are performed to determine the deficient factor. The failure to correct would require further investigation to exclude a further specific inhibitor or lupus anticoagulant (Figure 35.4).

The most frequent use of the APTT is to monitor heparin treatment and to adjust the infusion schedule, as illustrated in Table 35.3.

Thrombin time

The thrombin time is used as a rapid screen for abnormalities of fibrinogen and to assess whether heparin is the cause of a prolonged APTT. Thrombin is added to citrated plasma and the time taken for fibrin formation is measured (Figure 35.5).

A prolonged thrombin time may be due to:

- Dysfibrinogenaemias, which can be inherited or acquired, with a structurally abnormal fibrinogen molecule with altered functional properties.

- Low fibrinogen level (<1g/L).

- Raised fibrinogen degradation products (FDP) levels.

- Heparin therapy.

Table 35.3   This shows a heparin infusion regime, with laboratory monitoring of treatment using the APTT. The therapeutic range should be determined from the APTT range equivalent to a plasma heparin concentration of 0.2–0.4 IU/ml

Heparin infusion schedule		
i.v. bolus	5000 units	
i.v. infusion	15000 units/12 hours	
Check APTT after 2–6 hours		
• Acceptable range	1.5–2.5	
• In pregnancy	1.5–2.0	
Adjust heparin as follows:		
> 5.0	Stop for 1 hour	
	Decrease by 6000 units/12 hours	Recheck APTT in 2–6 hours
4.1–5.0	Decrease by 3600 units/12 hours	Recheck APTT in 2–6 hours
3.1–4.0	Decrease by 1200 units/12 hours	Recheck APTT in 2–6 hours
2.6–3.0	Decrease by 600 units/12 hours	Recheck APTT in 2–12 hours
1.5–2.5	No change	Recheck APTT within 24 hours
1.2–1.4	Increase by 2400 units/12 hours	Recheck APTT in 2–12 hours
<1.2	Increase by 4800 units/12 hours	Recheck APTT in 2–6 hours

Check APTT 2–6 hours after starting heparin.
Do not re-prescribe heparin for more than 24 hours.
Checking APTT on a daily basis is the mandatory minimum for all patients receiving intravenous heparin.
Monitor platelets after 4 days of heparin treatment.

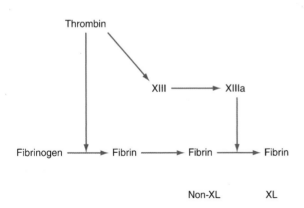

Figure 35.5   Thrombin time

The presence of heparin in a sample is confirmed by correction of the thrombin time with protamine sulphate, which neutralizes the anticoagulant activity.

Reptilase time

Reptilase is an enzyme from the venom of the snake *Bothrops atrox* (Per-de-lana), which clots human fibrinogen by cleaving fibrinopeptide A from fibrinogen. Reptilase is not inhibited by heparin or anti-thrombin III. A prolonged thrombin time and normal reptilase time is also in keeping with the presence of heparin in the sample. The reptilase time is prolonged in dysfibrinogenaemia and hypofibrinogenaemia.

Fibrinogen

While inherited disorders of fibrinogen are rare, acquired disorders are common in patients with consumptive coagulopathies, liver disease and following major surgery, including cardiopulmonary bypass. Furthermore, the association of high fibrinogen levels and increased risk for ischaemic heart and peripheral vascular disease is well recognized. Fibrinogen is also an acute-phase reactant, with increased levels commonly seen in inflammatory diseases. The interpretation of results is therefore difficult, and the most appropriate method is dependent on the reason for the investigation. Confirmation of low fibrinogen levels with a manual Clauss method is advisable. There are numerous methods used to measure fibrinogen, with clotting methods used most commonly to measure functional fibrinogen, based on fibrin formation. In the thrombin time method (Clauss), the thrombin time is proportional to the concentration of fibrinogen in the test sample. A calibration curve is prepared from known fibrinogen concentrations and used to convert the thrombin time to a fibrinogen concentration. There is little interference from FDPs or heparin, unless they are present in high concentrations.

A fibrinogen titre may be obtained using a series of dilutions of plasma, followed by the addition of thrombin. The dilution at which the fibrinogen is diluted out is a measure of the concentration of fibrinogen present. The test is usually run in parallel with protamine sulphate and E-aminocaproic acid (EACA) as indicators of FDPs and fibrinolysis, respectively. Physicochemical methods, used less commonly, measure the total fibrinogen and may not reflect the functional activity, while immunological methods measure factor-related antigen present both in fibrinogen and FDPs. The increased use of automated coagulometers has led to the automation of fibrinogen assays as a derived parameter from the prothrombin time, based on a turbidometric analysis using a spectrophotometer.

D-dimer assays and FDPs

D-dimer assays are used increasingly in the diagnosis of venous thromboembolic disease. The D-dimer fragments are produced during the degradation of thrombin-generated fibrin clots by plasmin. Assays are based on detection by antibodies specific for cross-linked fibrin fragments with no cross-activity with fibrinogen. These tests can, therefore, be performed on plasma samples. There are currently three main methods for D-dimer detection. An enzyme-linked immunosorbent assay (ELISA) is highly sensitive and provides quantitative results. The main disadvantage is that the technique is time consuming and therefore presents problems where this assay is used for rapid screening for venous thromboembolic disease. Latex agglutination assays are more rapid but have a lower sensitivity of 80%, requiring them to be used in conjunction with a clinical probability score as part of any screening procedure. Quantitative automated latex assays require special equipment to measure the decrease in light transmittance at 405 nm; this has the advantage of being sensitive and also rapid. Whole blood agglutination assays offer the most rapid assay, based on quantitative red cell agglutination, in which the monoclonal antibody for a D-dimer is linked to monoclonal antibody binding to red cells. These assays are rapid but operator-dependent, and do not give a quantitative result. These assays do have a high negative predicted value for venous thromboembolic disease, and are therefore commonly combined with a clinical predictive probability score in screening patients to exclude venous thrombosis. Raised D-dimer results are not specific for deep vein thrombosis and, particu-

larly in the more sensitive assays, low levels of fibrin are detected in a variety of conditions, such as infection inflammation, vasculitis, pregnancy and in particular for up to 3 weeks following surgery. Raised levels of D-dimers and FDPs are seen in disseminated intravascular coagulation and represent a helpful method in monitoring disease progress following *in vivo* plasmin activation. The assay may also be used to assess whether a fibrinolytic response to a therapeutic fibrinolytic agent, such as streptokinase or urokinase, has been achieved. As D-dimer assays are more specific and distinguish between fibrinogenolysis and fribrinolysis, they have largely replaced assays for FDPs.

FDPs increase following plasmin degradation of fibrinogen and non-cross-linked fibrin and result in prolonged thrombin time or reptilase clotting time. The most commonly performed FDP assays use a latex agglutination technique, in which an antibody that recognizes FDPs is coated on the surface of latex particles. The particles agglutinate in the presence of FDPs and the concentration is determined by the dilution that sustains agglutination. As antibodies used in this assay may cross-link the fibrinogen, the latter must be removed from the patient sample. This is accomplished by clotting the sample with thrombin or snake venom in the presence of a plasmin inhibitor to prevent *in vitro* generation of split products. These reagents are incorporated in special collection tubes.

Factor assays

Specific coagulation factor assays are based on either the prothrombin time or APTT. A range of dilutions of plasma standard are added to a specific factor-deficient plasma. The clotting times obtained show a linear relationship to the factor concentration when plotted on log paper. The activity of the factor in the test plasma can then be determined from the graph. These assays are particularly important in the identification of patients with inherited disorders and also in the monitoring of factor concentration replacement therapy. Factors II, V, VII and X are commonly assayed using a one-stage prothrombin time, while factors VIII, IX, XI and XII are based on an APTT method. Factor XIII deficiency is not detected by any of the routine coagulation tests, as it does not participate in the reaction leading to the formation of fibrin. A urea solubility test is a commonly used method to screen for factor XIII deficiency. A fibrin clot is formed and either acetone or urea added to the plasma sample, incubated at 37°C. Fibrin cross-linked by the action of factor XIII is insoluble in these solutions, but in the absence of factor XIII activity a fibrin clot will dissolve within an hour.

Natural anticoagulants

In vivo there is continuous low-grade activation of coagulation and there are natural inhibitors of activated coagulation factors. A deficiency of such factors may be associated with a prothrombotic tendency.

Anti-thrombin III

Anti-thrombin III is a major regulator of thrombin *in vivo*. Functional assays are preferred, as a variety of molecular forms are recognized that produce normal quantitation as measured by immunological techniques. Most functional assays measure neutralization of thrombin of factor Xa in the presence of added heparin.

Proteins C and S

Protein C is activated following thrombin generation. Thrombin binds to thrombomodulin on the surface of endothelial cells and binds and activates protein C. Thrombin in this situation loses its procoagulant activity and is no longer able to convert fibrinogen to fibrin. Activated protein C acts as a natural anticoagulant by degrading factors V and VIII, limiting further thrombin generation. Protein S serves as a co-factor for activated protein C. A further important finding is that activated protein C resistance may occur due to a defect of the factor V molecule, the factor V Leiden mutation. This is associated with an increased risk of venous thrombosis and is the most prevalent inherited prothrombotic risk factor known. PCR screen is recommended for patients with a prothrombotic history to exclude this factor. PCR screen for the G2020 prothrombin mutation is also routinely performed as part of a thrombophilia screen.

Fibrinolysis

Fibrinolysis results in the breakdown of the fibrin clot and it is initiated by the release from vascular endothelium of tissue-type plasminogen activator (tPA) and urokinase-type plasminogen activator (uPA). These activators convert plasminogen into the active enzyme plasmin, which degrades fibrin. There is also a natural inhibitor to plasmin, αII anti-plasmin and plasminogen

activator inhibitor type 1 (PAI-1) released by endothelium, which binds to and inactivates free tPA and uPA.

Markers of activated coagulation

Over the last few years there has been increasing interest in hypercoagulability and tests available for its detection. Assays for markers of coagulation activation have several potential uses, including characterizing patients with clinical conditions predisposing to thrombosis, aiding the diagnosis of acute thrombotic events and monitoring anticoagulant therapy. This may be achieved by measuring the enzymatic forms of coagulation zymogens generated during coagulation activation, or indirectly by measuring activation peptides generated when zymogens are activated. In addition, by measuring complexes that result from enzyme inactivation by naturally occurring plasma inhibitors, a further approach is available. A number of immunoassays are available to measure fragments generated from the activation of clotting factors such as factor IX and X activation peptides. Prothrombin fragment $1 + 2$, which results from thrombin-mediated activation of prothrombin, and fibrinopeptide A, cleaved from the α chain of fibrinogen by thrombin, are indices of thrombin generation and activity, respectively. Immunoassays for quantifying protein C activation peptide or activated protein C can be regarded as indices of thrombin and thrombomodulin function. Immunoassays are also available for the measurement of enzyme-inhibited complexes, such as thrombin, anti-thrombin, and other complexes that result from the inhibition of activated protein C by protein C inhibitor and anti-trypsin. Currently, the usefulness of markers of coagulation activation is better for assessing hypercoagulability than in the diagnosis of acute thrombotic events. For the latter purpose it is more effective to measure markers of fibrinolysis activation, such as D-dimer.

Automated coagulation

Recent advances in technology have heralded the introduction of automated instruments for coagulation screening. An increase in workload, the demand for greater specificity and the reduction in manual labour have ensured that most laboratories now have semi- or full automation. Most manual methods can be modified for instrumentation, although results vary greatly between instruments. All routine coagulation screening tests, including factor assays, can be analysed on automated instruments. More advanced instruments allow chromogenic assays for specialized coagulation tests. The early instruments involved detection of the fibrin clot through electrodes. An electrode moves in and out of the reagent/plasma. Calcium is added and, as soon as the first fibrin clot is formed, the electrical circuit is completed and the timer stopped. The majority of modern-day instruments involve photo-optical endpoint detection. As the clotting process takes place, the light scattered from a fixed beam increases. The clotting time is obtained from the coagulation curve as the time required for the sample to reach the preset percentage of the scattered light intensity. Full instrumentation includes robotic sampling, barcode reading of samples, automatic reagent dispensers and a data management system. However, as clotting times vary between different instruments, depending on the method of endpoint detection, results from automation are not strictly comparable. Therefore, manual techniques are still used as reference methods.

Further reading

Lugassy G, Shulman S. *Thrombosis and Anti-thrombotic Therapy.* 2001: Hartin Dunitz, London.

SECTION 6

CYTOGENETICS

36

Chromosome banding and analysis

Mervyn Humphreys

Introduction

Cytogenetics involves the study of human chromosomes in health and disease. In the human nucleus the genetic material (DNA) is chemically bound to proteins and packaged into distinct structures called chromosomes. Typically, human cells harbour a total of 46 chromosomes, or 23 pairs, one member of each chromosome pair being inherited from each parent. The DNA of each cell is packaged into chromosomes to facilitate the correct separation of the genetic material to both daughter cells at each cell division. When human gamete cells, sperms and eggs, are produced, the chromosome number is halved to 23 via meiotic cell division, so that when a new zygote is formed, by fusion of one sperm and one ovum, the cells should have the correct chromosome number 46. Historically, 1956 is considered to mark the beginning of modern human cytogenetics, as prior to this time the number of chromosomes in the normal human cell was thought to be 48.

Cytogenetic analysis enables the detection of chromosome abnormalities. These abnormalities may be numerical (extra or missing chromosomes) or structural (deletions, duplications, translocations, etc.). Chromosome preparations can be prepared and analysed from various body tissues, including peripheral blood, amniotic fluid, skin or bone marrow. Chromosome studies are an important laboratory diagnostic procedure in many clinical situations. For example, patients with multiple birth defects and/or mental retardation, abnormal sexual development or infertility and numerous types of malignancies may harbour cytogenetic abnormalities. It is

therefore very important that chromosome studies are carried out as part of the routine investigations in such patients.

Up to the early 1970s cytogenetic analysis was only carried out on non-banded, solid-stained chromosome preparations. Chromosomes could only be identified and sorted based on shape and size, and therefore only numerical abnormalities or large structural rearrangements could be detected. Some clear numerical abnormalities cannot be definitively characterized using solid staining alone (Figure 36.1). Solid staining is, however, still the method of choice for investigations of chromosome instability, following exposure of patients or cells to clastogens.

In the early 1970s the first chromosome banding techniques were introduced, which allowed much more accurate identification of each chromosome pair. This in turn enabled the detection of more subtle structural abnormalities associated with specific disease conditions. This chapter will describe and explain the underlying principles of the various chromosome banding techniques that are available and highlight their main applications in the laboratory. An overview of the procedure of cytogenetic analysis will also be given.

Chromosome banding

Since the first banded chromosome preparations were described in the early 1970s, there has been a rapid proliferation of chromosome staining techniques that has enabled the very precise characterization of the normal

The Science of Laboratory Diagnosis, Second Edition   Edited by David Burnett and John Crocker
© 2005 John Wiley & Sons, Ltd

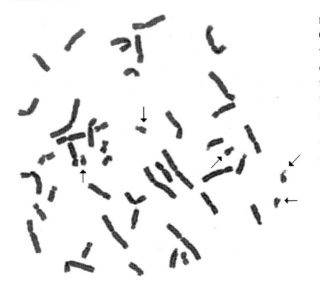

Figure 36.1 Solid-stained chromosome metaphase from a female patient with Downs syndrome (trisomy 21). Although chromosome 21 cannot be distinguished from chromosome 22 in solid-stained preparations, the five G group chromosomes present (21s and 22s) are arrowed

human karyotype. The Giemsa banding method, developed in the mid-1970s, is the most widely used technique for routine chromosome analysis. The numerous other banding methods are generally only utilized to aid the identification of specific chromosome abnormalities whose exact nature is uncertain following G-banded analysis.

Although the biochemical basis of chromosome banding is poorly understood, the various patterns obtained appear to reflect the highly organized fashion by which the enormous stretch of human DNA is packaged into the chromosomes. Chromosome banding techniques can be divided into two groups: (a) those that result in bands distributed along the length of the whole chromosome, such as G, Q and R-banding; and (b) those that stain a restricted number of specific chromosome regions, such as C-banding, NOR staining and DAPI staining.

Giemsa banding (G-banding)

Chromosomes may be G-banded by treating them with various chemicals that produce alternating bands of dark and light intensity along the length of the chromosomes. The most widely used method involves the digestion of chromosome preparations with the proteolytic enzyme trypsin, followed by Giemsa staining. Many G-banding

methods now utilize Leishmann's stain rather than Giemsa stain. Some methods involve pretreating slides with salt solution (2x SSC). Each chromosome exhibits a characteristic and consistent G-banding pattern, enabling the accurate identification of each chromosome pair and the detection of structural chromosome abnormalities, such as deletions, inversions and translocations.

It is essential that slides are aged prior to G-banding by either leaving them at room temperature for 3–4 days, heating them overnight at 60°C or pretreating them with hydrogen peroxide. The ageing of chromosome preparations strengthens the integrity of chromosomes, making them less vulnerable to over-digestion by trypsin (Figure 36.2).

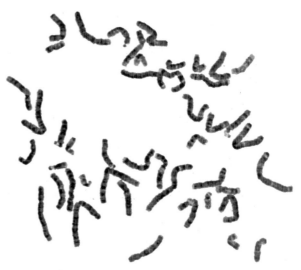

Figure 36.2 Normal female metaphase spread stained by G-banding

Mechanism

Although no satisfactory hypothesis has explained the mechanism of G-banding, it appears to be related to DNA composition and presumably involves the selective removal of proteins from different chromosome regions. Chromosomes are believed to contain a basic structure that is enhanced by the G-banding procedure. Each length of about 146 base pairs of human DNA is wound around a core consisting of eight histone protein molecules, to produce repeating units called nucleosomes or chromomeres. Successive nucleosomes are arrayed like beads on a string. This elementary fibre of linked nucleosomes is further coiled to form the chromatin fibre. Chromatin fibres are further looped and coiled into the final chromosome packages. It is believed that the dark G-bands may simply correlate with these bead-like chromomeres and the G-banding pattern therefore reflects the structural organization of chromatin along the chromosome length.

It has alternatively been suggested that the dark and light G-bands correlate with the differing functional content of the DNA in these chromosome regions. Replication studies have shown that regions of DNA with similar replication times are clustered together, with the DNA in the dark G-bands replicating late in S phase, compared to the light G-band DNA. *In situ* hybridization studies have shown a correlation between the G-banding pattern and the location of repetitive DNA sequences. Dark G-bands have been shown to be rich in L1-type repetitive DNA sequences that are relatively AT-rich and encode very few expressed genes. Light G-bands have similarly been shown to be rich in Alu-type repetitive DNA sequences that are relatively GC-rich and encode many expressed genes.

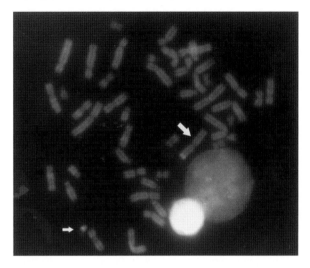

Figure 36.3 Q-banding. Metaphase spread from a male patient with an abnormal X chromosome, derived from a t(X;Y) rearrangement. Small arrow indicates the normal Y chromosome; large arrow indicates the abnormal X with Yq heterochromatin attached to Xp

Application

G-banding is by far the most widely used chromosome banding method for routine cytogenetic analysis in clinical investigations. This method enables the identification of each chromosome pair and the detection of the majority of numerical and structural chromosomal abnormalities. Cytogenetic laboratories that do not routinely use G-banding generally use R-banding. The other chromosome banding methods are generally only used when an initial G-banding analysis detects a chromosome abnormality requiring further investigation for its accurate characterization. The G-banding pattern is grossly similar to the Q-banding pattern.

Quinicrine banding (Q-banding)

Q-banding was the first chromosome banding technique, introduced in 1968, when chromosome preparations were stained with quinicrine mustard. Q-banding is nowadays generally produced using quinicrine dihydrochloride, which is less toxic. A series of bright and dull fluorescing regions are revealed along the chromosomes when viewed with fluorescence microscopy (450–500 nm). The Q-banding pattern strongly resembles the G-banding pattern, with the brightly fluorescing Q-bands corresponding to the dark-staining G-bands. Notable exceptions include the distal long arm of the Y chromosome, which shows extremely bright fluorescence. The

satellite regions of the acrocentric chromosomes (13–15 and 21–22) also show characteristic Q-banding patterns (Figure 36.3).

Mechanism

Because Q-banding and G-banding patterns show such similarities, the mechanisms are clearly influenced by the same parameters of chromosome composition (see G-banding). The Q-banding pattern is explained by the specification of nitrogen mustards for guanine. Quinicrine fluorescence is enhanced in DNA regions rich in AT sequences and quenched in GC-rich regions, thereby producing the Q-banding pattern. The varying AT/GC DNA content of the chromosome bands therefore explains differences in staining intensity when treated with quinicrine.

Applications

Q-banding requires a fluorescence microscope for analysis. Q-banded chromosome preparations are not suitable for routine cytogenetic investigations, as the fluorescence fades rapidly during analysis. This banding method is, however, useful for specific examination of the heteromorphisms associated with the Y chromosome and the satellite regions of the acrocentric chromosomes.

Q-banding patterns of short arm and satellite heteromorphisms can, for example, sometimes be used to determine the parental origin, and the stage of meiotic non-disjunction in trisomies involving the acrocentric chromosomes.

Reverse banding (R-banding)

R-banding of chromosomes is complimentary to Q- and G-bands and was first reported in 1971. Slides are incubated in phosphate buffer at 85–89°C, followed by staining with Giemsa or acridine orange, yielding a banding pattern which is the reverse of G- or Q-banding. When stained with Giemsa, the bands are pale and require phase contrast for analysis. This was the first non-fluorescent banding technique to be developed. Using acridine orange staining, the positive R-bands fluoresce green/yellow, while the negative R-bands fluoresce orange/red. R-banding is most successful when slides have been aged at room temperature for several days or at 60°C overnight. Freshly made slides require shorter incubation times in buffer (Figure 36.4).

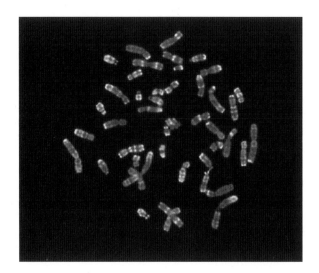

Figure 36.4 R-banding using acridine orange

Mechanism

As for G- and Q-banding, the R-banding pattern appears to reflect the structural and functional make-up of the chromosomes. The positive R-bands are GC-rich, early replicating, and contain housekeeping genes, while the negative R-bands are AT-rich, late replicating and contain no housekeeping genes. The R-banding pattern is produced by the differential denaturation of the GC- and AT-rich chromosomal regions. The AT-rich regions denature at a lower temperature and fluoresce red with acridine orange. Acridine orange intercalates between the base pairs of the double-stranded GC-rich regions and fluoresces yellow. It is not entirely clear-cut as to why Giemsa treatments also produce R-banding. It may be due to differential interaction of proteins with the AT-rich and GC-rich chromosomal regions. The fact that aged slides require shorter incubation times and yield better R-banding again suggests that, as slides are aged, their general structure becomes more stable and less vulnerable to degradation by various agents (see G-banding).

Application

Although the large majority of cytogenetic laboratories use G-banding for routine investigations, R-banding is the method used for routine chromosome analysis in many French laboratories. This banding technique generally reveals no new information that is not available following G-banding but on occasions may be used to more accurately delineate the breakpoints of structural abnormalities, particularly if terminal chromosomal breakpoints are involved.

Constitutive heterochromatin banding (C-banding)

The C-banding procedure involves treating chromosomes with acid (HCl), alkali (BaOH$_2$) and hot salt solution (2x SSC). C-banded chromosome preparations are overall lightly stained, except for dark staining of the regions of constitutive heterochromatin. These are located at the centromeres of all the chromosomes except the Y chromosome, where it is located on the distal long arm (Figure 36.5).

Mechanism

The harsh C-banding treatments are thought to facilitate preferential loss of DNA and protein from the non-C-band chromosome regions. Successive depurination and denaturation of the chromosomal DNA occurs during the acid and alkali treatments. Further small DNA fragments are lost during the salt treatment, leaving only the tightly compacted centromeric heterochromatin. Non-histone

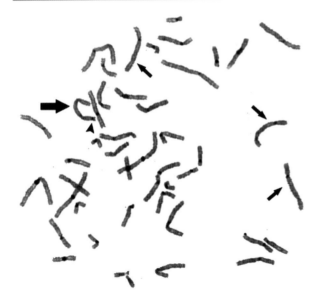

Figure 36.5 C-banding of a metaphase spread from a patient with an inversion of chromosome 4. The inverted chromosome 4 (large arrow) has its centromere position moved towards the short arm telomere end (arrowhead). The normal B group chromosomes (4 and 5) cannot be distinguished using C-banding only (small arrows)

proteins bound to the C-band regions may prevent the same DNA denaturation occurring at these loci.

Applications

The C-bands of all chromosomes, especially chromosomes 1, 9, 16 and Y, vary in size between homologues as well as between individuals. The extreme variation in size of the C-bands has no phenotypic effect, as these regions contain only constitutive heterochromatin and no important genes. If it is unclear whether an extra band or abnormal chromosome segment, detected by G-banding, represents a normal variation of a heterochromatic region or a euchromatic chromosomal abnormality of possible clinical significance, C-banded analysis may provide conclusive information. C-banding may on occasions enable the determination of the origin of non-disjunction in patients with trisomies. When the chromosome involved has a notable heterochromatic variant, then comparing C-banded preparations from the proband and both parents may indicate in which parent, and possibly in which stage of meiosis, the non-disjunction error occurred that caused the trisomy.

Nucleolar organizer region staining (NOR staining)

The ribosomal RNA genes that form and maintain the nucleolus in interphase nuclei are located on the short arms of the acrocentric, satellited chromosomes (13, 14, 15, 21 and 22). When chromosome preparations are treated overnight with silver nitrate solution, these nucleolar organizer regions (NORs) stain darkly (Figure 36.6). The satellites of the acrocentric chromosomes

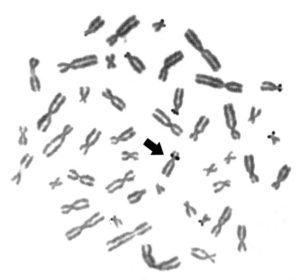

Figure 36.6 NOR-stained metaphase from a patient with a reciprocal translocation between chromosomes 7 and 14. The arrow indicates the abnormal chromosome 14 with chromosome 7 material translocated above the NOR

are often seen to group together within cells. This phenomenon, called satellite association, presumably reflects the common function of the different NORs in the organization of the cell's nucleolus.

Mechanism

NOR staining involves the extraction of DNA, RNA and histones from chromosomes. It is actually the residual non-histone proteins adjacent to the NORs, rather than the NORs themselves, that are selectively stained by this method. Studies have shown that this method only stains the active NORs that participated in the formation of the nucleolus in the preceding interphase of the cell cycle.

Application

The number of NORs detected per metaphase spread varies between individuals because only active NORs that participated in the formation of the nucleolus during the preceding interphase stage are stained. The NOR staining pattern of acrocentric chromosomes is consistent within an individual and is heritable. NOR patterns and the Q-banding appearance of acrocentric satellites are therefore useful for determining parental origin and/or the stage of meiotic non-disjunction involved in trisomies involving these chromosomes. NOR staining is useful for the characterization of small marker chromosomes, to confirm whether or not they are satellited and therefore derived from an acrocentric chromosome.

DA–DAPI banding

When chromosomes are stained with the fluorescent dye 4,6-diamino-2-phenyl-indole (DAPI) and treated with the non-fluorescent counterstain distamycin (DA), a subset of fluorescent C-bands are revealed. The heterochromatic regions of chromosomes 1, 9, 16 and Y and the proximal short arm of chromosome 15 are very brightly fluorescing. Using DAPI alone produces a banding pattern similar to Q-banding (Figure 36.7).

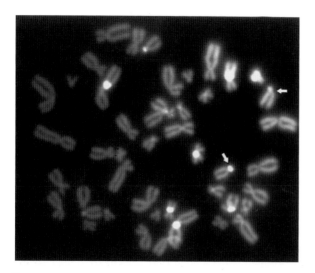

Figure 36.7 Male metaphase stained using DA/DAPI Banding. Arrows indicate the chromosome 15s with brightly fluorescencing short arms

Mechanism

DAPI binds to DNA but has an affinity for AT base pairs. DAPI binding alone therefore yields a weak Q-banding pattern. Although DAPI fluorescence is enhanced by both AT and GC base pairs, there is a significant enhancement of fluorescence in regions of AT-rich DNA. There is also some evidence that DAPI binds to AT clusters in the minor groove of the DNA double helix. DA also shows AT-specific DNA binding affinity. Although the two dyes used have similar base-pairing preference, they have non-identical binding affinities and dissimilar structures. The differential fluorescence obtained may be due to competitive binding between the two dyes, which bind at similar but not identical sites. Alternatively, DA may block DAPI binding in euchromatic regions, whereas DAPI binding sites remain available in heterochromatic regions.

Applications

DA/DAPI banding is used predominately for the interpretation of certain chromosome abnormalities detected using more routine banding methods (G- or R-banding), e.g. DA/DAPI banding may be of use where a structurally rearranged chromosome has a breakpoint close to a region selectively stained with DA/DAPI banding. DA/DAPI banding is particularly useful for studying small satellited marker chromosomes. This technique can identify those marker chromosomes involving the proximal end of chromosome 15. DAPI staining is also the most commonly used counterstain for routine fluorescence *in situ* hybridization of chromosome preparations.

Replication banding

A G- or R-banding pattern can be produced on chromosome preparations if they are grown in the presence of the thymidine analogue 5-bromo-2-deoxyuridine (BrdU) and stained with the fluorescent dye Hoechst 33258. This method utilizes the fact that different regions of the chromosome complement replicate at different stages during S phase. This method relies on the incorporation of label into DNA, so BrdU is added to living cells in tissue culture. By controlling the timing of when the pulse of BrdU is administered to cell cultures relative to the harvest time, either an early- or late-replicating banding pattern can be produced. If BrdU is added at culture initiation, but removed about 6 hours before harvest at 48 hours, a G-banding pattern is obtained. If

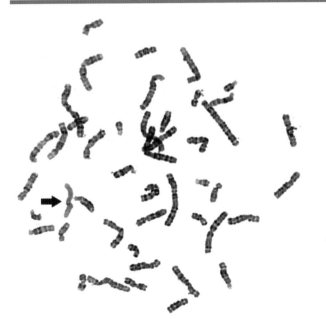

Figure 36.8 Metaphase spread after replication banding. This preparation was obtained from blood cultures to which BrdU was added 6 hours before harvesting. Chromosomes show an R-banding pattern. This patient carries a t(X;11) translocation. In this instance, the normal X is late-replicating. With late-pulse BrdU cultures utilized, the late-replicating X stains lightly (arrowed)

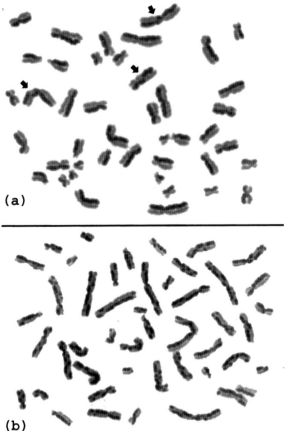

(a)

(b)

Figure 36.9 Metaphase spreads stained for sister chromatid exchanges (SCEs). (a) Metaphase from blood cultures with only three spontaneous SCEs arrowed. (b) Metaphase from blood cultures from the same individual, incubated with the cross-linking agent mitomycin C, showing a highly significant increase in the level of SCEs (>100/cell)

BrdU is only added about 6 hours before cultures are harvested, R-banding results (Figure 36.8).

If cells undergo two complete cycles of replication in the presence of BrdU, the sister chromatids of each chromosome are differentially stained. The harliquinization pattern obtained enables the detection of sister chromatid exchanges (SCEs), which are points along the length of chromosomes where the chromatid material is swapped between sister chromatids. SCE preparations are stained with the fluorochrome Hoechst 33258. They are then either viewed by fluorescence microscopy (360–400 nm) or, if they are first exposed to UV light and then stained with Giemsa stain [Fluorescence Plus Giemsa (FPG) staining], they can be analysed using light microscopy (Figure 36.9).

Mechanism

BrdU is a thymidine analogue that is readily incorporated into chromosomes. When chromosomes are stained with the fluorochrome Hoechst 33258 (which binds to AT-rich base pairs), chromosome regions that replicate in the presence of BrdU contain BrdU-substituted DNA. When BrdU is present at culture initiation, it is present for the early part of one cycle of DNA replication, and therefore chromosome regions which replicate early in S phase (R-bands) become BrdU-substituted and are therefore weakly fluorescing or light-staining with Giemsa. The G-bands replicate late in S phase, after the BrdU has been removed from the cultures, and therefore incorporate thymidine and are brightly fluorescing, or dark-staining with Giemsa (G-banding). Alternatively, if BrdU is only added to cultures about 6 hours before harvesting, it is only present for the late part of one DNA replication cycle and the early-replicating regions (R-bands) have already been replicated, incorporating thymidine, and fluoresce brightly or stain darkly with Giemsa. Only the late-replicating regions (G-bands) become BrdU-substituted and therefore fluoresce weakly or stain lightly with Giemsa (R-banding).

Although homologous chromosomes show similar replication patterns, in females the early- and late-replicating X chromosomes can be distinguished. The late-replicating X chromosome is darker staining with early pulse BrdU replication banding and lighter staining with late-pulse BrdU replication banding (Figure 36.8).

The harliquinized staining pattern obtained when BrdU is present in cell cultures for two cycles of replication reflects the asymmetric incorporation of BrdU into chromosomal DNA. By semi-conservative replication, each new strand of DNA consists of one original DNA strand and one newly constructed strand. After two cycles of replication in the presence of BrdU, one chromatid contains DNA with BrdU substituted into one DNA strand, while its sister chromatid contains two BrdU-substituted DNA strands. This chemical difference between the sister chromatids explains the difference in staining intensity obtained. The staining intensity is proportional to the amount of thymidine-containing DNA present in each chromatid. When chromosome preparations are stained using the fluorescence plus Giemsa method, more DNA is lost from the bifiliarly BrdU-substituted chromatid than its counterpart, thereby producing the characteristic harliquinized staining pattern.

Application

Apart from providing alternative methods for G- and R-banding, the staining patterns obtained after a pulse of BrdU is administered early or late in the cell cycle is mainly used for replication studies. In normal females one X chromosome is inactivated in each cell by a random process, and this inactivated X is always the last chromosome to complete its replication in each cell cycle. Replication banding is useful for investigating the pattern of X-inactivation in females carrying structural abnormalities involving the X chromosome, where the pattern of X-inactivation is generally found to be a non-random event. The illustrated example in Figure 36.8 shows a female patient carrying a t(X;11) balanced translocation. Replication staining showed that the normal X chromosome is late-replicating in all cells. This skewing of the normally random X inactivation pattern ensures that autosomal segments involved in such X–autosome translocations are not also inactivated, which would have a deleterious clinical impact.

The production of harliquinized chromosome staining patterns enables the detection of sister chromatid exchanges (SCEs). These are points along the length of chromosomes where there is exchange of material between the two sister chromatids of individual chromosomes, producing a checker-board appearance. Normal human cells show a mean frequency of 5–8 SCEs/cell, but SCE levels have been demonstrated to increase with exposure to many mutagens. The main application of this technique is therefore as a method for monitoring mutagen-induced chromosome damage, in patients or cells. In many cases, SCE has proved more sensitive for the detection of chromosome damage than measurement of chromosomal aberrations (Figure 36.9). However, not all test mutagens show a positive correlation between induced chromosomal breakage and induced SCEs, thereby indicating that these two parameters reflect different and independent expressions of mutagen-induced damage. This method is also used as a diagnostic test for the chromosome instability disorder Bloom syndrome, in which cells show a significant increase from the normal baseline level of spontaneous SCEs. SCEs can also be used to study cell kinetics by indicating the duration of the various stages of the cell cycle.

Chromosome analysis

The large majority of routine cytogenetic analysis is carried out by the examination of banded metaphase preparations (mostly G- or R-banded). Cytogenetic analysis is a highly skilled laboratory discipline and several years' training are required before a cytogeneticist becomes competent in recognizing the normal karyotype and detecting the variety of karyotypic abnormalities that may be encountered.

Classification of banded chromosomes and nomenclature

Chromosomes are identified, karyotyped and described using the guidelines proposed in the International System of Chromosome Nomenclature (ISCN). This is the report published by the Standing Committee on Human Cytogenetic Nomenclature. The basic terminology for describing human karyotypes was put forward by this group in 1971 (Paris nomenclature). The main features used to distinguish chromosomes are length, centromere position, presence of secondary constrictions (satellites) and banding pattern. The centromere is the primary constriction that divides each chromosome into a short arm (p arm) and long arm (q arm). The satellites are secondary constrictions located at the ends of chromosomes 13–15, 21 and 22. The autosomes are numbered in pairs by decreasing size from 1 to 22, leaving the sex chromosomes (X and Y). Based on length, centromere position and satellites alone, the chromosomes of the human karyotype can be sorted into seven groups, A–G (X chromosome included in C group/Y chromosome included in G group) (Figure 36.10).

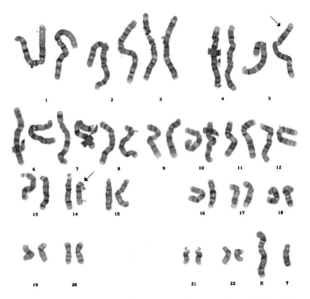

Figure 36.10 G-banded karyotype from a male patient with a balanced reciprocal translocation, involving the short arm of chromosome 5 and the long arm of chromosome 14. The abnormal chromosomes are arrowed

Based on centromere position, there are three types of chromosome: metacentric (centromere in the middle), acrocentric (centromere at one end) and sub-metacentric (centromere off-centre). Individual chromosome pairs can, however, only be accurately identified and sorted from their banding patterns. The ISCN includes a complete set of diagrammatic chromosome maps (ideograms). These ideograms illustrate each chromosome, dividing them into convenient segments (regions) of roughly equal length by defining several fixed points (landmarks). These landmarks include the chromosome ends (telomeres), the centromeres and other prominent bands. Each region is numbered sequentially, moving outward, in either direction, from the centromeres. For example, 1p3 represents chromosome 1, short arm,

region 3. Each major band within a region is also numbered in sequence, with band 1 being nearest the centromere. Therefore, 1p31 indicates chromosome 1, short arm, region 3, band 1. The quality of chromosome preparations has improved over the years, with more elongated chromosomes being produced. With this improvement, it was shown that certain bands, as seen in shorter chromosome preparations, actually resolved into several finer bands. For this reason, the ISCN has produced updates of the chromosome ideograms to match up with these longer chromosome lengths. Where chromosome bands were found to split into more bands, sub-band numbers have been assigned. By convention, a decimal point is placed before any sub-band and up to two new numbers added thereafter to describe the new sub-bands. Therefore, 1p31.2 describes chromosome 1, short arm, region 3, band 1, sub-band 2 (Figure 36.11).

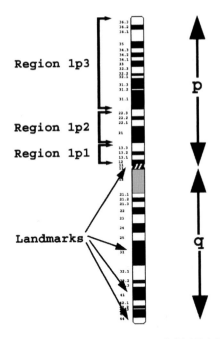

Figure 36.11 Ideogram of chromosome 1, highlighting the p and q arms, the chromosome regions on the p arm and landmarks on the q arm

The ISCN system enables the accurate description of breakpoints in all chromosome rearrangements. When using ISCN to describe karyotypic abnormalities, the cytogeneticist must utilize the most appropriate ideogram showing equivalent banding resolution to the chromosome being analysed.

Chromosome variation

In order to recognize any chromosome abnormality present in any human chromosome preparation, the cytogeneticist must be very familiar with the appearance of the normal human karyotype. This is complicated by the occurrence of considerable variation in certain heterochromatic regions, including centromeric and satellite polymorphisms. It is important that these regions of normal chromosome variation are recognized and distinguished from other clinically significant chromosome abnormalities.

Chromosome analysis

The majority of routine chromosome analysis is performed by microscopically examining banded metaphase preparations. Suitable metaphases are first located by screening banded slides, using low-power microscopy ($\times 100$ magnification). Suitable metaphases are then examined using higher magnification (usually $\times 1000$). For constitutional karyotype analysis, only five or six metaphases of suitable quality need be examined, except where a possible chromosome mosaicism may be expected, when more cells should be analysed. The quality of metaphases selected for analysis depends largely on the reason for carrying out the cytogenetic investigation. If checking for an obvious numerical abnormality (e.g. trisomy 21) then high-quality metaphases are not required. However, if a subtle abnormality may be present (small deletion or rearrangement involving small segments), then more elongated chromosome spreads must be examined.

If the cytogeneticist is satisfied that all chromosome pairs show the recognized normal banding pattern, a normal karyotype can be reported. Karyotypes are described using ISCN nomenclature. In general, this has the following order: total number of chromosomes, sex chromosome constitution, description of abnormality (if present), and each of these is separated by a comma. Thus, the normal female karyotype formula is 46,XX and the normal male karyotype is 46,XY. Where a chromosome abnormality is recognized, the appropriate karyotype formula is assigned. Each type of structural abnormality has an associated ISCN abbreviation, e.g. 't' for translocation, 'i' for inversion, etc. The chromosomes involved and any breakpoints are included in the assigned karyotypic formula, e.g. the abnormal karyotype illustrated in Figure 36.10 has the formula 46,XY,t(5;14)(p15.2;q24.1). This indicates that chromosome 5 is broken in the p arm at band 15.2, while chromosome 14 has been broken in the q arm at band 24.1). If the abnormality is indistinct or breakpoints are unclear by microscopic examination, the preparation of karyotypes may help characterize the exact nature of the abnormality. This would formerly have involved photographing the abnormal cells using photomicroscopy, developing the film, printing the film, cutting out and rearranging the chromosomes into the standard karyotype order. Nowadays, the production of karyotypes in diagnostic cytogenetic laboratories is made significantly easier by using dedicated image analysis systems. These systems link the microscope to a digital camera that is used to capture a digital image of the metaphase spread to be analysed. Specialized cytogenetic software then enables the arrangement of the chromosomes on a computer screen to produce a final karyotype, which can be printed out and/or stored electronically.

Chromosome analysis for acquired chromosome abnormalities

The cytogenetic analysis of malignancies (leukaemias and solid tumours) is routinely carried out to detect any associated acquired chromosome abnormalities. Detection of such abnormalities provides vital information in relation to disease diagnosis, patient prognosis and for monitoring response to therapy. Chromosome analysis for acquired chromosome abnormalities bears a few important differences from constitutional analysis. Acquired chromosome abnormalities are clonal, being confined only to the malignant cells. In addition metaphases obtained from malignant cells typically show inferior morphology (short and poor bands) compared to non-malignant cells. It is important, first, that the cytogeneticist analyses a larger number of cells to enable detection of small clonal abnormalities (i.e. not all cells detected may belong to the abnormal clone), and second, that a representative selection of all metaphases is examined to avoid the inadvertent selection of the better quality but possibly non-malignant cells.

Molecular cytogenetics

The most recent significant development in the field of routine diagnostic cytogenetics has been the introduction of molecular cytogenetic techniques in the 1980s. A wide range of commercially available probes are now available which can be used to highlight specific regions of the human karyotype by the fluorescence *in situ* hybridization (FISH) technique. FISH enables the detection of some very subtle abnormalities that are beyond the limits of any banding technique. FISH probes can also be utilized to quickly and accurately characterize complicated or unidentified chromosome abnormalities, detected using banding techniques. Furthermore, FISH probes allow specimens to be screened for important cytogenetic abnormalities, even when dividing metaphase spreads are not available. This has enabled rapid prenatal diagnosis, as amniotic fluid samples can be screened for specific abnormalities by FISH after 24 hours, rather than waiting for up to 2 weeks for enough cells to grow in culture to produce chromosome preparations. FISH is also particularly useful in malignancy studies where mitotic cells may be difficult to obtain.

All routine diagnostic cytogenetic laboratories now rely very heavily on these FISH tests, which complement the routine banding methods. In many instances FISH tests are actually more appropriate than the alternative full karyotype analysis.

Further reading

Benn PA, Tantravahi U. Chromosome staining and banding techniques. In *Human Cytogenetics Constitutional Analysis: A Practical Approach*, 3rd edn, Rooney DE (ed.). Oxford University Press, New York, 99–128.

Bickmore A, Sumner AT. Mammalian chromosome banding—an expression of genome organization. *Trends Genet.* 1989; **5**(5): 144–148.

Comings DE. Mechanisms of chromosome banding and implications for chromosome structure. *Ann Rev Genet* 1978; **12**: 25–46.

Cross I, Wolstenholme J. An introduction to human chromosomes and their analysis. In *Human Cytogenetics Constitutional Analysis: A Practical Approach*, 3rd edn, Rooney DE (ed). Oxford University Press, New York, 1–31.

Goldman MA, Holmquist GP, Gray MC *et al.* Replication timing of genes and middle repetitive sequences. *Science* 1984; **224**: 686–692.

Gustashaw KM. Chromosome stains. In *The AGT Cytogenetics Laboratory Manual*, 3rd edn, Barch MJ, Knutsen, T, Spurbeck JL (eds). 1997: Lippincott-Raven, New York.

Holmquist G, Gray M, Porter T, Jordan J. Characterization of Giemsa dark and light band DNA. *Cell* 1982; **31**: 121.

ISCN. *An International System for Human Cytogenetic Nomenclature*, Mitelman F (ed). 1995: S Karger, Basel.

Richardson AM. Chromosome analysis. In *The AGT Cytogenetics Laboratory Manual*, 3rd edn, Barch MJ, Knutsen T, Spurbeck JL (eds) 1997, Lippincott-Raven, New York.

Sumner AT. The nature and mechanisms of chromosome banding. *Cancer Genet Cytogenet* 1982: **6**: 59–87.

Verma RS, Babu A (eds) *Human Chromosomes: Manual of Basic Techniques*. 1989: Pergamon, New York.

37

Fluorescence *in situ* hybridization

Ivor Hickey

Fluorescence *in situ* hybridization (FISH) is a powerful technique that plays a significant part in several current areas of genetic research. It refers to a series of related procedures, in which single-stranded nucleic acid molecules (probes), tagged with chemicals that are either themselves fluorescent or can be detected by immunofluorescence microscopy, are used to identify specific target nucleic acid sequences in cytological preparations.

The technique derives directly from the original nucleic acid hybridization experiments first pioneered by Speigleman in the 1960s, which were adapted by several groups, using radiolabelled probes to identify nucleic acid sequences in fixed material on microscope slides. Early examples included the identification of ribosomal RNA genes in the nucleoli of *Xenopus* oocytes and centromeric satellite DNA in metaphase mouse chromosomes. Although protocols have developed greatly since then, the basic steps have remained largely unaltered. All variations of the technique include a nucleic acid probe, a cytological preparation and a detection system. The principal steps in the system will be described at this point, before variations and applications of the technique are encountered.

Choice of probe

In many cases a genomic clone of DNA can be used, although, as will be seen later, other sources of DNA can also be utilized for chromosome painting. In some applications RNA molecules may be used, although this is rarely done today. The probe must be labelled prior to use, in order to detect the hybridized material at the end of procedure. It is important to realize that a factor in probe detection is the length of a probe. Under the same labelling and detection systems, a smaller probe will always give a weaker signal than a longer probe. Although probes as small as 500 base pairs can be detected in certain circumstances, cosmids, vectors derived from bacteriophage λ, which contain approximately 40 kb of cloned DNA, are the most popular sources of probe. DNA cloned in vectors carrying larger inserts, such as bacterial artificial chromosomes (BACs), P1 artificial chromosomes (PACs) or yeast artificial chromosomes (YACS), will work well in all instances.

Labelling of probes

The most frequently used labels for probes in FISH experiments are modified deoxyuridine triphosphates. The modifications involve addition of haptens, immunoreactive groups such as digoxigenin or biotin, which are linked to the 5 position of the pyrimidine ring by a long spacer arm. These may be detected by indirect immunofluorescence techniques. Alternatively, probes may be labelled with nucleoside triphosphates containing a fluorochrome such as fluorescein, which can be detected directly by its own fluorescence. Probes can be labelled using any of the systems frequently employed elsewhere in molecular biology. These include polymerase chain reaction (PCR), nick translation and random primer labelling. Of these, nick translation is probably the most popular, since it will produce labelled DNA fragments of small size. The size of probe is important, as large probe molecules have difficulty in diffusing

The Science of Laboratory Diagnosis, Second Edition   Edited by David Burnett and John Crocker

through cytological material to reach their target DNA, and their use often results in high background fluorescence. The optimal size of probe is between 200 and 500 bases. Probes produced by PCR are increasingly important in the techniques of chromosome painting and fibre FISH, which will be described in detail later.

Hybridization

Here the procedures broadly follow those of other molecular nucleic acid hybridization protocols. Differences relate to attempts to maintain the morphology of the cytological preparation in good condition, and to prevent binding of the probe to repeated sequences distributed throughout the genome. To maintain the integrity of the cytological preparation, hybridization is usually carried out at reduced temperatures, typically 35–42°C, in 50% formamide. Most eukaryote genomes contain large amounts of dispersed repeated DNA sequences. For this reason, if genomic material is used as probe, it is likely to contain DNA sequences that are repeated elsewhere in the genome. This will result in a level of fluorescence across all regions of the chromosomes, which will reduce the specificity of the probe. To prevent this and thus to improve the quality and sensitivity of the final image, unlabelled DNA from the repetitive fraction of the genome (Cot 1 DNA) is usually added to the probe during hybridization.

Detection of hybridized probe

When probes are labelled directly with fluorescent nucleotides, detection simply requires observation of the material using a fluorescence microscope with appropriate filters. Since the signal is not amplified, this method will result in less intense fluorescence, but the level of background fluorescence is low. The use of coupled charge device (CCD) cameras to detect low-level fluorescence can make this method sensitive enough for use with small DNA targets. When probes are labelled with haptens, their presence is detected with antibodies conjugated to fluorochromes. Digoxigenin- and biotin-labelled probes may both be detected in this way, but biotin has the added advantage that it has an extremely high affinity for the egg-white protein, avidin. This allows the use of avidin conjugated with fluorochromes to be used in detection. The only shortcoming of this technique is where the target tissue contains enough biotin to give rise to background fluorescence. In the case of cytogenetics this is not a major problem.

Frequently the fluorescent signal from a target is amplified by using more than one layer of antibody in the detection process.

One of the major advantages of FISH technology is the fact that different fluorochromes can be used simultaneously in conjunction with a series of probes labelled with different haptens. The result is a two-colour FISH image. For example, two probes may be hybridized to the same chromosome preparation. If one is labelled with biotin and detected with fluorescein-conjugated antibodies, and the other is labelled with digoxigenin and detected using Texas red, then both loci will be detected simultaneously as areas of green or red fluorescence. This approach can be extended by also using directly labelled probes in the same experiment, or when probes labelled with a mixture of two haptens are used. If such probes are detected by antibodies conjugated to two different fluorochromes, the result is a signal of intermediate colour; red fluorescence by Texas red and green fluorescence from fluorescein will give an orange signal. A series of probes can be labelled with different ratios of the same two haptens. The resulting fluorescence can be converted to a digital signal in a CCD camera and dedicated software will recognize subtle differences in fluorescence. These will then be allocated false colours. This approach has led to the development of spectral karyotyping, which is described later.

After detection of the probes, it is necessary to detect the remaining areas of the chromosomes or nuclei to which probe has not hybridized. This is done using the fluorochromes 4,6-diamino-2-phenyl-indole (DAPI), Hoechst 33258 or propidium iodide. Combinations of DAPI and propidium iodide will produce a banding pattern that can be helpful in chromosome identification. However, due to the fact that it is excited by more than one wavelength and fluoresces at several different wavelengths, propidium iodide may cause problems where images are captured using monochrome CCD cameras.

Applications in basic research

Although this technology can potentially be used with all species of eukaryote, this chapter will concentrate on uses in human genetics. FISH can be used to detect genes or other DNA sequences from specific chromosomal regions. The precision required by the experiment determines the approach to be used. At the simplest level, the process can be used to identify whole chromosomes, a technique known as 'chromosome painting'. In this case it is necessary to isolate DNA from a single human chromosome in order to make a probe. This is carried out in one of two ways. Originally, rodent × human somatic cell hybrids were used as a source of DNA. In these cell hybrids it is possible to isolate clones containing only a single human chromosome. DNA is isolated from such clones and the human DNA is specifically amplified using primers complimentary to *alu* sequences. These represent a highly repeated sequence found in human but absent from rodent DNA.

It is now possible to isolate specific human metaphase chromosomes directly, using fluorescence-activated cell sorting (FACS). DNA from the pellet of purified chromosomes is amplified by PCR using degenerate primers. This is now the method of choice for commercial suppliers of chromosome paints. Chromosome painting is particularly useful for the study of translocations. This is well illustrated in Figure 37.1. Here chromosome painting is used to identify the chromosomes involved in a translocation that has arisen in a human tumour. Small translocated fragments of chromosomes are often only detectable using this approach.

Refinement of the chromosome painting principle has led to protocols in which each pair of chromosomes in a cell can be identified simultaneously. This is referred to as 'spectral karyotyping'. In this technique, paints for each chromosome pair are hybridized to the chromosomes in the same reaction. Each chromosome paint is a mixture of several different fluorochromes, combined in different ratios. This means that the fluorescence emitted by each chromosome has a specific spectrum. This is

detected by the sensor and the software attributes a different false colour to each spectrum. The result is a computer image in which all chromosomes can be detected by their own specific colour.

A more sophisticated use of FISH is required to map the chromosomal location of a specific gene sequence. For this task, DNA cloned in YACs, BACs or cosmids is normally used as probe. This provides sufficient fluorescence to be easily detectable. Examples are shown in Figure 37.1. The procedures involved are similar to those employed for chromosome painting, but a greater amplification of the signal may be required. FISH is much more successful for this task than the previously used radiolabelled probes, because of the reduced background and the short time required to complete the experiment (2 days as compared to several weeks needed for exposure of autoradiographs). As described earlier, more than one probe may be used simultaneously. This approach can be used in different ways. When attempting to localize a probe on a chromosome, it is often necessary to identify the chromosome unambiguously at the same time. This is done by using a probe for a centromeric DNA repeat sequence specific to the chromosome in question. To determine the order of closely linked genes along the chromosome, dual- or triple-colour FISH can be used. Because of the colours used, this process is often referred as 'traffic lighting'. The position of probe on a chromosome can sometimes be identified by the banding pattern, but is often expressed

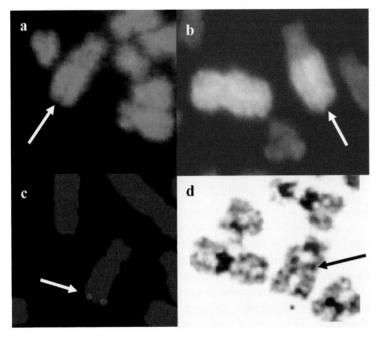

Figure 37.1 (a) Part of a metaphase from a human tumour cell stained with DAPI. A morphologically atypical chromosome is indicated by the white arrow. (b) The same chromosome from a metaphase that has been hybridized to chromosome paint for chromosome 2. Clearly, the distal region of the chromosome (arrow) is composed of material derived from chromosome 2. The brown chromosomal stain is propidium iodide and the paint is labelled with FITC. A normal copy of chromosome 2 is also present in the frame. A similar approach showed that the rest of the chromosome is composed of chromosome 17. (c, d) How FISH can be used to map the translocation point. A BAC that maps to the distal region of chromosome 17, 17q25.3, as shown in (c), was hybridized to the translocation chromosome in the tumour cell. The fact that it be seen in (d) maps the translocation to the extreme distal telomere of chromosome 17. (c) and (d) are digital images obtained using a CCD camera

simply as F/pter units. These represent the fractional distance from the telomere of the p arm of the chromosome, as compared to the length of the entire chromosome.

A serious limitation to the mapping of genes by FISH is caused by the relatively condensed state of mitotic metaphase chromosomes. This means that signals from genes lying within approximately 1–2 Mb of each other will overlap, and it is not possible to distinguish the two separate signals. A number of approaches have been used to overcome this problem. Chromatin is much less condensed during interphase, and sequences that could not be separated on metaphase chromosomes are often resolvable by hybridization of probes to the nuclei of non-dividing cells. A drawback in this system is that it is not possible to orientate genes in relation to the centromere. An alternative process that allows this is the use of meiotic chromosome preparations. These are considerably more elongated than mitotic chromosome preparations. However, they are not so convenient to prepare. One approach that has been used successfully to produce elongated mitotic chromosomes has been to use cytospin preparations of unfixed metaphases. A cytospin is a device frequently used in haematology to prepare slides of blood cells. It consists of a modified centrifuge in which cells are spun directly onto slides. When unfixed metaphases that have been swollen in hypotonic saline are treated in this way, the shear forces produced during centrifugation stretch the chromosomes up to twenty times their normal length. Even though this causes many of the metaphases to be disrupted and chromosomes to be deformed, it has an advantage over interphase analysis, in that individual chromosomes can be identified and the orientation of FISH signals to centromeres and telomeres can be observed.

The ultimate degree of resolution that can be obtained with FISH analysis is found in the technique of fibre FISH. Here the probe is hybridized to DNA that has been spread on a slide after removal of most or all of its chromatin packaging. No information at all can be obtained on the orientation of the signal to the chromosome, but the technique is extremely powerful for fine-scale analysis of small regions of the genome. Spreading of DNA can be achieved in a number of ways. Extended chromatin fibres can be obtained from nuclei of unfixed interphase cells treated on microscope slides with detergent and high salt to remove histones. This causes the looped structure of chromatin to untangle and the DNA extends to a length comparable with that of pure DNA. Such techniques are known as 'halo production' or DIRVISH (direct visual hybridization). These allow ordering of probes to a lower resolution limit of 3–5 kb. Purified DNA can also be spread on microscope slides

for use in fine structure analysis. The DNA may be entrapped in agarose plugs, such as those used for pulsed-field gel electrophoresis, which are melted and gently spread on the slide, or DNA in solution can be allowed to spread on silanated slides. In this case, the end of the molecule binds to the glass and the rest of the DNA is combed out into a pattern that is more or less linear by the meniscus as the solution evaporates.

Both of these protocols facilitate extremely fine-scale study. Typical examples include ordering of probes produced by PCR along DNA cloned in YACs or cosmids. This can be very useful in circumstances where a contig (a group of ordered overlapping cloned DNA fragments) is incomplete and the size of gaps need to be estimated.

Applications in medical genetics

As noted above, chromosome painting is particularly useful for detecting translocations that would be too small to be resolved unambiguously conventional G-banding. Other uses that can be made of FISH include detection of aneuploidy, particularly in amniocentesis. Here analysis of interphase nuclei can again be undertaken. Rather than using whole chromosome paints to detect numbers of homologues, probes specific to repeated DNA sequences found at the centromeres of different chromosomes are used. This can detect the presence of extra copies of the chromosomes involved in the common aneuploid syndromes, such as Down's, Edward's and Pateau's. The sex of an embryo can also be determined in amniotic cells using two-colour probes for X and Y chromosomes. In these procedures FISH allows for a result to be obtained in a much shorter time than conventional chromosome analysis, where cells must be cultured, and has the added advantage that, as only interphase cells are necessary, the number of cells scored can be very high. However it is more expensive and does not give as much information on the nature of any cytogenetic abnormality as G-banding, e.g. it will not distinguish between the presence of an intact extra chromosome and a fragment of the chromosome containing the centromere.

Applications in cancer diagnosis and research

It is in the study and accurate diagnosis of cancers and leukaemia that FISH currently makes its major contribution to medicine. In the vast majority of cases, malignant tissue shows at least some cytogenetic aberrations. Conventional cytogenetics can be applied only with some difficulty to these situations but FISH, particularly on interphase nuclei, can produce results accurately and in a short period of time, two criteria that are of obvious importance in patient management.

Although random translocations are common in tumour cells, many cancers, particularly leukaemias and lymphomas, carry specific translocations that can be used to make an accurate diagnosis. These often result in fusion between copies of two different genes, creating a novel gene. A classical example of this is the Philadelphia chromosome, which is detected in chronic myeloid leukaemia. Here, highly specific translocations between chromosomes 9 and 22 bring about fusion of the *abl* and *BCR* oncogenes to produce a novel tyrosine kinase. Here conventional G-banding is problematical. This is because the malignant cells may not provide significant numbers of metaphases *in vitro* and the quality of chromosome spreads is usually well below that obtained from normal lymphocytes. Chromosome painting can be applied even where the quality of chromosome preparations is poor, as the target chromosomes will be identifiable due to fluorescence, even though they may not be clearly detected by G-banding. The main advantage of FISH technology in this instance is again the ability to obtain cytogenetic information from non-dividing cells. The use of fluorescent probes, often cosmids, for regions on either side of the tumour-specific translocation will allow an accurate diagnosis. The two probes are labelled with different haptens, so that they can be detected as two different colours, usually red and green. In normal cells, where no translocation is present, two red and two green fluorescent spots will appear on the nucleus. The dots will be distributed randomly across the nucleus. In the presence of a translocation, one red and one green dot will be found in close proximity to each other in every tumour cell. Overlap will often occur and a yellow region of mixed signal will be observed. This approach allows a clear-cut detection of translocation in a large number of cells and can differentiate between normal cells and leukaemic cells in the sample. In addition to diagnostic work, this system can also be used to look for the presence of residual leukaemic cells in patients after therapy. Specific aneuploidies can be detected in leukaemic tissue by the same methods as described above for amniotic cells.

Cytogenetic analysis of solid tumours has always lagged behind that of blood cancers. This is in part a consequence of the greater difficulty of obtaining usable chromosome preparations. Despite this, many solid tumours have been found to carry specific chromosomal aberrations. These can be looked for by interphase FISH, either in touch preparations, where excised tumour material is 'touched' onto microscope slides to leave behind a film of cells, or by the use of cytological smears of small numbers of cells obtained in fine needle aspirates.

In addition to translocations and changes in chromosome number, tumours often contain multiple copies of oncogenes or genes conferring resistance to chemotherapeutic drugs. These arise either as elongate regions of chromosomes where the gene has ampified *in situ*, known as homogenously staining regions (HSRs), or in small extrachromosomal elements, referred to as 'double minutes' (DMs). Oncogene amplification is an important factor in prognosis. FISH allows for the detection of amplification in interphase nuclei of tumour samples. An example of this is screening of breast cancer biopsies for amplification of the oncogene *erbB-2* on chromosome 17. Normal cells in the biopsy will provide a control, showing two small fluorescent spots corresponding to the two unamplified copies of the gene present, whereas the area of fluorescence is much greater where amplification has taken place. Examples of this are seen in Figure 37.2.

A somewhat different application of FISH, in both cancer research and treatment, has been the development of a technique that will provide an overall estimate of specific gains and losses of chromosomes, or chromosome regions from a particular tumour. This is known as comparative genome hybridization. Here DNA is extracted from the tumour after removal from the patient. This DNA is labelled with a fluorochrome (green). It is mixed with DNA extracted from normal cells, which been labelled red, and the mixture hybridized onto normal metaphase chromosomes. The differently labelled probes compete for sites the chromosomes. If the tumour shows no gains or losses of chromosomal material, the resulting *in situ* hybridization will contain 46 chromosomes, all of which will fluoresce an even yellow. However regions of the tumour that have undergone amplification will be over-represented in the extracted DNA and will out-compete the red fluorescing DNA. Such regions will therefore appear green. Conversely, regions lost from the tumour, which are likely to contain suppressor genes, will fluoresce red. Analysis of this two-colour competitive hybridization requires sophisticated computer software, but it may become a major tool for providing a broad spectrum molecular analysis of individual tumours.

FISH appears to have an established role in molecular biology. How the technique evolves in future will depend on the increased understanding of genetic processes in this disease. In some of the applications to which it is put it may be replaced by non-cytogenetic techniques, such

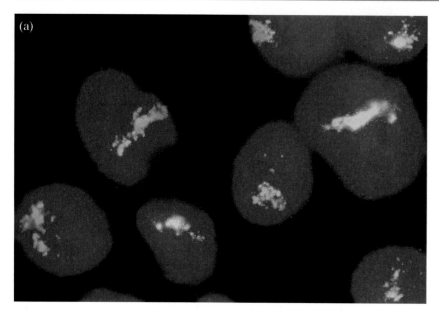

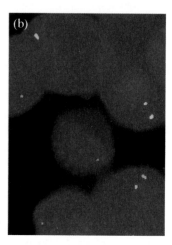

Figure 37.2 (a) Interphase cells from a fine needle aspirate of a breast tumour that have been hybridized with a probe for the oncogene erbB-2. In this case the cells show amplification of the oncogene, while in (b) the aspirate contains cells in which the oncogene has not been amplified, and each cell shows one or two spots, corresponding to the normal genes. In smear preparations made from fine needle aspirates the cells are not flattened, which explains why the erbB-2 signal is not in the same focal lane in each cell. In these examples the probe was directly labelled with FITC and the nuclei counterstained with DAPI. Courtesy of Dr Damien McManus, Royal Victoria Hospital, Belfast

as PCR. Areas where this may happen include the detection of cancer-specific translocations, or the determination of sex in amniotic cells. However, one of the most important advantages of FISH is that it does not destroy the cells on which it is carried out. In many areas this ability to obtain molecular genetic information while still being able to identify cellular and tissue structure is essential, e.g. in the molecular pathology of cancer. In addition, the coupling of molecular and cytological techniques provides a valuable control against erroneous results arising from contamination of samples. For these reasons, the technique is likely to remain of importance in both research and the applied biosciences for a considerable time.

Further reading

Haaf T, Ward D C. Structural analysis of a-satellite DNA and centromere proteins using extended chromatin and chromosomes. *Hum Mol Genet* 1994; **3**: 697–709.

Heiskanen M, Hellsten E, Kallioniemi O-P *et al*. Visual mapping by fibre—FISH. *Genomics* 1995; **30**: 31–36.

Kallioniemi A, Kaltioniemi O-P, Sudar D *et al*. Comparative genomic hybridization for molecular cytogenetic analysis of solid turnouts. *Science* 1992; **258**: 818–821.

Pardue M L, Gall J G. Chromosomal localization of mouse satellite DNA. *Science* 1970; **168**: 1356–1358.

Schrock E, duManoir S, Veldman T *et al*. Multicolor spectral karyotyping of human chromosomes. *Science* 1996; **273**: 494–497.

SECTION 7

CLINICAL CHEMISTRY

38

Acquisition, uses and interpretation of clinical biochemical data

William J Marshall

Introduction

Clinical biochemical investigations are used extensively in medicine for a variety of purposes (see Table 38.1). The majority of the more familiar investigations involve the measurement of a substance in a body fluid, usually serum (or plasma) or urine. Assays may also be made on other fluids, e.g. spinal fluid, fluid obtained by paracentesis, intestinal secretions and faeces, and on biopsy samples of body tissues.

The results of most clinical biochemical investigations are expressed quantitatively as a concentration or often, in the case of enzyme measurements, as an activity. Molecular genetic analysis, although increasingly part of the repertoire of clinical biochemical laboratories, is not discussed in this chapter.

The fact that results are expressed numerically affords them an apparent simplicity: they appear easy to assess and to compare with reference ('normal') ranges or with results obtained previously in the same patient(s). Whereas, for example, a subtle sign on a radiograph may be open to a variety of interpretations (or may be missed by an inexperienced observer), a serum sodium concentration of 143 mmol/l appears unequivocally 'normal' (the reference range is 135–145 mmol/l) and is clearly different from a value of 147 mmol/l, which is by definition 'abnormal'.

But is it? Let us examine these statements in some detail. A serum sodium concentration may be within the normal range, but that does not exclude the possibility that a subtle abnormality of sodium or water homeostasis is present, neither does it mean that the individual is necessarily healthy. Conversely, the finding that an individual has a serum sodium concentration of 147 mmol/l does not necessarily mean that a disorder of sodium or water homeostasis is present: indeed, the individual may be perfectly healthy. These statements follow from the fact that, as is discussed later in this chapter, 5% of 'normal' individuals would *be expected* to have values outside the reference range, although clearly the further a measured value is from the limits of the reference range, the more likely it is to be of pathological significance.

Comparison of a result with a reference range may be of value when the measurement is made in an individual for the first time. In practice, measurements are often made repeatedly, e.g. to determine the progress of a condition or response to treatment. A given measured value can then be compared with a previous one to see whether a significant change has occurred. But whether, for example, a serum sodium concentration of 145 mmol/l on one day is significantly different (i.e. truly represents a physiological or pathological change) from one of 147 mmol/l on the previous day requires a knowledge of the reliability of the data, not only in terms of analytical quality, but also of any biological variation that affects the concentration of sodium *in vivo*. Finally, any conclusions that are drawn will be unreliable if the sample to be analysed is not collected and handled prior to analysis in a way that does not affect sodium concentration.

The Science of Laboratory Diagnosis, Second Edition   Edited by David Burnett and John Crocker
© 2005 John Wiley & Sons, Ltd

Table 38.1   The uses of biochemical tests in medicine

Use	Example
Diagnosis	Blood glucose concentration (diabetes)
Assessment of severity	Serum creatinine concentration (renal failure)
Prognosis	Prothrombin time, severity of acidosis, etc. (acute liver failure)
Monitoring disease/ treatment	Glycated haemoglobin (diabetes)
Long-term follow-up	Some tumour markers (cancer)
Screening	Neonatal blood TSH (congenital hypothyroidism)
Detecting drug toxicity	Thyroid function tests (for patients treated with lithium)
Stratification for clinical trials	Plasma cholesterol concentration (for trials of cholesterol-lowering drugs)

Lest readers be concerned about whether any conclusions at all can be drawn from clinical biochemical data (or, and worse, be dismissive that these matters are trivial and of no consequence), it should be emphasized that laboratory personnel go to considerable efforts to ensure that the data that they provide are reliable, i.e. that they are accurate (are a true measure of the variable in question) and precise (are reproducible). It is also important that the analyte can be measured over a clinically useful concentration range, and that results are available sufficiently quickly to be used to inform clinical management. To achieve this requires appropriate methodology and instrumentation, and adherence to procedures designed to maximize quality.

Nevertheless, it is still important for the users of clinical biochemical laboratory data to be aware of the sources of error (not all of which are in the laboratory), and of pitfalls in the interpretation of results, if they are to obtain the maximum clinically useful information from them. Most of the rest of this chapter is divided into two sections: the first deals with sample collection and analysis; the second with the uses and interpretation of biochemical data.

Sample collection and analysis

Factors that can affect the quality of results are conventionally divided into pre-analytical, analytical and post-analytical, i.e. respectively arising before the sample is analysed, during the analysis, and once results have been generated.

Pre-analytical factors

Biochemical variables can be affected by many physiological variables (Table 38.2). In addition, all biochemical variables are subject to random biological variation.

Table 38.2   Examples of physiological factors affecting the results of biochemical tests

Factor	Test (all in serum or plasma)
Age	Cholesterol, urate, alkaline phosphatase
Sex	Gonadal steroids, gonadotrophins, HDL cholesterol
Body mass	Triglycerides
Time	Cortisol (diurnal variation)
	Gonadotrophins (catamenial variation in women)
	25-Hydroxycholecalciferol (seasonal variation)
Stress	Cortisol, prolactin, growth hormone, catecholamines, glucose
Posture	Renin, aldosterone, plasma proteins
Food intake	Glucose, triglycerides, phosphate

For some, particularly those that are subject to tight feedback control, e.g. plasma calcium concentration, this variation may be small, but for others it may be a significant factor to be taken into account when interpreting results.

The effect of drugs on biochemical variables *in vivo* is potentially a huge problem, although in practice the number of important examples is relatively small. The hypokalaemia that frequently occurs in patients treated with diuretics is one such. Biochemical measurements are also often made to assess the effect of drugs, e.g. measurement of glucose and glycated haemoglobin in patients with diabetes treated with hypoglycaemic agents. Drugs can also be a source of potential analytical error: e.g. prednisolone cross-reacts with cortisol in many immunoassays.

Finally, pre-analytical errors can occur because of incorrect sample collection, e.g. measuring glucose in a blood sample not collected in a container with fluoride to inhibit glycolysis, or handling, e.g. causing haemolysis or evaporation of water. All laboratories publish handbooks that should include information on the type of sample to collect and any special conditions that must be observed.

Exceptionally, errors can arise because of misidentification of samples. Extreme vigilance is necessary to prevent this. Request forms must be properly completed and matched to the patient, and samples positively identified at all stages of handling, e.g. if serum has to be transferred from the initial (primary) container to a secondary container for analysis. In many hospitals and clinics, blood and other samples are collected by trained nurses or phlebotomists. Many laboratories find that mistakes are more likely to occur if samples are collected by doctors. In laboratory medicine, as in clinical medicine, it is good practice to take as much care with apparently simple procedures as it is with complicated ones.

Analytical factors

A detailed discussion of laboratory procedures is beyond the scope of this chapter. It is a condition of accreditation by CPA(UK) Ltd (Clinical Laboratory Accreditation) that laboratories use acceptable internal quality control and external quality assurance procedures. Problems that can affect the quality of results are discussed in the chapters on individual analytical techniques.

Post-analytical factors

Once results have been generated and validated, errors may still arise before they reach patients' notes. With increasing use of electronic transmission of results from laboratory to ward or clinic, the risk of such errors has decreased considerably, but it can never be entirely eliminated. It is a particular risk if results are telephoned, as may be necessary if they need to be communicated to the doctor urgently. Ironically, these are just the sorts of results for which an error could have particularly harmful consequences.

The interpretation of laboratory data

Although biochemical data are extensively used in the diagnosis and management of patients, they rarely provide a complete diagnosis. More often, they reflect pathological processes rather than specific diseases, and may not even be specific for one process, although in a particular clinical situation or in the light of other investigations, one may be more likely than another. For example, a low serum albumin concentration has many potential causes, including decreased synthesis, increased volume of distribution or increased loss or catabolism, and each of these itself has several potential causes. In a patient known to have chronic liver disease, decreased synthesis would be likely to be the most important cause.

Biochemical results can be assessed in relation to various criteria, according to the reasons for performing the test: the reference range for comparable healthy people; the range of values expected in a particular condition; cut-off values or action limits, or results obtained previously in the same individual.

Normal ranges and reference intervals

The term 'normal' has several meanings. A normal (Gaussian) distribution describes a symmetrical distribution of data around a mean that can be described by a specific mathematical function. Statistically, the normal range is the range of values for such data from the mean minus two standard deviations to the mean plus two standard deviations, and encompasses approximately 95% of the values. For many people, however, normal means 'conforming to type' or, by implication, 'healthy', since normal ranges for human biological variables are usually based on measurements made on a sample of individuals from a 'normal' (in the sense of 'healthy') population.

There are many pitfalls in the use of normal ranges. Within the disciplines of laboratory medicine, it has been argued extensively that the term should not be used. Instead of 'normal population' the term 'reference population' is preferred, since this does not imply any specific characteristics (e.g. health) in the population. (Indeed, there is no reason why one should not attempt to define the ranges of test results characteristic of a reference population composed of patients with particular diseases.) The upper and lower values of the distribution are termed the 'reference limits' and the range between them the 'reference interval'. But worthy though this endeavour is to direct more objective analysis of data, the terms are not widely used outside laboratories and indeed, many laboratories continue to refer to 'normal ranges'. Furthermore, reference intervals are often based on the same data as were used to calculate normal ranges and are identical to them.

By definition, since the normal range encompasses only 95% of values from the population being studied, 5% of values will fall outside this range—2.5% above and 2.5% below. Thus, some values in healthy people will inevitably fall outside the normal range for the population, although common sense tells us that the further away a result is from the limits of the range, the more likely it is to be 'abnormal' in the sense of being pathologically significant. The more variables that are measured, the more likely at least one is to fall outside the relevant normal range. If 20 independent analytes were to be measured, the probability that one would be abnormal is 0.64, i.e. better than evens. Since automated analysers routinely measure this number of analytes, falsely 'abnormal' results are an inevitable occurrence.

Another problem in interpretation stems from the fact that the range of variation of a test result in an individual is likely to be less than the range seen in the population, since the population, even when comparable in terms of, for example, age, sex and ethnic origin, is composed of individuals who are genetically distinct. The normal range for plasma creatinine concentration in adult males is approximately 60–120 μmol/l, but the range of values that would be observed with repeated measurements in a single individual would be much less than this. An individual might have a result within the normal range as defined for the population that was actually abnormal for him.

There follow some specific examples where normal ranges are not appropriate standards against which to judge patients' results.

Example 1: a result within the normal range may falsely suggest normal function

Creatinine is measured in serum as an index of renal function, specifically of the glomerular filtration rate (GFR). Creatinine concentration is inversely proportional to the GFR (Figure 38.1) and in practice, the GFR may fall to half normal (equivalent to the loss of one functioning kidney) before serum creatinine concentration exceeds the upper limit of normal. Serum creatinine concentration is thus an insensitive index of early loss of renal function.

Example 2: a result within the normal range may falsely suggest no risk of disease

If plasma cholesterol concentrations are measured on a group of healthy people, it is possible to derive a normal range, but it is well established that increasing cholesterol concentrations are linked to an increasing risk

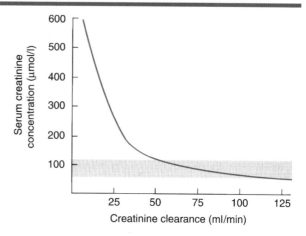

Figure 38.1 Serum creatinine concentration and creatinine clearance. Because clearance (a measure of the glomerular filtration rate, GFR) is inversely related to serum creatinine concentration, clearance may fall to half its normal value (approx. 120 ml/min) before serum creatinine concentration becomes abnormal. The shaded area shows the normal reference range for serum creatinine concentrations

of coronary heart disease, even within this range (Figure 38.2). For cholesterol, therefore, the concept of a normal range is misleading. Rather, we define ideal concentrations (which to some extent themselves depend on the presence of other risk factors for coronary disease) and threshold values for intervention and target values for treatment. The target value for secondary

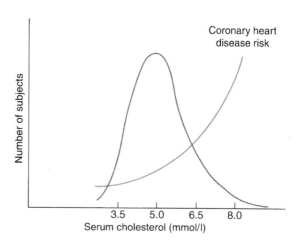

Figure 38.2 The distribution of serum cholesterol concentrations in healthy adult subjects and the risk of coronary heart disease. Approximately one-third of values exceed the current recommended ideal concentration (5.0 mmol/l) and are associated with a significantly increased risk of coronary disease

prevention of coronary disease in the UK is currently a total cholesterol concentration of less than 5.0 mmol/l (LDL less than 3.0), although there is evidence that even lower targets may be more appropriate.

Example 3: any concentration is abnormal

Since drugs are not physiological constituents of the body, drug concentrations measured in patients cannot be compared with normal ranges. In the context of therapeutic drug monitoring, 'therapeutic' and 'toxic' ranges are more appropriate (although even these terms should be interpreted with caution), whereas in the context of poisoning, 'action levels' are used to help to determine appropriate management.

Critical differences

The preceding discussion relates to the comparison of measured data with expected values based on observations on other people. When a measurement has been repeated, it is more relevant to consider it in relation to the previous value. The relevant question is whether the two values differ significantly.

This will depend on two factors: the innate variability of the parameter being measured, even when sampling conditions are identical (biological variation), and the analytical variation, i.e. the inevitable error attendant on any measurement (albeit, it is to be hoped, very small). Both of these can be determined from the results of repeated measurements of the same and a series of similar samples, and a function known as the critical difference (CD) calculated from the equation: $CD = 2.8 \times (SD_A^2 + SD_B^2)^{1/2}$, where SD_A and SD_B are the analytical and biological standard deviations, respectively. The CD indicates the least difference between two values that is unlikely to have occurred as a result of biological and analytical variation at a probability of 0.95 ($p = 0.05$). Whether any such change is clinically significant is another matter, but clearly a change cannot be considered to be of potential clinical significance if it is less than the CD.

The concept of critical difference is not widely understood outside laboratories, yet is fundamental to the use of laboratory data in monitoring the natural history of disease and response to treatment. Values for some CDs should be available from the local laboratory. Critical differences are independent of normal ranges. Indeed, two results may be critically different yet both be within the normal range. Consider, for example, an increase in

serum creatinine concentration from 80 to 100 μmol/l: the CD for creatinine in this range of concentrations is about 17 μmol/l. Thus, an increase of 20 μmol/l is of potential clinical signficance (implying a decrease in renal function), even though both values are within the normal range. This discussion emphasizes the fact that serial measurements in individuals can (and in practice frequently are) more informative than 'one-off' measurements.

Action limits, target values, cut-off points and predictive values

For some laboratory investigations, it may be appropriate to consider the results against *action limits*, i.e. values used to determine whether a specific action should be taken. Obvious examples include action limits of the concentrations of poisons to direct treatment, e.g. with serum paracetamol concentration to indicate whether treatment with N-acetylcysteine should be initiated (or continued) to prevent hepatic damage. Many laboratories have action limits to determine how they respond to a result—typically, when an abnormal value should be telephoned to the requesting clinician, or when a further investigation should be performed to provide further information, e.g. to trigger serum protein electrophoresis to look for a paraprotein when a patient's total globulin concentration is unexpectedly high.

Because for most laboratory data there is an overlap between the range of values that are usually seen in healthy people and those that occur in disease (particularly in the early stages of the latter, or when it is relatively mild), the selection of action points is particularly critical when tests are used for screening (detecting subclinical disease). Setting the action limit (more frequently called a *cut-off* value in this context) too low will mean that, while everyone with the condition will be diagnosed correctly using the test, this will be at the expense of a miscategorizing a significant number of healthy persons as possibly having the disease (false positives). Setting the cut-off value too high excludes all healthy inviduals, but some with the disease will be missed (false negatives; see Figure 38.3). In screening for a serious but potentially treatable condition, it is desirable to have no false negatives (missed cases). A classic example is the widespread neonatal screening programme for phenylketonuria and congenital hypothyroidism. It should be emphasized that screening tests are not diagnostic. Further, definitive, investigations are required to establish the diagnosis, and, in the false positives, to exclude it.

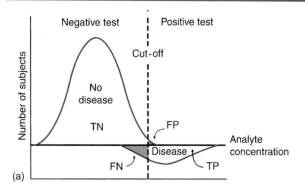

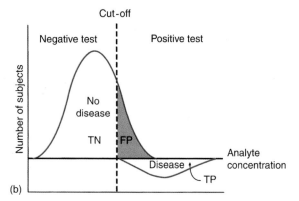

Figure 38.3 The effect of moving the cut-off point that determines the positivity/negativity of a test result. Hypothetical distributions for the concentration of an analyte in patients with and without disease are shown. Because these overlap, if the cut-off is selected to decrease the numbers of false positive results (and hence increase specificity) (a), there are significant numbers of false negative results (decreased sensitivity). If the cut-off is set lower (b), false negatives are eliminated (maximizing sensitivity) but at the expense of increasing the number of false positives (thus decreasing specificity). The distributions of values for individuals with disease have been shown below the horizontal axis for clarity

Table 38.3 Sensitivity, specificity and the predictive value of tests

		Test result	
		Positive	Negative
Disease status	Positive	True positive (TP)	False negative (FN)
	Negative	False positive (FP)	True negative (TN)

Sensitivity (positivity in disease) $= TP/(TP + FN)$
Specificity (negativity in health) $= TN/(TN + FP)$
Positive predictive value (PV^{+}) $= TP/(TP + FP)$
Negative predictive value (PV^{-}) $= TN(TN + FN)$

The numbers of true and false positive and negative results can also be used to calculate the predictive value (PV) of a positive or negative result, i.e. the probability that a positive (or negative) test will correctly classify the person being tested.

The concepts of sensitivity, specificity and predictive values can also be used to describe the performance of tests done for diagnostic purposes, but both in this case and in screening it is important to appreciate that they can only be applied reliably to patients who are similar to those on whom the data were derived. A test for, say, rheumatoid arthritis may appear to have high sensitivity and specificity when applied to a group of patients with established disease. However, the sensitivity would be likely to be much lower in a group of people in whom the disease had a very low prevalence, or who had much earlier disease. This is a major drawback to (and frequent source of error in) the use of these concepts.

The performance of screening tests can be measured by calculating functions known (in this context) as sensitivity (a measure of the ability of the test to detect people who have the disease) and specificity (a measure of its ability to identify people who do not have it) (Table 38.3). Such calculations require reliable identification of true and false positives and negatives, which in turn requires a 'gold standard' or definitive diagnostic test that unequivocally identifies the presence or absence of disease. Histological examination of tissue or molecular genetic analysis may provide the gold standard, but sometimes true positivity or negativity can only be determined in retrospect, by observing the outcome.

Likelihood ratios

These functions express the odds that a given finding, e.g. a certain test result, would occur in a person with, as opposed to without, a certain condition. The likelihood ratio (LR) for a positive result is given by $LR_{pos} = sensitivity/(1 - specificity)$. The odds that a negative result would occur in a person with, as opposed to without, a particular condition (LR_{neg}) is given by $LR_{neg} = (1 - sensitivity)/specificity$. Likelihood ratios can be used to convert pre-test probability (in a screening test, this will be the prevalence of the condition in the population being screened) into the post-test probability of the condition being present. Such data can be used to direct management and are potentially of great value in clinical audit.

Evidence-based clinical biochemistry

It will have been seen that biochemical and other laboratory test results must be interpreted with care. Many currently available tests provide less reliable information than is often appreciated or assumed, not usually because of analytical problems but, rather, because of poor sensitivity and specificity. New diagnostic tests are being developed and introduced all the time, and are usually enthusiastically promoted by the manufacturers of test kits, and supported by clinicians who are seeking improved diagnostic performance. Their evaluation, however, is often poor. Ideally, all laboratory tests should be evaluated with a similar rigour to that required before the introduction of new treatments, so that they can be used rationally, on the basis of scientifically sound evidence.

Conclusion

Biochemical tests have become an essential part of modern medical practice. They have many potential uses but, for many tests, the ease with they can be requested and performs belies their complexity. They should all be performed with care and interpreted through an appreciation of the underlying physiological and pathological principles, whatever the purpose for which they are to be used.

Further reading

Fraser CG, Fogarty Y. Interpreting laboratory results. *Br Med J* 1989; **298**: 1659–1660.

Jones R, Payne B. *Clinical Investigation and Statistics in Laboratory Medicine.* 1997: ACB Venture Publications, London.

Marshall WJ. The uses of biochemical data in clinical medicine. The acquisition of biochemical data. The interpretation of biochemical data. In *Clinical Biochemistry*, Marshall WJ, Bangert SK (eds). 1995: Churchill Livingstone, Edinburgh, 1–24.

Moore RA. Evidence-based clinical biochemistry: a personal view. *Ann Clin Biochem* 1997; **34**: 1–7.

Oxford Centre for Evidence-Based Medicine. Likelihood ratios. http://www.cebm.net/likelihood_ratios.asp

Price CP. Christenson RH (eds). Evidence-based Laboratory Medicine. 2003. Washington: AACC Press.

Read MC, Lachs MS, Feinstein AR. Use of methodological standardized in diagnostic test research: getting better but still not good. *J Am Med Assoc* 1995; **274**: 645–651.

Tape TG. Interpreting diagnostic tests. http://gim.unmc.edu/dxtests/Default.htm

39

Immunoassay in clinical biochemistry

Joan Butler and Susan M Chambers

Introduction

Immunoassay uses the antigen–antibody reaction as a means of quantitating either the antigen or the antibody. Most applications in clinical biochemistry have used the technique to quantitate the antigen, whereas in immunology and microbiology it is also used to quantitate (or detect) circulating antibody. Antibodies can be raised against a wide variety of substances. Small molecules can be made immunogenic by chemical coupling to a large molecule, such as albumin or polylysine, and are then referred to as haptens.

Assay design

Despite the apparent complexity of published methods, there are two basic assay designs, competitive or limited antibody methods, using antigen labelled with a tracer or reporter molecule and having the generic title 'immunoassay', and non-competitive or excess antibody methods, using labelled antibody and having the generic title 'immunometric assay'.

In a *competitive assay*, the analyte in the sample (or calibrant) competes with labelled analyte for the binding sites on a limited amount of antibody. It is essential that the amount of antibody is insufficient to bind all the labelled analyte, so that competition for binding sites must occur. At equilibrium the amount of labelled analyte bound to the antibody will be inversely related to the amount of unlabelled analyte in the sample or calibrant. Determination of the label in the bound fraction will provide a measure of the amount of analyte, by comparison with a calibration curve:

$$Ag + Ag^* + Ab \quad \rightarrow \quad AgAb + Ag^*Ab + Ag^*$$
$$\textit{initial state} \qquad\qquad \textit{final state}$$

In order to determine the amount of labelled analyte in the bound (or free) fraction, these fractions must be separated, except in the rare cases where the signal from the label is modified by binding of the labelled analyte to the antibody.

In a *non-competitive* or *immunometric assay*, the conditions are such that the analyte is allowed to react with an excess of labelled antibody. The unreacted antibody is then separated, and the amount of labelled antibody bound to analyte is measured:

$$Ag + Ab^* \quad \rightarrow \quad AgAb^* + Ab^*$$
$$\textit{initial state} \qquad \textit{final state}$$

This simple design is the basis for a number of more complex formats. Analytes that are large molecules may be reacted with another antibody, termed the capture antibody, directed against a different and spatially distinct epitope on the analyte molecule, and usually linked to a solid phase:

$$Ab_1 + Ag + Ab_2^* \quad \rightarrow \quad Ab_1AgAb_2^* + Ab_1 + Ab_2^*$$
$$\textit{initial state} \qquad\qquad \textit{final state}$$

where Ab_1 = capture antibody, Ab_2^* = labelled antibody.

This assay design is the so-called sandwich or two-site immunometric assay, and is the design currently most

The Science of Laboratory Diagnosis, Second Edition   Edited by David Burnett and John Crocker
© 2005 John Wiley & Sons, Ltd

used for assay of polypeptides. The analyte must be large enough for simultaneous binding by two antibodies. Antibody addition to the sample may be simultaneous (a one-step format) or sequential (with removal of the sample before addition of the labelled antibody, a two-step format). More than one capture or labelled antibody may be used, giving a multi-site assay.

In requiring two distinct but connected epitopes, the two-site assay design offers considerably greater specificity than a competitive single-antibody design. Although polyclonal antisera can be used in sandwich assays, this design came into general use only when monoclonal antibodies became available.

In immunometric assays for small analytes, the unreacted labelled antibody is usually removed by the addition of analyte coupled to a solid phase. Attachment to a solid phase impairs reactivity and the coupled analyte will therefore not compete with free analyte from the sample. Alternatively, antibody specific for the complex of hapten and anti-analyte antibody, and not reactive to either of these components separately (anti-immune complex or anti-metatype antibody), can be used:

$$Ag + Ab_1 \rightarrow AgAb_1 + Ab_1 \rightarrow +Ab_2^* \rightarrow AgAb_1Ab_2^*$$
$$\hspace{9cm} +Ab_1 + Ab_2^*$$
$$\textit{initial state} \hspace{3cm} \textit{final state}$$

where $Ab_1 = anti\text{-}Ag$, $Ab_2 = anti\text{-}(AgAb_1)$.

This format demonstrates the fundamental difference between competitive and antibody excess immunoassays, viz. that the former measures signal from antibody not bound to analyte and the latter measures signal from antibody bound to analyte or antibody occupancy. The latter is inherently more sensitive, since it is easier to distinguish a small number from zero than to distinguish a large number from a slightly larger number. Moreover, antibody excess methods are more rapid, affected less by variations in reagent quality and quantity and may have a wider working range. Figure 39.1 shows typical calibration curves for a competitive immunoassay and a two-site immunometric assay.

Assay conditions and calibrators

The concentration of antibody or antibodies is chosen to optimise the working range of the assay for its clinical purpose, in general lower concentrations of antibody being required for lower concentrations of analyte. The steep part of the standard curve and the range of highest precision should correspond to the concentration range

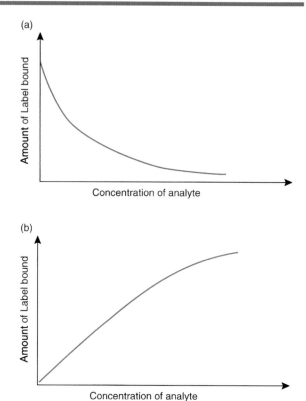

Figure 39.1 Typical standard curves for (a) a competitive immunoassay, (b) a two-site immunometric assay

over which values are required clinically. It follows that the working range has limitations, e.g. a human chorionic gonadotrophin assay designed for oncology will not be useful in determining concentrations in pregnancy.

Many factors other than amounts of reagents must be controlled within and between batches to maintain the optimization of an assay. Rate of reaction and position of equilibrium are dependent on temperature, pH and ionic strength. Cross-reactivity of structurally related molecules will also be affected by changes in these variables. As far as possible, these factors, especially the sample matrix, must be kept constant. If a reaction is not permitted to reach equilibrium, lack of constancy of timing can lead to drift, i.e. systematic error in the result according to the position of the sample in the batch. In automatic analysers these factors can be closely controlled, leading to consistency of results within and between laboratories.

Calibrants or standards can pose a special difficulty in immunoassay, since for many substances there is no practicable alternative assay system. In the case of polypeptide hormones, until the advent of recombinant

DNA technology it was not possible to prepare enough pure material for measurement by physicochemical methods to provide calibrators for immunoassay. For this reason, International Standards prepared for bioassays were adopted for immunoassays, with unitage assigned as the consensus of collaborative studies using a number of bioassay systems. These Standards contain a few micrograms of analyte with milligrams of albumin carrier and excipients, and absolute methods of analysis such as amino acid analysis cannot be used. Growth hormone and prolactin assays in the USA are inappropriately calibrated in mass terms.

The inherent heterogeneity of glycoprotein hormones is a major barrier to standardization, and has led to differing bioactivity/immunoactivity ratios in successive International Standards. Use of International Standards tends to minimize, but does not eliminate, differences between assays. Serum-based standard reference materials or certified reference materials cannot be used as primary calibrants, since immunoassays are subject to matrix effects. The ultimate aim is to calibrate protein assays in mass or molar terms, a severe challenge for many analytes. For discussion of the difficulties of calibration, see Bristow, 1998; Stenman, 2001.

Labels

Many different types of label or reporter molecule are in use. Labelling procedures are designed not to impair the binding of the labelled substance to its appropriate antibody or analyte. Measurement (detection) of the label may require further reagents and/or highly specialized equipment. Types of label in common use are given in Table 39.1.

Table 39.1   Types of label in common use

Radioisotopes
Chemiluminescence
    Enhanced chemiluminescence
    Electrochemiluminescence
Fluorescence
    Time-resolved fluorescence
Enzymes
    Colorimetry, rate colorimetry
    Fluorescence
    Chemiluminescence
    Amplification (cascades)

Radioisotopes are easily detectable, but have the disadvantage of being hazardous and requiring specific handling and disposal procedures. They also have a short 'shelf-life', as the labelled molecule is damaged by radioactive decay. With the advent of automation, they have become restricted to more specialized and low-volume assays.

Fluorescence polarization is only suitable for the estimation of small haptens and drugs, but other fluorescent methods are applicable to a wide range of analytes. Commonly used fluorophores include fluorescein, umbelliferone, luminol and rare-earth metals. Time-resolved fluorescence techniques use lanthanide chelates, which produce a relatively long-lived fluorescence; sensitivity is improved by taking readings after the short-lived background fluorescence produced by endogenous sample components has decayed. Sensitivity is also enhanced by the large Stokes' shift of lanthanide chelates (i.e. the difference in wavelength between the excitation and emission peaks) and their very narrow emission maxima, which reduce background fluorescence. Multiple labelling, using different lanthanides, is also possible, and offers great potential for multiplexed and miniaturized analysis. Lanthanide ions are also a component of cryptate labels; the ions are enclosed within a large organic 'cage-like' molecule, a cryptand, and the resulting cryptate is very stable and inert. The technique of time-resolved amplified cryptate emission is based on the amplified non-radiative transfer of energy from a fluorescent donor (the cryptate) to a spatially close acceptor molecule. Thus, bound and free label can be distinguished by their emission spectra, allowing a homogeneous assay system applicable to both large and small molecules.

In chemiluminescence, the excited molecule is produced by a chemical reaction; chemiluminescent substrates produce photons (light), usually by an oxidative reaction. In electrochemiluminescence, light emission is initiated electronically by applying a voltage to the reaction solution, eliminating problems associated with reagent addition and mixing.

Labelling with enzymes and detection with substrates giving colorimetric, rate colorimetric, fluorimetric or chemiluminometric endpoints gives greater sensitivity and a wider working range. This technique, when applied to fluorescence or chemiluminescence, is described as 'enzyme-enhanced' or 'enzyme-amplified'. One form of heterogeneous solid-phase assay that has gained widespread application to many antigen–antibody systems is the enzyme-linked immunosorbent assay, or ELISA. The sample is first incubated with a solid-phase antibody (typically on a microtitre plate), then any unbound antigen is removed by washing, after which a second, enzyme-labelled, antibody is added. Enzyme activity bound to the solid phase is proportional to the concentration of captured antigen (i.e. analyte).

The search for the 'ideal' label continues (see Kricka, 1994); recent developments include sub-micrometre-sized particulate labels coupled to specific binding agents, offering greater sensitivity.

Homogeneous assays

The term 'homogeneous' is used for immunoassays in which separation of bound and free label is not required. In such systems the signal is modified by antibody binding, with the result that bound and free label can be distinguished in the reaction mixture, e.g. binding of enzyme-labelled analyte to the antibody may inhibit the activity of the enzyme, either by steric hindrance or by inducing distortion of the active site. This system (EMIT[R], enzyme-multiplied immunoassay technique, Syva) can be used on a number of chemistry analysers and is widely used for the measurement of drugs. Fluorescence polarization is also used for drug assays. Another example is the turbidimetric immunoassay for small molecules, in which cross-linking of analyte-coated latex particles by antibody is inhibited by free analyte from the sample, causing a decrease in turbidity. If the analyte is a large molecule and in sufficiently high concentration, the formation of antigen–antibody complexes can be measured by nephelometry and no label is needed. Homogeneous assays for large and small analytes are feasible with the recently developed cryptates (see section on Labels). Some types of homogeneous assay available are given in Table 39.2. However, most of these techniques are not generally applicable, and most immunoassays are of the heterogeneous type, in which separation of bound and free label is required.

Table 39.2 Homogeneous immunoassays

Enzyme inhibition or de-inhibition (EMIT[R])
Fluorescence polarization
Non-radiative energy transfer (+ time-resolved fluorescence)
Nephelometry
Turbidimetry

Separation methods

Any technique used to separate bound from free analyte or antibody must not disturb the primary reaction.

The difference in molecular size between free and antibody-bound analyte was exploited in early systems such as protein precipitation with ammonium sulphate or polyethylene glycol and adsorption of free analyte with charcoal. Immunological separation through the use of an anti-species antibody proved much more reliable. For example, since antibodies are bi- or multivalent, if the primary antibody was raised in a rabbit, antibodies to rabbit immunoglobulins raised in a donkey will produce complexes with the rabbit immunoglobulins that are sufficiently large and insoluble to form a precipitate. Some serum or immunoglobulins from a non-immunized rabbit (carrier serum) is usually added to ensure precipitation. Such reagents are of general applicability. This separation system (in the example donkey anti-rabbit) is called a 'second antibody' and assays using it are called double-antibody methods, although this name is occasionally also used to mean a two-site assay. The formation of the second antibody precipitate is slow, assays usually being left overnight, but this stage can be shortened considerably by the addition of polyethylene glycol. After centrifugation, the supernatant is removed by aspiration or decantation, procedures requiring skill and experience with the very small precipitates produced.

Solid-phase separation methods

These techniques, which have largely superseded all other methods, involve attaching reagents to solid phases by covalent bonding or by absorption. The solid phase can be the wall of a plastic tube, the well of a microtitre plate or the surface of large beads or small particles. Particles with a magnetizable core offer exceptionally rapid and efficient separation. Separation is by simple and convenient decantation or aspiration of the liquid phase, usually followed by washing of the solid phase with buffer to ensure completeness of separation and to reduce non-specific binding (the apparent binding in the absence of antibody).

Simultaneous assay of two or more analytes is now feasible with instrumentation capable of separating mixtures of antibody-coated beads into analyte-specific colour-coded sets at the final stage of assay for separate measurement. Such a system would permit, for example, immunoassay of multiple analytes in a single Guthrie spot for neonatal screening.

The solid phase can be a multipurpose reagent, made by coating with second antibody or with streptavidin, one specific reagent being coupled with biotin, which has a very high affinity for streptavidin. Other pairs include fluorescein with anti-fluorescein. This technique has the additional advantage that the specific reactions occur in the liquid phase. Coupling to a solid phase diminishes the affinity of an antibody and the speed of reaction, and may alter other characteristics. Solid-phase techniques also permit variations of assay protocol from the basic form of simultaneous addition of all reagents to the sample. Such variations may result in increased specificity and other improvements. Reagents immobilized onto strips of paper form the basis of dipstick tests, e.g. for pregnancy testing. Other disposable point-of-care immunoassay devices include tests for cardiac markers and drugs.

Automation

Automation of immunoassays is technically very demanding because of the requirement for separation of bound and free label in most methods. Early instruments were batch analysers using a single assay format, usually a homogeneous assay, for a limited number of analytes. Present high-throughput, totally automated systems, available from the late 1980s, may be batch analysers or may offer random access with infrequent calibration (often at intervals of weeks or months) derived from a high level of stability of both instrument and reagents. Random access avoids the need to batch samples even for infrequently requested tests and gives short turnaround times. Different assay formats, but with a common measurement system, can be included on a single instrument. Precise timing permits short reaction times without incubation to equilibrium. Precision should always be better than that of manual assays but differs considerably between different types of instrument. Inherent disadvantages are complexity and inflexibility.

Miniaturization

Developments in other disciplines have permitted the miniaturization of immunoassay devices. The 96-well microtitre plate may be succeeded by high-density plates with many multiples of this number, requiring specialized liquid-handling systems for very small volumes of sample and reagents. Of particular interest in areas of medicine where large numbers of patients require identical sets of tests, as in drug or tumour marker screening, is the development of systems using microarrays of reagents. Such a microarray consists of multiple discrete microspots of reagent printed or otherwise formed on an inert support (e.g. a 5×5 array of spots on a 1×1 cm substrate or chip, or an 8×8 array in each well of a standard microtitre plate). For immunoassay the immobilized reagent will usually be a specific antibody, and each microspot may be a different antibody, allowing simultaneous estimation of a number of analytes. Incubation with sample and a mixture of the other specific reagents and the remainder of the immunoassay procedure are carried out in the usual way, and the signal (usually fluorescence or chemiluminescence) is detected or imaged by a camera device. Some microspots in the array may be designed to detect interferences in the sample, e.g. heterophilic antibodies, and to provide quality control of reagents, a level of quality inspection not easily achieved in simpler systems. These devices offer substantial savings of sample, reagents and time compared with conventional automated systems.

In the future, fully integrated immunoassay microchips may become available, containing microfabricated structures capable of carrying out all the steps from sample preparation to signal detection. For a description of achievements in microchip immunoassay, see Kricka and Wilding (1998), and for a literature survey of developments in miniaturization generally, see Kricka and Fortina (2001).

Calculation of results

Since the calibration curve for immunoassay (a plot of label bound vs. concentration of analyte) is not a straight line, fitting a curve to the data, with its attendant imprecision, is a matter of judgement. Various empirical manipulations have been employed to make some or all of the graph linear. Bound label (or percentage bound if the total amount of label added is known) vs. concentration or log concentration, log bound label vs. log concentration, and logit–log plots are commonly used [logit $= \log\{(B/B_o)/1 - (B/B_o)\}$] where $B_o =$ bound label in the zero calibrator). Lin–log, log–log and logit–log graph papers are available. Modern instruments designed for immunoassay have computer programs for curve fitting, including complex methods such as cubic spline or four-parameter log–logistic curve fits.

Accuracy and precision

The accuracy of the result of an assay is the closeness to the true concentration of the analyte, for many substances still the subject of research and debate. Precision is the variability of the result obtained, and imprecision can be minimized by the use of appropriate reagents e.g. a label with superior detectability, by reduction of the number of steps and by close control of technique. Internal quality control gives information only about imprecision. Manual assays are usually performed in duplicate. Imprecision varies with the concentration of analyte. A typical example is shown in Figure 39.2.

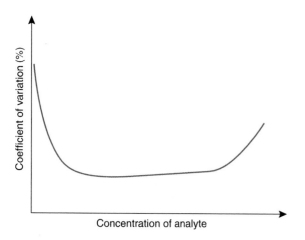

Figure 39.2   A typical precision profile

The concentration range of low imprecision should ideally match the range over which clinical results will be obtained, and the imprecision be appropriate for clinical utility of the results. Some workers define the working range of an assay as that over which the coefficient of variation (CV) is less than 10%.

The sensitivity or minimum detectable concentration can be defined in several ways, e.g. as the concentration corresponding to 2, 2.5 or 3 standard deviations (SDs) of the signal of the zero calibrator above (for immunometric assays) or below (for competitive assays) the mean value for the zero calibrator, the SD being obtained from, say, 20 replicates of the zero calibrator in a single batch. This is sometimes termed the analytical sensitivity. More realistic may be the use of between-batch SDs, and analyte-free serum, giving the 'biological detection limit'. Others use the concentration at which between-batch CV is 20% on biological samples, to give a value termed 'functional sensitivity'.

When the term 'sensitive' is used in the description of an assay, it implies not only that low concentrations of analyte can be distinguished from zero or absence of analyte, but also that precision at low levels is good enough for small changes in low analyte concentrations to be measured reliably. This is particularly important in the field of tumour markers.

Note that 'sensitivity' has alternative meanings; it is also the slope of the standard curve at any given concentration, and clinical sensitivity is a measure of the ability of a test to detect the presence of disease.

Quality control

Internal quality control (IQC) provides information about precision within and between assays and about the variability of reagent quality, but not about accuracy nor validity, or about errors with, or interference in, individual samples. IQC requires materials of similar composition (analyte and matrix) to clinical samples, in sufficient quantity for repeated use both within and between batches of an assay or for long-term use on an automated analyser. Liquid materials are usually stored frozen. Commercial QC materials are supplied lyophilized. During lyophilization (and subsequent storage) some components may be damaged, e.g. unstable analytes or binding proteins for steroids. The concentrations of the analyte chosen for the QC materials (usually low, middle and high values) should correspond to significant points of the assay, such as clinical decision points, but should avoid areas of high imprecision, which might make interpretation difficult. Commercial QC materials achieve the required values by the use of stripped serum and the addition of analyte, which may limit the similarity to clinical samples. Materials of human origin must be used.

Continuous recording of IQC results is essential; demonstration of acceptable performance is required for laboratory accreditation, and the records may also be invaluable in trouble-shooting (in-house or by the manufacturer). QC software is provided on automated instruments but may not be ideal, necessitating transfer of data to an alternative system or program. For rules on the application of QC results, see Westgard (2005) and Price & Newman (1997).

External quality assurance schemes (EQAS) seek to provide information about the comparability of methods and to investigate validity via recovery of added standard, linearity on dilution, specificity, performance with low-analyte serum, interference and other factors. Such schemes are available only for established assays, and it is common for laboratories assaying esoteric compounds, possibly infrequently, to exchange samples for comparison and reassurance.

Specificity, cross-reactivity and interference

The high specificity of the binding site of an antibody for its antigen is a major advantage of immunoassays. A single epitope on a complex molecule may involve amino acids spatially close only in the tertiary or quaternary structure of the molecule, and an antibody to such an epitope will therefore not react with denatured forms or fragments. However, a polyclonal antiserum will contain antibodies of differing affinities and specificities. If the antigen preparation used for immunization was impure, then the antiserum will contain antibodies to the impurities, and the resulting lack of specificity may compromise the validity of the assay, especially if the calibrant and label are also impure. Selection of monoclonal antibodies may minimize cross-reactivity, but closely related molecules may still be recognized by the antibody, especially in the case of small molecules, such as steroids and drugs.

Hyperspecificity of an assay may occur if a monoclonal antibody is directed to an epitope occurring in some but not all biologically active forms of a heterogeneous analyte.

Cross-reactivity in a competitive assay is usually defined arbitrarily as that concentration of cross-reactant giving 50% of the signal found in the absence of analyte, expressed as a percentage of the concentration of analyte giving the same signal. The measured cross-reactivity will vary at different points on the dose–response curve, and will also vary with the presence or absence of analyte, and with assay format and reaction conditions such as temperature and time of incubation. It is therefore impossible to calculate the true concentration of analyte in the presence of a cross-reactant, even if the cross-reactivity is known. Negative interference in certain assay designs from cross-reactants—including several drugs in common use—has recently been recognized as a potentially serious problem in digoxin monitoring (Valdes and Jortani, 2002).

In two-site immunometric assays, it is important to test potential cross-reactants in the absence and in the presence of analyte, since the cross-reactant may react with either or both antibodies. Reaction with both antibodies will give an increase in signal, whereas reaction with one antibody may produce a decrease in signal at high cross-reactant concentrations, which can be detected only in the presence of analyte.

Cross-reactivity of structurally related compounds, conjugates or metabolites is a particular problem with steroid assays. In some cases, e.g. cortisol and testosterone in plasma, a direct method is routinely used (although the limitations must be borne in mind). In others, e.g. cortisol in urine, a preanalytical extraction step is required in some assays, but there are cases in which this is essential, e.g. to remove potential cross-reactants when assaying 17-hydroxyprogesterone in infants in whom a diagnosis of congenital adrenal hyperplasia is suspected.

Interference from apparently unrelated substances in clinical samples may occur in several ways. The poorly characterized substance(s) termed digoxin-like immunoreactive substance, which occurs in the serum of patients with certain conditions, irrespective of digoxin therapy, gives falsely high results in digoxin assays, and appears to be fortuitous cross-reactivity. Autoantibodies may interfere by contributing to the assay analyte which *in vivo* is sequestered by the autoantibody and therefore biologically inactive, as in the case of macroprolactin. Alternatively, the autoantibodies may take part in the assay reaction; the effect on the result will depend on assay design (e.g. anti-triiodothyronine and anti-thyroxine in assays for free thyroid hormones). For some analytes, the occurrence of interference from autoantibodies is sufficiently frequent to require screening of samples, e.g. for thyroglobulin assay, or re-assay after removal of the autoantibody, e.g. prolactin.

Complement binding may lead to destruction of the antigen-antibody complex. This effect can be prevented by the addition of EDTA to chelate calcium ions. Antianimal antibodies, antibodies in human serum to immunoglobulins of other species, e.g. human anti-mouse antibodies (HAMA) and heterophilic antibodies, are now known to occur in a high proportion of patients, HAMA being present in large amounts in patients given monoclonal antibodies for imaging and therapeutic purposes. Anti-animal antibodies and probably also rheumatoid factor can bind to a single antibody, reducing its affinity for its antigen, or cross-link two antibodies, thereby mimicking antigen. Very high concentrations can produce negative interference in a manner analogous to the high-dose hook effect. These effects can be blocked by the addition of immunoglobulins from the same animal species as the reagent antibodies. Kit manufacturers now routinely include immunoglobulins from mouse and other species and specific antibody blockers in reagent antibody formulations.

A simple test for the presence of an interferant is examination of linearity on dilution with a diluent of similar matrix. Lack of linearity suggests a problem, although good linearity does not exclude one.

For a review of all types of interference, see Selby (1999).

High-dose hook effect

In a two-site immunometric assay with simultaneous addition of the two antibodies to the sample (a one-step assay), when the concentration of analyte is very high and the antibodies are no longer in excess, cross-linking of capture and labelled antibodies by analyte will be diminished, with binding sites on each antibody being occupied by separate molecules of analyte. The observed signal will therefore be reduced. At extremely high concentrations of analyte, the signal may fall below that of the top calibrator and a falsely low result will be read off (Figure 39.3). This phenomenon is known as

It is difficult to maintain constant vigilance for possible occurrence of this effect, but as an incorrect (perhaps apparently 'normal') result may lead to inappropriate and possibly harmful action being taken, every practicable effort should be made. Routine dilution of samples with values in the upper part of the standard curve, or those with appropriate clinical information, e.g. 'large pituitary tumour', is sometimes used. Individual devices, such as those for pregnancy testing, are also vulnerable. The hook effect can be avoided by using a two-step format, in which the sample is incubated with solid-phase capture antibody, excess analyte removed by washing and the labelled antibody added subsequently. In this format, very high concentrations will be read as 'greater than the top calibrator', with no indication of how much greater. However, the extra step increases the overall imprecision of the assay, a factor of some importance for tumour markers. Systems that can employ a kinetic reading very early in the reaction time enable an 'estimate' of the final result, automatic dilution and re-assay, virtually eliminating this problem.

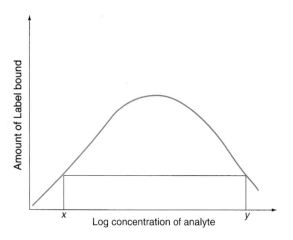

Figure 39.3 The high-dose hook effect. x = concentration of highest calibrator; y = concentration above which falsely low values will be obtained on undiluted samples

the high-dose hook effect, or bi-phasic response, and will be important only for those analytes that occur clinically in a concentration range of several orders of magnitude, as seen for tumour markers such as human chorionic gonadotrophin, α-fetoprotein and prolactin. The position of the hook is dependent on the concentrations of the antibodies.

Further reading

Bristow AF. Standardisation of protein hormone assays: current controversies. *Proc UK National External Quality Assurance Schemes Meeting* 1998; **3**: 66–73.

Kricka LJ. Selected strategies for improving sensitivity and reliability of immunoassays. *Clin Chem* 1994; **40**: 347–357.

Kricka LJ, Wilding P. Miniaturization of immunoassay devices. *Proc UK National External Quality Assurance Schemes Meeting* 1998; **3**: 166–171.

Kricka LJ, Fortina P. Microarray technology and applications: an all-language literature survey including books and patents. *Clin Chem* 2001; **47**: 1479–1482.

Price CP, Newman DJ (eds). *Principles and Practice of Immunoassay*, 2nd edn. 1997: Macmillan, London.

Selby C. Interference in immunoassays. *Ann Clin Biochem* 1999; **36**: 704–721.

Stenman U-H. Immunoassay standardization: is it possible, who is responsible, who is capable? *Clin Chem* 2001; **47**: 815–820.

Valdes R, Jortani SA. Unexpected suppression of immunoassay results by cross-reactivity: now a demonstrated cause for concern (Editorial). *Clin Chem* 2002; **48**: 405–406.

Westgard JO. 2005: http://www.westgard.com

Wild D (ed.). *The Immunoassay Handbook*, 2nd edn. 2001: Nature Publishing Group, New York.

40

Ion-selective electrodes

Alan D Hirst

Introduction

The basis of most conventional forms of clinical biochemistry measurement is the production of a coloured compound. Electrochemistry is different in that the measurement is based on production of a voltage (potential) or current, and the measuring system is a voltmeter or ammeter rather than a photometer.

An electrochemical detector, which responds specifically to a given analyte, is called an ion-selective electrode (ISE). The early electrodes responded to ions, hence the name, but more recently, electrodes have been developed that respond to metabolites such as glucose and urea although they are usually included in the same category because they share a common technology. Glucose sensors used in clinical areas are often ISE devices, and all critical care analysers are based on ISE technology.

The basis of ISEs is that they produce a potentiometric (voltage change) or amperometric (current change) response to changes in the analyte, i.e. there are two type of primary electrode. Secondary electrodes use other features, such as enzymes, to achieve specificity and release a product that can be detected by an ISE.

Electrodes are used in a number of clinical applications. The most frequently used electrodes are for:

- *Ions*: e.g. hydrogen (pH), sodium, potassium, chloride, fluoride, calcium, magnesium, lithium, ammonium (NH_4^+).

- *Gases*: e.g. oxygen, carbon dioxide, ammonia (NH_3).

- *Secondary or complex electrodes*: e.g. glucose, urea, lactate, creatinine.

The advantages of ISEs in clinical applications are that they are:

- Non-photometric, which means that an optically clear solution is not needed, i.e. whole blood can be used.

- Rapid and direct, allowing measurement of true concentration or biological activity.

Theory

A potentiometric cell and sources of potentials

Four elements are required to make a measurement with a potentiometric ISE:

- A measuring half-cell.

- A reference half-cell.

- A salt bridge or equivalent electrical connection.

- A measuring device.

A schematic view of this arrangement is shown in Figure 40.1.

A functional electrode (cell) is made up of two half-cells, a measuring electrode and a reference electrode. Each half-cell produces a potential, but a 'potential' as such cannot be directly measured. It is the potential difference (i.e. voltage) between the two half-cells that produces a measurable signal. The reference half-cell should be designed to have a constant potential, while

The Science of Laboratory Diagnosis, Second Edition   Edited by David Burnett and John Crocker
© 2005 John Wiley & Sons, Ltd

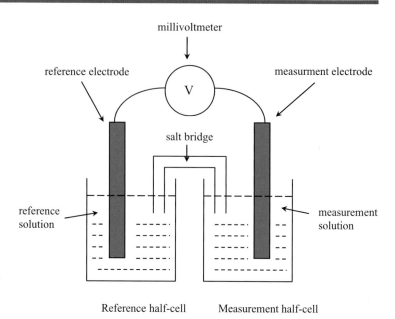

Figure 40.1   A simple electrode consisting of a measurement half-cell and a reference half-cell connected by a salt bridge

the measuring electrode has a potential, which varies with the concentration of the substance being measured, and so the potential difference, or voltage, will vary in a reproducible way with the concentration of the substance.

Measurement and reference half-cells (giving rise to electrode potentials)

The potential of each half-cell arises from a charge separation created by migration of ions as follows. At the electrode surface, or at any junction, liquid or solid, there will be a tendency for ions to pass from one phase into the other, e.g. if this is at the electrode surface, ions will go from the electrode into solution. If these ions are hydrogen ions, e.g. for a pH electrode, and they go into the solution without a corresponding negatively-charged ion, a charge separation will be created, with the solution becoming more positively charged (with hydrogen ions) and the electrode becoming more negatively charged (with electrons). As this process continues, the increasing charge separation produces an increasing potential between the electrode and the solution, which will oppose further ionic migration, until an equilibrium is reached, at which there is no further net movement of ions. This process is illustrated with a zinc electrode in Figure 40.2.

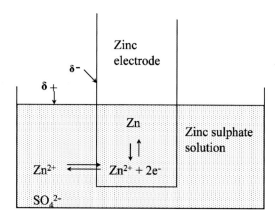

Figure 40.2   A zinc half-cell consisting of a zinc metal electrode in contact with a zinc sulphate solution; zinc ions will migrate from the electrode into the solution, leaving a small negative charge on the electrode and making the solution more positively charged

If the electrode is in contact with a solution with a low concentration of ions, there will be a relatively large outflow of ions from the electrode before equilibrium is reached, and a relatively large potential will be established. Conversely, a concentrated solution will tend to oppose migration of ions from the electrode and will produce a lower potential. In other words, the potential produced will vary inversely with the concentration of ions in the solution.

The reference electrode works in exactly the same way as the measuring electrode, but is in contact with a solution of constant concentration and should have a constant potential.

Salt bridge (giving rise to a junction potential)

To be able to measure the potential difference between the two half-cells there must be an electrical circuit, and to do this there must be electrical contact between the reference electrode solution and the measuring electrode solution. This is usually by direct contact or by a 'salt bridge', as shown in Figure 40.1.

There is ion migration between solutions in contact, similar to ion migration between electrodes and solutions. If the anions and cations in one of the solutions are a different size, they will migrate at different rates, as shown in Figure 40.3, and this will also result in a charge

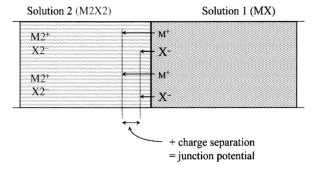

Figure 40.3 Illustration of junction potential. Solution 1 is a salt consisting of a relatively small metal ion (M) and a large anion (X). At the liquid junction, the smaller metal ion will diffuse into the other solution (NY) at a greater rate than the anion, causing a charge separation that is the junction potential

separation, which will produce a potential that will oppose further charge separation. All electrode systems have liquid junctions and therefore junction potentials. One of the main features of the design of a reference electrode is to minimize the size and variability of the junction potential. For this reason, the most common reference electrode is the 'calomel' (mercuric chloride) electrode. This is a chloride electrode that uses saturated potassium chloride as the reference electrode solution, because potassium ions and chloride ions have a similar ionic size and migrate at a similar rate. However, this does not entirely eliminate the junction potential, because the unknown solution it is in contact with has a variable composition.

The electrodes described so far are simple systems, with no element of selectivity, and low resistance, and are the basis of the common battery. For measurement purposes, a selective membrane needs to be introduced, and a typical working system is shown in Figure 40.4.

When the electrode is surrounded by a selective membrane—glass in this example—there is a further charge separation at the surface of the surface of the membrane. This is the 'membrane potential'. This is described in more detail in the next section.

Streaming potentials

Motion in one of the solutions, e.g. from a mechanical mixer or in a continuous flow analyser, can also produce a streaming potential. Most instruments take static readings to avoid this source of error.

Measuring system

The potential difference is measured with a millivoltmeter, as shown in Figure 40.4. Typical measuring voltages are 59 mV for each decade (ten-fold) change in concentration for a monovalent ion such as hydrogen and sodium, and 29.5 mV for a divalent ion such as calcium. A measurement error of 1 mV, from any source (e.g. junction potential), would result in a readout error of 4% for a monovalent ion and 8% for a divalent ion. This means that sensitive, stable millivoltmeters are required for the measurement.

The circuit must allow minimal current, because a large current would disturb the ion equilibrium at the electrode surfaces. Electrode membranes must be theoretically capable of electrical conductance, but in practice they have a very high resistance—of the order of 10^9 ohms. Similarly, the millivoltmeter must draw a minimal current from the circuit by having a very high input resistance. This requires special voltmeter design, and a standard voltmeter would not be adequate. Needless to say, in such a system, which requires high electrical resistance and negligible current to operate, cleanliness is very important, and systems need to be carefully sealed and insulated to give reproducible results.

Calibration

To make useful measurements with a working electrode system, as shown in Figure 40.4, the system must first be calibrated. The response of an electrode system is an

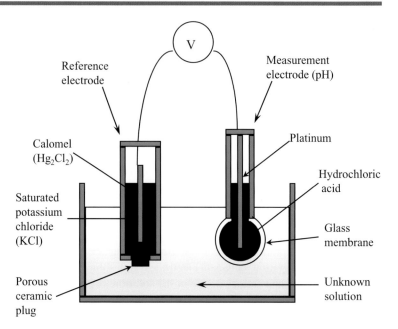

Figure 40.4 This is a typical working electrode system, consisting of a glass pH electrode and a calomel (mercurous chloride) reference electrode, both immersed in a solution whose pH is being measured. The porous ceramic plug forms the salt bridge and controls loss of the internal solution from the reference electrode

inverse logarithmic response defined by the Nernst equation:

$$\text{EMF (voltage)} = E_{\text{reference}} - E_{\text{unknown}}$$
$$= \frac{RT}{nF} \log_e \frac{(A_{\text{reference}})}{(A_{\text{unknown}})}$$

where A = Activity, R = the gas constant, T = absolute temperature, n = valency charge and F = Faraday constant. It can be seen from this that there is a complex inverse logarithmic relationship between the concentration (strictly, the 'activity') of an ion and the voltage produced by an electrode. This means that calibration of the system and producing a readout is not a simple matter, as it would be, say, for a colorimetric blood glucose system.

The usual approach is to measure the logarithmic 'slope' of the electrode, by measuring the voltage at two concentrations. Ideally this should be 59 mV for a 10-fold change in concentration. However, electrodes are rarely ideal, and the signal deteriorates with time, so the slope needs to be checked regularly.

Specificity—how electrodes are made selective

Ways of achieving specificity (how do you measure what you need?)

In simple electrodes, specificity for a particular ion is determined by a selective membrane surrounding the electrode, which acts by selective ion exchange, e.g. the pH electrode has a glass membrane, which acts as a hydrogen ion exchanger. Glass is a complex silicone crystal lattice, which contains charged ions (sodium for soda glass). At the surface there is a very thin hydrated layer where these ions can exchange with ions in the liquid in contact (Figure 40.5). Exchange of ions between the membrane and liquid will take place provided that the physical size of the ion and its electrostatic charge are compatible with the crystal lattice structure, but as membranes become more complex other factors play a more important part.

With standard sodium silicate glass, hydrogen ion exchange is favoured, but an 'alkaline error' occurs owing to interference from sodium ions at alkaline pH. At alkaline pH conditions, as the hydrogen ion concentration becomes very low, the relative contribution to the electrode response from sodium ions becomes more significant until it exceeds the hydrogen ion response. This is known as the 'alkali error'. Varying the composition of the glass can exaggerate these effects, so that the glass becomes a different electrode. Common variations in glass structure are shown in Figure 40.6.

In practice, no electrode is absolutely specific for a single ion, and the preference it shows for a particular ion is called the 'selectivity'. In this example, at neutral/acid pH the glass electrode is a hydrogen ion electrode with a high selectivity for hydrogen ions over sodium, but at alkaline pH it has the reverse characteristics. The prime objective of membrane design is to maximize

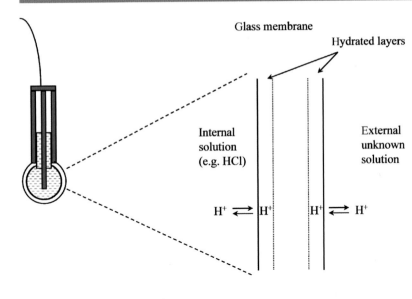

Glass membrane

Hydrated layers

Internal solution (e.g. HCl)

External unknown solution

$H^+ \rightleftarrows H^+$ $H^+ \rightleftarrows H^+$

Figure 40.5 A pH electrode operates on the principle of hydrogen ion exchange on both sides of the membrane. There is no transfer of hydrogen ions through the membrane—an equilibrium is established—although theoretically there must be electronic conduction for the electrode to form part of a measuring circuit. In practice the membrane will have a resistance of 10^9 ohms and there will be negligible current

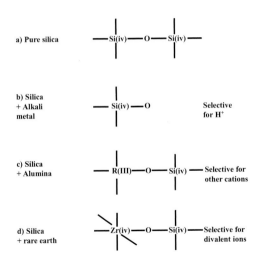

a) Pure silica   —Si(iv)—O—Si(iv)—

b) Silica + Alkali metal   —Si(iv)—O   Selective for H$^+$

c) Silica + Alumina   —R(III)—O—Si(iv)—Selective for other cations

d) Silica + rare earth   —Zr(iv)—O—Si(iv)—Selective for divalent ions

Figure 40.6 Different type of glass that are used for electrodes

By altering the glass composition, electrodes can be produced that respond to sodium and potassium. The best sodium electrode has a selectivity for sodium over potassium of 100:1 and this is clinically useful for biological fluids with high sodium concentrations and low potassium. However, the best glass potassium electrode has a selectivity for potassium over sodium of 20:1, which is not ideal for blood applications, where the sodium concentration is normally about 30 times the potassium concentration. For these applications, more selective membranes are needed.

Ion-selective membranes

The paradox in developing ion-selective membranes is that the membrane must be impermeable to water, so that there is negligible electrical conduction, which would short-circuit the electrode, but ions by their nature have a preference for solution in water. The membrane needs to have a component for which the ion has an equivalent preference, either by electrostatic attraction, as in the case of ion exchange, or by substitution of the hydration shell (provided by the water solvent), as in the case of neutral carriers. Living cells often use such carriers for transporting ions and water-borne nutrients across cell membranes, which are usually hydrophobic barriers, and this has provided models for the design of ISE membranes.

To have a functional membrane that uses an ion exchanger or neutral carrier, the membrane needs an inert support, which must be able to contain and retain

selectivity to avoid interference from other similar ions. In the case of halides, e.g. chloride, this can easily be achieved by using a silver chloride crystal membrane, in which only a chloride ion can fit easily into the crystal lattice. More difficult problems arise when trying to measure calcium in the presence of magnesium and vice versa (both being present in similar concentrations in blood), because the ions are similar in size. Even more difficult is the design of an electrode to detect lithium in blood at a concentration of 1 mmol/l against a background of 140 mmol/l of sodium.

Ionophore

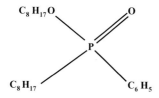

Alkyl Phosphate

Mediator

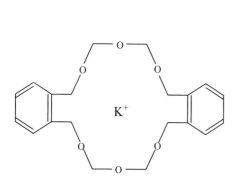

di-n-octylphenyl phosphonate

Figure 40.7   Calcium carrier

the ion carrier; this usually means it traps the solvent in which the carrier is dissolved.

In the case of calcium sensors ion-exchange materials have been found that bind calcium with a high selectivity (see Figure 40.7). The electrode consists of a calcium salt of an alkyl phosphate dissolved in di-*n*-octophenyl phosphonate—a solvent that is not volatile and not soluble in water. This is mixed with PVC dissolved in a volatile solvent, the mixture is poured onto a flat surface and the volatile solvent allowed to evaporate away. This leaves a thin PVC layer with the calcium exchanger trapped within it.

In an ideal electrode, the carrier would be completely insoluble in water, but in practice it is gradually leached away, leading to a gradual loss of response of the electrode, which is why electrode membranes usually have to be changed regularly.

Neutral carriers are an alternative to ion exchange, and the most widely used is valinomycin for potassium electrodes. Crown ether compounds are ring structures containing several oxygen atoms which can mimic the hydration shell of an atom, as shown in Figure 40.8. Valinomycin (Figure 40.9) is a similar large, complex ring compound containing six oxygen atoms within the ring structure. It is also able to complex potassium, i.e. the ion will exchange its aqueous hydration shell for valinomycin and migrate from an aqueous solution into a hydrophobic membrane.

One of the advantages of neutral carriers is that they tend to be less water-soluble than ion exchangers, which must of necessity have slight solubility. They make membranes, which have a longer life. Neutral carriers have been developed for a number of ions, including sodium, chloride, calcium, magnesium, lithium, ammonia (see Figure 40.10) and carbonate (see Figure 40.11).

The preceding account is all related to potentiometric electrodes, which have been used for illustration because they include all the problems related to electrochemistry.

Electrochemical reactions

The description of electrode potential given earlier is a simplification of the real situation to help illustrate how

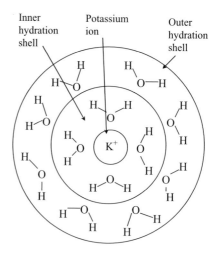

Figure 40.8   (a) An example of a crown ether compound (dicyclohexyl-18-crown-6) which acts as a substitute hydration shell for an ion such as potassium, and is able to transport the ion through a hydrophobic membrane. (b) A potassium ion in solution surrounded by an inner hydration shell and an outer hydration shell and an outer hydration shell of water molecules

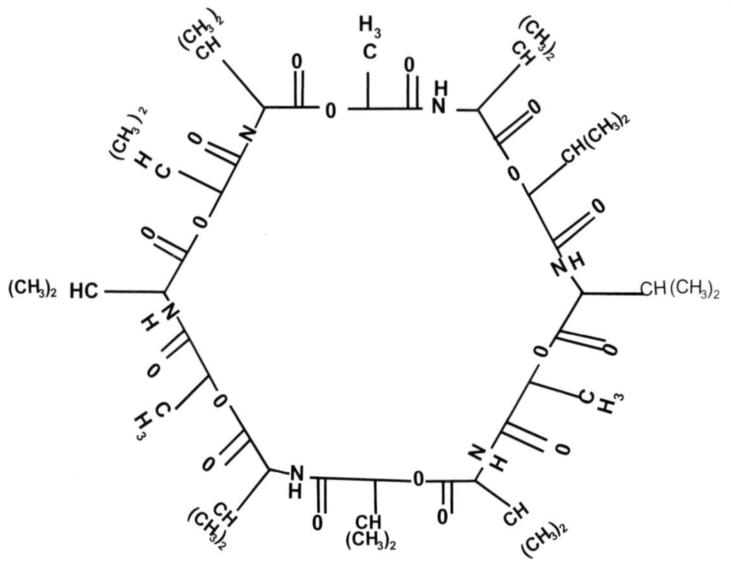

Figure 40.9 Structure of valinomycin

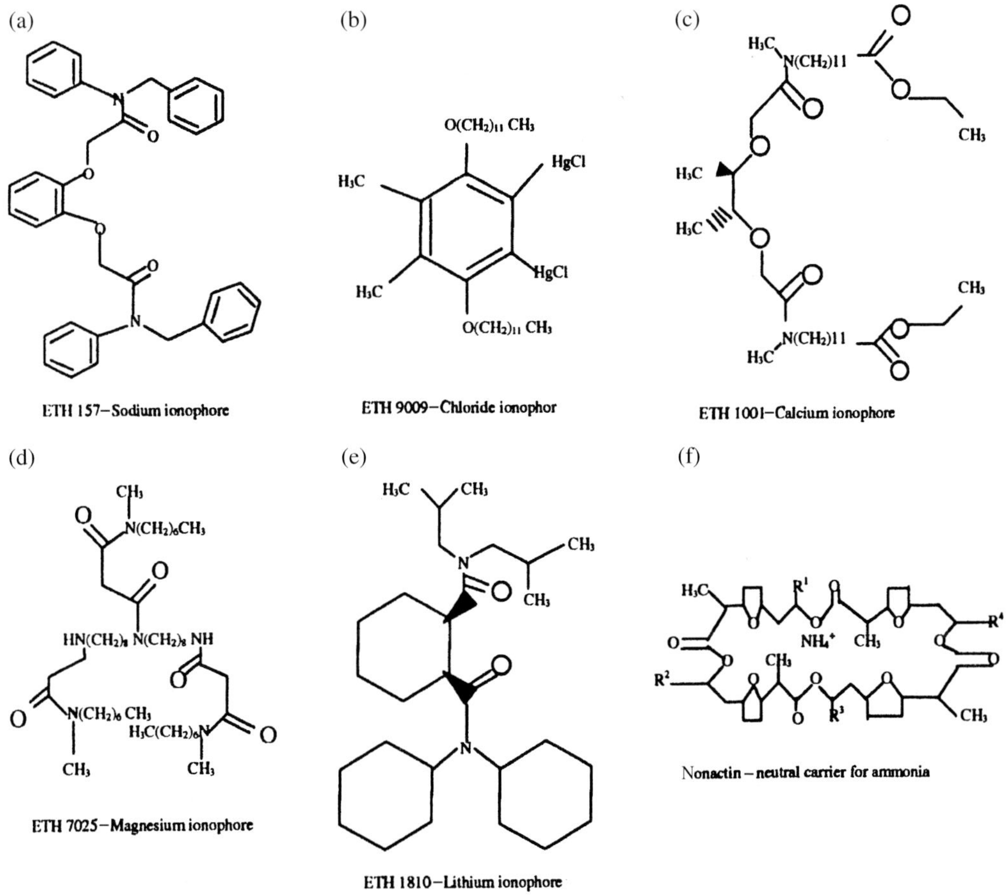

(a)

ETH 157–Sodium ionophore

(b)

ETH 9009–Chloride ionophor

(c)

ETH 1001–Calcium ionophore

(d)

ETH 7025–Magnesium ionophore

(e)

ETH 1810–Lithium ionophore

(f)

Nonactin – neutral carrier for ammonia

Figure 40.10 A group of ETH compounds used as ionophores on ISEs

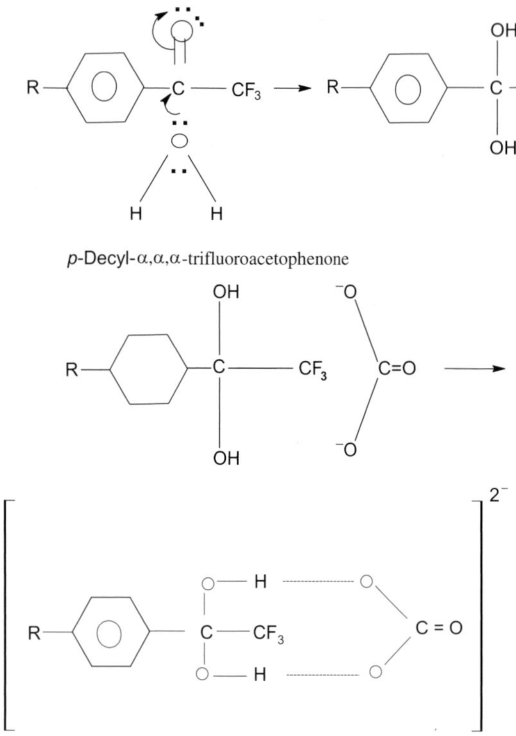

p-Decyl-α,α,α-trifluoroacetophenone

Figure 40.11 Ionphores used in a carbonate electrode

the electrode works. In fact, what is really happening at the electrode surface is that an electrochemical reaction is taking place to produce a charged species prior to the charge separation, e.g:

$$Zn \rightarrow Zn^{++} + 2e^-$$

In a conducting material such as a metal electrode, the electron structure is similar to a 'sea' in which the electrons are free to move throughout the solid. The energies of the electrons are filled to a level called the Fermi level. In the solution there is a different situation. The ions are surrounded by a hydration shell (Figure 40.8), which effectively separates them from the other ions, and the electrons are restricted to different (lower) energy bands. At the instant the electrode comes into the contact with the solution, the difference in energy levels favours a flow of electrons to equalize the energy and an equilibrium is quickly reached at the state of lowest free energy (known as the Gibbs' free energy level). This is the basis of the electrode potential.

This electrochemical reaction takes place spontaneously because of the property of the electrode material to be able to lose an electron and form an ion, and so the main application of these (potentiometric) electrodes is measurement of ions. The concept of electrochemical

reactions can be expanded to include other chemical reactions, which do not occur spontaneously but are promoted by an applied potential. This opens up the possibility of analysis of substances that do not necessarily exist as ions in solution but will give rise to an electrochemical reaction in suitable circumstances.

Amperometric electrodes

There is another class of electrodes, called amperometric electrodes because they produce a current rather than a voltage. This type of electrode is designed to measure an electrochemical reaction—a chemical reaction that produces or consumes electrons—by measuring an electrical current instead of measuring the voltage produced by a charge separation. The most common of these in clinical use is the oxygen (pO_2) electrode. In the case of the oxygen electrode the reaction is:

$$O_2 + 2H_2O + 2e^- \xrightarrow{-0.7 \, V} H_2O_2 + 2OH^-$$

For the related peroxide electrode, the reaction is:

$$H_2O_2 \xrightarrow{+0.7 \, V} 2H^+ + O_2 + 2e^-$$

The first reaction is used in the standard oxygen (pO_2) electrode, known as the Clarke electrode, while the second is used in some glucose electrodes, as described later, to measure peroxide produced by the enzyme glucose oxidase.

It can be seen from these electrochemical reactions that the reactions are facilitated by an applied voltage (0.7 V) and this voltage can add to the specificity of the electrode response. The main feature of these electrodes is that a constant voltage is applied to the measurement electrodes and the resulting current (in microamps) is proportional to the rate of the reaction. This is a direct linear relationship, in contrast to the complex inverse logarithmic response of potentiometric electrodes. Because current is being measured, these electrodes (e.g. a pO_2 electrode) do not need a reference electrode.

However, the reaction and current will also be related to the surface area of the electrode.

Polarography

This application of electrochemistry is also known as polarography. The voltage applied is a polarizing voltage, and the electrochemical cell is called a polarographic cell.

To get a measurement of the analyte concerned or, for example, pO_2 (the partial pressure of oxygen is not strictly speaking 'concentration' but is equivalent in gaseous terms), the rate of reaction should be constant, so the pO_2 should be constant. A key requirement of this type of system is that the electrode should not consume the oxygen at the electrode surface at a faster rate than oxygen can diffuse through the electrode solution to the electrode surface, otherwise the current will fall as the pO_2 in contact with it falls. To maintain a steady state to allow measurement, measuring cells must be designed so that the electrode at which the reaction takes place is very small (e.g. a needle point), so that a minimal amount of the analyte is consumed in the measurement. This means that a typical system will only produce a current of microamp proportions, which requires an ammeter specifically designed for such measurement.

Oxygen electrode

To have a functional electrode, the electrodes at which the electrochemical reaction takes place must be in contact with a constant solution—one with a constant resistance, so that there will be no variation in resistance, which would affect the applied voltage and hence the current produced. The Clarke oxygen electrode consists of electrodes in contact with an electrolyte solution, which is contained by a silicone rubber membrane. Gaseous oxygen can pass freely through the membrane, but the membrane is hydrophobic, not allowing water or dissolved electrolytes to pass through and change the composition and resistance of the electrolyte solution. This is shown in Figure 40.12.

Glucose electrodes

Glucose electrodes use a combination of a specific enzyme and a specific polarization voltage to provide a response that is specific for glucose. At the present time there are two different enzymes and three different electron transfer reactions in common use.

The simplest form of glucose electrode is to use the enzyme glucose oxidase in conjunction with an oxygen electrode. Glucose oxidase catalyses the reaction:

$$\text{glucose} + O_2 + 2H_2O \rightarrow \text{gluconic acid} + H_2O_2$$

The oxygen electrode can measure the fall in pO_2 as a measurement of glucose consumed in the reaction. Unfortunately, if the cell is open to the atmosphere, oxygen will be replenished from atmospheric oxygen,

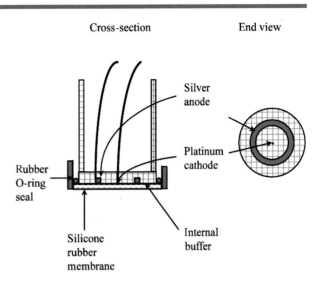

Figure 40.12 A Clarke oxygen electrode. This consists of a very small area platinum cathode suurounded by an annular silver anode. Both are in contact with an internal buffer enclosed within a hydrophobic silicone rubber membrane. Oxygen can diffuse freely through the membrane and dissolve in the internal buffer. The resulting electrochemical reaction at the platinum cathode is measured

and there will also be problems if whole blood is used because of the oxygen binding effects of haemoglobin. Because of these problems, better applications have been developed:

- The glucose oxidase/peroxide electrode. This is used to detect the peroxide produced by the reaction, with an applied potential of $+0.7$ V.

- The glucose oxidase/ ferrocene electrode. This electrode uses ferrocene as an electron transfer agent in the following electrochemical reaction:

Glucose $\xrightarrow{\text{glucose oxidase}}$ gluconolactone $\xrightarrow{80 \text{ mv } e^-}$
+ ferrocinium $\quad\quad\quad$ + ferrocene (Fe^{2+}) $\quad\quad$ + ferrocinium (Fe^{3+})

This is the basis of the Medisense® glucose stick assay, and is illustrated in Figure 40.13.

- The glucose dehydrogenase/ferricyanide electrode. This electrode works in a similar way, but with a different enzyme and electron transfer agent:

Glucose $\xrightarrow{\text{glucose dehydrogenase}}$ glucuronic acid $\xrightarrow{80 \text{ mv } e^-}$
+ $Fe(CN)_6^{3-}$ $\quad\quad\quad$ + $Fe(CN)_6^{4-}$ $\quad\quad$ + $Fe(CN)_6^{3-}$

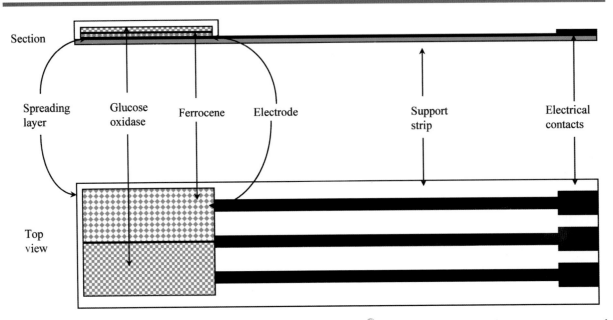

Figure 40.13 An example of a solid state glucose electrode—the Medisense® system. This system has three contacts—a central cmmon electrode, one in contact with the ferrocene alone (for non-specific reactions) and one in contact with glucose oxidase plus ferrocene. The difference in the two signals provides a measurement of glucose concentration

This is the basis of the Boehringer Mannheim Corporation (BMC) Advantage® glucose stick assay.

Drug interference

The three types of glucose electrode described above are in common use and are in general effective measuring devices, but it is known that a number of substances, including common drugs such as paracetamol, can interfere and give a signal with these systems. This is because most compounds can produce an electrochemical reaction, given a large enough polarizing voltage, and this includes most drugs. It is on this basis that therapeutic drugs and many other biological compounds can be measured by chromatography using a polarographic cell as an electrochemical detector.

Electrochemical detectors

These detectors are a development of the polarographic electrode for use as a detector in high performance liquid chromatography (HPLC). A typical laboratory application for this would be measurement of catecholamines (adrenaline, noradrenaline) for the detection of phaeochromocytoma. The electrochemical reaction is shown in Figure 40.14.

The electrodes described so far operate in stable conditions, e.g. they are in contact with a constant

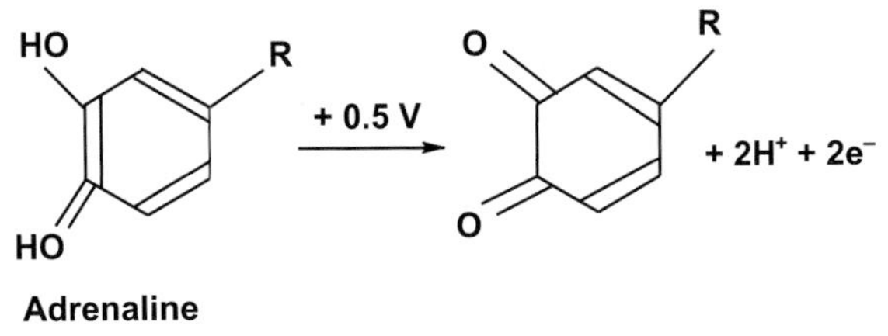

Figure 40.14 Electrochemical reaction for catecholamines

solution. In a chromatographic system, selectivity is provided by chromatographic (i.e. physical) separation of similar compounds, e.g. adrenaline and noradrenaline (as opposed to using a selective membrane), but the solvent systems used for the separation are variable, so the resistance of the solution in the measuring cell will vary, and that would affect the applied voltage. To overcome this problem, a third electrode is used in the HPLC measurement cell, which has the function of monitoring the applied voltage and holding it at a steady value through a feedback circuit.

Complex electrodes

These consist of an electrode within an electrode, and the most common example is the pCO_2 (carbon dioxide) electrode found in all blood gas analysers.

pCO₂ Electrode

This electrode consists of a standard pH electrode in contact with a weak bicarbonate buffer and encased in a polyvinyl chloride (PVC) membrane. This is shown in Figure 40.15.

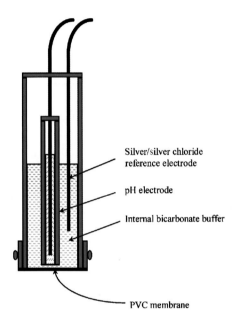

Figure 40.15 A pCO_2 electrode consisting of a pH electrode and an internal silver/silver chloride reference electrode. The CO_2 diffuses through the PVC and changes the pH of the internal buffer

The PVC membrane is permeable to gases, e.g. carbon dioxide, but impermeable to water. Carbon dioxide diffuses across the membrane and dissolves in the buffer and changes the equilibrium of the bicarbonate buffer.

$$CO_2 + H_2O \rightleftharpoons H_2CO_3 \rightleftharpoons HCO_3^- + H^+$$

In doing so the pH of the buffer will change, and this is measured by the pH electrode.

Ammonia electrodes are made in exactly the same way, with a pH electrode immersed in a buffer. The differences are that the buffer is different:

$$NH_3 + H_2O \rightleftharpoons NH_4^+ + OH^-$$

and that the membrane contains the neutral carrier nonactin (see Figure 40.10f) to assist the transfer of the ammonia.

Other complex enzyme-mediated electrodes

Lactate electrode

This is commonly used in critical care units, and by athletes testing for anaerobic status after exercise. It works in the same way as a glucose electrode (it is usually a modified glucose electrode) using a different enzyme–lactic oxidase:

$$Lactate + O_2 + H_2O \rightarrow pyruvate + H_2O_2$$

The peroxide formed is measured with a peroxide electrode.

Urea electrode (Roche Diagnostics)

This is a more complex electrode that uses the enzyme urease. This splits urea to form carbon dioxide and ammonia; the latter is converted to ammonium ions, which are then detected with an ammonium electrode:

$$Urea + H_2O \xrightarrow{Urease} \begin{cases} CO_2 + H_2O & \longrightarrow & H^+ + HCO_3^- \\ + & & \\ 2NH_3 + H_2O & \longrightarrow & NH_4^- + OH^- \end{cases}$$

Unlike the ammonia electrode, the ammonium electrode has poor selectivity, but is used because the urease enzyme can only work at a low pH, at which the ammonia is converted to ammonium ions. The ammonium electrode suffers from interference from potassium, so the electrode is used in an array with a compensating potassium electrode. This is shown in Figure 40.16.

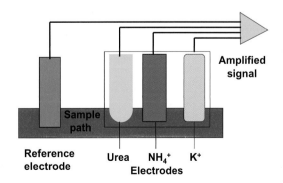

Figure 40.16 Schematic diagram of the analytical principles of a potentiometric sensor for urea measurement

Creatinine electrode (Nova Biomedical, UK)

This electrode uses a complex array of enzymes:

$$Creatinine + H_2O \xrightarrow{\text{creatinine amidohydrolase}} creatine$$

$$Creatine + H_2O \xrightarrow{\text{creatine amidohydrolase}} sarcosine + urea$$

$$sarcosine + O_2 + H_2O \xrightarrow{\text{sarcosine oxidase}} formaldehyde + glycine + H_2O_2$$

The peroxide is measured with a peroxide electrode.

Point of care testing (POCT)

Ion-selective electrodes (ISEs) are widely used in POCT instruments, principally because they can utilize whole blood, rather than serum, and because they can produce a result in less than 1 minute.

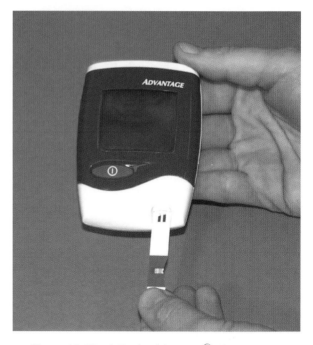

Figure 40.17   A Roche Advantage® glucose meter

Glucose meters

These are used by nurses and doctors and by many patients. They are inexpensive ($\sim$ US $20) and easy to use. The principles of the ISE components of such meters were described on p. 389. Figure 40.17 shows a typical meter (Roche Instruments plc) and measurement strip. The latter are disposable.

Critical care analysers

These are more complex instruments, used in most critical care units, e.g. accident and emergency departments, intensive care/therapy units, special care baby units, coronary care units and delivery suites. They contain an array of electrodes and other sensors, usually in groups, as shown in Figure 40.18.

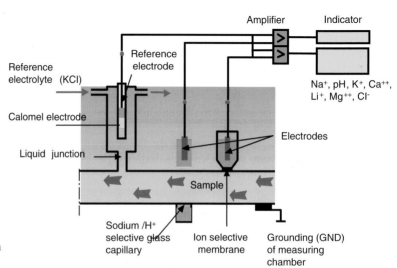

Figure 40.18   An electrode array as used in a typical critical care analyser

- Blood gases: pH, pO_2, $pa\ CO_2$. This group measures the blood acid–base status as an index of renal and respiratory function.

- Ions: sodium, potassium, chloride, calcium, and magnesium. This group is used in critical care units for assessment of conditions such as body fluid volume and renal and cardiac function.

- Metabolites: glucose, urea, creatinine, lactate. This group is used for assessing conditions such as renal and liver function.

- Co-oximetry: haemoglobin, oxyhaemoglobin, carboxyhaemaglobin. These components are measured using spectrophotometry rather than ISEs. They are combined with the other tests because they give additional information, particularly on respiration.

Safeguards

Network connection

Point-of-care instruments produce results which directly affect patient care. The early instruments were stand-alone and all record-keeping was manual and inconsistent. This has been identified as a major risk management issue, and has led to a new generation of instruments, which can be connected via a network to a central data manager. This has several advantages:

- Data is collected and stored centrally. This includes test results, patient ID, operator ID and date/time, i.e. a full audit trail.

- Operator ID can be controlled so that only trained operators can use instruments.

- The instrument performance can be monitored centrally.

It is important that critical care instruments are always operational. Network control enables laboratories to provide 24 hour support for these analysers.

One of the early problems with network control was that companies were using different communications systems, which were incompatible. This problem was solved when the diagnostics companies formed CIC (Communications Industry Consortium) to resolve the problem. CIC produced a set of communications standards, which were adopted by the National Committee for Clinical Laboratory Standards (NCCLS) as Standard NCCLS-POCT-IA.

Policy

One of the main applications of ISEs is point-of-care testing, (POCT), where the tests will be done by nurses and clinicians without formal laboratory training. As there are numerous problems that can occur with ISE measurements, there must be safeguards built into the whole process (not just the measurement system) for this application to be acceptable, and they should be made clear in a hospital policy on POCT. Without this safeguard, patients are placed at risk and the institution has a risk control issue.

The main input of the laboratory is the production of the specification that the instrument must meet (i.e. instrument performance). The specification should address issues such as selectivity of the electrodes. Fortunately, modern technology allows us to build in suitable safeguards, as outlined below.

Instrument checks

Modern instruments are operated by computers, which check electrode performance of functions such as electrode signal (e.g. slope: mV/decade) and response time, and other checks such as temperature, air bubbles, membrane leaks, etc. For a laboratory-based instrument, where the staff should understand the electrode characteristics, it is acceptable to have a high-level override facility to produce measurements in an emergency situation. For POCT applications, if an electrode response falls outside specified limits, the test must be disabled until the problem is resolved.

There are other useful functions, which are enabled with a computer-controlled instrument:

- *Operator identification*. Training is an important feature of POCT, and an operator function can be used so that only those trained to operate the instrument are allowed to use it.

- *Remote lockout*. This is a facility whereby the instrument is connected to the laboratory computer, which monitors the quality control performance of the instrument, and locks the instrument if the QC falls outside predefined limits. The laboratory computer then alerts laboratory staff to the problem.

- *Quality control (QC) and Quality assurance (QA).* Quality control is real-time checking of the instrument. This involves analysing material of known composition and checking that the results obtained are within clinically significant limits, as defined by the professional bodies (such as the national quality assurance bodies). Quality control should be performed regularly by the operators (e.g. nurses and clinicians) doing the tests, and an essential part of their training is the significance of doing quality control, recording results and what action to take should the QC check fail. This training should be given by experienced laboratory professionals.

Quality assurance is a retrospective examination of instrument performance, usually done as part of an external QA scheme. The UK laboratory accreditation agency, CPA(UK) Ltd, requires that laboratories participate in a recognized EQA scheme and maintain an adequate performance. If POCT instruments are under the control of the main laboratory, the laboratory accreditation is applied to the POCT service, provided that it is operated to an acceptable standard. This approach is recommended as the best way of providing quality patient care at minimal risk.

- *Maintenance.* Maintenance checks are usually planned preventative maintenance such as replacing tubing, seal, electrodes, etc. These tests are best done by experienced laboratory professionals, but if they are done by non-laboratory staff, rigorous training on the significance of the checks is vital.

- *Training.* Training of all users is an essential feature of a hospital POCT policy. For modern instruments, the training need not be in great depth or time consuming, provided that adequate safeguards have been built into the instrument. Training should include not only operation of the instrument, but an understanding of all error signals, the significance of results, and the importance of recording results and QC procedures.

Acknowledgements

I would like to thank Roche Diagnostics for their help with provision of a number of diagrams, and in particular Christoph Ritter, Nova Biomedical UK for information on electrodes, and Andrew St John for the use of several diagrams. Also many thanks to Janet Gourlay for all the typing and preparation.

Further reading

Hirst AD, Stevens JF. Electrodes in clinical chemistry. *Ann Clin Biochem* 1985; **22**: 460–488.

Crompton RG, Sanders GHW. *Electrode Potentials*. Oxford University Press, Oxford.

Ed Van Ysek P. *Modern Techniques in Electroanalysis*. 1996: Wiley, Chichester.

Accreditation and point of care testing. *Ann Clin Biochem* David Burnett 2000; **37**: 241–243.

Price CP, Hick JM (eds). Point of care testing. 1999: AACC (www.aaccdirect.org)

Kost GJ (ed.). *Principles and Practice of Point of Care Testing*. 2002; Lippincott, Williams & Wilkins, Philadepphia, PA.

Management and use of IVD point of care test devices. *MDA Device Bull* 2002; **3**. (www.medical-devices.gov.UK)

Annexe D of ISO 15189—Medical Laboratories. Particular requirements for quality and competence. ISO (International Standards Organisation), Geneva (Annexe D, which relates to quality management of point of care testing, is under discussion at the time of going to press, but should be agreed by the time of publication).

Structures of ionophores. *Fluka catalogue*. 2003: Sigma-Aldrich Company Ltd (www.sigma-aldrich.com)

41

Light absorption, scatter and luminescence techniques in routine clinical biochemistry

Bernard F Rocks

Introduction

Few of the chemical constituents of blood, plasma or urine can be measured directly. Analytical chemists have, however, developed indirect means of detecting and measuring quantitatively many of the constituents of clinical interest. Frequently the method involves adding to the diluted sample a substance (the reagent) that chemically reacts specifically with the particular component to be quantitated (the analyte) to form a product that is measured relatively easily. Whenever possible, the assay conditions are such as to produce a product whose quantity is proportional to the original concentration of the analyte.

When light strikes matter of any kind, the interaction may change the intensity, direction, wavelength or phase of the incident light. Light absorption, scatter and luminescence are three of the many optical effects that have been most often exploited for analytical purposes. The majority of quantitative measurements made in clinical biochemistry laboratories are based on the production of coloured reaction products, so that most frequently photoelectric absorbance devices such as colorimeters or spectrophotometers are used. Other light measurement-based methods in widespread use include turbidimetry, nephelometry, fluorimetry and measurement of chemiluminescence. The essential features of these techniques are discussed in this chapter.

Light absorption techniques

Absorption photometry forms the basis for most of the quantitative analyses carried out in clinical biochemistry laboratories. The primary reasons for this are ease of measurement, satisfactory accuracy and precision, and instrumentation that is stable, reliable and relatively inexpensive.

Photometers and spectrophotometers

Absorptiometers may be divided into two basic types, the single-beam and the double-beam instrument. In each type, although the light paths are different, many of the basic components are similar. A simple single-beam photometer is illustrated in Figure 41.1. Clinical biochemists often refer to this type of photometer as a colorimeter.

The light source provides radiant energy over the wavelengths of interest. For work in the visible range, it is now common to use tungsten–quartz–halogen lamps. These lamps may also be used for near-infrared and near-ultraviolet measurements (340–800 nm). For work at shorter UV wavelengths, a deuterium discharge lamp is normally used. Below 360 nm these sources provide a strong continuum which, together with fused silica cuvettes, fulfils most needs in the UV region. The power supply to the lamp must be of high stability.

The Science of Laboratory Diagnosis, Second Edition   Edited by David Burnett and John Crocker
© 2005 John Wiley & Sons, Ltd

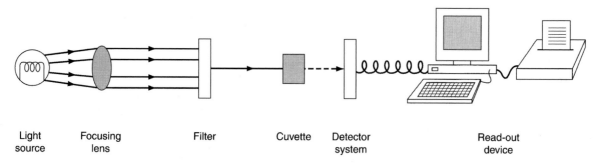

| Light source | Focusing lens | Filter | Cuvette | Detector system | Read-out device |

Figure 41.1 Basic components of a photometer

The wavelength appropriate for the particular assay is usually selected by using narrow-bandwidth, high-transmittance interference filters. Interference filters are expensive and some inexpensive colorimeters use filters of coloured glass or dyed gelatin (sandwiched between layers of glass). Spectrophotometers generate monochromatic light by means of a prism or grating monochromator, rather than by use of filters.

The cuvette is a transparent vessel that holds the solution being measured. The design of the cuvette and the means of admitting the sample to it and subsequently removing it vary with instrument and analyser type. The sample solution, held in the cuvette, absorbs a proportion of the incident radiation; the remainder is transmitted to a light detector, where it generates an electrical signal.

Many different types of photodetectors are in use. Various solid-state photodiodes and diode arrays are now frequently used in visible light and near-infrared instruments. These detectors are sturdy, inexpensive and have a linear response over several decades of light intensity. However, they give a low response to UV light. Where high sensitivity is required, and for UV work, vacuum photomultiplier tubes are used. The output from the detector may need amplifying and will need to be expressed as its logarithm in order for it to be linearly related to concentration. Both of these operations are conveniently carried out by means of a logarithmic amplifier. The signal, after any necessary transformations (most often analogue to digital), may be displayed by a meter, printed or stored.

Single-beam instruments

In single-beam instruments a blank (e.g. a cuvette containing water) is used to set zero, then the standards and samples are read. Interferences from variations in sample turbidity and source intensity changes and other instrument fluctuations are not automatically compen-

sated for. In some modern designs, a second detector is used to monitor the intensity of the light source and to electronically compensate for lamp drift. Single-beam instruments are well suited for quantitative absorption measurements at a single wavelength. Easy maintenance and low cost are distinct advantages of this type of photometer, which is to be found in the majority of automated clinical chemistry analysers.

Double-beam spectrophotometers

A double-beam instrument has two light paths, both originating from the same source. One beam passes through the sample cuvette and the other through the blank or reference cuvette. This is usually achieved by directing the light beam from the monochromator towards a rapidly rotating mirror or 'chopper' that alternately directs light through the reference cuvette and the sample cuvette. Light emerging from each cuvette is then reflected towards the detector. The detector output is consequently an alternating signal with an amplitude proportional to the ratio of the intensities of the sample and reference beams. The resulting electrical signals are processed electronically to give the absorbance on a readout device. Double-beam systems automatically correct for changes in light intensity from the light source, fluctuations in instrument electronics and absorption by the blank. An instrument of this kind is often provided with a motor-driven monochromator, so that automatic scanning and recording of an entire spectrum is possible. This enables their use for qualitative (e.g. drug identification) and quantitative analysis.

Beer's law

The mathematical basis for quantitative measurements is based on the experimentally derived Beer–Lambert relationship. Lambert's law states that the proportion of radiant energy absorbed by a substance is independent of the intensity of the incident radiation. Beer's law states that the absorption of radiant energy is proportional to the total number of molecules in the light path. It is not possible to measure directly the amount of radiation absorbed by a substance and it is usually determined by measuring the ratio of incident radiation falling on the sample, I_o, and the transmitted radiation that finally emerges from the sample, I. Using these measurements, the Beer–Lambert law can be expressed as:

$$\text{Log}_{10}(I_o/I) = ecI$$

where c is concentration of the substance in moles/litre, I is the optical path length in centimetres and e is the molar absorption coefficient for the substance, expressed as litres/mole/centimetre. The values for I and I_o cannot be measured in absolute terms and measurements are most conveniently made by expressing I as a percentage of I_o. This value is known as the percentage transmittance T, and gives a linear relationship with concentration if the logarithm of its reciprocal is used. This reciprocal logarithmic function of I and I_o, is known as absorbance (A):

$$\%T = (I/I_o) \times 100$$
$$A = \log_{10}(100/T) = -\log_{10}(I_o/I)$$

Absorbance is a most convenient parameter since, from Beer's law, it is directly proportional to the concentration of the absorbing species.

Spectrophotometers are usually linear over the range 0–2 Å, and chromophores can be measured at concentrations as low as 10^{-6} mol/l. Test values are usually calculated by comparing the absorbance readings of the test samples with readings obtained from assaying a series of standards or calibrators of known value.

Applications

The majority of determinations carried out in clinical biochemistry laboratories rely on photometric methods. A typical hospital laboratory would report about 5000 photometric assays/day and may include measurement of some of the following analytes: albumin, bilirubin, calcium, cholesterol, creatinine, glucose, iron, phosphate, total protein, urea, uric acid and many enzymes, e.g. acid phosphatase, alkaline phosphatase, alanine transaminase, creatine kinase and lactate dehydrogenase.

Turbidimetry and nephelometry

These related techniques are commonly employed in clinical laboratories as the means of conducting certain immunoassays. Both are based on the measurement of particle-induced light scatter. When light is directed through a solution containing suspended particles, some of the light will be scattered, some will be absorbed and the remainder will be transmitted through the liquid. This interaction can be used to measure the concentration of particles in suspension by measurement of light transmitted (turbidimetry) or by measuring the scattered light (nephelometry).

Light scatter involves a direct interaction between light and the particle it strikes. When a light beam strikes a particle, its electric field moves the particle's electrons in one direction relative to the nucleus. The electrons move back and forth in phase with the frequency of the incident light wave. This produces an oscillating dipole, the size of which depends on the electric field strength (related to frequency) and polarizability of the particle's electrons. The oscillating dipole becomes a source of electromagnetic radiation and radiates light, of the same frequency as the incident light but in all directions. The amount and distribution of scattered light also depends on particle size and concentration, and on the polarization of the light beam.

For particles smaller than one-tenth of the wavelength of the incident light, the re-radiated light waves are in phase and reinforce each other, resulting in a symmetrical, although not spherical, pattern of scattered light. This is termed Rayleigh scattering. Larger particles, (e.g. immunoglobulin–antigen complexes) act as a number of randomly spaced point sources, and destructive interference between light arising from different sites within the particle will occur, resulting in a maximum and minimum pattern of re-radiated light. This is known as Rayleigh–Debye scattering and, together with Rayleigh scattering, is illustrated in Figure 41.2. More light is scattered forward as the particle size increases and measurement of asymmetric light scatter can be used to measure particle size. Short-wavelength light (blue) is scattered much more than longer-wavelength light (red).

Applications

Immunoassays involving nephelometric and/or turbidimetric detection systems are used to measure certain analytes for which no specific colorimetric reagent is available, e.g. C-reactive protein (CRP), complement components C_3 and C_4, and individual

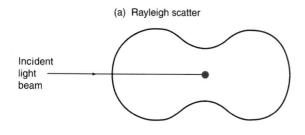

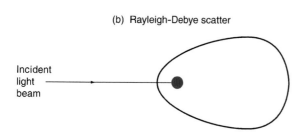

Figure 41.2 Two-dimensional angular distribution patterns for: (a) Rayleigh light scatter from a small particle; (b) Rayleigh–Debye light scatter from a larger, immunoglobulin-antigen-sized, particle

immunoglobulins. The protein solution and appropriate antibody are mixed together and allowed to react to form large complexes that scatter more light than the antibody or protein alone. Sensitivity is typically in the low mg/l range. The large light scatter produced when cetylpyridinium chloride is added to urine containing mucopolysaccharides is an example of a non-immunological use of turbidimetry.

Turbidimeters

In theory, turbidimetry can be measured by any standard photometer or spectrophotometer. Because a small change in transmitted light is measured in the presence of a large background signal, instruments with a high signal:noise ratio are desirable. A simple dedicated turbidimeter would consist of a quartz halogen light source, a narrow-band interference filter, a sample cuvette holder and a photodiode or photomultiplier (Figure 41.3). Use of short-wavelength light offers the advantage of increased scatter and thus a larger signal, but in biological solutions absorption of the light will also increase. Consequently antigen–antibody complex formation is usually measured in the range 340–400 nm. For good precision, timed reagent addition, mixing and

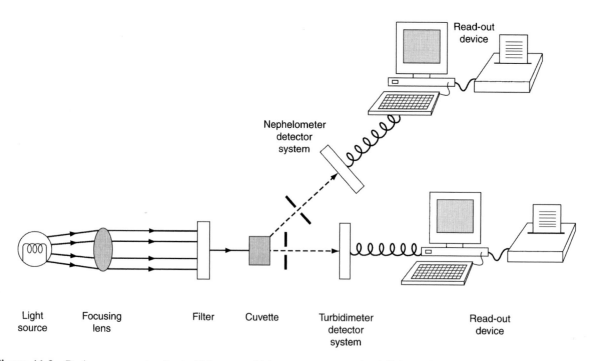

Figure 41.3 Basic components of a turbidimeter, which measures transmitted light, and a nephelometer, which measures scattered light

reading are necessary. When particle size increases slowly with time, the rate of decrease in transmitted light is best calculated from multipoint measurements. Automated discretionary photometric analysers are widely used for turbidimetric immunoassays.

Nephelometers

Nephelometers usually comprise a light source, an incident light filter, a sample holder and a detector set at an angle, so as to avoid direct transmitted light. Provided the filters (or monochromators) for incident and emitted light are set to the same wavelength, fluorimeters, in which the scattered light is measured at 90°, can be used, although with limited sensitivity. Light scatter measured at 90° is weaker than forward light scatter. Theoretically, the best sensitivity is attained by placing the detector angle as close to 180° as possible. This requires a tightly focused incident light beam and excellent optics. In practice, clinical nephelometers use detector angles between 90° and 170° to the axis of incident light (see Figure 41.3). Nephelometric measurements made at angles other than 90° to the incident light are best made from round- rather than square-faced cuvettes. At these detector angles, round cuvettes minimize reflection of the measured light by the cuvette walls. Nephelometers are often fitted with a cut-off filter to prevent fluorescent light from reaching the detector.

A tungsten quartz halogen bulb is frequently used. Alternative sources include xenon lamps, mercury-arc lamps, light-emitting diodes and lasers. The helium neon laser is especially useful for nephelometry because it has a high-intensity, narrow beam that does not require focusing or collimating optics. Unfortunately, the long wavelength red light (632.8 nm), is not scattered as much as short-wavelength light. The detector must be well shielded to minimize interference from stray light. For maximum sensitivity, dedicated nephelometers use low-noise photomultiplier detectors.

The wavelength for optimum scatter by fully formed antibody–antigen complexes is about 460 nm. However, in kinetic immunoassays it has been shown that the optimum wavelength changes as the immune complexes grow. For these widely used assays, monochromatic light is undesirable and incident light over a broad band (typically 450–550 nm) provides more reproducible peak rates.

The Beckman Immage® is a well-established example of a clinical laboratory nephelometer. Automated sample dilution, antiserum addition and antigen excess checking are some of the features of this type of dedicated analyser. Electronic differentiation of the light signal is used to identify and record the maximum rate of reaction and, through a stored calibration curve, relate it to concentration.

Nephelometry or turbidimetry?

In general, nephelometry has the potential to be slightly more sensitive and give faster results than turbidimetry. Turbidimetry, on the other hand, does not require a special detector and can be carried out on many of the currently available automated clinical analysers employing photometric measurement.

Luminescence

Luminescence is the emission of light or radiant energy when an electron returns from an excited or higher energy level to a lower energy level. There are several types of luminescence phenomena, including fluorescence, phosphorescence and chemiluminescence. Although luminescence phenomena differ in how an electron is activated to the excited state, they result in similar emissions of radiant energy.

Fluorescence

When light impinges on a molecular substance, enough energy at a specific wavelength may be absorbed to cause the substance to alter its electron configuration and place some of the electrons in an excited state. This state is short-lived and the excited electrons quickly return to the ground state. If the substance is of a particular chemical structure, the transition may be a multi-step process, with the major step resulting in the release of emitted light of lower energy than the excitation light. The other steps in the transition to the ground state are mostly vibrational energy loss, due to electron collisions. Emitted light that is produced as the substance passes from an excited state to the ground state is called fluorescence. Many molecules demonstrate fluorescence (fluorophores) and this property provides the basis of a sensitive method of quantitation. In general, most compounds that exhibit fluorescence contain multiple conjugated bond systems with associated delocalized π electrons. Most fluorophores that fluoresce intensely have rigid planar structures and electron-donating groups. For dilute solutions, the intensity of fluorescence is directly proportional to the concentration of the fluorophore. The wavelength maxima of absorption and emission are also useful in the identification of substances. The difference between the excitation and emission wavelength maxima is known as the Stokes' shift, and the quantum efficiency is a measure of the quantity of light emitted. If the Stokes' shift is large, it is easier to measure the emitted light without interference from the incident light. Also, if the quantum efficiency is high, the signal is stronger and the assay more sensitive. Analysis of blood and urine for porphyrins is a good example of the qualitative and quantitative use of fluorescence.

Fluorescence vs. photometry

Fluorescence measurements are more sensitive than absorbance and light scatter measurements. The magnitude of absorbance of a chromophore in solution is determined by its concentration and the path length of the cuvette. The magnitude of fluorescence intensity of a fluorophor is determined by its concentration, the path length and the intensity of the light source. For dilute solutions, fluorescence intensity is directly proportional to the concentration of the fluorophore. Through the use of more intense light sources, digital signal filtering techniques and sensitive emission photometers, the sensitivity of fluorescence measurements can be 100–1000 times greater than the sensitivity of absorbance measurements.

Fluorescence applications

Assays using fluorescence measurement techniques are routinely used in the clinical laboratory to determine porphyrins, drugs, hormones, specific proteins and antibodies, and for cell phenotyping. Methods used include direct measurement of emitted light and a variety of immunoassays using techniques such as fluorescence polarization, time-resolved fluorescence, laser-induced fluorescence/flow cytometry and, in serology laboratories, fluorescence microscopy.

Fluorimeters

Figure 41.4 illustrates the optical arrangement in a simple fluorimeter. The appropriate excitation wavelength is

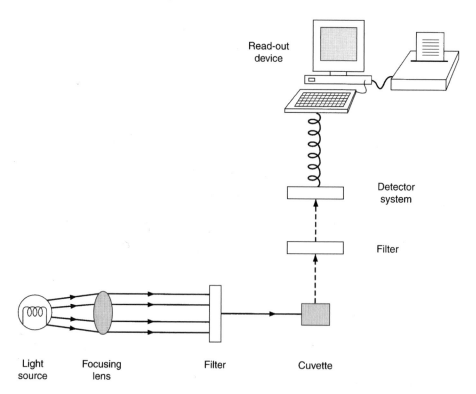

Figure 41.4 Basic components of a fluorimeter

filtered from the source and is directed into the solution held in the cuvette. The resulting fluorescent light is emitted in all directions, but it is usual to monitor the emerging light at right angles to the incident beam, the unabsorbed part of which passes through the cuvette and enters a light trap. The emission wavelength is selected from the emitted or secondary light and the beam is directed onto the detector, usually a photomultiplier. The output from this is amplified and processed as needed. If the amplifier gain and the excitation source are constant, the fluorescent output reading is linearly related to the concentration. A spectrofluorimeter employs monochromators instead of filters for wavelength selection.

First-generation fluorimeters often employed mercury vapour lamps. These lamps have their output concentrated into a relatively small number of sharply defined bands that limit the choice of excitation wavelength. A high-intensity source with a nearly continuous spectrum is the xenon arc. However, this source generates ozone and runs very hot. Most fluorimeters aimed specifically at the clinical market use either a tungsten halogen bulb or, for greater sensitivity, a rapidly firing xenon flash tube.

Double-beam spectrofluorimeters In these instruments, the beam of light from the source is chopped and split between the sample cuvette and a reference cuvette. The fluorescence produced by each cuvette is monitored by a single photomultiplier tube electrically phased with the chopper. The difference signal allows subtraction of the fluorescence produced in the reference cuvette and also compensates for lamp drift and flicker.

Fluorescence polarization analysers These instruments are basically filter fluorimeters to which a set of excitation and emission light polarizers have been fitted. Fluorescence intensity is measured both parallel and perpendicular to the plane of the excitation beam. The degree of fluorescence depolarization depends on molecular rotation, which is related to molecular size. This technique has been applied to homogeneous (nonseparation) immunoassays. In these applications, typically, a competitive binding immunoassay is performed in which an antigen and a fluorescent-labelled antigen compete for binding sites on an antibody. The binding of the fluorescent label to the large antibody, which rotates slowly, will cause the fluorescent light to remain highly polarized. Conversely, the unbound fluorescent-labelled antigen is free to rotate more rapidly and will produce depolarized fluorescence.

Some clinical fluorimeters of this type are dedicated to the measurement of only one fluorescent species. For example, the Abbott TDx® analyser system uses fluorescein-labelled immunoassay reagents exclusively. Because fluorescein absorbs in the visible region, a tungsten halogen light source can be used. Compared with other fluorimetric techniques, sensitivity is low and is applicable only to the assay of small molecules. The TDx® polarization analyser is relatively simple to operate and is widely used for therapeutic drug monitoring.

Time-resolved fluorimeters A problem often encountered with fluorescence-based immunoassays (particularly homogeneous assays) is the high background fluorescence caused by some of the components in blood samples (e.g. serum proteins, bilirubin and NADH). The use of time-resolved measurements and labels with long fluorescence decay times (> 500 ns) have ameliorated this limitation. Using this technique, the fluorescence from the analyte is monitored only after the background fluorescence has decayed. Automated systems using highly fluorescent lanthanide chelates are commercially available for a wide range of immunoassays. In the Perkin-Elmer AutoDELFIA® system, measurement is with a time-resolved fluorimeter which, for europium chelates, supplies 1000 pulses of light/second. The detector switches on 400 microseconds (μs) after each citation pulse and collects emitted light, at 613 nm, for 400 μs (see Figure 41.5). Detection limits as low as 10^{-14} mol/l of lanthanide chelates are possible.

Chemiluminescence

Chemiluminescence differs from fluorescence in that the excitation event is caused by a chemical or electrochemical reaction and not by photolumination. The physical event of light emission is similar to fluorescence, in that it occurs from an excited singlet state, and the light is emitted when the electron returns to the ground state. Chemiluminescence usually involves the oxidation of an organic compound, such as luminol, acridinium esters or luciferin, by an oxidant (e.g. hydrogen peroxide, hypochlorite or oxygen); light is emitted from the excited product formed in the oxidation reaction. These reactions are usually carried out in the presence of catalysts such as enzymes (e.g. alkaline phosphatase, horseradish peroxidase), metal ions or metal complexes.

Luminometers

Because chemiluminescence immunoassays depend on the use of luminescent compounds that emit light during

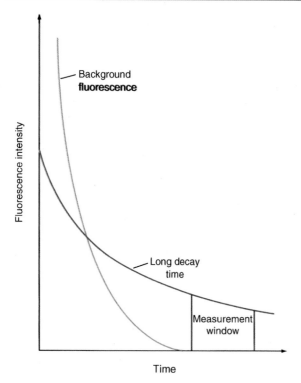

Figure 41.5 Principle of time-resolved fluorimetry. The long decay time from the label is measured after the background fluorescence has died away

the course of a chemical reaction, there is no need for an incident light source. The only signal emanates from the luminescent molecules and consequently, because of the high signal to noise ratio, these assays are potentially very sensitive. In principle, instrumentation is relatively simple, consisting of a reaction cuvette and a sensitive light measuring device contained within a light-proof compartment.

Application of chemiluminescence

The nature of light emission from chemiluminescence assays demands precisely timed reagent additions and very reproducible mixing procedures. Therefore, their application, at least in the routine laboratory, is confined to use on special automated immunoassay analysers. Their use as labels in immunoassay now dominate this important sector of the global diagnostic market. Examples of specific commercially available chemiluminescence techniques are given below. Chemiluminescence immunoassays are widely used to measure hormones,

specific proteins and certain drugs. For an account of immunoassay, the reader is referred to Chapter 39.

Direct chemiluminescence Acridinium esters are chemiluminescent labels that can be attached directly to antigens or antibodies and incorporated into different immunoassay strategies. At the signal-generation stage of the assay, the ester linkage is cleaved under alkaline conditions to release the unstable compound *N*-methylacridone, which decomposes with the emission of a flash of light. The maximum intensity occurs 0.4 seconds after initiation and the decay half-life is 0.9 seconds. This is the principle used in the Bayer ACS180® and Centaur® systems.

Enhanced chemiluminescence The addition of certain chemicals can dramatically enhance the output of light, e.g. horseradish peroxidase, in the presence of hydrogen peroxide, causes oxidation of luminol with the emission of light. The output of light is increased more than 1000-fold in the presence of substituted phenols and naphthols. Enhanced luminescence is a glow rather than a flash of light and persists for hours, although signal reading normally takes place after a few minutes. This type of signal generation is exploited in the Vitros ECi® immunodiagnostics system (Ortho-Clinical Diagnostics).

Chemiluminescence enzyme immunoassays There are substrates that give rise to luminescent end points for all of the commonly used enzyme labels, e.g. adamantyl 1,2-dioxetane arylphosphate is used with alkaline phosphatase as a label. Cleavage of the phosphate group produces an unstable anion that decomposes with the emission of light, e.g. as used in the DPC Immulite® analyser.

Electrochemiluminescence Electrochemiluminescence differs from conventional chemiluminescence in that the reactive species that produce the chemiluminescent reactions are electrochemically generated from stable precursors at the surface of an electrode. Electrochemiluminescence processes have been demonstrated for many different molecules by several different mechanisms, including an oxidation–reduction-type reaction with ruthenium (Ru^{2+}), tris(bipyridyl) and tripropylamine. This principle is employed in the Roche Elecsys® and E-170® analysers.

When an electrical potential is applied, the ruthenium label is oxidized and simultaneously tripropylamine is also oxidized to an unstable cation that spontaneously loses a proton. The resulting tripropylamine radical reacts with oxidized ruthenium, producing an excited ruthenium label that decays with the emission of a photon. Subsequent light emission is then measured by a photomultiplier and processed as appropriate for the quantitation.

Further reading

Skoog DA, Holler FJ, Nieman TA. *Principles of Instrumental Analysis*. 1997: Thomson Learning, Philadelphia, PA.

Wild DG (ed.). *The Immunoassay Handbook*, 2nd edn. 2001: Stockton Press, New York.

42

Analytical atomic spectrometry

Andrew Taylor

Introduction

Analytical atomic spectrometry is the term used to include a number of techniques that are extensively applied to the determination of individual elements in body fluids and tissues. The most important are atomic absorption spectrometry and inductively coupled plasma–mass spectrometry, with atomic emission, atomic fluorescence and X-ray fluorescence spectrometry having useful roles also. The major applications are to the measurement of essential minerals and trace elements, e.g. sodium, magnesium, zinc and copper, and toxic substances such as aluminium and lead. These techniques allow for accurate measurements of very low concentrations in complex biological samples.

Principles

Spectroscopy is the study of interactions between matter and electromagnetic radiation; when applied to quantitative analysis, the term *spectrometry* is used. Different types of spectroscopy are concerned with various regions of the electromagnetic spectrum (e.g. X-rays, UV light, infrared radiation), properties of the matter with which the interactions occur (e.g. molecular vibration, electron transitions) and the physical interactions involved (i.e. scattering, absorption or emission of radiation).

Quantitative analytical atomic spectrometric techniques include atomic absorption (AAS), atomic emission (AES), atomic fluorescence (AFS), inorganic mass spec-

trometry and X-ray fluorescence (XRF). AAS, AES and AFS exploit interactions between UV and visible light and the outer shell electrons of free, gaseous, uncharged atoms. In XRF, high-energy particles collide with inner shell electrons of atoms to initiate transitions that culminate in the emission of X-ray photons. For inorganic MS, a magnetic field separates ionized analyte atoms according to their mass: charge ratio.

Atomic emission, absorption and fluorescence

Every element has a characteristic *atomic structure*, with a positively charged nucleus surrounded by the number of electrons necessary to provide neutrality. These electrons occupy discrete energy levels but it is possible for an electron to be moved from one level to another within the atom by the introduction of energy (Figures 42.1, 42.2, 42.3). This energy may be supplied by collisions with other atoms or with free electrons, or as photons from light. Such transitions will occur only if the available energy is equal to the difference between two levels (ΔE). Uncharged atoms may exist at the lowest energy level or *ground state*, or at any one of a series of *excited states*, depending on how many electrons have been moved to higher energy levels, although it is usual to consider just the first transition. Energy levels and the ΔEs associated with electron transitions are unique for each element.

The ΔE for movements of *outer shell electrons* in most elements correspond to the energy equivalent to UV-visible radiation and it is these transitions which are

The Science of Laboratory Diagnosis, Second Edition   Edited by David Burnett and John Crocker
© 2005 John Wiley & Sons, Ltd

used for AA, AE and AF spectrometry. The energy (E) of a photon is characterized by:

$$E = h\upsilon \qquad (1)$$

where h = the Planck constant and υ = the frequency of the waveform corresponding to that photon (the dual concept of light as waveform and discrete particles is not considered further here). Furthermore, frequency and wavelength are related, as:

$$\upsilon = c\lambda \qquad (2)$$

where c = the velocity of light and λ = the wavelength. Therefore:

$$E = hc/\lambda \qquad (3)$$

and it follows that a specific transition, ΔE, is associated with a unique wavelength.

Under appropriate conditions, outer shell electrons of vaporized, ground-state atoms within the analytical system may be excited by *thermal energy* (i.e. collisions with other atoms). As these atoms return to the more stable ground state, energy is lost, some of which will be in the form of emitted light, which can be measured with a detector (Figure 42.1). The intensity of this light is

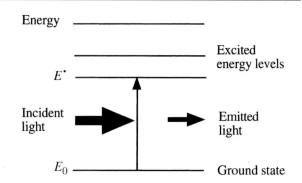

Figure 42.2 Partial energy level diagram showing absorption of light energy as the atom moves from ground state to an excited level. Light transmitted to the detector has been attenuated

loss of light is proportional to the number of atoms and is understood as *atomic absorption spectrometry* (AAS).

Some of the **radiant energy** absorbed by ground-state atoms can be emitted as light as the atom returns to the ground state. This emission is described as resonance fluorescence and, again, its intensity is proportional to the number of atoms in the light path. The technique is known as *atomic fluorescence spectrometry* (Figure 42.3).

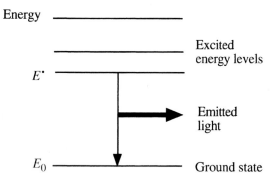

Figure 42.1 Partial energy level diagram showing emission of energy as light as atom drops from an excited level to the ground state

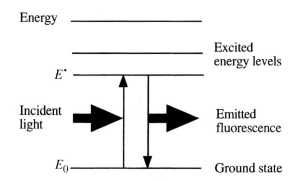

Figure 42.3 Partial energy level diagram showing absorption of light energy as the atom moves from ground state to an excited state, followed by emission of energy (light) as the atom drops back to the ground state

proportional to the number of atoms present and the process is *atomic emission spectrometry* (AES).

When *light (radiant energy)* of a characteristic wavelength enters an analytical system, outer shell electrons of corresponding atoms within the light path will be excited as energy is absorbed (Figure 42.2). Consequently, the amount of light transmitted through the system from a source to the detector will be attenuated. The

It follows from equations (1) and (2) that the wavelengths of the absorbed and emitted light are the same and are unique to a given element. It is this which makes AAS, AES and AFS *specific*, so that one element can be measured even in the presence of an enormous excess of a chemically similar element.

The Boltzmann equation (Haswell, 1991) relates the energies associated with different states to the atomic structure and, from the equation, the proportion of an atom population present as excited atoms compared with ground-state atoms can be calculated. The proportion is influenced by two features—temperature and the element. At the typical operating temperatures of around 2000°C, the ratio is at least $10^{-6}:1$ for most elements, and AAS and AFS afford superior *sensitivity* to AES. With systems that provide higher temperatures (see below, Instrumentation), the proportion changes and AES may be favoured. The atomic structures of the alkali metals (e.g. sodium, potassium, lithium) are such that the ΔEs are relatively small, corresponding to longer wavelengths, and although at about 2000°C the proportion of excited atoms is not high (10^{-4}–$10^{-6}:1$), the concentrations of sodium and potassium in biological specimens are sufficient that flame AES (also called flame photometry) is a suitable and well-established technique for measuring these metals in clinical laboratories.

Atomic absorption spectrometry can be used for the determination of more than 60 elements with instrumentation that is comparatively cheap and simple to operate, and it affords sufficient sensitivity to measure many of these elements at the concentrations present in clinical specimens (Haswell, 1991). A similar range of elements can be measured by atomic emission spectrometry. Flame photometry is convenient for the alkali metals at high concentrations, but AES is most useful with high temperature energy sources (see below, Instrumentation) when multi-element analysis can be undertaken. Effective atomic fluorescence requires intense, stable light sources and these are difficult to construct reliably. Most success has been with electrodeless discharge lamps for the metalloid elements of Groups 4–6 of the periodic table. Very low detection limits are achieved for these elements by AFS.

X-ray fluorescence

When high-energy photons, electrons or protons strike a solid sample, an electron from the inner shells (K, L or M) of a constituent atom may be displaced. The resulting orbital vacancy is filled by an outer shell electron, with an accompanying emission of an X-ray photon, its energy being equal to the difference between the energy levels involved. This emission is known as *X-ray fluorescence* (XRF). The energy of the emission, i.e. the wavelength, is characteristic of the atom (element) from which it originated, while the intensity of the emission is related to the concentration of the atoms in the sample. According to the type of spectrometer used to measure the emission, XRF is characterized as wavelength-dispersive (WDXRF) or energy-dispersive (EDXRF). Total

reflection XRF (TXRF) is usually described as a separate technique, although it may be seen as a variation of EDXRF.

Inorganic mass spectrometry

As samples are taken to high temperatures, organic components are destroyed and some or all of the inorganic elements are ionized. When these ions are directed into a mass spectrometer, they may be separated by passing through a magnetic field established by a quadrupole or some other mass filter. The ions, separated according to mass: charge (m/z) ratio, are detected and counted using an electron multiplier. This process is generally described as *atomic* or *inorganic mass spectrometry*.

Various ion sources have been employed, but for clinical analysis most recent work uses an inductively coupled plasma (ICP–MS). The technique is truly multi-element and affords detection limits that are in the μg/l range or, especially for elements with high atomic mass numbers, even lower. Elements that have hitherto been unable to be determined can now be quantified with confidence. The other major feature of mass spectrometry is the ability to measure different isotopes of the same element.

Instrumentation

Atomic absorption

An atomic absorption spectrometer consists of the following modules:

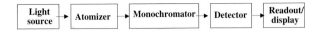

where the monochromator, detector and display are similar to those of other spectrometers. The essential feature of a good *light source* for AAS is to provide high-intensity monochromatic output, which is achieved with hollow cathode lamps. The lamps are constructed with the element to be measured as a major component of the cathode, so that the emitted light is of the same wavelength as is required for atomic absorption by the sample. Consequently, a different lamp is required for each element to be measured and, because of the costs involved, a comprehensive range of lamps is generally maintained at only a few specialist laboratories.

The *atomizer* is any device which will generate ground-state atoms as a vapour within the instrumental light path. If we consider calcium in a specimen of serum, the element is present in solution, bound to protein, complexed with phosphate and with some as the inorganic Ca^{2+}. Formation of the atomic vapour (atomization) requires the following steps:

- Removal of solvent (drying).

$$\downarrow$$

- Separation from anion or other components of the matrix $\rightarrow Ca^{2+}$.

$$\downarrow$$

- Reduction: $Ca^{2+} + 2e^- \rightarrow Ca^\circ$.

The energy necessary to accomplish these steps is supplied as heat from either a flame or an electrically heated furnace. Finally, within the atomizer there is absorption of the radiant energy.

Flame atomizers

The typical arrangement involves a *pneumatic nebulizer*, premix chamber and an air–acetylene laminar flame with a 10 cm path length (Figure 42.4). The high-speed auxiliary airflow causes sample solution to be continuously drawn through the capillary, due to the Venturi effect. The sample emerges from the nebulizer as an aerosol with a wide range of droplet sizes and is mixed with the flame gases and transported to the flame for atomization. However, only droplets less than 10 μm actually enter the flame, because those of larger size fall to the sides of the premix chamber and run to waste. Consequently, no more than about 15% of the sample enters the flame. Thus, with the pneumatic nebulizer, the original sample undergoes dilution with the flame gases, losses in the premix chamber and considerable thermal expansion (i.e. further dilution) within the flame. In addition to dispersion of sample through the flame, there are losses of atoms due to the formation of oxides or other species in the margins of the flame. The nebulizer sample uptake rate is usually about 5 ml/min and aspiration for several seconds is necessary to achieve a steady-state signal.

The advantages and disadvantages of the pneumatic nebulizer–flame atomization system are shown in Table 42.1. Because of its simplicity, speed and freedom from interferences, this approach is preferred wherever the analyte concentration is suitable. The lowest concentrations that can typically be determined are approximately 1 μg/ml. Air–acetylene burns at about 2000°C, while the hotter nitrous oxide–acetylene flame is approximately 3000°C and is used for elements which

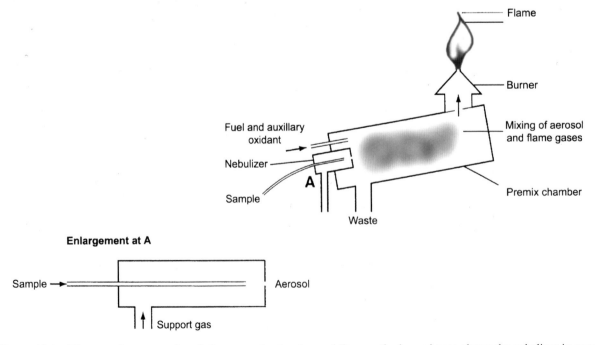

Figure 42.4 Diagram of a pneumatic nebulizer, premix chamber and Burner; the lower image shows the nebulizer in more detail

Table 42.1 Features of pneumatic nebulization with flame atomization

Rapid	Only about 15% of sample enters the flame
Reproducible	Wide range of droplet sizes
Few interferences	Low atomic density of sample in the flame
Steady-state signal	Burner conditions impose limitations on nebulizer

form refractory oxides and have no effective atomization in an air–acetylene flame.

Improved sensitivity is obtained with devices that overcome the limitations of pneumatic nebulizers listed above. These (a) trap atoms to give a greater density within the light path; (b) bypass the nebulizer, so that 100% of the sample is atomized; and (c) introduce the sample as a single, rapid pulse, rather than as a continuous flow. Some employ a combination of these features. Devices used in a flame, e.g. the slotted quartz tube and Delves' cup, are most effective with more volatile elements, such as zinc, cadmium and lead. These three approaches to improved sensitivity also feature in other atomizers used in AAS, AES, AFS and in ICP–MS.

Hydride generation

Certain elements, such as arsenic, selenium and bismuth readily form gaseous hydrides, e.g. arsine (AsH_3). Using simple additional instrumentation, a reductant such as sodium borohydride is added to the reaction flask containing acidified sample. Hydrogen is formed, which reacts with the analyte, the gaseous hydride is evolved and is transferred by a flow of inert gas to a heated silica tube positioned in the light path. The tube is heated by an air–acetylene flame or an electric current and the temperature is sufficient to cause dissociation of the hydride and atomization of the analyte (Figure 42.5). Thus, there is no loss of specimen, all the atoms enter the light path within a few seconds, and are trapped within the silica tube, which retards their dispersion. Hydride generation AAS allows the detection of a few nanograms of analyte from whatever sample volume is placed into the reaction flask. Variations to the instrumentation are possible to give a continuous-flow arrangement, which is simpler to automate.

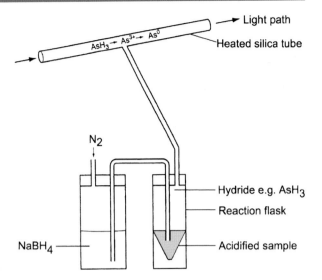

Figure 42.5 Diagram of a system for hydride generation and atomization

Mercury vapour generation

Mercury forms a vapour at ambient temperatures and this property is the basis for cold vapour generation. A reducing agent is added to the sample solution to convert Hg^{2+} to elemental mercury. Agitation or bubbling of gas through the solution causes rapid vaporization of the atomic mercury, which is then transferred to a flow-through cell placed in the light path (Figure 42.6). As with hydride generation, the detection limit is a few nanograms and common instrumentation to accomplish both procedures has been developed by some manufacturers.

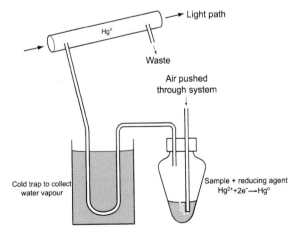

Figure 42.6 Diagram of a system for mercury vapour generation

Electrothermal atomization

Most systems use an electrically heated graphite tube; this technique is often called *graphite furnace atomization*, although different materials are sometimes employed. Electrical contact is made with the furnace and a voltage is applied. Resistance to the flow of current causes the temperature of the furnace to increase (as with the element of an electric fire). A programmed temperature sequence (Figure 42.7) can be set up so that

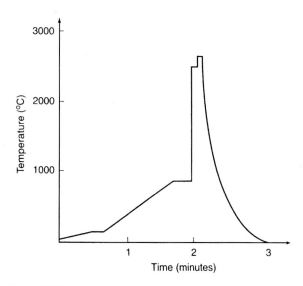

Figure 42.7 An example of a simple heating programme for electrothermal atomization

solution placed inside the furnace is carefully dried, organic material is then destroyed and the analyte ions dissociated from anions. With a rapid increase in temperature, ions are reduced to ground-state atoms for absorption of light. A small further temperature increase ensures that the graphite tube is clean for the next sample.

The atomization temperatures achieved by this technique can be up to 3000°C, so that refractory elements such as aluminium and chromium can be measured. Typically, only 10–50 μl of sample is injected into the furnace, so very small specimens can be accommodated and, because all the sample is atomized within a small volume, a dense atom population is produced in the light path. The technique is therefore very sensitive, allowing measurement of μg/l concentrations. Although slow

compared with flame AAS, the analysis can be automated and modern instruments will shut down at the end of a run so that unattended overnight operation is possible. Electrothermal atomization AAS (ETAAS) is subject to greater interferences than flame AAS and various procedures to eliminate or compensate for these are necessary. Similarly, different forms of graphite materials (electrographite, pyrolitically coated graphite and total pyrolytic graphite) are used, and the design of furnace and how it is heated may be optimized to promote atomization and reduce interferences. Establishing the methodological detail and careful attention when the instrument is set up each day are necessary to obtain accurate and precise results. Surveys of laboratory performance demonstrate that such expertise is usually found in centres where trace element analysis is a major activity.

Interferences

Most of the techniques may be considered to be reasonably mature, in that interferences are understood and there are procedures to overcome them. Devices that involve flow of solutions, such as nebulizers or flow injection systems, will give erroneous results if the samples and calibrants have unmatched viscosities, causing different rates of introduction into the analyser. Where this occurs, strategies such as internal standardization, standards additions or the addition of reagents to equalize flow rates provide for accurate determinations. Chemical interferences are those that influence the rate of atomization. Calcium bound to phosphate in serum is not entirely separated at 2000°C and will give a lower signal than an equivalent concentration of an aqueous calibrant. Addition of a release agent, such as La^{3+}, which binds preferentially to the phosphate, avoids this interference. Chemical interferences also occur within the graphite furnace, such as the sample matrix causing analyte atoms to be volatile and lost during the ashing phase. Chemical modifiers are typically added to stabilize the atoms and/or facilitate the removal of the matrix at an early stage of the heating cycle. The most difficult interferences are those that cause non-atomic absorption of the light beam and are usually a result of the complex nature of biological fluids. Compensation for non-atomic absorption is provided by using chemical modifiers to promote destruction of the organic matrix, devices to establish isothermal atomization conditions and by background correction techniques (Table 42.2).

Table 42.2   Approaches to eliminate non-atomic absorption

Technique	Rationale	Examples
Chemical modifiers	Promote the destruction of sample matrix Delay atomization of analyte	O_2, $Mg(NO_3)_2$, $(NH_4)_2HPO_4$ Pd^{2+}, Ru^{2+}
Isothermal atomization	Reduce vapour phase interactions by delaying atomization until furnace reaches constant temperature	L'Vov platform, graphite probe, novel furnaces
Background correction	Separately measure total and non-atomic absorption; difference = atomic absorption	Deuterium BC, Zeeman-effect BC, Smith–Heijfte BC

Atomic emission

Instrumentation for atomic emission includes:

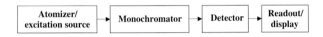

As indicated above, the heat source for atomization and excitation to a higher energy level can be a flame. Historical alternatives include arcs and sparks, but modern instruments use argon or some other gas in an ionized state, which is called a *plasma*.

Inductively coupled plasmas

The plasma is initiated by seeding from a high voltage spark to ionize the atoms:

$$Ar + e^- \leftrightarrow Ar^+ + 2e^-$$

and is sustained with energy from an induction coil connected to a radiofrequency generator. This is known as an *inductively coupled plasma* (ICP).

Plasmas exist at temperatures of up to 10 000°C and in the instrument have the appearance of a torch (Figure 42.8). Samples can be introduced via a nebulizer or, as for AAS, by hydride generation, cold vapour generation or electrothermal vaporization from a graphite atomizer. The main feature of AES is that it permits multi-element analysis. Optical systems direct the emitted light either via a monochromator to a single detector or to an array of monochromators and detectors positioned around the plasma. With the first arrangement, a sequential series of readings can be made with the monochromator driven to give each of the wavelengths of interest in turn. Simultaneous readings can be made with the second arrangement, as each of the monochromators is set to transmit light of predetermined wavelengths. A sequentially reading instrument is less expensive than a simultaneously reading instrument, but more sample is required to take a series of readings. For most elements, the analytical sensitivity for ICP–AES is similar to that obtained with flame AAS.

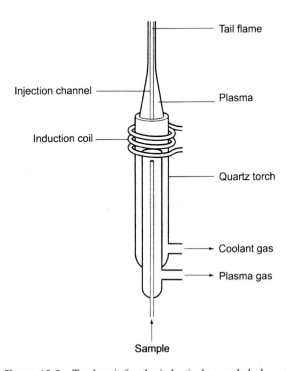

Figure 42.8 Torch unit for the inductively coupled plasma

Interferences

At the high operating temperatures of the ICP, many energy transitions take place, giving rise to the potential for spectral interferences, where emission of light from different elements occurs at wavelengths that are too close together to be separated by the spectrometer bandwidth. Most of these are documented, so that where an interference is suspected an alternative resonance line may be used for the measurement.

Atomic fluorescence

Few commercial instruments for AFS are available and these are confined to the measurement of hydride-forming elements and mercury. The components are similar to those for AAS. Electrodeless discharge lamps are used for the light source and the optical path is modified so that only the emitted, fluorescent light reaches the detector. Certain interferences are common to hydride generation, whatever detector is used. If one hydride-forming element is present in the sample in large amounts, it will consume the reducing agent so that other elements may not be detected. High concentrations of transition elements also inhibit hydride formation. Where this may be a problem, the analyte can be separated from the matrix, e.g. by chelation and solvent extraction or by chromatography.

X-ray fluorescence

Specimens are irradiated by high-energy photons, usually the polychromatic primary beam from X-ray tubes. However, it is the use of radioactive isotopes such as ^{244}Cm, ^{241}Am, ^{55}Fe and ^{109}Cd sources that is of interest for clinical applications. The latter is particularly important as the source in portable instruments developed for *in vivo* XRF (see below, Applications).

As sample matrix contributes considerably to signal intensity, calibration can be difficult, usually requiring the use of different reference materials and/or internal standardization. Fewer problems are encountered with samples prepared as very thin films and in TXRF. Together with the effect of the matrix, sensitivity is also influenced by wavelength, such that lighter elements present a difficult analytical challenge.

In WDXRF, high-intensity X-rays are used to induce the fluorescence emission, which is dispersed into individual spectral lines by reflection at an analyser crystal.

The diffracted beams are collimated and directed onto a photon detector. As with ICP-AES, spectrometers may operate sequentially, with a number of interchangeable crystals to permit the measurement of the full range of elements, or in a multichannel (simultaneous) mode, usually preset for specific analytes. Detection limits for light elements are 10–100 times lower than with EDXRF. Resolution is good, although less so at shorter wavelengths. Sequential instruments require long analysis times to measure several elements, compared with simultaneous instruments or EDXRF technology.

For EDXRF, X-rays emitted from the sample are directed together into a crystal detector. A pulse of current is generated with a height that is proportional to the energy of the X-ray photon. The different energies associated with the various atoms (elements) in the sample are sorted electronically. Lower energy sources (a low-power X-ray tube or an isotopic source) are used. The detector has to be maintained at a very low temperature and in a clean vacuum. Analysis times are 10–30 times longer than with WDXRF but, as a truly multi-element technique, the total time is not necessarily any greater.

When a collimated beam of X-rays is directed against an optically flat surface at an angle of around 5' (5/60 of a degree), total reflection will occur. This is the principle of TXRF, in which the sample is exposed to both primary and total reflected beams and is excited to fluoresce. Emitted radiation is resolved and measured as an ED spectrum. As there is effectively no absorption by the matrix, measurement and calibration are much simpler and sensitivities are greater than with other X-ray techniques.

Inorganic mass spectrometry

The modules required for inorganic mass spectrometry include:

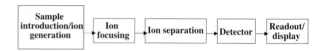

Ion sources

As mentioned above, there are a number of ion generation devices but the most widely used is the ICP. Samples are usually introduced to the plasma via a nebulizer or by chemical vaporization (hydride generation and mercury cold vapour generation). Electrothermal vaporization and vaporization caused by laser ablation of a solid sample are sometimes used.

Mass analysers

The inductively coupled plasma torch is interfaced to the mass analyser via two metallic cones (skimmer and sampler), through which ions are extracted into the ion-focusing unit, where a system of ion lenses direct ions to the mass analyser. Several analyser configurations are commercially available. Those with a quadrupole system have a limited resolution power, allowing the separation of species on a m/z unit basis. To exploit the full potential of the technique, the ICP source has to be coupled to a high-resolution sector field mass analyser, which can achieve much greater resolution and with higher sensitivity than with quadrupole ICP–MS. Time-of-flight mass spectrometers are particularly useful for the analysis of rapid, transient signals, such as those generated by electrothermal vaporization.

Interferences

ICP–MS is subject to many spectral interferences caused by overlapping isotopes, either of different elements or ions formed from matrix components and the plasma gas. Examples important for clinical analyses include $^{40}Ar^+$ on ^{40}Ca, $^{31}P^{16}O_2^+$ on ^{63}Cu, $^{40}Ar^{+35}Cl^+$ on ^{75}As and $^{40}Ar_2^+$ on ^{80}Se. Sector field ICP–MS is not subject to most of these interferences, although loss of sensitivity is seen when high resolution is employed. This may lead to problems with some applications. A relatively new development in quadrupole instruments is the use of collision cells, where a gas-filled cell is included in the focusing unit. Collisions between polyatomic ions and the filler gas cause the former to dissociate and spectral interferences are greatly reduced. Another approach involves separation of analyte ions from those involved in the formation of polyatomic species. Separation may be achieved by vaporization of the sample, e.g. by hydride generation or by electrothermal vaporization, or pre-analytically by chromatography or some similar technique. The addition of nitrogen, helium or methane to the carrier gas or organic solvent to the diluent has been found to reduce some of the argon-based interferences.

Non-spectral interferences, associated with sample introduction, plasma fluctuations, etc., are effectively eliminated by using an internal standard. This should be an element not present in the original sample, not subject to spectral interferences and with a mass and ionization energy close to those of the analyte(s). Often used for biological specimens are scandium, for masses up to 80 atomic units (amu); indium, for 80–150 amu; and iridium, for masses above 150 amu.

Applications

Measurements of minerals and trace elements are required for many different clinical investigations (Taylor, 1996). Certain groups may have poor nutritional intakes of essential elements, e.g. the elderly, deprived children and women during pregnancy, and deficiencies of iron, zinc and selenium are not uncommon in these groups. Essential trace element deficiency also can occur during total parenteral feeding, and protocols for regular monitoring of patients are generally recommended. In other situations, iatrogenic poisoning can occur. Serum aluminium concentrations are regularly measured in patients with chronic renal failure, because of the use of oral aluminium-containing phosphate-binding agents and also from possible contamination of dialysis fluids. Dialysis fluids can become contaminated with other elements, and toxic events associated with copper and zinc have been reported. The diagnosis and monitoring of inborn errors of trace element metabolism usually require measurements of the element involved.

Increased exposure to minerals and trace elements can cause morbidity and some are carcinogenic (Baldwin and Marshall, 1999). While the function of many organs may be perturbed by accumulation of metals, the kidney, liver, nervous, intestinal and haemopoietic systems are more likely to be involved. Accidental (or even deliberate suicidal or homicidal) exposures to trace elements feature in the differential diagnosis when considering signs and symptoms involving these sites. Undue exposure may be consequent on sources within the environment or in the home, associated with hobbies or from unusual cosmetics and remedies.

In an occupational setting, there may be increased exposure to materials with recognized toxic potential. Determination of concentrations in appropriate specimens is a statutory requirement for lead and biological monitoring is also important in the implementation of the UK Control of Substances Hazardous to Health (COSHH) Regulations.

The usual specimens for analysis are body fluids—blood, serum and urine (Walker, 1998; www.sas-centre.org). Hair and nails are occasionally taken to investigate situations of over-exposure. The clinical conditions in which *tissues* are most likely to be analysed are Wilson's disease and haemochromatosis, the concentrations of copper and iron, respectively, in liver being such that even biopsy specimens can be investigated. Larger specimens of tissues removed during surgery or post mortem may be analysed for special investigations.

Many clinical investigations are concerned with measurements of just one or two elements in a specimen; either the symptoms are suggestive of, or there is known perturbation of exposure to, that element. In these situations AAS and AFS are ideal, being sensitive and accurate techniques. Scenarios where multi-element analyses would be helpful are now becoming more common. AES is often not appropriate for analysis of biological fluids but does provide multi-element analysis for specimens such as tissues and foods, where concentrations are higher. For studies requiring multi-element analysis of blood and/or urine, e.g. possible nutritional inadequacy, release from prosthetic implants and unidentified poisonings, ICP–MS provides the simplest, most cost-effective and often the most sensitive technique.

Results may be more informative when presented as the concentrations of the element in specific proteins or some other complex or molecule, rather than as the total concentration in the sample. Several techniques for speciation have been described and some can be directly coupled to the spectrometer in a tandem arrangement for analysis. Atomic fluorescence, ICP–AES and ICP–MS are generally used for detection.

The additional facility of ICP–MS, to determine individual stable isotopes, is exploited for metabolic studies such as measurements of intestinal absorption. Tracer doses with an enriched content of one isotope can be administered without exposing subjects to potentially harmful radioactivity, as occurs when radioisotopes are used for such work. For elements, such as lead and strontium, whose isotopes were partly generated by the radioactive decay of other elements, the ratios between isotopes are characteristic for different geographic locations. From measurement of isotope ratios in biological and environmental materials, sources of exposure may be identified.

XRF does not have a major role in measurements of trace elements in clinical investigations but recent developments have opened some interesting possibilities. Suitable instruments have been designed to be used to analyse tissues close to superficial surfaces of the body, such as the bones in the knee, fingers and the skull. *In vivo* measurements of lead have been undertaken to assess cumulative exposures in lead workers, and to investigate removal from bone stores into the circulation during pregnancy.

Quality Assurance

Apart from the actual analysis, adventitious contamination is the factor that has the greatest impact on the quality of results. Contamination can occur during collection and storage of specimens, the preparative procedure and the spectrometric measurement. Scrupulous attention to cleanliness and to methodological detail are essential to obtain meaningful results. Data from external quality assessment schemes indicate that, while some general hospital laboratories obtain good results, it is the specialist trace element centres that tend to maintain the highest standards of performance. This observation reflects the continuing application of practices to minimize contamination and their expertise and experience in ensuring optimal functioning of equipment. Such centres also accumulate experience with unusual clinical cases and are well placed to provide advice and interpretation.

Because of the stability of inorganic analytes and the purity with which standard materials can be prepared, there are reasonable numbers of reference materials available for use in validating methods and for internal and external quality control. Unlike many other clinical laboratory procedures, and partly as a consequence of the wide use of certified reference materials, accuracy is a straightforward concept and is not defined in the context of particular methodologies.

Conclusions

With recent improvements in the reliability of equipment and developments to reduce interferences, ETAAS and ICP–MS are the most suitable techniques for the measurement of minerals and trace elements in clinical samples. For certain specific applications AES, AFS and XRF are particularly suited. The clinical importance of flame photometry is decreasing with the introduction of sodium and potassium ion selective electrodes.

Accounts of the principles of atomic spectrometric techniques and detailed considerations of instrumentation and applications are given in many textbooks (e.g. Haswell, 1991; Sneddon, 2002). A valuable information source describing current developments in analytical atomic spectrometry for clinical and biological materials, foods and beverages is given in an annual review, part of the Atomic Spectrometry Update series (Taylor *et al.*, 2003).

References

Baldwin DR, Marshall WJ. Heavy metal poisoning and its laboratory investigation. *Ann Clin Biochem*, 1999; **36**: 401–407

Haswell S (ed.). *Atomic Absorption Spectrometry. Theory, Design and Applications* 1991: Elsevier, Amsterdam.

Sneddon J (ed.). *Advances in Atomic Spectroscopy*, vol. 7, 2002; Elsevier, Amsterdam.

Taylor A. Detection and monitoring of disorders of essential trace elements. *Ann Clin Biochem* 1996; **33**: 486–510.

Taylor A, Branch S, Halls DJ, Patriarca M, White M. ASU: clinical and biological materials, foods and beverages. *J Anal Atom Spectrom* 2004; **19**, 505–556.

Walker AW (ed.). SAS trace element laboratories. In *Clinical and Analytical Handbook*, 3rd edn. 1997: Royal Surrey County Hospital, Guildford, UK.

43

Dry reagent chemistry techniques

JA Schroeder, JC Osypiw and **GS Challand**

Introduction

Dry reagent chemistry, thin film chemistry, reagent strip chemistry and solid support analytical chemistry are all synonyms. They describe techniques based upon the incorporation of one or more chemical reagents into a convenient portable unit, which can then be used to carry out chemical analyses without the necessity to make up and transport reagents in liquid form. Probably the earliest and most familiar example is litmus paper, still used in school chemistry departments, analytical laboratories and for in-the-field use testing soil pH. Made by incorporating a vegetable pigment derived from moss (first described in English in 1502) into interstices between the cellulose fibres of paper, it was used by Peacham to colour paper blue in 1606 (OED, 1989) and is likely to have been in use as an indicator ('the acid test') for at least 300 years.

A profound stimulus to the development of thin film chemistry techniques was the invention of photography. The property of silver halides to change colour on exposure to light was first noted by Fabricius in 1556, and the first photographs may have been produced by Schultze in 1727 (Stenger, 1939). The first practical photographic films and paper were developed in the nineteenth century, and today a modern instant colour print film may have as many as 15 discrete layers, each involving a distinct chemical reaction or physical function, all incorporated into a single, stable, portable unit.

The first application of these techniques for clinical biochemistry appeared in the mid-1950s, with the development of reagent strips for the measurement of glucose in urine (Adams *et al.*, 1957). A comparatively untrained analyst, nurse or patient could dip the reagent strip into a urine sample, and within a couple of minutes could obtain a semi-quantitative measurement of the concentration of glucose by comparing the colour developed by the strip with a pre-printed colour chart. This, together with the subsequent application of similar technology to blood glucose analysis (Marks and Dawson, 1965), revolutionized the monitoring of diabetic patients.

Accurate quantitation was improved with the development of simple photometers to measure reflected light for reading blood glucose reagent strips (Mazzaferri *et al.*, 1970)—so-called glucose meters—and further major developments occurred in the 1970s, when the technology of photographic film manufacture was applied to clinical chemistry analyses. Today, many hundreds of analyses are available in thin-film format, and machines have been developed that are capable of measuring colours or other signals developed on a wide range of reagent strips and producing an accurate and precise result every few seconds.

The technology has the potential to revolutionize clinical chemistry practice, both in reducing the requirement for traditional analytical skills in common analyses, and in the capability for analyses to be simply and rapidly performed outside an analytical laboratory, e.g. in wards or clinics, in family practitioner's offices and in a patient's own home. Walter and Boguslawski (1988) have reviewed the field and described the range and technology of available assays.

The Science of Laboratory Diagnosis, Second Edition   Edited by David Burnett and John Crocker
© 2005 John Wiley & Sons, Ltd

Principles of Methodology

In their simplest form, thin-film chemistry analyses consist of a pigment or other reagent trapped within the cellulose fibres of a strip of paper. These produce a visible reaction when an analyte diffuses into the matrix, either in liquid form, e.g. litmus paper and other indicator papers for the estimation of the pH of a liquid, or in gaseous form, e.g. ferrous hydroxide paper for the detection of hydrogen cyanide; mercuric bromide paper for the detection of arsine (Curry, 1988).

More complex systems consist of a series of layers (see Specific Examples, below), each of which has one or more functions. From the base, these are as follows:

1. *A support layer.* This is the foundation for the dry reagent elements. It is usually thin plastic, which may either transmit or reflect light.

2. *A reflective layer.* Its purpose is to reflect back to the eye or mechanical detector as much as possible of the light emitted by the chemistry of the reagent layer(s). This may be included with the support layer by using a reflective plastic. Alternatively, it may be a layer of a pigment, such as titanium dioxide, or a reflective material, such as metal foil.

3. *One or more analytical layers.* These usually consist of thin porous gelatine films within which one or more reagents have been included during manufacture of the film. The reagents must be stable once the gelatine layer has dried. A single layer is adequate when the incorporated reagents do not interact with each other in the absence of an analyte. Multiple layers (each one of which is dried before the next is applied) are necessary to separate reagents that interact with each other in the absence of an analyte. As well as gelatine, fibrous materials such as cellulose can be used. These may function as filters (e.g. to separate red blood cells from plasma) or as molecular sieves, to separate one reaction product from another. Alternatively, reagents can be introduced by immersing the fibrous material in an appropriate solution, then drying.

4. *A spreading layer.* This usually consists of a fibrous material or a membrane. When a drop of sample is applied, it rapidly spreads the sample out laterally and enables a uniform diffusion into the analytical layers.

Complex reagent strips require very accurate manufacture, particularly for the analytical layers, in which the concentration of reagents in the gelatine, the pore size of the gelatine, the thickness of each layer, and the extent of drying of each layer must be carefully controlled (e.g. Bevan, 1996). However, once manufactured, each strip contains all the analytical steps required to carry out an assay. No prior reconstitution of reagents is needed, the strip is portable and can be stable for weeks or months, and the analyst need only apply the sample to initiate the analysis.

Semi-quantitative results can be obtained by matching the colour developed after a fixed time to pre-printed colour charts. In daylight or good artificial light, an experienced analyst with normal colour vision should generate results within $\pm 25\%$ of the true value. For reactions monitored by UV or fluorescence detection, and where more accurate quantitation is needed, a meter is required to measure the colour or other signal. Most dry reagent chemistries are monitored by diffuse reflectance photometry (Kortum, 1969); front-face fluorescence (Pesce *et al.*, 1971) can also be used.

Monitoring of reactions

It may not be obvious, other than to an artist, photographer or physicist, that the properties of reflected light are different to those of transmitted and absorbed light familiar to analysts. But the so-called primary colours of paints and other pigments (red, yellow and blue) are not the same as those of transmitted light (red, yellow and green). In an art gallery, we usually look at a painting from the front, with the painting being illuminated from above. If a painting is illuminated directly from the front, colouring and detail are lost to the observer because of non-coloured reflected light scattered from its surface. We are dealing with the laws of reflectance photometry.

Some light falling on a reagent strip will simply be reflected from its surface (specular reflection). Since this has not interacted with chromophores within the analytical layers, it has the same properties as light from the origin, and cannot be used to monitor a reaction. Some light does enter the analytical layers and can interact with chromophores before being returned by the reflectance layer in the strip. Light scattering and reflection without chromophore interaction can also take place within the analytical layers. The light returned after transmission through the analytical layers (diffuse reflection), which contains a mixture of interacted and scattered light, is used to monitor a reaction. It is detected by measuring the light returned at an angle away from the main specular reflection beam.

After reaction, the concentration of analyte in a sample can be calculated by comparing the amount of diffuse reflected light with that of a standard. The relationship is governed by the equation:

$$R_u = R_s \cdot I_u / I_s$$

where R_u is the percentage reflectivity of the sample, R_s is the percentage reflectivity of the standard, I_u is the intensity of the reflected light from the sample, and I_s is the intensity of the reflected light from the standard. Percentage reflectivity measurements, like transmittance, are not linear with respect to concentration, and in practice linearizing algorithms, such as that of Williams and Clapper (1953), are used to convert a measurement of percentage reflectivity to concentration.

Fluorescent products of a reaction can be monitored using front-face fluorimetry. Monochromators are used to separate fluorescent light emitted by the analytical layers from reflected light. If quenching within the reagent strip is negligible, the measured fluorescence is linear with respect to fluorophore concentration.

Specific Examples

Dry reagent chemistries can be used to measure many hundreds of urine analytes, blood metabolites and proteins. Some can be carried out using a single analytical layer, others require multiple layers and/or the incorporation of physical structures into the analytical layers. Even trace quantities of analytes, such as hormones and drugs, can be measured by utilizing immunoassay techniques within the analytical layers. Later developments using monoclonal antibodies and immunometric assay systems are now widely used. Most of these have been developed by commercial companies, and patent considerations have forced the development of many different solutions to the same problems: typically, in linkages binding antibodies to solid supports; and the choice of reagents to develop a final coloured signal. A selection of specific examples is described below.

Glucose

Glucose was the first biological analyte to be measured using dry reagent techniques (Adams *et al.*, 1957; Marks and Dawson, 1965) because of its presence in comparatively high concentration, the relative simplicity of the reaction used and its importance in monitoring patients with diabetes mellitus. Modern glucose methods rely on

Surface layer	Semipermeable spreading layer
Analytical layer	Paper: buffer, glucose oxidase (GO), peroxidase (P) and indicator (I).

| Glucose + O_2 | Gluconic acid + H_2O_2 |
| H_2O_2 + I reduced | H_2O + I oxidized |

Support layer	Reflective transparent plastic

Figure 43.1 The structure of a Dextrostix® glucose reagent strip (adapted from Walter and Boguslaski, 1988)

enzymatic assays, which generally utilize the enzyme glucose oxidase. A typical example is the three-layer Dextrostix® reagent strip, illustrated in Figure 43.1. A blood sample is applied to the surface layer, which both acts as a spreading layer and is a semi-permeable membrane that separates blood cells from plasma. Plasma from the sample diffuses into the paper analytical layer, which contains the buffered enzyme reaction system, activated by plasma water. Within the analytical layer, glucose and atmospheric oxygen are acted on by the glucose oxidase to produce hydrogen peroxide and gluconic acid. In the presence of peroxidase, also contained within the analytical layer, hydrogen peroxide oxidizes a redox indicator to produce a visible colour change. The plastic support layer also acts as a reflective layer, and after blood cells are wiped from the surface, the colour developed can be read from the top, either visually (by comparing with a pre-printed colour chart) or by using a glucose meter.

Many alternatives to this simple reagent strip for glucose have been developed, e.g. the Fuji® strip (Kobyashi *et al.*, 1982) incorporates a masking and reflective layer containing the white pigment titanium dioxide between the spreading and analytical layers. The support layer is transparent rather than reflective plastic, and the colour change is read from below. This removes the need to wipe blood cells from the strip.

Alanine aminotransferase

Many plasma enzymes can be measured using dry reagent techniques, although analytical systems are more sophisticated, because enzymes are large molecules that do not readily diffuse through matrices. Also, the measurement of enzymes frequently relies on multi-step reactions that are themselves enzymatic. Careful manufacturing control of both the enzyme reagents and

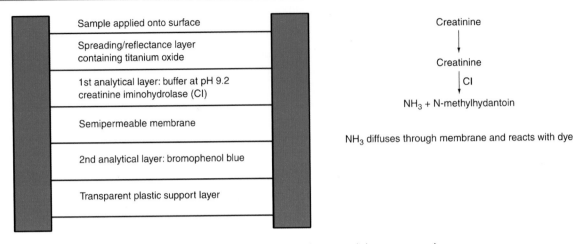

Figure 43.2 The structure of a Vitros creatinine reagent strip

other participating reagents, such as co-factors, are therefore necessary. Some dry reagent layers for enzyme analysis have open lattices that allow serum enzymes to enter the reagent layers of a strip, e.g. Walter *et al.* (1983a, 1983b), while others have closed lattices which retain the enzymes on the surface layer of a slide.

A typical example of a closed lattice system is the Vitros (formerly Ektachem®) method (Eastman Kodak Co., 1992) for alanine aminotransferase (ALT). The spreading layer, which is semi-permeable and retains the serum enzyme, also contains the ALT substrates L-alanine and sodium α-oxoglutarate. ALT catalyses the transfer of an amino group from L-alanine to α-oxoglutarate to produce pyruvate and glutamate. Unchanged reagents and reaction products diffuse into the analytical layer, which contains lactate dehrogenase (LDH) and NADH. Pyruvate produced by ALT in the sample is acted on by LDH to produce lactate, while NADH is converted to NAD^+. The change of absorbance at 340 nm is measured from below using reflectance photometry.

In this system, the spreading layer is also used to initiate the reaction, and the activity of ALT can be measured without the enzyme itself entering the traditional analytical layer. Although pyruvate in the sample can itself participate in the reaction, the concentration in serum is usually too low to cause significant interference.

Creatinine

Serum creatinine can be measured using a multi-layered slide that has an internal separation layer (Sunberg *et al.*,

1983). The structure of a typical reagent strip is shown in Figure 43.2.

For this strip, the spreading layer contains titanium dioxide, which allows it also to serve as the reflectance layer. When serum is applied, creatinine enters the first analytical layer. Here, ammonia is produced from creatinine by the specific enzyme creatinine iminohydrolase, which is incorporated within the layer. The gas-permeable membrane below the first analytical layer allows ammonia to diffuse into the second analytical layer, but constituents such as buffers and hydroxyl ions, which could interfere with the subsequent reaction, cannot traverse the membrane and are trapped in the first analytical layer. The second analytical layer contains an indicator, bromophenol blue, which changes colour in response to ammonia. Viewed from below, the colour change in bromophenol blue can be related to creatinine concentration. Ammonia can interfere, but the concentration in serum is usually too low to give erroneous results.

Potassium

Electrolytes can be measured using ion-selective electrodes (Chapter 40, this volume) constructed as a reagent strip. In a typical ion-selective electrode, an electrically conducting membrane separates the sample from an internal solution of constant composition. A difference in concentration produces an electrochemical gradient across the membrane, which gives rise to a potentiometric difference. An internal reference electrode, usually silver/silver chloride, is also immersed in the filling solution. The change in potential at the internal

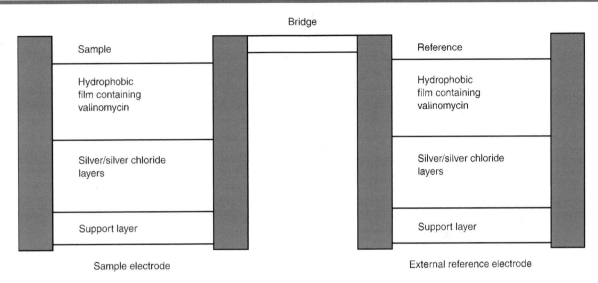

Figure 43.3 The structure of a Vitros potassium ion-selective electrode strip

reference electrode is measured by comparison with an external reference electrode (Russell and Buckley, 1988).

Figure 43.3 shows the structure of a Vitros ion-selective electrode reagent strip. Like a conventional ion-selective electrode, the concentration of an ion is measured from the potentiometric difference between two electrodes; the bridge forms a stable liquid junction connecting the two electrodes. Unlike a conventional ion-selective electrode, a solution of known composition is applied to the second (external reference) electrode, so the sample is referenced directly to a standard solution. Different ions can be measured using different ion-selective membranes. For potassium measurement, each electrode includes a hydrophobic film containing a high concentration of valinomycin. This permits the passage of potassium ions but excludes other cations and anions. A potentiometric difference then solely reflects any difference in potassium concentration between the sample and the standard solution.

Ions such as potassium can also be measured using more conventional dry reagent chemistry. The analytical layer typically contains a hydrophobic organic phase, which excludes all ions except those whose passage is mediated by an ionophore, such as valinomycin for potassium. The ionophore mediates a cation–H^+ interchange between the aqueous (sample) and organic phases. The resulting change in pH within the organic phase causes a change in colour of a redox dye incorporated within the analytical layer (Charlton et al., 1982). A similar approach is also used for the measurement of 'specific gravity' in urine analysis reagent strips—actually a measure of total ionic activity.

Human chorionic gonadotropin

Probably the most widely used dry reagent chemistry strips are those for the measurement of human chorionic gonadotropin (HCG). Designed for visual reading and available over-the-counter, they can be sensitive enough to permit the diagnosis of pregnancy within a few days of conception.

Classic techniques for the measurement of trace quantities of hormones such as HCG relied upon the immunoassay techniques developed in the 1960s. Such techniques relying on limited quantities of an antibody and subsequent differentiation between bound and free antigens have been adapted for thin-film methodology. The structure of a typical format for hormone measurement, the assay of total serum thyroxine, is shown in Figure 43.4 (Nagatoma et al., 1981). The first analytical layer incorporates peroxidase-labelled thyroxine, which is carried with serum thyroxine into the second analytical layer. The second analytical layer consists of an antibody to thyroxine, covalently bound to the matrix. Diffusion of the sample through this layer gives partition between thyroxine in the sample and peroxidase-labelled thyroxine: the greater the concentration of thyroxine in the former, the lower the concentration of peroxidase-labelled thyroxine which is bound, and the greater the concentration of free peroxidase-labelled thyroxine that is available to diffuse through the third analytical layer (containing glucose) into the fourth analytical layer, which incorporates glucose oxidase to generate hydrogen peroxide from glucose and atmospheric oxygen. Peroxidase from free peroxidase-labelled thyroxine

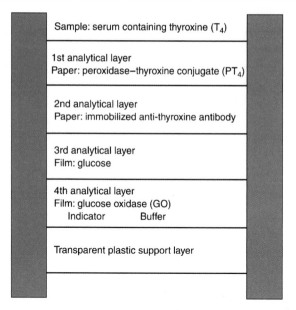

| Sample: serum containing thyroxine (T$_4$) |
| 1st analytical layer |
| Paper: peroxidase–thyroxine conjugate (PT$_4$) |
| 2nd analytical layer |
| Paper: immobilized anti-thyroxine antibody |
| 3rd analytical layer |
| Film: glucose |
| 4th analytical layer |
| Film: glucose oxidase (GO) |
| Indicator   Buffer |
| Transparent plastic support layer |

Figure 43.4   The structure of a Fuji® thyroxine reagent strip

then catalyses the oxidation of a redox dye, which results in a colour change proportional to the amount of free label, which is in turn related to the amount of thyroxine in the original sample.

Such reagent strips are complex to manufacture, and because classic immunoassay techniques require long incubation times, the sensitivity of these methods in dry reagent formats (perhaps 10 µmol/l) is inadequate to detect trace quantities of hormones such as HCG in early pregnancy. Most modern pregnancy test kits analyse urine and utilize immunometric techniques, in which an excess of antibody is present and for which short incubation times are possible. Early versions used a mixture of wet and dry reagent techniques. A monoclonal antibody to the α-subunit of HCG was covalently bound to a matrix. The sample was added first, any HCG present binding to antibody-linked matrix. A solution containing an enzyme-labelled antibody to the β-subunit of HCG was added and incubated for a short time, allowing the interaction to proceed in which intact HCG was sandwiched between matrix-bound antibody and labelled antibody. After adding a buffer solution to wash surplus sample and free enzyme-labelled antibody from the strip, a third solution was added, containing a dye substrate for the enzyme label, which generated a coloured product. In the absence of HCG from the sample to form the sandwich, no coloured product bound to the matrix was developed. A convenient positive control for the reaction could be incorporated

by binding in one area of the strip the first antibody that had already been allowed to react with intact HCG. This area of the strip then gave a positive reaction, even in the absence of HCG in the original sample.

Later versions of immunometric assay technology have included all the components of monoclonal antibody reactions in a dry reagent format. Some have used particle agglutination techniques, relying on the ability of particles, such as those containing a gold sol, to change colour when bound together in the presence of HCG. Others have relied on a region of immobilized HCG antibody covalently bound to a reagent strip. Urine (travelling along the strip rather than through it) mobilizes buffered coloured particles linked to a different HCG antibody. In the presence of HCG in the urine sample, these form a sandwich and produce a discrete coloured region over the immobilized antibody. Again, a positive control can be incorporated within the strip by including a region of immobilized antibody already bound to HCG.

Cardiac troponin T

Troponin T is a so-called cardiac marker, which is now widely used to 'rule in' or 'rule out' myocardial infarction in patients presenting with chest pain (Collinson *et al.*, 2001). Because of the speed with which results can be obtained and the ease of use in a point-of-care environment, thin-film chemistry techniques have been widely adopted for its measurement. A typical example is the GLORIA^{TM} immunoassay developed by Roche, which uses whole blood. A glass fibre spreading layer traps blood cells. Two monoclonal antibodies to different sites of troponin T are contained in the first analytical layer. One of these antibodies is conjugated to biotin, the other to gold particles. The antibodies form a complex in the presence of troponin T. The second analytical layer contains support-linked streptavidin, which binds to biotin and thus immobilizes any troponin T complex. The accumulation of gold particles in the troponin T complex causes the formation of a purple colour, which can be read either visually or using a reflectance meter (Wilding and Ciaverelli, 1999).

Drugs of abuse

'Urinalysis,' the use of a single reagent strip to measure several different urinary constituents, has been in use for several decades. The selection of different chemistries for use in such reagent strips has been governed more by technical achievability than by clinical utility: a good example is the incorporation of a bilirubin-sensitive reaction pad within such multi-strips. Still very widely used, their clinical utility within a hospital environment is controversial (NICE, 2003).

A more modern application of such multi-strip technology is the development of systems for the detection of drugs of abuse in urine. A major driving force in this has been requirements to screen subjects pre-employment or during employment in a very wide range of settings. Such systems have also found use in hospital accident and emergency departments, essentially to screen out the presence of drugs of abuse, which may contribute to altered mental consciousness. Many variants of the technology exist, but all basically use two monoclonal antibodies to each drug or drug group, one capable of linking to a solid support, and the other capable of generating a coloured signal (Wilding and Ciaverelli, 1999). A typical drug panel incorporated into such a multi-strip includes tests for drug groups, such as barbiturates, benzodiazepines, opiates; sympathomimetic amines, such as amfetamine and tricyclic antidepressants; and specific drugs or metabolites, such as cocaine, methadone and tetrahydrocannabinol.

Technically, the development of such strips poses great problems. These include minimizing interference by closely related drugs; ensuring an appropriate sensitivity limit even when faced with one of a group of drugs, each of which may have different cross-reactivity to the incorporated antibody (the benzodiazepine group is an obvious example); and distinguishing between over-the-counter or prescribed drugs and drugs of abuse (e.g. pseudoephedrine and amfetamine). Even with built-in positive and negative controls, such strips are capable of being misread, particularly when used by inexperienced or untrained staff in settings far removed from an analytical laboratory. The finding of a positive result by such a screening procedure must therefore always be followed by verification by another independent method (Wilding and Ciaverelli, 1999).

Quality Control of Dry Reagent Chemistry

Controlling the quality of results given by reagent strips poses different problems to those of traditional wet chemistry analyses. For the latter, new reagents can be made up, and the concentrations of reagents used in the assay can be modified by the analyst. It is therefore comparatively easy to change assay ingredients in response to unacceptable performance. But dry reagent strips cannot be modified by the analyst, and it is seldom obvious from inspection of the strip itself that analytical performance is unacceptable. A major quality control problem is therefore identifying poor performance and determining its cause. In practice, the cause is seldom the reagent strip itself.

For the manufacturer and the analyst, dry reagent chemistries pose a further problem, because the long-term stability of each batch of strips can only be predicted from the stability of previous batches. In practice, there is always some batch-to-batch variation in stability, even when reagent strips are stored in ideal conditions. As part of a quality control programme, it is therefore necessary to monitor long-term trends in performance, so that appropriate action can be taken before quality control becomes unacceptable.

Identification of unacceptable performance— extra-laboratory semi-quantitative assays

At present, the main area of clinical use for semi-quantitative dry reagent use is in urine testing. A wide range of reagent strips is available, which may include just one analyte (e.g. for glucose or protein), or a range of analytes, the colours of each reagent pad having to be matched visually in strict time sequence to a pre-printed colour chart (see Figure 43.5). Although semi-quantitative assays for blood glucose have been largely superseded by the use of reagent strips read in blood glucose meters, these assays pose similar quality control problems. In addition, many new extra-laboratory reagent strip tests have recently been introduced, which range from the measurement of whole blood lipid fractions to the detection of drugs of abuse in urine or saliva. These semi-quantitative assays can be carried out in a wide range of settings: wards, clinics, primary case practices, schools and the home. Little attention has been paid to performance, because there is a widespread belief that such assays are foolproof, and in a hospital setting they are often delegated to the most junior member of ward staff, who may have no experience of analytical chemistry and who may receive no training.

The first survey of the performance of urine analyses on hospital wards (Challand, 1987) showed that the correct result (i.e. matching to the right colour pad) was obtained in only about 50% of analyses. Around 5% of all measurements gave grossly aberrant values. Similar findings have since been obtained in studies from many different locations.

With quantitative assays, it is comparatively easy to define acceptable performance numerically, either in terms of analytical achievability [the approach of most

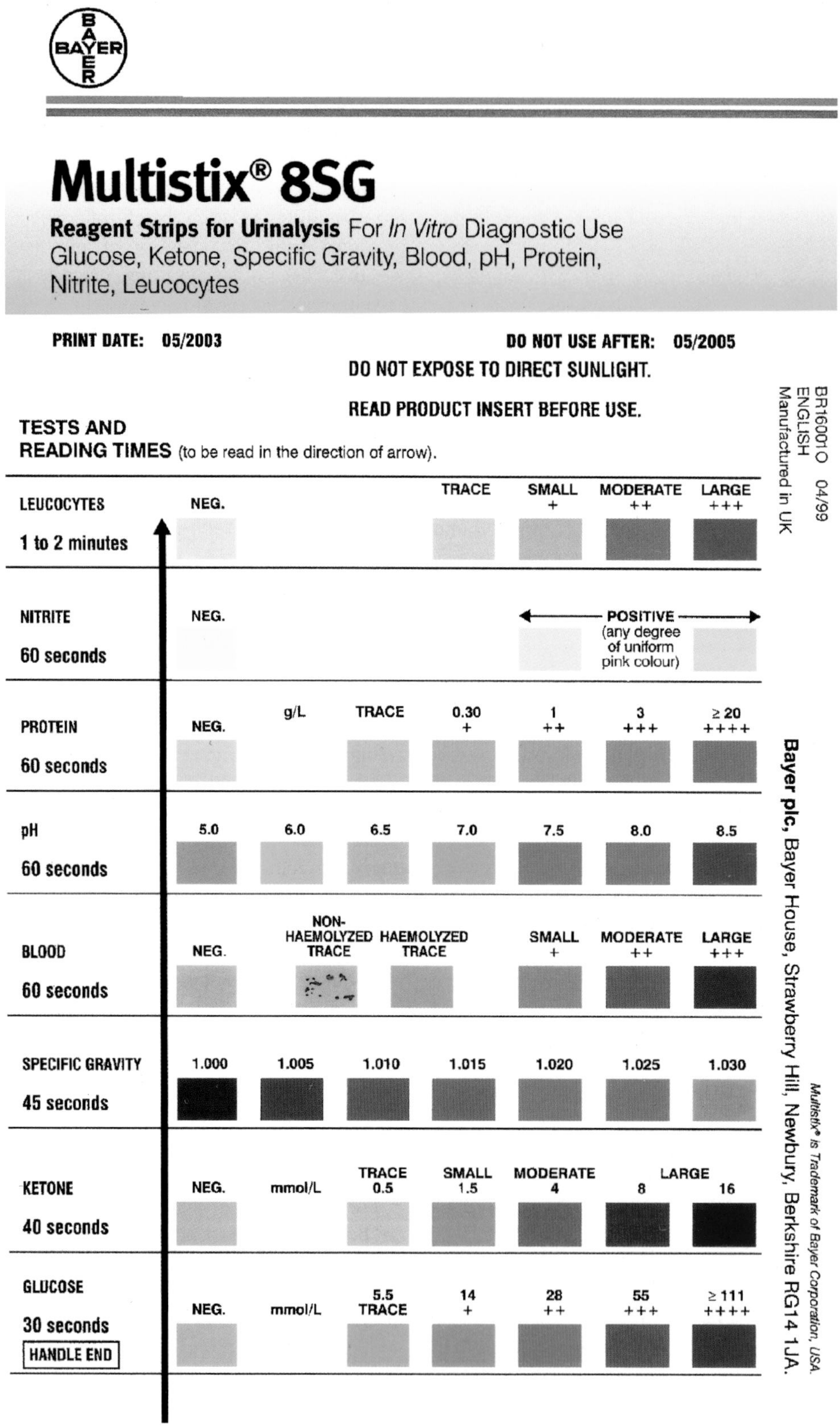

Multistix® 8SG

Reagent Strips for Urinalysis For *In Vitro* Diagnostic Use
Glucose, Ketone, Specific Gravity, Blood, pH, Protein,
Nitrite, Leucocytes

PRINT DATE: 05/2003   **DO NOT USE AFTER: 05/2005**

DO NOT EXPOSE TO DIRECT SUNLIGHT.

READ PRODUCT INSERT BEFORE USE.

BR16001O 04/99
ENGLISH
Manufactured in UK

TESTS AND
READING TIMES (to be read in the direction of arrow).

					TRACE	SMALL +	MODERATE ++	LARGE +++
LEUCOCYTES 1 to 2 minutes	NEG.							

NITRITE 60 seconds	NEG.			◄─ POSITIVE ─► (any degree of uniform pink colour)		

	g/L	TRACE	0.30 +	1 ++	3 +++	≥ 20 ++++
PROTEIN 60 seconds	NEG.					

	5.0	6.0	6.5	7.0	7.5	8.0	8.5
pH 60 seconds							

	NEG.	NON-HAEMOLYZED TRACE	HAEMOLYZED TRACE	SMALL +	MODERATE ++	LARGE +++
BLOOD 60 seconds						

	1.000	1.005	1.010	1.015	1.020	1.025	1.030
SPECIFIC GRAVITY 45 seconds							

	NEG.	mmol/L	TRACE 0.5	SMALL 1.5	MODERATE 4	LARGE 8	16
KETONE 40 seconds							

	NEG.	mmol/L	5.5 TRACE	14 +	28 ++	55 +++	≥ 111 ++++
GLUCOSE 30 seconds **HANDLE END**							

Bayer plc, Bayer House, Strawberry Hill, Newbury, Berkshire RG14 1JA.

Multistix® is Trademark of Bayer Corporation, USA.

Figure 43.5   The pre-printed colour chart for a Bayer Multistix® 8SG urine analysis reagent strip. Reproduced by permission of Bayer Health Care, LLC

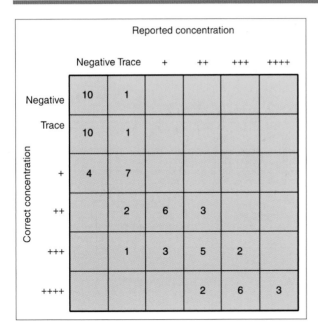

Figure 43.6 Bias in urine protein reagent strip assays. Six pre-prepared urine samples with protein concentrations corresponding to a different colour block were distributed 'blind' to 11 nurse analysts. The figure compares the known protein concentrations with the number of analysts reporting each colour block. As well as the expected scatter of results, a systematic bias exists, analysts tending to underestimate the true protein concentration by one colour block

Table 43.1 Some identified causes of poor performance in carrying out manual reagent strip assays

- Use of out-of-date reagent strips
- Keeping reagent strips in conditions that shorten shelf-life
- Leaving the top off the strip container, or removing the dessicant
- Cutting the strip in half to save money
- Using an unsuitable sample container (e.g. a bleach container for a urine sample)
- Failure to dip a urine reagent strip completely into the sample
- Insufficient sample applied to a blood reagent strip
- Carrying out the test at the wrong temperature
- Reading the colour pad too soon, or too late
- Reading the wrong colour pad on a multi-analyte reagent strip
- Poor lighting conditions
- Poor colour vision in the analyst
- Wrongly transcribing a result on to a report form
- Using the wrong units when reporting

external quality assurance (QA) schemes] or in terms of clinical utility (Fraser *et al.*, 1993, 1997). Semi-quantitative assays do not lend themselves to an easy numerical approach. One cannot use the mean value obtained from QA distributions as the best estimate of the true value, since this often has a bias, introduced either by approximation to the nearest colour match or through deficiencies in technique (e.g. Figure 43.6). Samples distributed as part of a survey or a QA programme are therefore usually synthetic, with weighed-in constituents defining the true value (although this is difficult for some analytes, such as bilirubin or red blood cells). When the weighed-in value corresponds to the concentration required to match exactly one pre-printed colour block for each analyte, in practice only around half the people carrying out the analysis achieve the correct match: approximately 95% achieve a match within one colour block of the correct figure. Results outside this range can be taken to be unacceptable performance. An alternative approach is to weigh in amounts of constituents that produce a colour half-way between two colour blocks. Results corresponding to either of the two adjacent colour blocks are regarded as acceptable: in ward surveys, 10–20% of returns are unacceptable by the rather tighter criterion (Tighe P, personal communication). When unacceptable performance is identified, a cause needs to be found: some of the possible causes are listed in Table 43.1. Almost all of these are due to deficiencies in understanding, in training, or in technique (all of which can be remedied locally). The cause is seldom due to manufacturing deficiencies in the reagent strip, although it has to be said that exaggerated claims for the likely accuracy of these reagent strips in a point-of-care testing environment are sometimes made by manufacturers.

Assessment of long-term trends—quantitative assays

Automated instruments using dry reagent chemistries have been available for several years. These can carry out many different analyses on small quantities of serum, with throughput and precision of analysis matching more traditional wet chemistry analysers. Reagent slides are typically bought in single batches sufficient to last 6 months. If stored in ideal conditions, each batch may need just a single calibration before use, the stability being good enough to maintain quality for the lifetime of the batch. However, in practice, storage conditions may not be ideal (temperature differences between the floor and ceiling of a cold room have been sufficient to change stability) and the very slow deterioration of reagent strips is not identical from batch to batch. Quality control is therefore aimed at ensuring that the initial calibration is adequate, then monitoring slow drift to identify the point at which either a second calibration is required, or at which unused slides should be discarded.

Conventional quality control sera can be used for both purposes, but suffer from disadvantages. They are expensive; matrix effects particularly relating to viscosity and subsequent diffusion through the layers of a slide may make their behaviour different to samples from patients, and the results for some analytes may change markedly in the first few hours following reconstitution. We find that the results obtained from patients' samples can give more reliable QC information. Although patients' results are obviously more scattered than the results of a conventional QC serum, more data are available for statistical analysis. For most analytes, parameters such as the mean patient result (after exclusion of extreme values) and the number of results falling outside a pre-set limit (such as an automatic 'telephone limit' for serum sodium concentration) are sufficiently sensitive and provide almost all of the necessary QC information. Initial calibration can be judged by the comparability of a patient daily mean following previous calibrations. A drift in daily mean can be used to judge the point at which re-calibration or new slides are necessary. Figure 43.7 shows a daily patient mean plot for serum sodium analyses, showing the period before and after re-calibration.

Quality control statistics based on patients' samples can be used to ensure long-term comparability of results within a laboratory, but do not ensure that results are comparable to those produced by other laboratories. Participation in external quality assurance schemes can provide this information, and gives more reliable information than, for example, the results obtained by analysing a quality control sample of known composition. External quality assurance schemes are now available for thin-film chemistry analyses carried out in a point-of-care environment (Bullock, 1999), and are probably most widely used for ward blood glucose analyses; participation in such schemes is now required for laboratory accreditation in the UK (Burnett, 2000).

The temperatures of the dry reagent strip and the sample affect both the speed of diffusion of sample and the rate of reaction within the strip. Good temperature control is essential. The overall performance, as judged by external QA data, of two reagent strip analysers over a 2 year period is shown in Figure 43.8. Temperature control in the laboratory in which they were situated

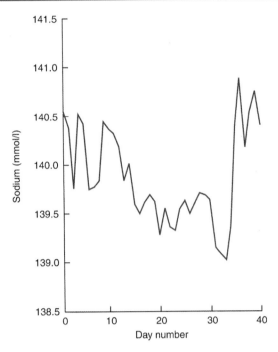

Figure 43.7 Daily patient means, sodium analyses. The plot shows successive daily mean values for serum sodium analyses carried out using a Vitros analyser following calibration. A fall in results is apparent, which averages ca. 0.04 mmol/l each day. Re-calibration was carried out after day 34

was less than ideal, and the deterioration in performance over the hot months of summer is obvious.

Automatic analysers, using both dry and wet reagent chemistry, on occasion produce 'fliers'—apparently correct but aberrant results. The prevalence of these is likely to be less than 0.2%. Short of analysing all samples in duplicate, such errors can only be detected by comparing results with previous results from the same patient or by being alert for discrepancies between results and the clinical information provided.

Summary

The technology of dry reagent chemistry has now advanced to the point at which almost all conventional liquid reagent clinical chemistry analyses can be reproduced in dry reagent format. Although reagent costs are usually higher for the latter, they offer significant advantages. Sample volumes are usually low, sensitivities are comparable to conventional techniques, precision can be at least as good, the techniques are rapid and

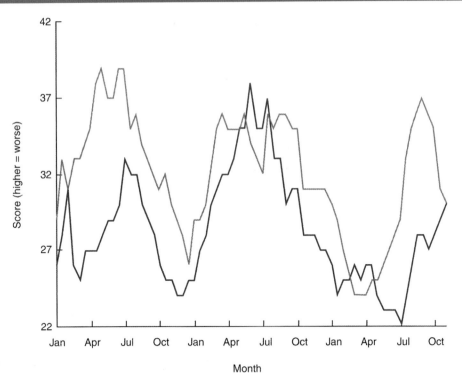

Figure 43.8 Overall external QA results—seasonal trends. The overall mean running variance index score (OMRVIS, an index of imprecision) for two identical Vitros analysers housed in the same laboratory over a 2 year period. The precision in summer months is significantly worse than in winter months, probably due to inadequate temperature control in the laboratory

reliable, and carrying them out requires little specific analytical skill. They are therefore appropriate in a clinical chemistry laboratory, where their use frees scarce technical and scientific resources for development of new assays and new techniques. They are also easily adapted to a near-patient environment, e.g. on wards, in clinics, in primary care and for use by patients themselves.

Despite its apparent simplicity, this technology is not foolproof. Without careful attention to detail in ensuring the identity of the patient, the appropriateness of the sample, the correct procedure of analysis, including timing, temperature and quality control, and the accurate and appropriate recording of the reaction, analyses can give dangerously misleading results. With an increasingly wide utilization of the technology, there are major benefits to the patient and to the clinician in the speed with which results can be obtained. The challenge to the manufacturer is continual development, not only in introducing new assays but also in simplifying current assays and ensuring that they are as accurate and as free from interference as possible. The challenge to the analytical laboratory is in ensuring that wherever this

technology is used, the analyst is trained in the appropriate analytical procedures and educated to be aware of both the strengths and limitations of the technique.

Further reading

Adams EC Jr, Burkhardt CE, Free AH. Specificity of glucose oxidase test for urine glucose. *Science* 1957; **125**: 1082–1083.

Bevan D. Case study. Better comparability means better business for Kodak. *VAM Bulletin*. 1996; **15**: 10–12. Laboratory of the Government Chemist, Teddington, UK,

Bullock D. Point of Care Testing, Price C, Hicks J (eds). 1999: AACC Press, Washington, 157–174.

Burnett D. Accreditation and point-of-care testing. *Ann Clin Biochem* 2000; **37**: 241–243.

Challand GS. Is ward biochemical testing cheap and easy? *Intens Care World* 1987; **4**: 9–11.

Charlton SC, Zipp A, Fleming RI. Solid-phase colorimetric determination of potassium. *Clin Chem* 1982; **28**: 1857.

Collinson PO, Boa FG, Gaze D. Measurement of cardiac troponins. *Ann Clin Biochem* 2001; **38**: 423–449.

Curry AS. *Poison Detection in Human Organs*, 4th edn. 1988: Charles C Thomas, Springfield,IL, 79, 103.

Eastman Kodak Co. *Test Methodology. Kodak Ektachem Clinical Chemistry Slides (ALT)*. Publication No. MP2-36 4/92. 1992: Eastman Kodak Co, Rochester, NY.

Fraser CG, Hytolft Petersen P. Desirable standards for laboratory tests if they are to fulfil medical needs. *Clin Chem* 1993; **39**: 1447–1455.

Fraser CG, Hytolft Petersen P, Libeer J-C, Ricos C. Proposals for setting generally applicable goals based solely on biology. *Ann Clin Biochem* 1997; **34**: 8–12.

Kobyaŝhi N, Tuhata M, Akui T, Okuda K. Evaluation of multi-layer film analytical elements in plasma and in serum by Fuji dry chem slide GLU-P. *Clin Rep* 1982; **16**: 484–487.

Kortum G. *Reflectance Spectroscopy: Principles, Methods, Applications.* 1969: Springer, New York.

Marks V, Dawson A. A rapid stick method for determining blood glucose concentration. *Br Med J* 1965; **1**: 293–294.

Mazzaferri EL, Lanese RR, Skillman TG, Keller MP. Use of test strips with colour meter to measure blood glucose. *Lancet* 1970; **i**: 331–333.

Nagatoma S, Yasuda Y, Masuda N *et al.* Multilayer analysis component utilising specific binding reaction. European Patent Application No. 81108365.8, 15 October 1981.

NICE. *Preoperative Tests. The Use of Routine Preoperative Tests for Elective Surgery.* Clinical Guideline 3. June 2003: National Institute for Clinical Excellence, London.

OED. *Oxford English Dictionary*, 2nd edn. Litmus, Litmus paper. 1989: Clarendon Press, Oxford.

Pesce AJ, Rosen CH, Pasby TL. *Fluorescence Spectroscopy.* Dekker, New York, 1971.

Russell LJ, Buckley BM. Ion-selective electrodes. In *Principles of Clinical Biochemistry: Scientific Foundations*, 2nd edn, Williams DL, Marks V (eds). 1988: Heinemann Medical Books, Oxford, 201–214.

Stenger E. *The History of Photography.* 1939: Mack Printing Co, Easton, PA, 1.

Sunberg MW, Becker RW, Esders TW *et al.* An enzymatic creatinine assay and a direct ammonia assay in coated thin films. *Clin Chem* 1983; **29**: 1267.

Walter B, Berreth L, Co R, Wilcox M. A solid-phase reagent strip for the colorimetric determination of serum aspartate aminotransferase (AST) on the Seralyser®. *Clin Chem* 1983a; **29**: 1267.

Walter B, Boguslaski R. Solid-phase analytical elements for clinical analysis. In *Principles of Clinical Biochemistry. Scientific Foundations*, 2nd edn, Oxford, Williams DL, Marks V (eds). 1988: Heinemann Medical Books, 150–265.

Walter B, Co R, Makowski E. A solid-phase reagent strip for the determination of serum alanine aminotransferase (ALT) on the Seralyser. *Clin Chem* 1983b; **29**: 1168–1169.

Wilding P, Ciaverelli C. Hand-held sensor systems. In *Point of Care Testing*, Price, C, Hicks J (eds). 1999: AACC Press, Washington, DC, 41–66.

Williams FC, Clapper FR. Multiple internal reflections in photographic colour prints. *J Opt Soc Am* 1953; **43**: 595–599.

44

Separation techniques

Roy Sherwood

Why separate?

Most of the analyses carried out in clinical laboratories involve the detection and quantitation of individual compounds in body fluids, usually blood or urine. For this purpose, specific chemical or immunological methods are used for the compound of interest. Whilst such assays account for the bulk of analyses in the clinical laboratory, in some instances a family of closely related compounds may need to be measured. Although specific assays could be developed for each compound of the family group, this approach is often economically or practically less viable then using a technique that can separate and quantitate all the compounds simultaneously. A wide variety of separation techniques are used in clinical laboratories, but the vast majority are based on the principle of chromatographic or electrophoretic separation. Chromatography in all its various guises, e.g. thin-layer chromatography (TLC), high-performance liquid chromatography (HPLC) or gas chromatography (GC), can be used to separate many different types of compounds from small molecules, such as amino acids and drugs to proteins such as glycated haemoglobin. Electrophoresis, on the other hand, is typically used for the separation of proteins, either coarsely (e.g. serum proteins), or specifically to identify variants of a particular protein (e.g. inherited variants of haemoglobin).

Chromatography

Chromatography was 100 years old in 2003. M. S. Tswett of Warsaw University first described the use of adsorption to separate leaf pigments in March 1903. The principle of all the different types of chromatography is the interaction of molecules of interest between a mobile phase (liquid or gas) and a stationary phase (solid). Those molecules which interact with the stationary phase will move more slowly across a plate or through a column than those which do not interact, therefore resulting in a separation of molecules from within a mixture. Control of these interactions, and hence separation, is achieved by exploiting subtle differences in certain physical properties of the different molecules in samples, e.g. their solubility in either water or organic solvents, net charge and size. Table 44.1 details the molecular properties that govern separation in the various forms of chromatography.

Thin-layer chromatography (TLC)

Principles

TLC superseded paper chromatography in the 1960s and is now itself largely being superseded by HPLC. In TLC the stationary phase (commonly alumina, silica gel or cellulose) is coated onto a glass, plastic or metal plate. A solvent mixture (mobile phase) applied to one end of the plate travels along the plate by capillary attraction and results in chromatographic separation of the solutes in a sample applied to the plate. Unless they are fluorescent, most compounds will require derivatization (chemical modification) to enable them to be visualized: this is achieved typically by spraying with, or dipping the plate into, chromogenic reagents. Qualitative information can be gained simply by viewing the plate and identification

The Science of Laboratory Diagnosis, Second Edition   Edited by David Burnett and John Crocker

Table 44.1 Molecular properties that govern separation in various forms of chromatography

Property	Type of chromatography
Adsorptive properties	TLC, HPLC
Partition	GC, HPLC
Antigen–antibody or enzyme–substrate interactions	Affinity
Molecular size and shape	Gel filtration
Ionic charge	Ion exchange

of individual spots can be achieved by measurement of the retention factor (Rf, distance travelled by the spot divided by the total distance travelled by the solvent front). Greater resolution can be obtained by running the plate a second time, but with the solvent direction at 90° to that in the first run (two-dimensional TLC). The disadvantage of 2-D TLC is that only one sample can be applied to each plate. Quantitation either requires the use of a densitometer that can scan the plate, or elution of the spot from the stationary phase followed by colorimetric measurement. 2-D TLC has, however, undergone a resurgence of interest with the developments in the field of proteomics. Following 2-D TLC, the pattern of spots corresponding to individual proteins is compared between individuals with a particular disease and controls, and spots differing in intensity between the groups are eluted from the plate to identify the specific protein involved.

Applications

TLC is predominantly used now as a screening technique as it is relatively quick, cheap and easy in comparison to other chromatographic methods. The applications for TLC in a clinical laboratory include assays of amino acids, drugs and carbohydrates.

Amino acids

Neonatal screening programmes exist in many countries for the early detection of children with phenylketonuria. Although specific spectrophotometric or HPLC methods exist for phenylalanine, many screening laboratories prefer to use a 1-D TLC method that separates the basic, neutral and acidic amino acids, because this has the potential for indentification of other amino acid disorders, e.g. tyrosinaemia, maple syrup urine disease,

etc. Confirmation of the identity of an abnormally raised amino acid can then be achieved by 2-D TLC or HPLC, e.g. the characteristic pattern of abnormally raised branched-chain amino acids (leucine, isoleucine and valine) in maple syrup urine disease. Recent advances in technology associated with liquid chromatography, in particular in combination with mass spectrometry (LC–MS; see later), have led to a reduction in the use of TLC in neonatal screening programmes.

Drugs

Urine drug screening is complicated by the diversity of drugs available for 'recreational' use or taken in deliberate or accidental overdose, which include basic, neutral and acidic compounds. In the unconscious or non-cooperative patient, little information may be available about the consumption of specific drugs. TLC is often the technique of choice for initial screening, and commercial systems, e.g. Toxilab®, are available. These tend to have separate plates and solvent systems for acidic and basic drugs, with the neutral drugs included in either one of the systems. Sequential spraying of different chromogenic reagents results in different drugs staining different colours, thus permitting easier identification. In recent years, however, there has been a significant move towards the use of enzyme immunoassays on automated analysers for first-line screening for drugs of abuse.

Carbohydrates

TLC is the technique of choice for initial screening of urine or faecal samples from symptomatic infants for disorders of carbohydrate metabolism, e.g. fructosuria, etc. Only qualitative results are required for this application, but the development of tests for gastrointestinal tract function and integrity using orally administered sugars has resulted in the need for quantitative TLC of sugars. An example is the use of a mixture of mono- and disaccharides (xylose, rhamnose, 3-o-methylglucose and lactulose), which cross the wall of the gastrointestinal tract via different mechanisms, to assess the permeability of the gut for the differential diagnosis of gastrointestinal tract disease. Reduction in the surface of the gut available for absorption (e.g. coeliac disease) leads to a progressive reduction in monosaccharide absorption, while damage to the integrity of the gut wall (e.g. in Crohn's disease) leads to an increase in disaccharide absorption.

High-performance liquid chromatography (HPLC)

Principles

HPLC is the commonest form of chromatography used in the clinical laboratory. Enhanced performance is achieved by containing the solid phase in narrow columns (typically 150×5 mm) and pumping the mobile phase through the column under pressure (typically $1.5–2.0 \times$ atmospheric pressure). Although ion-exchange or size exclusion mechanisms of separation are occasionally used in HPLC, most methods are based on the adsorption of the molecules to the solid phase. In normal-phase HPLC, hydrophilic binding groups on the surface of a silica packing material attract hydrophilic but not hydrophobic molecules, the opposite being true for reverse-phase HPLC. Thus, in normal-phase HPLC a mobile phase of increasing polarity will more effectively remove polar molecules from the solid phase, while in reverse-phase HPLC increasingly hydrophobic (organic) mobile phases will more readily remove non-polar molecules from the solid phase. Reverse-phase HPLC is, therefore, particularly suited to the separation of uncharged molecules, which predominate in biological fluids.

Equipment for HPLC

The components of an HPLC system comprise: a pump(s), sample introduction system (syringe injector or autosampler), column, detector and data collection system (chart recorder or computer). For most applications, a single liquid phase can be used throughout at a constant flow rate (typically 1–2 ml/min), i.e. isocratic elution. However, in some complex applications where the compounds being separated are similar in structure, it may be necessary to vary the composition of the liquid phase during the analysis, i.e. gradient elution. An example of gradient elution is the separation of amino acids in blood or urine.

The choice of the method of detection for HPLC is dependent on the type of analyte, with ultraviolet (UV), fluorescent and electrochemical (EC) detection being routinely used. UV detection predominates in reverse-phase HPLC but is seldom used in normal phase methods, as the high concentration of organic solvent in the mobile phase results in a large background absorption between 190 and 230 nm. Fluorescence detection has high sensitivity but requires compounds either to have native fluorescence or to be chemically modified to induce fluorescence. Electrochemical detection is based on the oxidation of compounds at a carbon or metal electrode and can offer excellent sensitivity and specificity for particular compounds.

Mass spectrometry (MS) has been used as a mode of detection in combination with gas chromatography for many years. The large volumes of liquid flowing through a typical LC system with a flow rate of 1 ml/min prevented the combination of LC and MS initially. The introduction of microbore LC (<1 mm internal diameter) and developments in the production of very fine liquid aerosols (electrospray) have resulted in LC–MS becoming a viable technique. LC–MS or tandem MS (MS–MS) are probably the fastest-growing separation techniques in the clinical laboratory.

Sample preparation for biological samples

A complication of analysing biological samples using HPLC is the high protein content in many body fluids (approximately 70 g/l in plasma and serum). This can produce background interference and can lead to column clogging, so some form of sample preparation is usually required prior to analysis. The exact form of sample preparation will vary with the specific application, but usually deproteinization and/or extraction of the compound of interest is carried out. Both liquid–liquid and solid-phase extractions are used for HPLC methods involving blood samples. When urine is used, interference in UV or fluorescent detection methods can occur if coloured or fluorescent pigments are present, and some form of extraction will often be necessary, either liquid–liquid or solid phase.

Applications

The majority of applications of HPLC in laboratory medicine fall into the field of clinical biochemistry, although haematologists also use the technique. Groups of compounds that are regularly analysed by HPLC in the clinical laboratory include biogenic amines, amino acids, porphyrins, drugs, vitamins, haemoglobin and carbohydrates. Many other specific applications have been described for research purposes, including nucleosides, collagen degradation products and steroids, but these have not often become part of the routine repertoire of tests.

Biogenic amines

The catecholamines, adrenaline, noradrenaline and dopamine and their metabolites, are measured in plasma and urine samples for the detection of tumours of neural crest origin—phaeochromocytoma and neuroblastoma. Phaeochromocytomas secrete large amounts of adrenaline and/or noradrenaline, which is further metabolized to 4-hydroxy-3-methyl-mandelic acid (HMMA). Increased concentrations of both the catecholamines and HMMA can be detected in urine from patients with phaeochromocytoma using reverse phase HPLC with electrochemical detection. This technique can also be used to detect the abnormally high amounts of dopamine and its metabolite homovanillic acid (HVA), produced by neuroblastomas in children.

Serotonin (5-hydroxytryptamine, 5-HT) is synthesized from tryptophan and metabolized to 5-hydroxyindole acetic acid (5-HIAA) by monoamine oxidases. Carcinoid tumours secrete abnormal amounts of 5-HT and measurement of blood/urine serotonin concentrations or urinary 5-HIAA excretion is useful in the detection of tumours and in monitoring therapy. Methods for the simultaneous determination of HMMA, HVA and 5-HIAA by reverse-phase HPLC are in routine use in clinical laboratories.

Amino acids

The use of TLC for qualitative identification of abnormalities of amino acid metabolism has been described previously. Quantitation of specific amino acids is often necessary, particularly for monitoring therapy in disorders such as phenylketonuria, tyrosinaemia or maple syrup urine disease. The first specialist HPLC system was the amino acid analyser, which is based on the separation of amino acids by cation exchange chromatography, with spectrophotometric detection following post-column reaction with ninhydrin to produce coloured derivatives. Many alternative derivatization methods have now been described to separate amino acids by reverse-phase HPLC with UV, fluorescent or electrochemical detection (see Further Reading).

Porphyrins

The porphyrins are cyclic tetrapyroles that are formed by oxidation of the porphyrinogens, the intermediates of the haem biosynthetic pathway. A class of inherited disorders exists (the porphyrias) in which specific enzyme deficiencies lead to accumulation of the precursors. The clinical presentation of the porphyrias is diverse, ranging from chronic photosensitivity to acute abdominal pain and, although some idea of the exact diagnosis can be gained from the symptoms, characterization of the type of porphyria requires identification of the pattern of porphyrins in blood, urine and faeces. This can be achieved by liquid–liquid extraction of the porphyrins, followed by reverse phase HPLC with either UV or fluorescent detection, since the porphyrins have native fluorescence. An example of porphyrin separation by HPLC is shown in Figure 44.1.

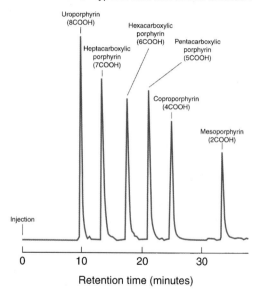

Figure 44.1 HPLC of a standard mixture used for urinary porphyrin analysis. Peaks correspond to uroporphyrin (8 COOH), heptaporphyrin (7 COOH), hexaporphyrin (6 COOH), pentaporphyrin (5 COOH), coproporphyin (4 COOH) and mesoporphyrin (2 COOH). Column, 0.8×15 cm SAS-Hypersil (5 μm). Gradient elution and UV detection (400 nm)

Drugs

Immunoassay techniques have now replaced HPLC as the routine method for many of the established anti-convulsants, e.g. phenytoin, phenobarbitone, valproate and carbamazepine. However, the newer generation of anticonvulsants, including lamotrigine, vigabatrin, gabapentin, topiramate, leviteracetam and oxcarbazepine, are measured by reverse-phase HPLC with UV detection. Therapeutic drug monitoring is, however, considered to be less important for many of the newer anticonvulsants compared to the earlier drugs, as they have wide therapeutic windows (lamotrigine, topiramate and leviteracetam) or their plasma concentration is poorly correlated to clinical efficacy (gabapentin, vigabatrin). Monitoring is, therefore, primarily carried out in suspected noncompliance with therapy.

Other drugs

Assays for many thousands of other drugs in biological fluids have been developed. Readers seeking further information should consult the Further Reading section at the end of this chapter. The use of separation techniques including LC is of particular relevance where a drug has an active metabolite that needs to be measured alongside the parent drug, e.g. amiodarone, dothiepin, etc.

Vitamins

The vitamins are a diverse group of compounds, but virtually all have been measured in blood or urine by HPLC (see Further Reading for details).

Haemoglobins including glycated haemoglobin

Over 400 structural variants of haemoglobin are known, most of which have no clinical sequelae for the individual. However, some variants are associated with disease, e.g. HbS (the haemoglobin of sickle cell disease). A definitive diagnosis requires the identification of the variant present. Until relatively recently, separation of haemoglobins was achieved by electrophoresis, but several commercial dedicated HPLC systems based on ion-exchange chromatography have now appeared. These have a faster sample throughput and are useful in population screening for haemoglobinopathies. Modifications to these systems enable them to be used to quantitate the glycated fraction of the haemoglobin, HbA_{1c}, with an analytical cycle time of 4–8 minutes. A HPLC version of the boronate gel affinity chromatography method is also available, which has the benefit of being unaffected by the presence of inherited haemoglobin variants. A reference method for HbA_{1c} measurement has been established that involves the cleavage of haemoglobin into peptides by endoproteinase Glu-C, followed by separation and quantitation of the hexapeptides by HPLC-electrospray ionization–mass spectrometry (ESI–MS) or HPLC-capillary electrophoresis.

Carbohydrates

Screening for inherited disorders of carbohydrate metabolism is usually carried out by TLC, as previously described. Quantitation of specific carbohydrates is often not necessary, but the development of intestinal sugar absorption/permeability studies has necessitated accurate measurement of specific sugars in urine, e.g. lactulose, rhamnose, xylose, when quantitation is required. Separation can be achieved using ion exchange chromatography but detection has been difficult, as carbohydrates have neither usable UV nor fluorescent properties. The advent of pulsed amperometric electrochemical detection has improved the situation vastly, although progress has been slow.

Gas chromatography (GC)

Principles

In GC, the compounds of interest are separated by the partition between the solute in an inert carrier gas stream (nitrogen, argon or helium) and a liquid of low volatility held on an inert support (hence its former name, gas–liquid chromatography, or GLC). The inert support is usually glass microbeads or synthetic halogenated polymers and a derivatized polyalcohol or silicone. Conventional GC columns are typically 1–3 m long with a 2–6 mm internal diameter, but the majority of clinical applications use capillary columns, which can be up to 40 m in length with an internal diameter of 0.2–0.5 mm. The benefits of capillary GC are generally improved resolution and shorter run times. The detection systems available for GC are: flame ionization (FID), electron capture (ECD) and mass spectrometry (GC–MS). A comparison of normal vs. capillary GC and details of the mode of action of the types of detectors is given in a review by Lewis and Sampson (1994).

Applications

Compounds that can be separated by GC must be volatile or capable of being converted to a volatile state by derivatization. These include alcohols, steroids, drugs, organic acids and bile acids.

Alcohols

Ethanol and methanol are volatile compounds readily measurable by GC with FID. A normal GC column can be used, as the extra resolution of capillary GC is unnecessary. Ethylene glycol measurements in suspected toxicity are also feasible.

Steroids

Urine steroid profiling provides information on the production and metabolism of steroids from the adrenal gland, testes and ovaries. It is particularly important in assessing children of uncertain gender or with precocious sexual development. There has also been considerable interest in measuring steroids to detect anabolic steroid abuse in athletes. Using capillary GC with FID following derivatization of the steroids, up to 25 steroids and metabolites can be detected and quantitated in one run (Figure 44.2). The wider availability and reduction

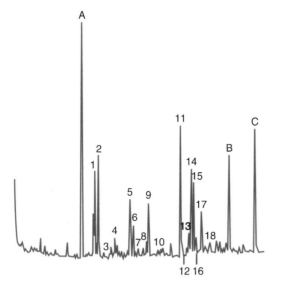

Figure 44.2 Typical chromatogram from capillary GC analysis of methyl oxime-trimethylsilyl ether (MO-TMS) derivatives of steroids in urine from a normal adult female. The peak identities are as follows: A, B, C, internal standards; 1, androsterone; 2, aetiocholanolone; 3, dehydroepiandrosterone; 4, 11-oxo-aetiocholanolone; 5, 11β-OH androsterone; 6, 11β-OH aetiocholanolone; 7, 16α-OH dehydroepiandrosterone; 8, pregnanediol; 9, pregnanetriol; 10, androstenetriol; 11, tetrahydrocortisone; 12, tetrahydro-11-dehydrocorticosterone; 13, *allo*-tetrahydrocorticosterone; 14, tetrahydrocortisol; 15, *allo*-tetrahydrocortisol; 16, α-cortolone; 17, β-cortolone; 18, α-cortol

in cost of GC–MS instruments has progressively led to the replacement of conventional capillary GC of steroids with GC–MS.

Drugs

Drugs that are not easily measured by HPLC, e.g. valproate, the tricyclic antidepressants, etc., are often assayed by GC, either for therapeutic drug monitoring or for toxicological purposes. Most systems use normal GC columns with FID, but GC–MS has a particular role in confirming positive drugs of abuse screens obtained using TLC, EMIT or other immunoassays. Specific methods for many drugs can be found in the book by Ghosh (1992).

Organic acids

Inherited diseases that produce changes in organic acid excretion include specific diseases, e.g. propionic acidaemia, and families of diseases such as those associated with abnormalities of the urea cycle. Urinary organic acid measurements are usually carried out using capillary GC–MS. The added benefit of MS as the detector is the positive identification of any unusual compounds.

Electrophoresis

Principles

Electrophoretic separation is based on the differential migration of charged molecules under the influence of an applied electric potential. Molecules that can be separated by electrophoresis must either carry a net positive or negative charge in their native state, e.g. many proteins and amino acids, or must be able to accept a charge, e.g. carbohydrates complexed with borate ions. The chemical environment around the molecule, the electrolyte solution, must be capable of conducting an electric current, but also has a critical role in determining the state of ionization and hence the charge on any molecule in contact with it. The choice of electrolyte and its pH is critical to achieving optimal mobility and separation. Movement of the charged particle is brought about by the action of the electric force. The migration velocity is dependent on the relationship between the applied potential and the distance between the electrodes—greater migration can be obtained by increasing the voltage applied or decreasing the distance between electrodes. The passage of an electric current will inevitably generate heat, and optimal conditions will have to balance with maximizing separation. A retarding force, which is a function of the size of the molecule and the viscosity of the solution, counteracts the forward migration induced by the electric field. The rate of migration is therefore directly proportional to the field strength and the net charge of the molecule and inversely proportional to the size of the particle and the viscosity of the solution.

Electrophoretic separation can be achieved in free solution but usually some form of solid support medium is used, such as paper, cellulose acetate, agar gel or polyacrylamide gel. In the past 10 years, much interest has focused on carrying out electrophoresis in narrow capillaries at high voltage, i.e. capillary electrophoresis.

Applications

Electrophoresis was first used in the clinical laboratory in the 1950s for the separation of serum proteins. Since then, applications have been developed to separate serum proteins, isoenzymes (e.g. creatine kinase, alkaline phosphatase, etc.), haemoglobin variants and DNA fragments following the polymerase chain reaction (PCR). As for chromatography, many other applications exist, such as the separation of lipoproteins, but these have tended to remain in the research domain and have not become routine tests.

Serum protein electrophoresis

The principal use of electrophoretic separation of serum proteins is the identification of monoclonal gammopathies, although it continues to be used to demonstrate the (non-specific) changes associated with a variety of conditions, e.g. nephrotic syndrome. The early methods for serum protein electrophoresis used cellulose acetate as a support medium, but this produced limited resolution of serum proteins and has largely been superseded by agarose gel electrophoresis. Serum proteins are separated into the main bands corresponding to albumin, α_1-globulins, α_2-globulins, β-globulins (β_1 and β_2) and γ-globulins. If plasma is used rather than serum, an additional band from fibrinogen is present, usually between the β- and γ-globulin regions (Figure 44.3). Visualization following staining with Ponceau red or Coomassie brilliant blue stains is usually adequate to detect gross abnormalities, but densitometric scanning can be used if quantitative data on the individual fractions is required, i.e. if a paraprotein is present. Even

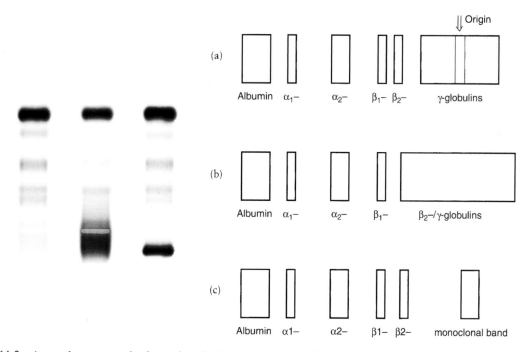

Figure 44.3 Agar gel serum protein electrophoresis: (a) normal pattern; (b) polyclonal increase in γ-globulins due to cirrhosis of the liver; (c) monoclonal gammopathy (IgG) with immune paresis

greater resolution can be obtained using polyacrylamide gels but this is seldom of value in routine clinical use. Automated systems for serum protein electrophoresis are now available.

Isoenzymes

Many of the enzymes that are routinely measured in serum exist as a mixture of isoenzymes, each of which may be produced by a different organ system in the body, e.g. creatine kinase (CK) in serum is a mixture of CK-MM (from skeletal muscle), CK-MB (predominantly from the heart) and CK-BB (from brain). Electrophoresis can differentiate whether the cause of a raised total CK is damage to cardiac or skeletal muscle. Separation is achieved using agar gels that are overlaid with a synthetic substrate to the enzyme that produces a fluorescent compound visible under UV light when acted on by CK. Although measurement of the cardiac-specific troponins has largely replaced CK-MB measurements in many laboratories, electrophoresis remains the only method capable of detecting the presence of macro-CK complexes. Electrophoresis is also used to separate alkaline phosphatase into the liver, bone, placental and intestinal forms and to determine the pattern of isoenzymes of lactate dehydrogenase.

Haemoglobin

Until the recent introduction of HPLC methods for the identification of haemoglobin variants, electrophoretic methods were in common use, based on the different overall charge on the haemoglobin molecule caused by the amino acid substitutions. Cellulose acetate was normally the support medium for screening methods, with citrate agar gel electrophoresis used for positive identification of any abnormal variants seen on screening. The separation of haemoglobin variants by citrate gel electrophoresis relies on the interactions of the substituted amino acids with agaropectin. Those variant haemoglobins with substitutions near the surface, e.g. HbS and HbC, are retained, while those with deeper substitutions, such as HbD and HbG, are not. Complex combinations of electrophoresis or isoelectric focusing are required to identify rare haemoglobinopathies.

DNA fragments following PCR

Whilst outside the scope of this section, it is worth remembering that many of the molecular techniques now being introduced into the clinical laboratory include the electrophoretic separation of the restriction fragments of DNA, following PCR and treatment with restriction enzymes. Agar gel is the support medium used in the vast majority of applications in molecular biology, with visualization either by radiolabelling or by staining with ethidium bromide. An example of the use of such techniques is the detection of the two mutations in the HFE gene associated with genetic haemochromatosis: C282Y and H63D.

Capillary electrophoresis (CE)

Although electrophoresis in a narrow capillary was first described in 1937, it has only been since 1985 that the technique has come into its own. Capillaries 25–100 μm in diameter and 25–100 cm in length are used, the ends of which are placed in buffer vials, which also contain the electrodes. Very high voltages (10–30 kV) are applied to produce the electroendosmotic flow within the capillary. The type, pH and ionic strength of the buffer filling the capillary are critical to achieving the desired separation.

There are four major modes of separation by capillary electrophoresis: capillary zone electrophoresis (CZE) or free solution separation; micellar electrokinetic capillary chromatography (MECC); capillary isoelectric focusing (CIEF) and capillary isotachophoresis.

The principles of these different modes of separation and potential applications in laboratory medicine have been reviewed recently. A commercial instrument using CE for serum protein electrophoresis has been developed (Beckman Instruments). This uses a number of capillaries in parallel to achieve high throughput and includes identification of paraproteins using the technique of immunosubtraction. CE became the dominant methodology in the Human Genome Project and is the basis for the current generation of bench-top DNA sequencers.

Further reading

Chace DH. Mass spectrometry in the clinical laboratory, *Chem Rev* 2001; **101**: 445–477.

Ghosh MK. *HPLC Methods in Drug Analysis*. 1992: Springer Verlag, Berlin.

Lehmann R, Voelter W., Liebich HM, Capillary electrophoresis in clinical chemistry, *J. Chromatogr B* 1997; **697**: 3–35.

Lewis J, Sampson D. Chromatography for the clinical biochemist. *Clin Biochem Rev* 1994; **15**: 56–63.

Sherwood RA. Liquid chromatography: applications in clinical analysis. In *Encyclopaedia of Analytical Science*, 2nd edn. 2004: pp. 267–76 Academic Press, London.

SECTION 8

IMMUNOLOGY

45

Protein assays

David Burnett

Introduction

Qualitative and quantitative techniques for protein analysis are essential tools in the routine immunology laboratory, whose remit includes the analysis of some proteins in blood and other body fluids. Specifically, the proteins of major interest to the immunologist include the immunoglobulins (antibodies), the proteins of the complement system and, most recently, cytokines, which have a role in the immune system. The purpose of this chapter is to describe briefly the principles of the methods used for routine protein analysis. Although some of the methods described are used for the study of proteins of the complement system, the nature of that system demands special considerations for accurate interpretation. Assays for complement proteins are therefore described in detail in Chapter 46. Similarly, assays for autoimmune antibodies are addressed in the chapter on immune complex disease and cryoglobulins (Chapter 48).

The main purpose of the routine laboratory is to detect, characterize and measure the quantity of:

1. Deficiencies of specific proteins, such as in immunoglobulin deficiency.

2. Abnormal or inappropriate expression of proteins, e.g. in monoclonal gammopathies, autoimmune disease or atopy.

Methods for the analysis of proteins rely on a variety of principles. For most routine assays such as those which are described in this chapter there are, however, really only two basic properties utilized:

1. Individual proteins have a characteristic electrical charge, which means that different specific proteins can be separated by electrophoresis.

2. Each specific human protein has a unique structure and this can be used to produce antibodies to that protein, polyclonal antibodies by immunizing animals with that human protein, or monoclonal antibodies by hybridoma technology. Antibodies specific for a protein are the basis of immune assays.

The selection of an appropriate assay method will depend upon whether a qualitative or quantitative result is required. Furthermore, the concentration of the protein of interest will be crucial to the choice of test, e.g. the detection or measurement of oligoclonal and monoclonal immunoglobulins in CSF and urine may require sample concentration or the choice of a method more sensitive than that required for serum specimens.

A short historical perspective

The principles of electrophoresis, the method of separating molecules in an electric charge, had been known for some time when the Swede, Arne Tiselius, in 1930, suspecting the complex nature of blood proteins, began experimenting with the electrophoresis of serum in a liquid buffer medium. In 1937 he identified several

The Science of Laboratory Diagnosis, Second Edition ˙Edited by David Burnett and John Crocker
© 2005 John Wiley & Sons, Ltd

discrete protein zones, which could be seen after the electrophoresis of serum; these he designated *albumin*, *α-globulin*, *β-globulin* and *γ-globulin*, albumin having the fastest mobility towards the anode and γ-globulin the slowest. This basic nomenclature is still in use today (see below). In the 1950s paper began to be used as a support medium, followed in later years by the use of cellulose acetate and gels such as agar, agarose and polyacrylamide. Today, liquid phase electrophoresis has been reintroduced for routine tests (see below).

As early as 1905, Bechhold showed that a protein *antigen* and an antibody to that antigen could form a precipitate. It was 1946, however, before Oudin described a useful development of this principle and in 1948 Elek and Ouchterlony introduced 'double diffusion' in a gel independently. This simple method, which is still used (described below), continues to be referred to as the 'Ouchterlony method'. Grabar and Williams, in 1953, combined electrophoretic separation of serum proteins with immunoprecipitation (qualitative immunoelectrophoresis), using polyclonal antibodies to whole serum, and the true nature of the heterogeneity of serum proteins was recognized. As specific proteins began to be purified and antibodies to them raised in animals, specific quantitative immune assays became possible. Radial immunodiffusion (the Mancini technique) was introduced in 1965 and this, too, is still used routinely (see below). The sensitivity of quantitative protein assay has since been improved, with radio-immunoassays and enzyme-immunoassays allowing realistic measurements down to the order of several ng/ml.

Qualitative techniques

Electrophoresis

Serum protein electrophoresis, although giving limited resolution, is a fundamental method for analysing samples for gross protein abnormalities. The support medium for gel electrophoresis is usually a cellulose acetate membrane or agarose gel. Buffers vary but usually are based on barbitone, with a pH of about 8.5. Gels or membranes for routine electrophoresis are available commercially and these are frequently used to minimize preparation time and to ensure consistent results. The support membrane is placed on an electrophoresis tank, connected at each end to buffer solution. The sample to be analysed is loaded at the cathode end and an electric current applied for 30 minutes to 1 hour. The proteins in the sample migrate in the current at rates proportional to their charge. After completion of electrophoretic separation, the gel or membrane is removed and the proteins insolubilized by fixation, usually in acetic acid solution, and visualized by staining with an appropriate protein dye (Figure 45.1). The gel can be semi-quantitated by *densitometry*; i.e. the gel is scanned using a densitometer, which measures the density of staining (Figure 45.1).

Only proteins with a concentration of 0.1–0.5 g/l or greater will contribute to the serum protein bands seen, of which usually six are represented. These are designated, in order of electrophoretic mobility, as:

1. The albumin band (represented by serum albumin).

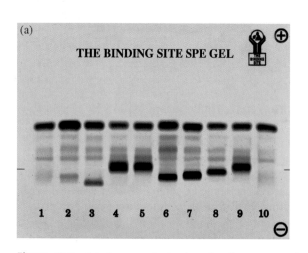

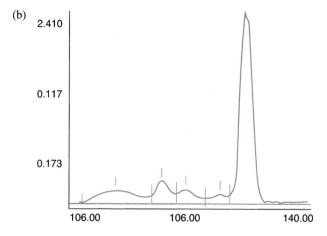

Figure 45.1 (a) Agarose electrophoresis of serum samples, stained for protein. The samples were loaded at the cathode (bottom). The band at the top of each lane represents albumin. The heavily stained bands at the cathode end represent paraproteins. (b) Densitometry scan of agarose electrophoresis of serum from a healthy subject. The tall peak on the right represents albumin

2. The α_1 band (represented usually by α_1-antitrypsin, orosomucoid and α-lipoprotein).

3. The α_2 band (represented by haptoglobin and α_2-macroglobulin).

4. The β_1 band (represented by transferrin).

5. The β_2 band (represented by complement proteins and β-lipoprotein).

6. The γ band (represented by the immunoglobulins IgG, IgM and IgA).

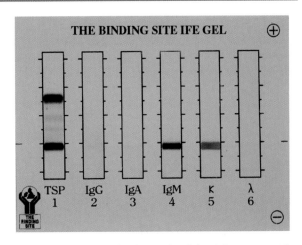

Figure 45.2 Immunofixation and staining of serum proteins following electrophoresis. The lane labelled TSP shows the staining pattern for all proteins. The band at the top is albumin. The band nearest the bottom is a paraprotein. Immunofixation with antibodies to human IgM, IgA and IgM reveals that the paraprotein is IgM. Fixation with antibodies to κ and λ light chains show that the paraprotein is IgMk

Most serum proteins, being present in blood at concentrations below the threshold for this method, do not contribute to the bands seen. Nevertheless, for the immunologist perhaps the most relevant information obtained from electrophoresis is the detection of immunoglobulin deficiency or monoclonal gammopathies. Because immunoglobulins usually represent many different antibody molecules, they are by nature heterogeneous and are not represented by a discrete γ band. Rather, this band is seen as a broad smear *unless* there is a monoclonal (or 'M') band. In cases of monoclonal gammopathies, there is production predominantly by a single expanded clone of immunoglobulin-producing cells, of immunoglobulin of one isotype (IgG, IgM or IgA) with discrete specificity. These immunoglobulin molecules are thus essentially identical and produce a discrete γ or M band (Figure 45.1). The identification of the nature of the monoclonal M protein in serum and free light chains (Bence–Jones proteins) in urine can be carried out using *immunofixation* by precipitating the protein in the support medium, after electrophoresis, with a specific antibody to each isotype. Non-precipitated proteins are washed out and the remaining precipitate visualized by staining with a protein dye (Figure 45.2). The M protein can also be characterized by immunodiffusion or immunoelectrophoresis and the concentration measured by quantitative immunoassay (these methods are described below). By contrast, a reduced γ band suggests an immunoglobulin deficiency and this should be investigated further by quantitative assay (see below).

Just as DNA sequencing in gels has been largely replaced by capillary systems, protein electrophoresis can now be performed in capillaries containing a liquid phase. The Beckman-Coulter paragon CZE 2000 is one example. It has been designed to allow the rapid analysis of many specimens—70 samples in 90 minutes. The resolution is similar to that of gels. Indeed, the result,

which has the format equivalent to a gel densitometry scan, can be 'reversed' to give the simulated image of a stained gel.

Ouchterlony immunodiffusion

Immunodiffusion is carried out usually in agar or agarose gels. Classically, a rosette of wells is cut into the gel with a well also cut at the centre of the rosette (Figure 45.3). The central well is filled with test specimen and each surrounding well in the rosette with an antiserum of different specificity. The gel is incubated in a humid atmosphere for several hours. The proteins in the central well and those from the rosette diffuse into the gel. If the specimen contains a protein to which one of the antisera is raised, a precipitate begins to form; this precipitate is insoluble at concentrations of 'equivalence'. The gels can be washed, dried and stained for archiving. Using this method, the presence of several proteins can be detected simultaneously in the test specimen. Alternatively, several test samples can be analysed for the presence of a specific protein by putting a specific antiserum in the central well and a different test sample in each of the surrounding wells. Commercially supplied 'Ouchterlony' plates are available, e.g. to identify the isotype and subclass representing a paraprotein in a serum sample.

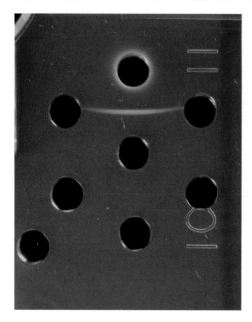

Figure 45.3 Ouchterlony immunodiffusion showing the classic 'rosette' pattern of wells cut into agarose gel. An antibody (raised in an animal such as rabbit or sheep) was put into the central well and serum samples into the surrounding satellite wells. The serum in the well at the top contained the protein of interest. The antibody molecules have diffused radially through the gel and where it met the protein diffusing from the bottom well. The protein (antigen) molecules have been bound by antibody molecules, resulting in a visible, insoluble precipitate

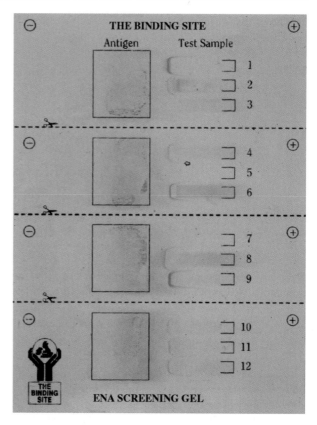

Figure 45.4 Countercurrent electrophoresis. This example is a commercial kit designed to detect autoantibodies. The target antigen is in the square sections at the left (cathode) and the patient's serum applied at the anode (right side of this picture). Under the influence of an electric current, the antigen and the patient's immunoglobulin molecules migrate towards each other. An immunoprecipitate, stained with a protein dye, indicates the presence of autoantibodies to the antigen

Countercurrent immunoelectrophoresis

Countercurrent electrophoresis is similar, in principle, to immunodiffusion but the antigen and antibody are electrophoresed towards each other in the gel (Figure 45.4). The use of electrophoresis rather than diffusion means that results are obtained more quickly. It has been recommended that countercurrent immunoelectrophoresis should be used as a rapid initial screening method (e.g. for detecting antibodies to extractable nuclear antigens) and positive results confirmed by other methods, such as Ouchterlony immunodiffusion.

Immunoelectrophoresis

Qualitative immunoelectrophoresis (described originally by Grabar and Williams) begins with electrophoresis in cellulose acetate, agar or agarose. A trough is cut in the membrane or gel, adjacent to the electrophoresis track.

Following electrophoresis, antiserum is placed in the trough and the membrane/gel is incubated in a moist atmosphere for several hours. During this time, the electrophoretically separated proteins and the antibody molecules from the trough diffuse through the support medium. If antibodies to the separated proteins are present, an immunoprecipitate forms in the gel, which is insoluble at a point of 'equivalent' concentrations. These precipitates are often visible in the unstained 'wet' gel but sensitivity can be increased after the gel is washed, fixed and stained (Figure 45.5). An antiserum raised to whole serum reveals precipitate arcs representing all the proteins present to which there are antibodies in the antiserum. The absence of a precipitin arc (when compared to a reference specimen) indicates a protein deficiency. Monoclonal paraprotein will also be evident

(a)

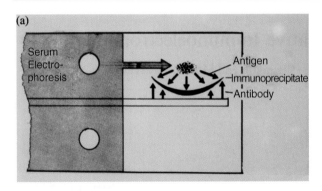

(b)

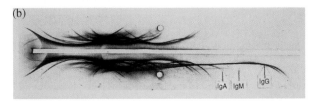

Figure 45.5 (a) Diagram showing the principle of qualitative immunoelectrophoresis. The patient's sample is placed in a well cut into the gel and the proteins separated by electrophoresis. After electrophoresis, antiserum is put into a trough running parallel to the separated proteins. The gel is left in a moist atmosphere to allow the separated proteins and the antiserum molecules to diffuse into each other. The presence of proteins to which antibody molecules are present results in an arc-shaped precipitate. (b) Immunoelectrophoresis of two serum samples. The two sample application wells are at the centre of the gel, separated by a trough that contained sheep antiserum raised against human serum proteins. Electrophoresis was carried out with the cathode to the right. The immunoprecipitate arcs in the serum at bottom show a normal pattern; those for IgG, IgA and IgM are labelled. Note the absence of these immunoprecipitates in the upper sample, indicating that this patient was deficient in all three immunoglobulins

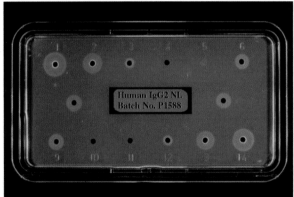

Figure 45.6 Single radial immunodiffusion. This example shows an agarose gel into which is dissolved an antiserum to human IgG_2. Human serum samples were put into the wells that were cut into the gel. The plate was incubated to allow the proteins in the samples to diffuse through the gel. The IgG_2 molecules were bound by antibodies to IgG_2, resulting in the visible insoluble precipitate rings. The area of a precipitate ring is proportional to the concentration of IgG_2 in the sample. Note the absence of rings in some samples, showing IgG_2 deficiency

because of abnormally shaped or pronounced precipitates. The presence or identity of a specific protein, such as a paraprotein, can be confirmed by putting a specific antiserum (e.g. antiserum specific for human IgG, IgA or IgM heavy chains or κ or λ light chains) into the trough.

Quantitative methods

Radial immunodiffusion (Figure 45.6)

This method is also known as 'single radial immunodiffusion' or 'the mancini method'. Agar or agarose, melted in a suitable buffer, is cooled to about 55°C and precipitating antiserum specific for the protein to be measured is added to the appropriate concentration. The antiserum-containing gel is poured onto a glass or plastic plate or tray and allowed to cool, whereupon the gel solidifies. Wells are cut into the gel and each of these is filled with several microlitres of test serum. A series of wells is each filled with reference serum (or reference solution) containing known concentrations of the protein to be assayed. The plate is left in a humid atmosphere to allow the proteins within the samples and reference solutions to diffuse into the surrounding antiserum-containing gel. As the protein molecules being assayed diffuse into the gel they form precipitates with the antiserum molecules. These precipitates are partially soluble as long as the antigen (protein) concentration remains in excess of that of antiserum. Thus, some protein molecules continue to diffuse radially from the sample well until the antigen concentration is 'equivalent' to that of the antibodies. At this point an insoluble precipitate ring is formed around the sample well. The area (and therefore the diameter) of the ring is directly proportional to the concentration of the protein in the test sample. Indeed, provided the antiserum concentration in the gel and the sample protein concentrations are within appropriate limits and the diffusion process has been allowed to run to completion, the immunoprecipitate ring area is *linearly proportional* to protein concentration. This requires that the test system be titrated by experimentation. It also means that the plates may have to be left for a considerable time (perhaps several days) for diffusion and precipitate formation to run to completion. These constraints may be inconvenient and too slow for some routine laboratories but commercial radial immunodiffusion plates are now available for the measurement of clinically relevant proteins, including the immunoglobulin isotypes, subclasses and light chains. These commercial plates are produced to within such fine tolerances that accurate and precise results are obtained before the diffusion has run to completion (the Fahey and McKelvey method), giving results in only a few hours. Indeed, the antiserum concentrations are incorporated so accurately that, with a small and usually irrelevant loss of accuracy, protein concentrations can be interpolated, from the ring diameters to standard reference curves supplied with the kit, without using standard reference solutions. The limit of sensitivity of a radial diffusion assay will depend largely upon the quality of the antiserum but is usually in the order of about 5 mg/l. Some commercially developed plates can measure proteins down to as low as 0.2 mg/l.

Turbidimetry and nephelometry

The quantitative methods described above rely upon the formation of insoluble protein–antibody complexes that can be visualized by eye in supporting gel media. If the precipitate is formed by a protein and antibody at low concentrations in a liquid medium, a finer precipitate is formed in suspension. This property can be used to measure the protein concentration. The presence of a precipitate will impede the passage of a light beam passed through the suspension (turbidimetry). Alternatively, the light scattered by the suspension can be detected at an angle to the incident light (Figure 45.7). This method is called nephelometry. The amount of immunoprecipitate, at a constant antibody concentration, will increase in proportion to protein concentration, until all of the antibody has been bound to antigen. The measurement of light scattering must therefore be made in conditions of antibody excess. This is done either as an 'end-point' or by a rate analyser that measures the increase in scattering as the precipitate forms. Clearly this approach, unlike even more 'low-tech' methods such as radial immunodiffusion, requires dedicated apparatus but does offer a degree of automation and large throughput of specimens. Some laboratories use centrifugal analysers in which reagents are mixed during centrifugation and this reduces assay time. The limit of sensitivity of this methodology, as with most immunoassays, will depend upon the specific

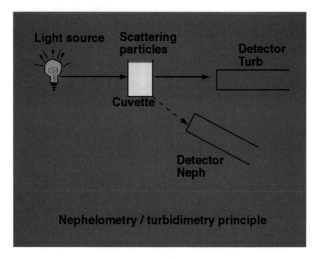

Figure 45.7   A simplified schema showing the principles of turbidimetry and nephelometry (see text for explanation)

system and, especially, the quality of antiserum, which must be polyclonal. In a good system, the limit is about 10 mg/l but this can be improved by about two orders of magnitude using 'particle-enhanced' nephelometry, when the antibodies are bound to tiny polystyrene beads. Reagents for turbidimetry and nephelometry of clinically important proteins, such as immunoglobulin isotypes and subclasses, are available commercially.

Enzyme-linked immunosorbent assays

Enzyme-linked immunosorbent assays (ELISA), also called enzyme-immunoassays (EIA), represent a versatile and sensitive principle for protein measurement that has largely replaced radio-immunoassays. They can measure proteins down to a concentration of about 1 μg/l. They are convenient assays to use if the protein of interest is present at low concentration. These assays are performed in 96-well plastic plates and reagent handling is usually done by means of multi-channel pipettes or even automated pipetting stations. The ELISA is eminently suited to automation or semi-automation and therefore, even if the protein being measured is at high concentration, necessitating sample dilution, if large numbers of samples are being processed this technique may be more convenient than other simpler methods, such as radial immunodiffusion. Many laboratories construct their own in-house ELISA systems but commercially available kits are available for a wide range of applications, including assays to measure clinically important serum proteins, cytokines, microbial antigens

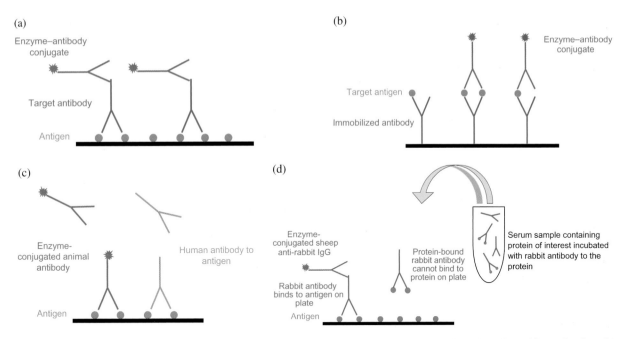

Figure 45.8 (a) Indirect ELISA. The figure shows the principle of this technique for the detection of specific antibodies. (b) Direct sandwich ELISA to detect a specific antigen in a sample. (c) Competitive ELISA to detect or measure a specific antibody to a known antigen. The method relies on an (enzyme-conjugated) antibody, raised in an animal such as rabbit or sheep, which recognizes the same antigen as the 'target' antibody to be measured. The specimen is mixed with the conjugated antibody, which competes for binding to the antigen immobilized on the ELISA plate. (d) Competitive ELISA to detect or measure a protein (antigen). The sample being tested is incubated with an antibody produced to the antigen of interest (in this case a rabbit antibody). The rabbit antibody binds to the target antigen in the sample, which prevents those antibody molecules from subsequently binding to the antigen-coated ELISA well. Any rabbit antibody that has not bound antigen in the pre-incubation is able to bind to the ELISA well and is detected by the addition of an enzyme-conjugated antibody to rabbit IgG (in this case, sheep anti-rabbit IgG). The amount of enzyme–substrate product measured will be inversely proportional to the amount of target protein in the original sample

(e.g. *Chlamydia trachomatis*; Hepatitis B virus antigens), IgE antibodies to allergens and antibodies to pathogens.

Different assay systems do vary in detail but the essential principles remain similar. The simplest forms are the 'indirect ELISA' for detecting specific antibodies and the 'direct sandwich ELISA' for detecting antigens.

The indirect ELISA for antibody detection (Figure 45.8a) is based upon microtitre plate wells coated with an appropriate target antigen (e.g. protein from a pathogen). The samples being tested are applied to the wells, followed by an enzyme-conjugated antibody to human immunoglobulin. The enzyme is usually horseradish peroxidase (HRP) or alkaline phosphatase. The choice of the anti-human immunoglobulin will allow the detection of all isotypes (by using antiserum raised against to human immunoglobulins IgG, IgA and IgM), or of a specific isotype (e.g. IgE antibodies to

allergens). After further washing to remove unbound conjugated antibody, a suitable substrate is added to the wells. A coloured product, detected using an ELISA reader collecting at the appropriate wavelength (450 nm for HRP; 492 nm for alkaline phosphatase), demonstrates target antibody in the original specimen. These assays can be quantitative.

For direct sandwich ELISA for detecting antigens (Figure 45.8b), the wells of 96-well microplates (also obtainable as eight-well strips) are coated with an antibody to the protein being detected or measured. This need not be a precipitating antibody and monoclonal antibodies are often used. Each well is filled with a test sample or one of a range of reference solutions of known concentrations. The wells are incubated for an appropriate time (usually about 1 hour), after which the wells are washed to remove material that has not been captured by the antibody on the well surface. The wells are then filled with a solution of another antibody to the protein being measured. Clearly, if the primary antibody was a monoclonal, the same monoclonal antibody might not be effective in this step because the target protein might have only one antigenic determinant (*epitope*) recognized by that antibody. This is where some experimentation is needed, to identify a second antibody that will recognize the protein after it has been captured by the primary one immobilized on the plate wells. This second antibody is conjugated to enzyme. The plate is incubated again to allow the second, enzyme-conjugated antibody to bind to captured protein. The plate is washed further and the substrate to the conjugating enzyme is added to the wells. The substrate produces a soluble, coloured reaction product. Since the amount of enzyme-conjugated antibody that binds will be proportional to the amount of protein captured by the primary antibody, it follows that the amount of enzyme reaction product will be proportional to the protein concentration in the original sample. The amount of reaction product is measured using an ELISA plate reader, which passes light through each well at a wavelength that is absorbed by the reaction product and, for quantitation, results are interpolated from those obtained with the reference solutions.

Another type of ELISA is competitive. An example is shown in Figure 45.8c. This demonstrates a competition ELISA for the detection of specific antibodies. The wells are coated with antigen that will be recognized by the antibody molecule of interest. The patient samples are added to the wells together with antibody molecules, raised in experimental animals, with specificity for the same antigen as that recognized by the antibody being assayed. There will therefore be competition for binding to the antigen. The more antibody molecules in the patient's sample, the less will be the binding of the conjugated antibodies. Figure 45.8d demonstrates the rationale for a competitive ELISA for the detection or measurement of an antigen. In this case, the wells are coated with the antigen of interest. The patient's sample is pre-incubated with, or added together with, an enzyme-conjugated antibody to the antigen. Any antigen in the sample will occupy antigen-binding sites on the antibody and decrease its binding to antigen coating the well.

There are many permutations on these basic ELISA styles and some of those are described in the list of further reading at the end of this chapter.

Conclusion

Routine immunology laboratories have at their disposal a range of methods for protein analysis from which to choose. The methods employed will be dictated by considerations including the nature of the specimens, the identities of the proteins being measured and their concentrations in the specimens. Also, the numbers of specimens routinely processed will dictate whether automated systems need to be used. Many of the methods used today have changed only in detail since specific proteins began to be identified and measured and some of these will probably continue to be employed long after we are gone. Others, such as ELISA, represent newer technologies and will displace those with technical or practical disadvantages, such as radio-immunoassay. There have been many developments in protein characterization, especially in the field of data analysis, such as for proteomics. If, when and how routine 'protein' laboratories adopt any of those or other new approaches, we will have to wait to find out.

Acknowledgement

I should like to thank Roger Drew of The Binding Site Ltd. for some of the figures.

Further reading

Chapel H, Haeney M. *Essentials of Clinical Immunology*, 3rd edn. 1993: Blackwell Scientific, Oxford.

Crowther JR. *The ELISA Guidebook*. Methods in Molecular Biology Series, vol 149. 2002: Humana, Totowa, NJ.

Rose NR, Hamilton RG, Detrick B. *Manual of Clinical Laboratory Immunology*, 6th edn. 2002: ASM Press, Washington, DC.

Sheehan C. *Clinical Immunology. Principles and Laboratory Diagnosis*, 2nd edn. 1997: Lippincott, Philadelphia, PA.

46

Complement assays

J North and K Whaley

Introduction

Complement is a system of serum proteins and cell receptors that has several functions, the majority of which help the host prevent or fight infection. Originally described as a heat-sensitive substance that could, together with specific antibody, lyse certain bacteria, we now know that complement proteins act through two main pathways. Activation of these pathways leads to the deposition of a potent opsonin on the surface of microorganisms, as well as producing an inflammatory response by releasing vaso-active and chemotactic factors. Further components can damage the surface of cells, and yet another group of components control the spontaneous and potentially harmful activation of these pathways.

Complement protein levels can be assayed by several methods and it is also possible to determine the functional activity of the majority of components. To fully appreciate the conditions required for these assays, it is important to understand the process that is occurring. Accordingly, a brief overview of complement is given in the following section, with more detailed descriptions to be found in the individual assay sections.

The classical pathway

The first pathway to be described is termed the 'classical pathway' and the components in this system are prefixed with 'C' and comprise C1q, C1r, C1s, C4 and C2 (the numbers being ascribed at the time of the components' definition, not the sequence of activation). The classical pathway can be activated by IgG or IgM which has

bound antigen. C1q binds to such antibody and, once attached, activates C1r, which in turn activates C1s. Activated C1s is a protease whose substrate is C4, which becomes cleaved. Cleaved C4 (C4b) will bind C2 and C1s will then activate C2 (to form C2a) by limited proteolysis. The active C4b2a complex (classical pathway C3 convertase) activates C3, again by limited proteolysis. Calcium and magnesium ions are both required for activation of the classical pathway. Activated C3 (C3b) will bind covalently to surfaces and act as a high-affinity ligand for C3b receptors on phagocytes.

This pathway can also be activated by C1q binding to C-reactive protein, which is an acute phase protein, similar in shape to IgM, that binds to the carbohydrate on some bacteria. Mannan-binding lectin (MBL) is a functionally similar protein that resembles C1q itself and MBL forms a macromolecular complex with MBL-associated serine proteases 1 and 2 (MASP1 and MASP2), which have much the same properties as C1r and C1s. The MBL–MASP complex can therefore activate the classical pathway through C4 when it binds to a suitable carbohydrate, such as mannose, N-acetylglucosamine, glucose or fucose.

The alternative pathway

C3, factor B, factor D and properdin are the components of the alternative pathway of complement activation. Activation of this pathway does not rely on any specific triggering factors but on a constant, low level of spontaneous activation. A small proportion of circulating C3 becomes hydrolysed and this form of C3 can bind to

The Science of Laboratory Diagnosis, Second Edition Edited by David Burnett and John Crocker
© 2005 John Wiley & Sons, Ltd

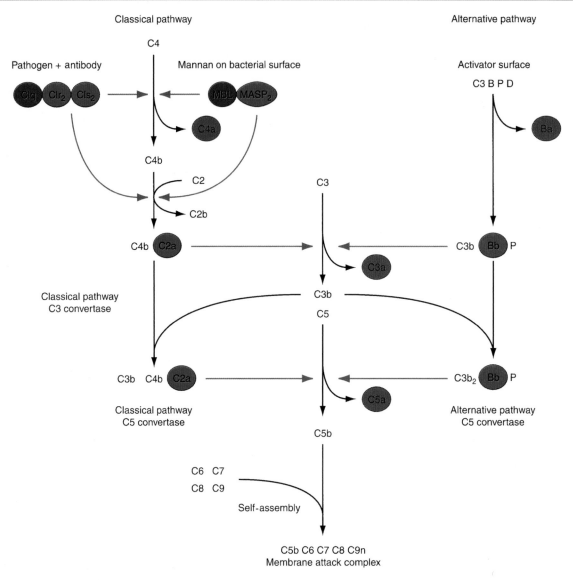

Figure 46.1   The classical and alternative pathways of complement activation. Components with protease activity are shown in green, collectins in blue and anaphylatoxins in red

factor B in the presence of magnesium ions. Bound factor B is cleaved by factor D to give Ba and C3Bb, and the latter can activate further C3 to form C3a and C3b. C3b can bind to surfaces and, once attached, bind more factor B. C3b bound to the surface of microorganisms is resistant to the regulatory activity of factors H and I, so activation is favoured. In the same way that factor B bound to circulating C3 is cleaved, factor B bound to C3b on surfaces is cleaved by factor D to give C3bBb. This complex is stabilized by properdin and both C3bBb and C3bBbP can cleave further C3 molecules, thus amplifying the process. Another function of the

C3dBbP complex is that it can bind to and activate C5 (see below).

The two pathways are shown in Figure 46.1.

The membrane attack complex

The complement components C5, C6, C7, C8 and C9 form the terminal pathway. C5 can be activated by either the classical or alternative pathway C5 convertases (C4b2a and C3bBbP, respectively). Activated C5 binds to C6 and the remaining components, C7, C8 and C9, bind in turn. Six molecules of C9 will bind to this complex and form a pore in the membrane of a cell on which it is present. This can lead to lysis of the cell and is a property used in the haemolytic assays described below.

Biologically active products of complement activation

One of the main functions of the complement system is to deposit C3b on the surface of microorganisms and, as described above, this can occur by either the classical or alternative pathways. C3b present on the surface of microorganisms increases their uptake by phagocytes, such as neutrophils, via receptors for C3b, and also stimulates the cells. Activation of the classical pathway by immune complexes of antibody and antigen increase the solubility of such complexes and aids their removal from the circulation by complement receptors on red blood cells.

As mentioned above, complexes of C5b–C9 can cause lysis of microorganisms by the insertion of C9 polymers into the cell membrane. Lysis of bystander cells may occur unless they are protected by the C3 receptor CR1, decay accelerating factor (DAF), membrane co-factor protein (MCP) and CD59, which prevents the polymerization of C9. The activation of C4, C2, C3, factor B and C5 results in relatively small fragments being released. The two most important are the anaphylatoxins C3a and C5a, which are vasoactive and release histamine from mast cells. C5a is also a powerful chemotactic agent that activates neutrophils and monocytes.

Control of complement activation

Spontaneous activation of complement needs to be controlled to prevent an inflammatory response occurring unnecessarily. The classical pathway is regulated by the serum proteins C1 inhibitor (C1-inh), C4bp and factor I and by the cell surface molecules membrane co-factor protein (MCP), decay accelerating factor (DAF, CD55) and CR1. The alternative pathway is regulated by factors H and I and MCP, DAF and CR1. All these factors accelerate the decay of one or more of the activated complement proteins or complexes, and hence complement activation will only occur if the activating stimulus can generate enough active products to overcome the inhibitory mechanisms.

Assay of serum complement levels

Specimen preparation and storage

Incorrect storage of samples for complement assay can result in decreased levels as some components are extremely labile. For assays of individual components in serum, blood samples should arrive in the laboratory as soon as possible after venepuncture. Blood should be allowed to clot at room temperature for 30 minutes, then the sample placed on ice for 1 hour for clot retraction to occur before separating the serum at 2–4°C. Samples should be aliquoted and stored at −70°C as quickly as practicable. For use, samples should be thawed at 37°C, then immediately placed on ice: repeated freezing and thawing will decrease the haemolytic activity of components. Blood collected into EDTA (which prevents further complement activation by chelating calcium and magnesium, and hence such samples are suitable for activation product assays) should be kept on ice for as short as time as possible before being spun to produce platelet-poor plasma, which is stored as for serum. Samples from tissue culture may benefit from the addition of proteinase inhibitors, such as PMSF.

Immunochemical assays

These assays utilize antibodies that are specific for individual complement components and are readily available commercially and can be used for nephelometric, ELISA or immunodiffusion assays. The choice of antibody is critical, as polyclonal antibodies may recognize breakdown products of the component under investigation and the resulting value obtained may not reflect the level of functional protein present.

The type of assay system used depends on the number of assays being performed, the level of sensitivity required, the level of the analyte and the quality of the available antibody. For instance, nephelometry is used in routine clinical immunology laboratories for measuring C3, C4, C1-inh and C1q in patient samples where levels are 50 μg/ml or above. For cell culture studies, however, levels may be as low as 1 ng/ml and ELISA, although being more labour-intensive and taking longer to perform, is more practical. Radial immunodiffusion and gel rocket techniques, although time consuming and not especially sensitive, are relatively simple and can be useful in identifying degradation products, e.g. double-decker rocket immunoelectrophoresis for the detection of C3d, and abnormal forms of complement components, e.g. Ouchterlony immunodiffusion of normal human serum (NHS) and C8-deficient serum against anti-C8 may reveal lines of partial identity suggesting C8β chain deficiency. The buffers used in these types of assay are those that are optimal for antibody binding and phosphate buffered saline (PBS) is usually used.

Haemolytic complement assays

CH50 assays

Lysis of red blood cells by complement will occur if the MAC is assembled on the cell membrane and C9 polymers inserted. The assays depend on the presence of all the necessary components and suitable conditions for complement activation. The simplest of these assays

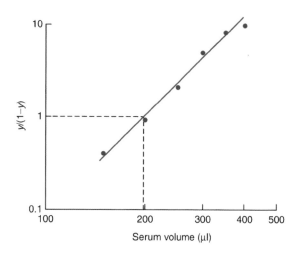

Figure 46.2 Log-log plot of $y/1-y$ against volume of diluted serum in a CH50 assay. At the point of 50% haemolysis, $y(1-y) = 1$ and the volume of diluted serum giving this is shown by the vertical line. $y =$ proportion of cells lysed. Redrawn from Whaley (1985), with permission from Elsevier

any concomitant activation of the classical pathway whilst permitting activation of the alternative pathway.

These assays need to be controlled with samples known to contain all the components, e.g. fresh NHS (positive control), and by buffer alone (negative control) to measure spontaneous lysis of the erythrocytes. Quantitation of the assay can be performed by comparing the amount of haemolysis (measured by the optical density of the cell supernatant, which is proportional the amount of haemoglobin released) to a known normal NHS in a one-tube method, or by diluting out the test sample to obtain a range of percentage haemolysis. Using the von Krogh equation, which describes the curve obtained by plotting the percentage lysis against the sample dilution, the sample dilution required to obtain 50% haemolysis is calculated and, after taking the initial sample dilution into account, this value is translated into CH50 units/ml. The CH50 unit obtained depends on the amount and nature of the antibody used to sensitize the cells, the erythrocyte concentration and fragility, the ionic strength, divalent cation concentration and pH of the buffer, reaction time and temperature.

CH50 and APH50 assays are used to determine whether or not a patient is genetically deficient in a complement component. A zero value in a CH50 assay, but not APH50, indicates a lack of C1, C4 or C2, while for a normal CH50 result and zero APH50, a deficiency of properdin or factor D may be present (factor B deficiency has not been described). Absence of lysis in both assays indicates lack of C3, C5, C6, C7 or C8. Low levels of lysis may occur in C9 deficiency. Low values above zero suggest that the level of one or more complement components is decreased, due either to consumption in a disease process, such as systemic lupus erythematosus, or may indicate a heterozygous deficiency state (although complement levels can be variable in these individuals, as many components are acute phase proteins).

Haemolytic assays for individual components using complement-deficient sera

Assays for the presence and functional activity of individual components can be performed using EA and a serum deficient in the chosen component. Serial dilutions of a test sample are added and lysis of EA will occur only if the tested-for component is present and functional. Other components are present in excess, so lysis is proportional to the amount of test component. Deficient sera can be obtained commercially but can also be prepared in the laboratory if such assays are

is the CH50 (Figure 46.2), which is a quantitative procedure that depends on a sample containing all the classical and terminal complement components, and on the components being functionally active. The assay is performed in the presence of calcium and magnesium ions (required for classical pathway activation) and the pathway is initiated by the presence of IgM on the surface of sheep red blood cells (EA).

A similar assay for the alternative pathway, the APH50, uses rabbit erythrocytes, which provide a surface for C3bBb binding. The addition of EDTA, by chelating calcium but not magnesium ions, will prevent

performed regularly. Such assays are of lower sensitivity than those described below and are not suitable for regulatory components (C1-inh, factors H and I, properdin).

Haemolytic assays for individual components using pre-sensitized EA

Erythrocytes can be pre-sensitized with early pathway components up to that under test. By adding a sample containing a component under investigation, this component can be activated or bound by those already present. Addition of the remaining components will result in lysis if the test component is present and functional. By ensuring that all other components are in excess, the degree of lysis is proportional to the amount of test component. Functionally pure components can be prepared in the laboratory but most are commercially available. The most commonly used pre-sensitized EAs are EAC1, EAC4 and EAC14. EAC1s are prepared by adding C1 (e.g. from 5 mM CaCl precipitated guinea-pig serum) to EA in a low ionic strength buffer that contains calcium and magnesium. Adding human serum in the presence of EDTA will result in the binding of C4 and C2, and subsequent incubation at 37°C will cause decay of C1 and C2 from the cells, leaving EAC4. EAC14 cells are prepared by adding further C1, again in the presence of calcium and magnesium.

EAC4 cells are used to assay C1 activity by adding dilutions of the test sample followed by guinea-pig C2. Haemolysis is achieved by adding the remaining components, usually in the form of rat serum containing EDTA (C^{rat}-EDTA). The concentration of effective molecules of the component under test is measured by plotting the Z value [$-\ln(1 - \%$ lysis)] against the dilution of the component under test (Figure 46.3). The straight-line plot obtained results from the 'one-hit theory,' in that a single effective complement molecule (C1–C9) results in cell lysis. One unit of complement is taken as that which gives 63% lysis in an assay for that component. If a straight-line plot is not obtained, then the concentration of one or more components under test is limited.

C4 is assayed using EAC1 by adding dilutions of the test sample, guinea-pig C2 and C^{rat}-EDTA as for C1, while C2 activity is measured using EAC14. In this case, the T_{max} time for the cells (time for maximum C4b2a formation) must be known. The T_{max} varies from batch to batch of EAC14 because it depends upon the amount of C4b present on the cells. In order to assay C3 activity,

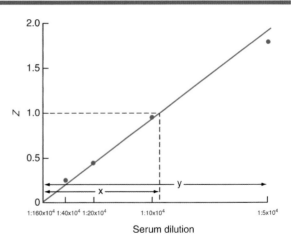

Figure 46.3 The number of functional molecules per cell (Z) is plotted against the serum dilution in a typical haemolytic titration of an individual complement component. The concentration of the component in this instance is given by $y/x \times 50\,000$. Redrawn from Whaley (1985), with permission from Elsevier

it is necessary to form EAC142. The C4b2a complex on these cells is more unstable than most, hence EAC14^{oxy}2 are prepared to provide increased haemolytic activity of C2 (see Figure 46.4).

EAC14 forms the starting point of functional assays of alternative pathway components. C2 and C3 are added to form EAC1423, with subsequent removal of C1 and C2 by incubation in EDTA buffer. The resultant EAC43b

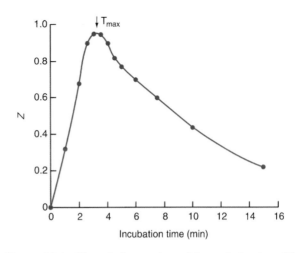

Figure 46.4 Plot of the number of haemolytic sites (Z) against the incubation time at 30°C in a T_{max} assay. T_{max} is indicated by the arrow. Redrawn from Whaley (1985), with permission from Elsevier

forms an alternative pathway, C3 convertase if factor B, factor D and properdin are added. Haemolysis is achieved by adding C^{rat}-EDTA. Activity of factor B, factor D or properdin is measured by omitting the respective pure component and replacing it with dilutions of the test sample although this method is not suitable for assaying serum factor D, only pure preparations. Terminal components are assayed by adding C3 and the terminal components up to the one under test to $EAC14^{oxy}$ 2. EAC1-8, used for measuring C9 activity, however, will undergo spontaneous lysis so must be used as soon as they are prepared.

Other assays of complement function

Measurement of the classical pathway activity is possible using commercial kits. Some of these are ELISA based and serum complement is activated by immune complexes present in the well. Measuring the amount of a terminal component neoantigen, usually C9, generated, assesses activity. An automated system uses liposomes that contain an enzyme (G6PDH), which is released when antibody reacts with antigen on the liposome only when the entire classical pathway is present. Reaction of the enzyme with a substrate in the reagent mixture gives a colour change that is proportional to the activity of the classical pathway. The authors are unaware of any automated methods for APH50. MBL can be assayed functionally by coating sheep RBC with mannan and performing the rest of the assay as for a CH50. An alternative functional assay that measures the ability of MBL to activate C4 has been described. Mannan is coated to an ELISA plate and the amount of C4c generated from added serum is measured, a high salt concentration in the buffer preventing classical pathway activation.

Functional assays of complement control proteins

C1 inhibitor activity can be assayed by commercial kits which utilize the ability of C1 inhibitor to inhibit a C1s analogue in a colorimetric reaction. C1 inhibitor activity can also be measured by testing the ability of the test sample to inhibit a given level of exogenous C1 added to sensitized EA. If serum is being tested then C1 first has to be removed, e.g. by precipitating C1 out using

phosphate buffer. C1 inhibitor can be allowed to bind to C1, either in the fluid phase before adding to EAC4 with C2 or on EAC14, prior to the addition of C2. For haemolytic inhibitor component assays, a 'solo' reaction containing no inhibitor is run in parallel. The inhibitory activity of the test sample is expressed in Z' units and assumes that the inhibition of lysis follows the same 'one-hit' theory as lysis. I is taken as the proportion of C1 lysis which is inhibited, and therefore: $I = 1 - e^{-z}$. Hence $Z' = \ln(1 - I)$ or:

$$Z' = \ln \frac{y \text{ in test sample}}{y \text{ in solo}}$$

When Z in the solo tube is between 0.5 and 1.5, Z' varies linearly with the dilution of C1 inhibitor. As for the calculation of Z, Z' is calculated from the graph of serum dilution against Z', taking the initial dilution into account.

Factor H levels can be assayed by measuring the ability of serum to accelerate the decay of the C3 convertase. EAC4b3bBbP are prepared by adding properdin, factor B and factor D to EAC4b3b and the amount of haemolytic activity remaining after a decaying the C3 convertase is compared to a solo tube. Factor I activity can be assayed by incubating the test sample with factor H added to EAC43 and then adding factors B and D and testing for residual haemolytic activity.

Detection of complement activation products

Several serum complement proteins are acute phase proteins, so during complement consumption, which can occur in conditions such as some types of bacterial infection or immune complex diseases, serum levels may remain normal. Increased complement turnover can be assessed by measuring products of complement activation, using antibodies that distinguish activation products from the native molecule. Commercial kits are available but in-house assays for activation products are easily established, provided that appropriate antibodies are used. ELISAs for C3a, C4a and C5a can be established, provided that standards can be obtained, but the clinical usefulness of these assays is limited. Of more help to clinicians are assays for C1s-C1-inh, C3bBbP or C5b-C9, increased, levels of which indicate activation of the classical, alternative or terminal pathway, respectively.

The latter assays use an antibody against one component, e.g. C1s, to bind the complex to an ELISA plate and an antibody against another component of the complex, e.g. C1-inh, to detect the complex.

Detection of complement receptors

Antibodies to complement receptors are available commercially and can be used in flow cytometry to detect the presence of receptors on cell suspensions. Some antibodies are also suitable for immunohistochemistry of tissue sections or cytospin preparation if cell morphology is required.

Further reading

Whaley K (ed.). *Methods in Complement for Clinical Immunologists*. 1985: Churchill Livingstone, Edinburgh. This text book provides a comprehensive, detailed account of the majority of complement assays, including the preparation of purified components.

Dodds A, Sims R (eds). *Complement. A Practical Approach*. 1997: Oxford University Press, Oxford. This is an up to date laboratory manual for all aspects of laboratory complement work.

Phimster GM, Whaley K. *Measurement of complement*. In *Clinical Immunology. A Practical Approach*, Gooi HG, Chapel H (eds) (1990). Oxford University Press, Oxford. This chapter provides guidance as to clinical indications for complement assays as well as methodologies.

47

Cellular immunology

Aarnoud Huissoon

Introduction

Cellular immunology is the study of the cells of the immune system. These tests are usually performed in the context of investigating possible defects of the immune system, e.g. in patients with recurrent infections or infants with failure to thrive in whom rare inborn immunodeficiencies may be suspected.

For convenience, peripheral blood leukocytes are usually assessed, but cells from other sources, such as lymph nodes and tissue biopsies, can also be used (usually in the research setting). Lymphocytes and neutrophils are most frequently studied, but other cell types, such as basophils, can also be tested in some circumstances.

In order to assess the cells of the immune system, information regarding the numbers of cells present, their phenotype and their functions may be required. A wide range of tools is available for these analyses, and many techniques are emerging into the routine clinical arena from research applications. Cellular immunology is therefore a rapidly evolving science. Conversely, several tests in current use have been largely unchanged for decades. These have proved to be robust and reliable in clinical use, and newer techniques have been slow to supersede them.

Qualitative and quantitative tests

At the simplest level, the actual number of circulating lymphocytes and neutrophils provides useful information about the immune system. These are readily avail-able from the automated white cell differential count. The lymphocyte population is divided into T, B and NK cells, which are themselves further divided into subsets. Abnormalities and deficiencies have been described affecting virtually all of these populations, and analysis of lymphocyte subsets and phenotypes is a valuable diagnostic tool.

Lymphocyte subsets are measured by labelling them with monoclonal antibodies. A wide range of antibodies has been developed, which identify an increasing range of lymphocyte subpopulations. Some of the commoner antibodies used to dissect these subpopulations are given in Table 47.1.

Formerly, lymphocyte subsets were enumerated by manually counting fluorescent antibody-labelled cells under the microscope. Now the flow cytometer provides a far more accurate tool for examining large numbers of lymphocyte markers in great detail.

Flow cytometry

In a flow cytometer, individual cells carried in a thin stream of fluid pass rapidly through a laser beam. Photomultipliers detect the scattering of laser light by the cell and measure the light emitted by any fluorescent markers that have been added to the cell (Figure 47.1). From this information, the size and granularity of the cell, as well as the level of expression of cell surface or cytoplasmic antigens that have been labelled with fluorescent antibodies, can be measured. Many thousands of cells per minute can be analysed in this way, so that a large amount of data regarding cell populations can be rapidly collected.

The Science of Laboratory Diagnosis, Second Edition   Edited by David Burnett and John Crocker
© 2005 John Wiley & Sons, Ltd

Table 47.1 Commonly used lymphocyte subset markers

	Major subsets		Other subsets		Other markers
Lymphocytes CD45⁺	T cells CD3⁺	T helper cells CD4⁺	Naïve T cells CD45RA⁺		Activation antigens HLA-DR, CD69, CD25
		T cytotoxic cells CD8⁺	Memory/effector T cells CD45RO⁺		Co-stimulatory molecules CD28, CD134 (OX40)
	NK cells CD16/CD56⁺ (CD3⁻)				
	B cells CD19⁺ or CD20⁺	Naïve B cells IgD⁺/CD27⁻	B-1 cells CD5⁺		B cell subsets and lymphoma
		Memory B cells IgD⁻/CD27⁺	B-2 cells CD5⁻		IgM, IgG, κ/λ Ig light chains, CD23

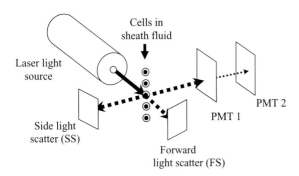

Figure 47.1 Simplified layout of a flow cytometer. Cells pass singly through a laser beam. For each cell, scattered light is measured by the forward and sideways light sensors. Fluorescent antibodies on the cell are excited by the laser light and emit light at different wavelengths, which is measured by the photomultipliers (PMT). On larger flow cytometers, two lasers and many photomultipliers, each measuring emitted light of a different wavelength, enable many different cell molecules or other properties to be examined simultaneously

Lymphocytes, monocytes and granulocytes can be approximately distinguished by their light scatter characteristics, alone or in combination with CD45 expression (Figure 47.2a). Fluorescent antibodies can then distinguish between the different populations of lymphocytes (Figure 47.2b).

It is usually necessary to know not only the proportions of lymphocyte subsets present, but also the absolute numbers of each subset in the original sample. Good age-related reference ranges are available for the major subsets. This quantitative result can be derived from

either dual- or single-platform methods. In the former the absolute lymphocyte count is obtained from a flow cytometric white cell differential count and the total leukocyte count from a standard haematology analyser. A single-platform method may be more accurate, especially where there is a very low proportion of the population of interest (e.g. CD4⁺ T cells in the acquired immunodeficiency syndrome, AIDS). Single-platform quantitation can be achieved by adding a known quantity of beads to a known volume of blood at the outset of the test. The beads and the antibody-labelled lymphocytes are then analysed simultaneously by the flow cytometer, and absolute lymphocyte subset counts can be calculated. An alternative approach is offered by counting the lymphocytes in a fixed volume of blood passed through the analyser, but this is dependent on the reliability of the flow cytometer's fluidics. Whole blood antibody-staining and lysis methods (rather than staining separated leukocytes) must be used for quantitative lymphocyte analyses.

Uses of lymphocyte subset analysis

Monitoring HIV infection/AIDS

This is the commonest indication for requesting lymphocyte subsets. Accurate quantitative results are essential. Typically, CD4⁺ T helper cell numbers are low, and the ratio of CD4⁺ to CD8⁺ T cells is inverted (it is about 1.5:1 in healthy adults). However, it cannot be used to diagnose HIV infection, since T cell subsets may be entirely normal in a HIV-infected individual, and there are also many other causes of perturbations of

(a)

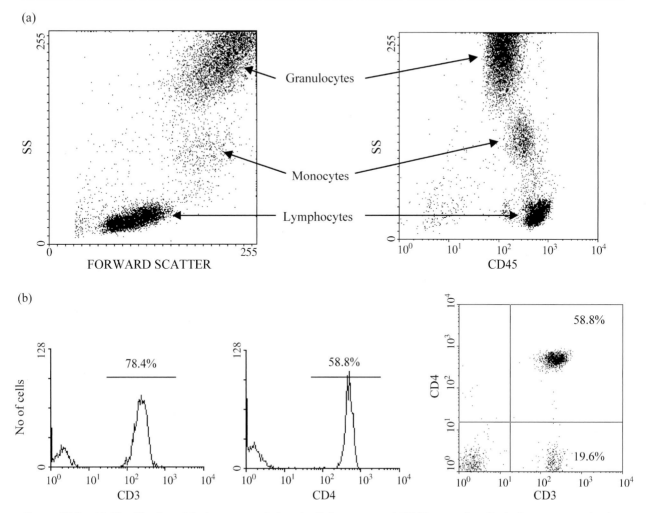

(b)

Figure 47.2 (a) Identification of leukocyte populations by light scatter and CD45 expression. Each dot represents the data collected from a single cell. Lymphocytes have moderate forward scatter (an index of size), low side scatter (SS, an index of cell complexity or granularity) and high CD45 expression. (b) CD3 and CD4 expression on the lymphocyte population. The cells have been labelled with fluorescein-conjugated CD3 antibodies, detected on PMT1, and phycoerythrin-conjugated CD4 antibodies, detected on PMT2. Having selected the lymphocyte population, expression of CD3 and CD4 can be viewed either singly, as histograms, or combined in a dot-plot. The dot-plot gives additional information, showing that CD4$^+$ cells are a subset of CD3$^+$ cells

lymphocyte subsets, e.g. stress, treatment with steroids, intercurrent infection or normal diurnal variation. Once HIV infection is diagnosed with serological or molecular biology tests, CD4 counts (in conjunction with measures of viral load measured by PCR) are essential in monitoring disease. They are used to indicate the level of immune suppression and when treatment with antiretroviral agents and prophylactic antimicrobials should be started. The performance of CD4$^+$ T cell monitoring for

HIV in the UK is subject to external quality control by NEQAS.

Investigation of immunodeficiency

Many primary immunodeficiency diseases are associated with abnormalities of lymphocyte subsets. Some examples are given in Table 47.2. While a low total

Table 47.2 Examples of some primary immunodeficiency syndromes with characteristic laboratory findings

Diagnosis	Infections	Immunoglobulins	Lymphocyte numbers	Typical lymphocyte subset analysis	Functional studies
X-linked (Bruton's) agammaglobuli-naemia	Bacterial	Low/absent	Normal	Absent B cells	Normal proliferation to mitogens
X-linked SCID	Viral, fungal and bacterial	Absent	Low	Absent T and NK cells	Absent proliferation to mitogens
HLA class II deficiency	Viral, fungal and bacterial	Normal/low	Normal	Reduced CD4$^+$ T cells Absent HLA-DR expression on B cells	Normal proliferation to mitogens, but reduced antigen-specific responses
X-linked hyper-IgM syndrome	Bacterial/proto-zoal	Raised/normal IgM; low/ab-sent IgG, IgA	Normal	Absent CD154 on activated T cells	Normal proliferation to mitogens, but reduced antigen-specific responses

lymphocyte count is often the first clue to the diagnosis of severe immunodeficiency, detection of the pattern of deficiency can help diagnosis, e.g. the absence of T and B cells with preserved NK cells may suggest a deficiency of RAG-1 or RAG-2 (genes that are involved in the generation of T and B cell antigen receptors). Functional studies are usually required in addition to lymphocyte subset analysis in the investigation of severe congenital immunodeficiencies (see below).

In some immunodeficiency diseases the absolute numbers of lymphocyte populations are normal, but subtle abnormalities can be detected with more detailed analyses, e.g. many patients with primary antibody deficiency (common variable immune deficiency) have entirely normal numbers of T, B and NK cells. However, their B cells show abnormal proportions of naïve and memory populations, suggesting a defect in peripheral B cell maturation or homeostasis as the cause for their failure to produce a normal antibody repertoire. T cells from patients with the hyper-IgM syndrome fail to express CD154 (formerly called CD40 ligand). CD154 is not normally expressed on resting peripheral blood T cells, and it is necessary to first stimulate the T cells in vitro and then measure expression of the molecule by flow cytometry.

Leukocyte adhesion deficiency (LAD) is caused by failure of neutrophils (and other white cells) to express the β2 integrins (CD11–CD18 heterodimers). As a result, the patient's neutrophils do not migrate from the blood stream to the site of an infection, and recurrent severe infections (with little or no pus formation) result. Wound healing is also impaired. This condition can be diagnosed by simply measuring neutrophil expression of CD18 and CD11a, b and c by flow cytometry.

Diagnosis of lymphoid malignancies

The quantitation and phenotype analysis of peripheral blood (or marrow) lymphocytes is essential in the diagnosis of B and T cell lymphoproliferative diseases. B cell clonality in these conditions is often detected by abnormal expression of immunoglobulin light chain on the B cell surface. T cells do not express any clonal markers on the cell surface, so that malignancies are detected by abnormal expression (loss or aberrant expression) of other surface markers (e.g. CD7, CD5, CD25). While many of these conditions are characterized by marked increases in peripheral blood lymphocyte numbers, some (particularly T cell neoplasms) may be clinically subtle in their presentation and have a normal lymphocyte count. In all cases, the lymphocyte immunophenotype has to be interpreted in the context of the patient's other clinical findings and the phenotype of the cells on microscopy.

Other inflammatory conditions and infections

Abnormalities of peripheral blood lymphocyte subsets and phenotypes have been described in a vast range of infectious and inflammatory diseases. However these abnormalities are rarely diagnostically helpful, and never specific.

Lymphocytes from sites other than blood and bone marrow

It is occasionally useful to analyse lymphocytes from other sites, such as cerebrospinal fluid and bronchoalveolar lavage fluid. In the latter case, the predominant lymphocyte populations may help to distinguish different interstitial lung diseases. In the former, the main purpose would be to exclude lymphoma involving the central nervous system.

Functional studies

T lymphocytes

In the course of an immune response, normal T cells exhibit several functions that can be assessed *in vitro*. These include proliferation, upregulation of cell surface antigens, cytokine production and apoptosis.

Proliferation

Measurement of T lymphocyte proliferation is a well-established method of assessing their immune competence. Previously, changes in the appearance of the cells on microscopy were used to assess the activation and proliferation response to various stimuli—hence the term 'lymphocyte transformation', which is often applied to this test. For several decades this process has been more accurately quantified by measuring radiolabelled ^{3}H thymidine incorporation into the DNA of proliferating cells. The tritiated thymidine is added to the cell culture for the last 16 hours of a 2–7 day culture, and the cells are then harvested to a paper filter. The amount of incorporated radioactivity, as detected by scintillation counting, is proportional to the DNA replication occurring in the proliferating cells (Figure 47.3a). Both the absolute incorporated radioactivity (in disintegrations or counts per minute, after correction for background counts) and the stimulation index (counts from stimulated cells divided by counts from unstimulated cells) should be reported.

Alternative methods of measuring lymphocyte proliferation have also been developed, although none of these has so far supplanted thymidine incorporation as the standard technique in clinical laboratories. These include flow cytometric detection of activation antigen expression (e.g. CD25, CD69, Ki67), bromodeoxyuridine incorporation, or dilution of the intracellular dye carboxy-fluorescein diacetate succinimidyl ester

(a)

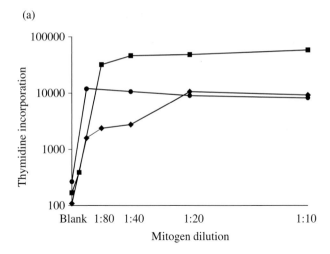

(b)

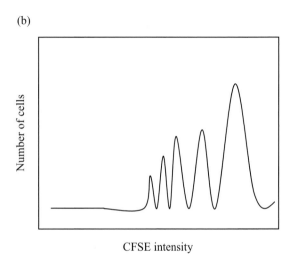

Figure 47.3 (a) Lymphocyte proliferation in response to the mitogens PHA 250 μg/ml (■), PWM 100 μg/ml (●), and OKT3 1 μg/ml (◆). ^{3}H Thymidine incorporation is indicated in disintegrations/minute. Reproduced from Huissoon *et al.* (2002), by permission of Blackwell Publishing Ltd. (b) Histogram representing the principle of CFSE dilution to measure cell proliferation. Cells are loaded with CFSE at the start of the procedure. This is a cytoplasmic dye that does not interfere with cellular function. Cells are incubated with mitogen or antigen for a number of days and CFSE intensity is analysed by flow cytometry. In the representation above, the right-hand peak represents cells that have not undergone cell division, and therefore contain the full starting amount of CFSE. With each cell division dye intensity is halved, so that each round of division can be identified as a new peak to the left of the non-proliferating cells. Co-labelling the cells with lineage-specific antibodies can identify which cell types have responded to the stimulus and which have not

(CFSE), by activated and proliferating T cells (Figure 47.3b). These methods have the advantage of not requiring the use and measurement of radioisotopes.

T cells can be stimulated to proliferate in response to a range of stimuli, and these are usually used in a range of concentrations to demonstrate a dose–response (Figure 47.3a). The induction of calcium flux by ionomycin and a calcium ionophore will stimulate many cell types, and this activation is totally independent of the normal cell signalling pathways. Phytohaemagglutinin, a plant lectin first identified for its ability to agglutinate red blood cells, and concavalin A, will stimulate all T cells through a range of surface receptors. Infants with inherited severe combined immune deficiency (SCID) fail to proliferate in response to these mitogens. Pokeweed mitogen stimulates both T and B cells. A more 'physiological' approach is to mimic the normal route of T cell stimulation through the T cell receptor. This can be achieved by cross-linking the receptor with anti-CD3 antibodies (which will activate all T cells) or by adding antigen to the culture. Antigens will be taken up by the blood monocytes and T cell stimulating peptides are presented to the T cells in the context of MHC class II molecules. Such antigen-specific proliferation will activate only a small proportion of the total peripheral blood T cells (about 1 in 10^4), and accordingly the amount of proliferation detected will be less than that seen with mitogen stimulation. Rarely, patients are detected with grossly normal T cell function but with subtle defects on more detailed testing, e.g. in chronic mucocutaneous candidiasis, the patient's T cells respond well to all mitogenic and antigenic stimuli with the exception of *Candida*. This remarkable 'hole' in the immune repertoire is unexplained.

Cytokine production

Cytokine production in response to mitogenic and antigenic stimuli can also be measured. Because cytokine production is an important function of T cells, detection of defective cytokine production to certain stimuli can be of clinical importance. Diseases caused by defective cytokine production are now beginning to be described (e.g. IL-12 deficiency). T cell cytokine production can be measured either in the culture supernatant by ELISA, by the Elispot technique, or by direct detection of intracellular cytokines in individual T cells by fluorescent antibody staining. In the Elispot assay, stimulated T cells are placed in flat-bottomed plastic culture wells that have been coated with antibodies against a specific cytokine (e.g. interferon-γ). Any cytokine secreted by

the T cells is bound by the antibody on the well. After a period of incubation, the cells are washed off and the bound cytokine is detected by a second antibody against that cytokine. This is visualized by a chromogenic enzyme–substrate reaction, and each spot on the well represents a cytokine-secreting T cell. The intracellular detection of cytokines by flow cytometry is less sensitive than the Elispot method, but does allow further characterization of the individual cytokine-producing cells using surface markers. T cells are stimulated by antigen or mitogen, and towards the end of the incubation brefeldin A or monensin is added to block cytokine transport from the endoplasmic reticulum. This results in the accumulation of sufficient intracellular cytokine to be detected by direct antibody labelling. The cells are then labelled with fluorescent antibodies against appropriate surface antigens, e.g. CD3 and CD69, and the cell membrane is fixed and permeabilized. This allows the intracellular cytokine to be labelled with specific antibody (Figure 47.4).

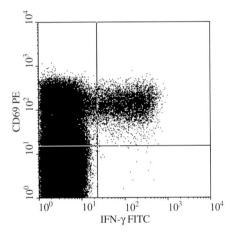

Figure 47.4 Interferon-gamma (IFN-γ) expression in T cells stimulated with staphylococcal enterotoxin B. CD69 (on the vertical axis) identifies activated T cells, and about 10% of these are seen to express IFN-γ. Reproduced from Huissoon *et al.* (2002), by permission of Blackwell Publishing Ltd

Apoptosis

Apoptosis (programmed cell death) is an important function of T cells, both in lymphocyte ontogeny and as part of the involution of a normal immune response. The autoimmune lymphoproliferative syndrome (ALPS) has been described where the ability of lymphocytes to undergo apoptosis is impaired. With each immune response the proliferation of lymphocytes is not balanced by a corresponding death of lymphocytes when the infective stimulus is gone. Such patients have raised serum immunoglobulins, autoimmune diseases with demonstrable autoantibodies, enlarged lymph nodes and a high peripheral blood lymphocyte count with an abnormal accumulation of CD4$^-$/CD8$^-$ T cells. There are a number of causes of this clinical picture, all related to defects in the cell surface or intracellular signalling mediators of apoptosis. The commonest type of ALPS is caused by mutations in the Fas protein (CD95). To detect defects in Fas-mediated apoptosis, the patient's T cells are first stimulated *in vitro* to render them susceptible to Fas-mediated apoptosis. An antibody against the Fas molecule is added to the culture. In normal individuals a high proportion of T cells undergo apoptosis in response to Fas ligation in this assay. In patients with ALPS this is markedly impaired. Apoptosis thus induced can be measured by a number of techniques, but most conveniently by flow cytometry. Features of apoptotic cells that may be measured include nuclear condensation (detected by propidium iodide staining), annexin V binding to externalized phosphadityl serine, DNA nucleosomal fragmentation (detected by fluorescent terminal nucleotide end-labelling), or caspase activation using the fluorescent caspase substrate Phi-Phi Lux.

In vivo tests

In vivo tests of T cell function are also possible. Delayed (Gell and Coombs type IV) skin reactivity to recall antigens is a good indicator of T cell immune competence. These tests are cheap and quick, but are not suitable for use in small children. A small amount of the antigen is injected into the dermis, and the reddening and swelling reaction after 2–5 days indicates a positive immune response to that antigen. This response is mediated mainly by T cells and macrophages. It is suppressed in malnutrition, HIV infection and sarcoidosis, and by corticosteroids or other immunosuppressive therapy. However, it is routinely performed only for contact and immunity testing for tuberculosis (the Heaf test or Mantoux test). Interpretation of a negative test is difficult if prior exposure or BCG vaccination status is not known. Other ubiquitous antigens, such as mumps, *Candida* and tetanus toxoid, can also elicit such responses, but are not used in routine clinical practice.

Natural killer cells

Cytotoxicity is a function of both CD8$^+$ T cells and NK cells. CD8$^+$ T cell cytotoxicity is antigen-specific and is not measured in routine clinical practice. NK cell cytotoxicity can be conveniently assessed by measuring lysis of the K562 cell line. K562 cells lack HLA class I expression, and so are a natural target for NK cells. The cells are loaded with intracellular radiolabelled ^{51}chromium and co-incubated with the patient's lymphocytes (containing the effector NK cells). Cytotoxic lysis of the target cells is identified by release of chromium into the culture medium. It is also possible to assess killing of K562 cells by flow cytometry. The target cells have to be labelled with a fluorescent lipophylic dye before incubation with the patient's leukocytes, so that they can be distinguished from the patient's own lymphocytes. Cytotoxic killing is identified by their permeability to propidium iodide, which is excluded by viable cells. With either method, killing should be assessed over a range of target: effector cell ratios. Defects of NK killing are seen in rare immunodeficiencies associated with partial albinism (e.g. Chediak–Higashi and Griscelli syndromes) and in familial haemophagocytic syndromes.

B lymphocytes

B cell function is most easily assessed by measuring the patient's serum immunoglobulins and antibodies against specific infectious agents and/or vaccines. If low antibody levels are found, the response to vaccination can be tested, and this is an excellent global indicator of B cell function. B (and T) cell proliferation can be stimulated by pokeweed mitogen, but this gives no information about immunoglobulin production. This can be tested by a reverse plaque assay, where stimulated B cells are plated into agarose containing immunoglobulin-binding erythrocytes. Complement is added and the red cell-bound immunoglobulin fixes the complement and induces haemolysis. Thus, each immunoglobulin-producing cell can be identified by the surrounding plaque of haemolysis. This assay is time-consuming and is now rarely performed, since it gives little additional information that is not obtained from serum antibody tests.

Neutrophils

Neutrophils are short-lived cells that actively ingest and kill organisms. The commonest neutrophil defect is reduced numbers of these cells. This can be congenital (e.g. Swachmann's syndrome or Kostmann's syndrome), but is most often acquired secondary to marrow failure (e.g. caused by drugs or neoplasms). Functional defects of neutrophils are relatively rare, but can be readily investigated *in vitro*.

In order to eliminate an invading organism, neutrophils must first migrate from the circulation into the tissue. This involves the ability to respond to chemotactic stimuli and adhere to vascular endothelium. Tests of neutrophil adhesion and chemotactic migration are available. Adhesion to materials such as glass wool, plastic culture dishes and cultured endothelial cells can be measured. However, the defects detected by such tests are all due to leukocyte adhesion deficiency syndromes and are more easily diagnosed by measuring leukocyte integrin expression by flow cytometry (see above). Neutrophil chemotaxis can be measured by microscopical observation of neutrophil movement towards stimuli such as casein and F-met-leu-phe. This can be performed using a Boyden chamber, where neutrophils are separated from the chemotactic stimulus by a micropore filter, and the leading front of neutrophils migrating through the filter is measured. Alternatively, a neutrophil suspension and chemotactic stimuli are placed in adjacent wells cut into agarose gel, and the movement of neutrophils under the agarose towards the stimulus is measured. Disorders of neutrophil migration have been described in primary immune deficiency states, including the hyper-IgE syndrome and Chediak–Higashi syndrome, as well as in some other diseases. However, the abnormalities are not diagnostic or consistent.

Having migrated to the site of infection, neutrophils eliminate their target organisms by phagocytosis and intracellular killing. Both of these functions can be tested using *Candida* as the target organism. Cultured *Candida* spores are incubated with isolated neutrophils and normal donor serum (which opsonizes the *Candida*). Tritiated uridine is added to the culture, and this will be incorporated only by viable extracellular *Candida*. The neutrophil/*Candida* cultures are harvested to filters and incorporated ^{3}H uridine is measured by beta counter. High counts (compared with normal control neutrophils) indicate impaired neutrophil phagocytosis. Assuming that phagocytosis is normal, intracellular killing of *Candida* can be measured by lysing the neutrophils and assessing *Candida* viability, either by ^{3}H-uridine incorporation or by methylene blue exclusion. *Staphylococcus aureus* is an alternative target for neutrophil killing assays. In this instance, killing is measured by plating the supernatant from lysed neutrophils on growth medium and counting the resulting bacterial colonies. A flow cytometric assay measuring phagocytosis of fluorescein-labelled, opsonized *Escherichia coli* has also been described.

By far the commonest cause of failure of neutrophil intracellular killing is chronic granulomatous disease. Despite its rather unhelpful name, this is a primary immunodeficiency disorder caused by deficiency of one of the enzymes of the NADPH oxidase chain that is responsible for the generation of microbiocidal superoxides and peroxide. These products of the 'respiratory burst' are released into the neutrophil phagolysosome and kill the phagocytosed organisms. The classic test for detecting the integrity of this function is the nitroblue tetrazolium (NBT) reduction test. NBT is a soluble yellow dye that is added to whole blood. Neutrophils are stimulated with phorbol myristate acetate (PMA), and the resultant reduction of the NBT to an insoluble blue product can be seen microscopically—the normal neutrophils contain blue granules. Failure of the neutrophils to reduce NBT (they therefore appear yellow) indicates a diagnosis of chronic granulomatous disease. Other techniques exist to measure the neutrophil respiratory burst. Light emission by chemiluminogenic substrates, such as luminol and lucigenin, activated by the neutrophil respiratory burst, can be measured by a luminometer. A simple flow cytometric method based on the oxidation of dihydrorhodamine is gaining wide acceptance, as it is highly sensitive and more easily detects carriers of defective genes (Figure 47.5).

Basophils

Basophils bind IgE antibodies via their FcεRI receptors. Cross-linking of this bound IgE by allergens results in activation of the basophil, with induction of CD63 expression and release of histamine and other products. This forms the basis of a novel means of allergy diagnosis. For many allergens, skin-prick testing and determination of allergen-specific IgE in serum are useful aids to the diagnosis of allergy. However, skin tests are not always possible, and *in vitro* assays for specific IgE are not available for all possible allergens (especially when the suspected allergen is a drug). Therefore, an alternative means to detect an allergic response *in vitro* is to add the suspect allergen to the patient's blood, and measure either histamine release into the supernatant or the expression of CD63 on activated basophils. These assays are becoming available commercially, but have not yet been widely validated in clinical practice.

The future of cellular immunology

This is a field that will undoubtedly continue to expand. An increasing number of techniques is coming through

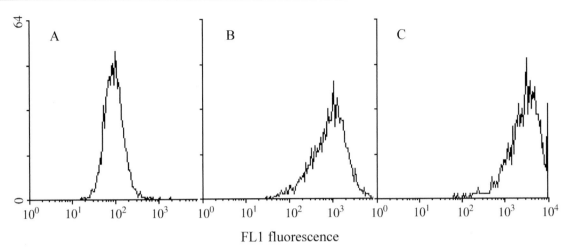

Figure 47.5 Respiratory burst measurement by dihydrorhodamine oxidation. Neutrophils in whole blood are stimulated by *E. coli* (B) or PMA (C), and dihydrorhodamine (DHR) is added. The oxidative burst converts DHR to rhodamine, with a resulting increase in fluorescence measured on FL1 compared to unstimulated neutrophils (A). Neutrophils from patients with chronic granulomatous disease do not oxidize DHR, and the shift in the population fluorescence is not seen. Healthy carriers of defective genes of the NADPH oxidase pathway usually demonstrate both normal and abnormal neutrophils, resulting in two fluorescence peaks

from research applications to the routine clinical laboratory. The applications of the flow cytometer continue to increase e.g., methods are now available to combine conventional flow cytometric measurements with *in situ* molecular biology, and new non-antibody reagents increase the scope of the properties of cells that can be assessed by this powerful method. Functional cellular assays in particular derive from recent advances in our understanding of basic immunology and disease processes. As with all diagnostic laboratory methods, these tests must be carefully evaluated and appropriately controlled, but the nature of functional assays makes these difficult to standardize. The interpretation of functional assays is also fraught with difficulties, and laboratories offering such assays must have sufficient experience and throughput of work to ensure quality. Close liaison with clinical staff is also essential to understand the significance of abnormalities observed.

Further reading

Rose NR, Conway de Macario E, Folds JD *et al.* (eds). *Manual of Clinical Laboratory Immunology*, 5th edn. 1997: American Society for Microbiology, Washington.

Baugarth N, Roederer M. A practical approach to multicolour flow cytometry for immunophenotyping. *J Immunol Methods* 2000; **243**: 77–97.

Brando B, Barnett D, Janossy G *et al.* Cytofluorometric methods for assessing absolute numbers of cell subsets in blood. European Working Group on Clinical Cell Analysis. *Cytometry* 2000; **42**: 327–346.

United Kingdom National External Quality Assessment Service (UKNEQAS) immune monitoring scheme. 2003: http://www.ukneqas.org.uk/Directory/LEUCO/immmon.htm

Comans-Bitter WM, de Groot R, van den Beemd R *et al.* Immunophenotyping of blood lymphocytes in childhood. *J Paediatr* 1997; **130**: 388–393.

Primary Immunodeficiency Diseases—Report of an IUIS Scientific Group. *Clin Exp Immunol* 1999; **118**(S1): 1–28.

48

Immune complex diseases and cryoglobulins

Siraj A Misbah

Introduction

Immune complexes (IC) are formed whenever antibody encounters antigen. This is a dynamic physiological process which enables potentially harmful exogenous antigens to be cleared by the host's mononuclear phagocytic system (MPS). Failure to clear complexes successfully may lead to immune complex deposition in the capillary basement membranes of glomeruli, skin, synovium and choroid plexus, where they trigger an inflammatory response. Inflammation induced by immune complexes is dependent on the ability of complexes to activate complement (determined by immunoglobulin isotype), with the consequent generation of potent proinflammatory mediators (C5a). C5a is a powerful chemoattractant which draws circulating polymorphonuclear leukocytes and monocytes to the site of immune complex deposition, thus serving to amplify tissue damage. The site of immune complex deposition depends partly on the size of the immune complex, as exemplified in the kidney, where small immune complexes are able to pass through the glomerular basement membrane but large complexes are unable to do so and accumulate between the endothelium and the basement membrane.

Several mechanisms ensure that immune complex deposition does not take place in health. These include: (a) phagocytosis of IC by the MPS—the size of the immune complex is a critical factor in this regard, since the MPS is only able to clear small complexes; (2) integrity of the complement pathway—proteins of the complement system play a vital role in maintaining IC in

solution by coating complexes with C3b (opsonization). This prevents the formation of large immune complex lattices and immune precipitation; in addition IC coated with C3b interact with the C3b receptor (CR1, CD35) on circulating red cells, which act as an efficient transporter of immune complexes to the MPS in the liver and spleen (Figure 48.1). Given the vital role of complement proteins in clearing IC, it is not surprising that patients with primary complement deficiency (especially of early complement components C1, C4, C2) have a high incidence of immune complex disease.

Other factors that influence immune complex deposition include physicochemical properties of antigen and antibody, including electrical charge, valency, avidity of antigen–antibody interaction and immunoglobulin isotype, e.g. IC containing cationic antigens bind tightly to the anionic glomerular basement membrane, causing tissue injury.

Although circulating immune complexes occur in a large number of diseases (Table 48.1), in the majority of cases these complexes are an epiphenomenal or incidental finding. This chapter is confined to those diseases where there is good evidence to support a pathogenetic role for immune complexes: serum sickness, systemic lupus erythematosus (SLE) and mixed cryoglobulinaemia.

Irrespective of the underlying cause, immune complex diseases share several common features which are of clinical significance: (a) multisystem involvement due to deposition of complexes in the capillaries of the kidney, skin, synovium and choroid plexus; (b) hypocomplementaemia during periods of active disease; (c) reduction in

The Science of Laboratory Diagnosis, Second Edition   Edited by David Burnett and John Crocker
© 2005 John Wiley & Sons, Ltd

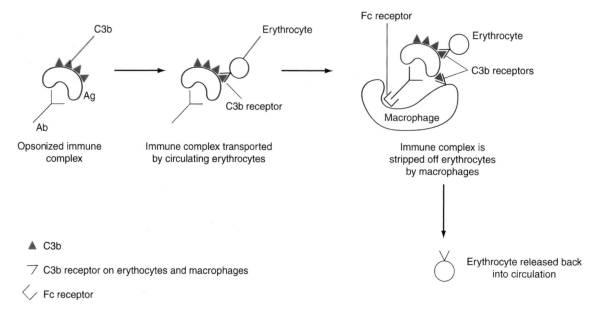

Figure 48.1   Transport of immune complexes by erythrocytes to mononuclear phagocytes in liver and spleen

Table 48.1   Disorders associated with circulating immune complexes

Immunological	Systemic lupus erythematosus
	Rheumatoid arthritis
	Mixed cryoglobulinaemia
	Felty's syndrome
	Ankylosing spondylitis
	Scleroderma
	Serum sickness
Infections	
Bacterial	*Staphylococcus aureus*, *Pseudomonas aeruginosa*, *Streptococcus* sp.
Mycobacterial	*M. tuberculosis*
Parasitic	Trypanosomiasis, onchocerciasis
Malignancy	All forms
Physiological	Normal healthy individuals Pregnancy

circulating immune complex levels by therapy (drugs, plasmapheresis) leads to improvement in disease activity.

Assays for circulating immune complexes

Over 30 assays for the detection of circulating immune complexes were described in the 1970s with the expec-

tation (subsequently unfulfilled) that they would be clinically useful in the diagnosis and management of immune complex disease. These assays were divided broadly into physical methods designed to differentiate between monomeric immunoglobulin and immune complexes, and biological methods dependent on the interaction of cell surface receptors or complement with immune complexes (Table 48.2).

The inherent problems with physical methods was exemplified by the polyethylene glycol (PEG) precipitation assay. In addition to precipitating immune complexes, PEG, even at low concentrations, also precipitates a variety of serum proteins, including IgG, thus causing major difficulties in the interpretation of results. Biological methods for the detection of immune complexes based on the recognition of complexes in humoral or cell receptor systems have proved equally unreliable. The Raji cell assay, which used a lymphoblastoid cell line derived from a patient with Burkitt's lymphoma, was used widely in the 1970s. Since the assay is based on the ability of lymphoblastoid cells (which possess surface receptors for C1q, C3b, C3d but no surface immunoglobulin) to bind serum immune complexes that have also bound complement, an unacceptably high rate of false positives was found in patients with antilymphocyte antibodies, as in SLE. Although a joint working group of the World Health Organization and the International Union of Immunological Societies (IUIS) in 1981 found four assays

Table 48.2 Immune complex assays

Physical methods—assays dependent on physicochemical properties of complex	Polyethylene glycol precipitation Cryoprecipitation Analytical ultracentrifugation
Biological methods—assays dependent on	
(i) Reaction with antiglobulins (subject to interference by endogenous rheumatoid factors)	Polyclonal rheumatoid factor assay Monoclonal rheumatoid factor assay[*]
(ii) Complement–protein interactions	^{125}C1q binding[*] Conglutinin (a bovine protein that binds immune complexes)-dependent assay[*]
(iii) Cell surface receptors	Raji cell radioimmunoassay[*]

[*]Assays found to be analytically acceptable by the WHO/IUS working group

analytically acceptable, none of the assays has withstood critical evaluation of its clinical usefulness, on account of their highly variable sensitivity, specificity and poor predictive value. In addition, the inability of most assays to detect specific antigen within immune complexes was a significant drawback. The joint WHO/IUIS working group concluded that detection of circulating immune complexes is not essential in any human disease and, more importantly, that the demonstration of circulating immune complexes was not specific for immune complex disease. As a result, most clinical immunology laboratories have abandoned immune complex assays and to date there is no evidence to suggest that immune complex assays should be re-introduced into routine clinical practice. In those cases where immune complex disease is suspected, demonstration of immunoglobulin and complement deposits on a biopsy of affected organs (e.g. skin, kidney) is taken as implicit evidence for the presence of immune complex deposits. Assays for circulating immune complexes are a poor substitute for direct immunohistological examination and immune complex disease should under no circumstances be diagnosed primarily on the demonstration of complexes in serum.

Serum sickness

Serum sickness is a good model to explain immune complex diseases. Von Pirquet in 1908 delineated serum sickness as a distinct entity in children repeatedly immunized with antidiphtheria serum derived from horses. Serum sickness was clinically manifest as widespread urticaria, fever, lymphadenopathy, arthralgia and proteinuria 8–12 days after the injection of horse serum. The latent period of 8–12 days reflected the time

necessary for patients to produce antibodies against horse proteins. Once a sufficient concentration of antibody complexes with circulating antigen, the resultant immune complex load overwhelms the control mechanisms of the body, leading to immune complex deposition and hypocomplementaemia. Clinical improvement is dependent on clearance of circulating complexes, which occurs spontaneously after 2–3 weeks in many patients; a minority may require treatment with steroids to expedite recovery.

More recently, serum sickness has been studied extensively in patients with aplastic anaemia receiving horse anti-thymocyte globulin (ATG). The clinical syndrome described in these patients is virtually identical to that described by Von Pirquet, with high levels of circulating immune complexes and hypocomplementaemia coinciding with the occurrence of skin rash and arthralgia. Immunofluorescent studies of biopsied skin revealed abundant deposits of immunoglobulin and C3 in the walls of small blood vessels.

With the decline in use of ATG, drug hypersensitivity reactions are at present the commonest cause of serum sickness. A wide range of drugs may act as haptens and bind to plasma proteins with the ensuing drug–protein complex triggering an immune response, e.g. penicillin, sulphonamides and thiouracils. Drug-induced serum sickness is usually self-limiting, provided that the offending agent is withdrawn.

Investigation

The diagnosis of serum sickness is usually self-evident by the characteristic clinical presentation in a patient with antecedent drug ingestion. Drug challenges are usually not required and should not be performed

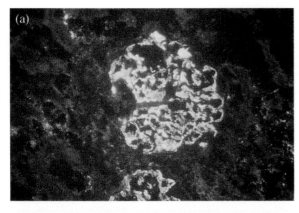

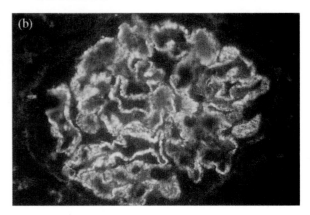

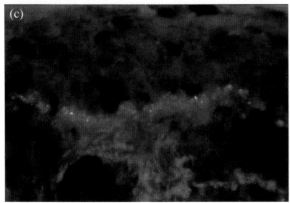

Figure 48.2   Immunofluorescence of renal and skin biopsies in a patient with SLE. (a) Glomerular IgA deposits in a membranous distribution. (b) Glomerular C1q deposits in a membranous distribution. (c) Granular IgG deposits at the dermo–epidermal junction (lupus band). Courtesy of Dr W. Merchant, Leeds General Infirmary. (a) and (b), courtesy of Dr P. Harnden, Leeds General Infirmary

routinely. The role of laboratory investigation is limited; while immune complex measurements are likely to show high levels in the circulation, this is seldom performed or required. During the acute stage of the disease, marked hypocomplementaemia (reduced C3, C4) is a feature and provides a useful pointer to systemic immune complex deposition. Tissue biopsies may be required in cases of diagnostic uncertainty and characteristically show immunoglobulin and C3 deposition on direct immunofluorescence of the skin and kidneys.

Systemic lupus erythematosus

Systemic lupus erythematosus (SLE) is a common human immune complex disorder with a prevalence of 200 cases per 100 000 population in the UK. In its most florid form, SLE affects the skin, kidneys, joints and central nervous system, although many patients may have only single organ involvement at first presentation. Patients presenting with predominant neurological disease pose difficult diagnostic problems, which are dealt with later in this chapter. Much of the organ damage in lupus is linked directly to the widespread deposition of

immune complexes that occurs in the skin, kidneys and choroid plexus. As in serum sickness, immunofluorescence of skin and kidney biopsies shows deposits of immunoglobulin and complement (Figure 48.2), while circulating immune complexes are found in a high proportion of patients with active disease. In keeping with the key role of the complement system in processing immune complexes, a range of complement abnormalities are seen in patients with SLE (summarized in Table 48.3).

Investigation of patients with suspected SLE

SLE is associated with a multitude of laboratory abnormalities, including polyclonal hypergammaglobulinaemia, leucopenia, hypocomplementaemia and a plethora of autoantibodies in blood. While the polyclonal increase in serum immunoglobulins is a non-specific marker of immune system activation, it results in a raised ESR, which acts as a useful diagnostic clue when combined with a normal CRP. Although the inability to mount an acute phase protein response in the face of active disease has long been recognized as a

Table 48.3 Abnormalities of the complement system in SLE

Primary	Total deficiency of early complement components C1q, C1r-1s, C4, C2 associated with high incidence of SLE
	Partial deficiency of C4 with one to two C4 null alleles is seen in approximately 15% of patients with SLE
Secondary	Decreased expression of CR1 is a feature of advanced SLE
	Increased activity of classical and alternative pathway reflected as hypocomplementaemia ($\downarrow$C3, $\downarrow$C4)
	Antibodies to C1q are associated with severe disease, particularly glomerulonephritis

Table 48.4 Causes of a positive ANA

Connective tissue disease
SLE
Sjögren's syndrome
Polymyositis
Rheumatoid arthritis
Vasculitis
Liver disease
Autoimmune chronic active hepatitis
Primary biliary cirrhosis
Alcoholic liver disease
Drugs
Infection
Malignancy
Healthy individuals

feature of SLE, this is not invariable. Patients with active serositis, chronic synovitis and concomitant bacterial infection are an exception to this dictum.

Autoantibodies as markers of disease

The presence of circulating antibodies to nuclear antigens is the hallmark of active lupus. The ensuing paragraphs will outline the principles and the clinical utility of the assays used to detect these antibodies.

Antinuclear antibody (ANA)

In clinical practice, the detection of antinuclear antibodies (ANA), as demonstrated by indirect immunofluorescence, is the single most useful sign for the diagnosis of SLE. ANA are detected by overlaying rodent tissue or tissue culture cells derived from a human epithelial cell line (HEp-2) with test serum, followed by a second antibody, anti-human IgG conjugated to fluorescein. Using rodent tissue, approximately 95% of patients with active untreated disease have high-titre ANA (>1 in 80). HEp-2 cells exhibit an even higher degree of sensitivity, with approximately 98–99% positivity in patients with untreated disease. Recent authoritative guidelines from the American College of Rheumatology, the College of American Pathologists, the Clinical Immunology Society and the National Institutes of Health recommend the use of HEp-2 cells as the best substrate for ANA screening (Kavanaugh *et al.*). With the widespread use of HEp-2 cells, the existence of

ANA-negative lupus as a diagnostic entity has been called into question (Cross *et al.*). Conversely, the likelihood of untreated SLE in a patient with negative ANA on HEp-2 cells is of the order of <1%. A positive ANA result, however, is not specific for SLE, since it occurs in a variety of other diseases (Table 48.4).

Several distinctive patterns of ANA are recognized on HEp-2 cells: homogeneous, nucleolar, speckled, peripheral and centromere (Figure 48.3). With the exception of the centromere antibody, which is a specific marker of the CREST syndrome (calcinosis, Raynaud's phenomenon, oesophageal dysfunction, sclerodactyly, telangiectasia) and scleroderma, none of the other ANA patterns is a reliable indicator of antigenic specificity. In view of this and the occurrence of ANA in many other disease states, it is essential to characterize a positive ANA further in terms of its antigenic specificity. In SLE, a positive ANA by indirect immunofluorescence reflects the presence of antibodies to nuclear antigens such as DNA, histones and a group of extractable nuclear antigens (ENA), known individually as Ro, La, Sm and U1-RNP (uridine ribonuclear protein).

Antibodies to extractable nuclear antigens (ENA)

Ro, La and Sm were named after the patients in whom they were first characterized: Robert, Lane and Smith. In conjunction with U1-RNP (uridine ribonuclear protein), these proteins are responsible for splicing and processing mRNA. In contrast to ANA, antibodies to ENA are specific for lupus and related disorders and are therefore helpful in the diagnosis. In addition, individual

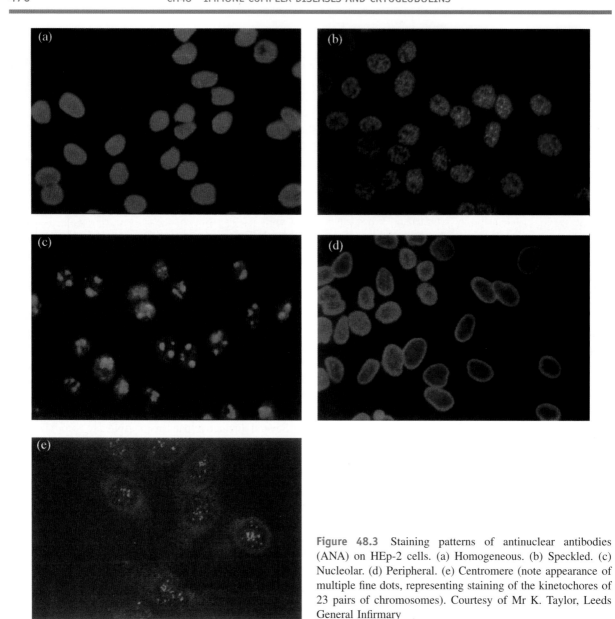

Figure 48.3 Staining patterns of antinuclear antibodies (ANA) on HEp-2 cells. (a) Homogeneous. (b) Speckled. (c) Nucleolar. (d) Peripheral. (e) Centromere (note appearance of multiple fine dots, representing staining of the kinetochores of 23 pairs of chromosomes). Courtesy of Mr K. Taylor, Leeds General Infirmary

antibodies tend to correlates with certain clinical manifestations; anti-Ro occurs in lupus and Sjögren's syndrome and correlates with cutaneous disease. It is important to recognize that anti-Ro antibodies may occur in the absence of ANA. The ANA-negative, Ro-positive profile occurs in a minority of patients with lupus (<1% on HEp-2 cells as substrate); on rodent tissue substrate, however, this figure rises to 5%, since the Ro antigen is poorly represented in rodent tissue. In 5–25% of pregnant women with lupus, anti-Ro antibodies cross the placenta to cause transient cutaneous lupus in the neonate; more seriously, 1–3% of babies born to anti-Ro positive mothers develop permanent congenital

heartblock, requiring pacemaker insertion. While anti-Ro antibodies occur in isolation in approximately 30% of lupus patients, they are accompanied by anti-La antibodies in 15% of cases. In the latter situation patients are less likely to have renal disease.

In addition to the clinical correlates discussed above, the ANA negative anti-Ro positive profile also acts as a marker for underlying primary complement deficiency affecting early complement components. Surveys of patients with homozygous C4 and C2 deficiencies reveal anti-Ro positivity in approximately 50–70% of cases. While the precise mechanism responsible for the association of SLE with primary complement deficiency has not been established, the existence of a hierarchy of disease severity in relation to the missing complement component is well documented; disease severity is greatest in patients with C1q deficiency, closely followed by total C4 deficiency. Disease severity in patients with C2 deficiency is comparable to that seen in patients with intact complement pathways.

Anti-Sm antibodies are highly specific for lupus but their prevalence varies with the ethnic background of the patient; 30% of Afro-Caribbean patients are anti-Sm-positive, in contrast to 10% of Caucasians. In view of the shared peptide sequences between Sm and U1-RNP, antibodies to Sm and U1-RNP tend to occur together.

The presence of anti U1-RNP antibodies in isolation was thought to identify a group of patients with lupus overlap syndromes, with additional features of polymyositis and scleroderma. Sharp and colleagues introduced the term 'mixed connective tissue disease' (MCTD) to characterize these patients, who were felt to have a better prognosis in view of the lower risk of renal and neurological disease. Long-term follow-up of the original cohort has questioned the existence of MCTD as a distinct benign entity, since many of the patients have subsequently developed renal and neurological disease.

Methods of detection

Immunoprecipitation assays   Antibodies to ENA may be detected by several methods. Initially, many laboraties used countercurrent immunoelectrophoresis (CIE) or the Ouchterlony double diffusion method to demonstrate the presence of antibodies. CIE is performed on agar gels, allowing antibody and antigen to migrate in opposite directions to meet in the centre of the slide, where immunoprecipitation occurs at the appropriate pH (Figure 48.4). The Ouchterlony double diffusion technique, too, is based on immunoprecipitation; antigen is placed in the centre well of an agar slide, while control and patient's sera are placed in the wells that surround the centre well. After 24–48 hours of incubation, precipitin lines are formed, denoting the presence of an antigen–antibody reaction. Precipitin identity is established by comparison with precipitin lines produced by previously characterized reference serum. Both CIE and double diffusion are qualitative techniques suitable for detecting high concentrations of specific antibodies (0.1–1.0 µg/ml). Occasionally the results of double diffusion tests may be difficult to interpret. False negative results may occur if the concentration of antigen is not adjusted to produce a zone of equivalence with

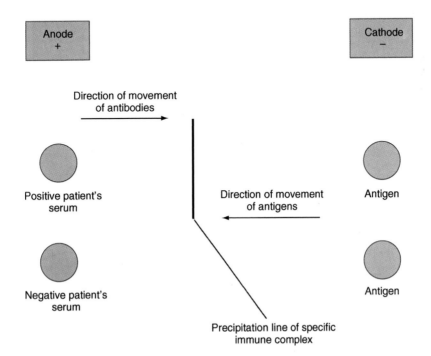

Figure 48.4   Countercurrent immunoelectrophoresis. Reproduced from Chapel *et al.* (1999) by Kind permission of Blackwell Scientific

the concentration of antibody in patient serum, and multiple precipitin lines of unknown specificity may interfere with identification of clinically significant antibodies. In contrast to double diffusion, CIE exhibits relatively greater sensitivity, speed and the ability to handle more samples. It is, however, technically demanding and the results less clear-cut.

Enzyme immunoassays　More recently, sandwich immunoassays have been developed to detect antibodies to ENA. Briefly, the method involves the addition of patient's serum containing antibody to microtitre plate wells coated with purified or recombinant individual ENA. Antibodies bound to antigen are detected by the addition of a polyclonal or monoclonal anti-human immunoglobulin antibody conjugated with an enzyme or luminescent molecule. The concentration of antibody in patient serum is directly related to the intensity of coloured or fluorescent product. Enzyme immunoassays are more sensitive (analytical sensitivity 1–10 ng/ml) than either CIE or double diffusion. Consequently, false positive results may occur in hypergammaglobulinaemic sera as a result of increased non-specific binding.

Immunoblotting　An additional method for detection of antibodies to ENA is the qualitative technique of immunoblotting (Western blot) (Figure 48.5). Briefly, antigens from a nuclear extract are separated according to molecular weight by sodium dodecyl sulphate electrophoresis (SDS–PAGE). The separated antigens are then transferred (blotting) to nitrocellulose paper, which is cut into single strips and incubated with patient's serum (commercial strips precoated with individual antigens are also available). Bound antibodies are detected by incubating the strips with an enzyme-labelled anti-human immunoglobulin. In a recent quality control exercise carried out by the Arthritis Foundation and the US Centres for Disease Control, immunoblotting was used to reanalyse anti-ENA specificities in reference sera previously characterized by immunofluorescence and double diffusion (Smolen *et al.*). The results of immunoblotting were largely in keeping with double diffusion, although differences in individual laboratories were noted in relation to the reporting of additional unspecified bands. This is a recognized phenomenon with immunoblotting, due to minor differences in techniques employed by individual laboratories. Immunoblotting is not at present used routinely in clinical immunology laboratories. In view of its specificity, it tends to be reserved for the investigation of patient samples producing discrepant results by standard assays. In those rare patients with compelling clinical evidence

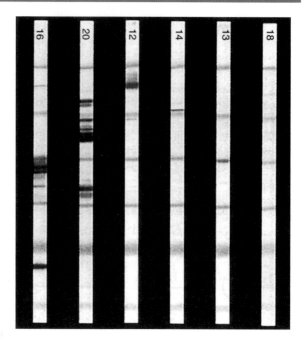

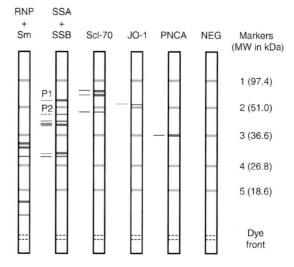

Figure 48.5　Classic profiles of antibodies to extractable nuclear antigens on immunoblotting. Modified with permission from Biodiagnostics Ltd. SS-A and SS-B are alternative terms for anti-Ro, La antibodies, respectively. P1 and P2 refer to individual subunits of Ro. Additional antibodies included are anti-Scl 70 (marker for scleroderma), anti-Jo1 (marker of polymyositis with interstitial lung disease), anti-PCNA (proliferating cell nuclear antigen; seen in 2–10% of cases of SLE)

of lupus or lupus overlap disorders, in whom conventional assays fail to detect antibodies to DNA and ENA, immunoblotting offers the potential of detecting antibodies to previously uncharacterized antigens.

Antibodies to double-stranded DNA (anti-dsDNA)

Antibodies directed against double-stranded DNA (anti-dsDNA) play an important role in the pathogenesis of organ damage in SLE, particularly in the kidney. Complexes of dsDNA and IgG anti-DNA antibodies have been demonstrated in eluates of renal biopsies. In keeping with this finding, levels of anti-dsDNA antibodies tend to correlate well with overall disease activity in SLE. In most patients, a rise in anti-dsDNA levels in serum is predictive of a disease flare. Occasionally a fall in previously elevated anti-dsDNA levels may presage lupus nephritis, presumably a reflection of immune complex deposition in the kidney. While antibodies to dsDNA are highly specific for SLE, occurring in 75–95% of patients with untreated disease, antibodies to single-stranded DNA (ssDNA) are non-specific, occurring in a variety of other disorders (rheumatoid arthritis, chronic active hepatitis, healthy elderly) in addition to lupus.

Methods of detection

Of the many methods available for detecting anti-dsDNA, most clinical immunology laboratories will use one of the following three assays.

Farr assay The Farr assay employs the use of radiolabelled dsDNA (^{125}I is commonly used as the radioisotope) as antigen. Incubating test serum containing anti-dsDNA with ^{125}I–dsDNA leads to the formation of immune complexes, which are precipitated using a saturated solution of ammonium sulphate. The amount of anti-dsDNA is directly proportional to the amount of radioactivity in the precipitate. The concentration of anti-dsDNA in test samples is derived by measuring the amount of ^{125}I-labelled DNA in the presence of a reference standard serum containing known amounts of antibody. A WHO standard serum designated Wo/80 is available for assay standardization. Since ammonium sulphate disrupts immune complexes containing antibodies of lower avidity, the Farr assay predominantly detects antibodies of high avidity which correlate well with the presence of severe lupus associated with renal disease. The Farr assay, however, does not detect low-avidity anti-dsDNA antibodies, which occur in patients with relatively mild lupus.

ELISA A number of commercial ELISA assays that utilize purified dsDNA (either recombinant or from calf thymus extract) are available for the detection of DNA antibodies. Since dsDNA does not bind directly to plastic wells, most assays utilize DNA complexed to poly-L-lysine or protamine to coat microtitre plates. In contrast to the Farr assay, ELISA assays detect both low- and high-avidity DNA antibodies. Consequently, the ELISA assay exhibits a higher degree of sensitivity for diagnostic purposes than the Farr assay; however, its relatively lower specificity results in the generation of a significant number of false positive DNA antibody results in patients without lupus, e.g. infections, chronic liver disease.

Indirect immunofluorescence using *Crithidia luciliae* Since the large mitochondrion (kinetoplast) of the haemoflagellate *Crithidia luciliae* is composed almost entirely of double-stranded DNA, indirect immunofluorescence studies using *Crithidia* as the antigen exhibit a high degree of sensitivity and specificity for the detection of anti-DNA antibodies in lupus. Commercial slides containing fixed *C. luciliae* are incubated with appropriately diluted test serum, followed by the addition of anti-human immunoglobulin antibody conjugated to fluorescein. Samples producing fluorescence confined to the kinetoplast are considered positive (Figure 48.6). Occasional samples may produce nuclear fluorescence as well, but this should be disregarded, since the nucleus contains many other antigens in addition to DNA. Although some workers have expressed concern that the kinetoplast may contain histones (basic proteins that bind DNA), leading to false positive results in anti-histone antibody-positive serum, this has not been confirmed. In most cases where contamination with histones is a concern, it is possible to perform immunofluorescence on *Crithidia* slides pretreated with hydrochloric acid, a procedure that removes histones. In view of the difficulties associated with standardization of immunofluorescent assays, the *Crithidia* assay is unreliable for serial monitoring of antibody levels.

Which anti-DNA assay to choose?

The ideal assay should be sufficiently sensitive and specific for the diagnosis of lupus, in addition to reflecting disease activity reliably. All three assays described (Table 48.5) fulfil the first criterion, with sensitivities >90% in patients with active disease. With regard to specificity, the *Crithidia* and Farr assays (specificity >90%) are superior to ELISA. ELISA assays, by virtue of their propensity to detect low-avidity antibodies, are known to produce false positive DNA antibody results in a significant minority of patients without lupus. Despite

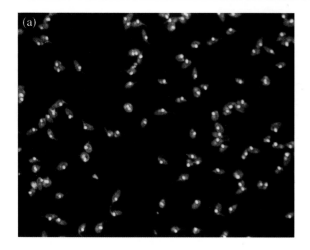

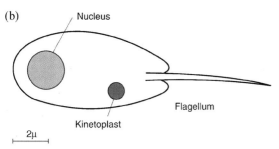

Figure 48.6 (a) Fluorescence confined to the kinetoplast of *C. luciliae* using serum containing high levels of anti-DNA antibodies from a patient with active SLE. (b) Diagrammatic representation of the anatomy of C. luciliae. Reproduced from Rose *et al.* (1992) by permission of the American Society for Microbiology

the development of disease flares, particularly involving the kidney. In a recent randomized Dutch study, patients with a 25% rise in anti-dsDNA levels receiving pre-emptive increases in immunosuppressive treatment had a significant decrease in relapses compared to the control group, who were treated conventionally (Bootsma *et al.*). A small proportion of lupus patients may relapse without an accompanying rise in DNA antibodies; similarly, a minority of patients may be clinically stable or asymptomatic despite the presence of persistently elevated antibody levels by all three assays.

Lupus and the antiphospholipid syndrome

Antibodies to phospholipids (APA) act as markers of thrombosis and occur in a third of patients with lupus. The term 'antiphospholipid syndrome' (APS) was coined to delineate those patients with thrombosis and elevated levels of phospholipid antibodies (Table 48.6). In contrast to other thrombophilic states, which result predominantly in venous thrombosis, patients with APS may develop thromboses of both arterial and venous

Table 48.6 Criteria for the diagnosis of the anti-phospholipid antibody syndrome[*]

Clinical	Venous and/or arterial thrombosis
	Recurrent fetal loss
	Persistent thrombocytopenia
Laboratory	Persistent elevation of IgG and/or IgM cardiolipin (β_2GPI-dependent) antibody[†]
	Lupus anticoagulant

[*]At least one laboratory and one clinical criterion should be present; laboratory tests should be positive on at least two occasions more than 3 months apart
[†]Measurement of cardiolipin antibody may soon be replaced by direct measurement of antibodies to β_2GPI

this drawback, ELISA assays are used increasingly in clinical practice in view of their high sensitivity, ease of automation, ability to quantify results reliably (useful for serial monitoring) and the lack of radioisotopes in the assay.

The Farr assay is equally suitable for disease monitoring and may indeed be superior to ELISA in predicting

Table 48.5 Comparison of three commonly used anti-dsDNA assays in SLE

	Farr	Crithidia	ELISA
Sensitivity	High	High	High
Specificity	High	High	Moderate
Detection of high-avidity antibodies	+++	++	++
Detection of low-avidity antibodies	+	++	+++
Ability to identify individual antibody isotypes (IgG, IgA, IgM)	No	Yes	Yes
Suitability for monitoring disease activity	Yes	No	Yes

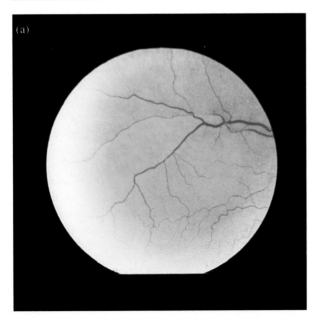

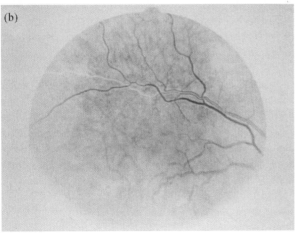

Figure 48.7 (a) Branch retinal artery occlusion in a patient with SLE and the anti-phospholipid syndrome; the defect is more pronounced in the subtraction angiogram shown in (b)

reagent. The inability of current ELISA assays to distinguish between thrombosis-associated and non-thrombosis-associated APA has led to difficulties in interpreting the clinical significance of elevated APA levels. The distinction is important, since patients with thrombosis-associated APA require intensive long-term anticoagulant therapy, probably for life. Recent evidence suggests that thrombosis-associated APA is directed largely against β_2 glycoprotein I (β_2GPI, a serum protein co-factor which binds phospholipids) rather than phospholipids *per se*. Two sources of β_2GPI are found in current assays: human serum test samples and bovine serum used to block ELISA plates. It is thought that the interaction of immobilized cardiolipin with β_2GPI alters its conformation, rendering it immunogenic. In view of the inability of conventional ELISA assays to differentiate between thrombosis-associated and non-thrombosis-associated APA, there is much interest in assays using purified β_2GPI as antigen. Although their presence is not currently included in the diagnostic criteria for the antiphospholipid syndrome, anti-β_2GPI antibodies are stronger predictors of thrombosis than conventional cardiolipin antibodies detected by ELISA.

APA which interfere with phospholipid-dependent clotting assays recognize a phospholipid–prothrombin complex and are termed lupus anticoagulants (LAC), in recognition of their occurrence in lupus patients. The term LAC is a misnomer, since it is associated with thrombosis *in vivo* rather than haemorrhage. The presence of LAC is suspected from a prolonged APTT which does not correct with the addition of normal plasma, thus suggesting the presence of an inhibitor. Since the demonstration of LAC antibodies indicates functional derangement of clotting, these antibodies correlate more closely with thrombosis than APA demonstrated by ELISA. Most patients with lupus will have LAC as well as cardiolipin antibodies (70%), although a minority of patients will have either cardiolipin antibodies or LAC (15% in each category).

vessels. Clinical manifestations are dependent on which organ is rendered ischaemic (Figure 48.7). APA may be detected by ELISA or by the prolongation of phospholipid-dependent clotting assays (activated partial thromboplastin time—APTT). APA detected by ELISA using cardiolipin, an acidic phospholipid, as antigen may not always act as a true marker of thrombosis, since many false positives have been described in patients with infection (bacterial, viral, protozoal), drug therapy and other connective tissue diseases. Indeed, the historical false positive VDRL is due to the presence of APA directed against cardiolipin present in the VDRL

Neuropsychiatric systemic lupus erythematosus (NPSLE)

The role of laboratory investigation

Neurological involvement in SLE is a major problem, affecting up to two-thirds of patients at some point in their illness. Whereas approximately 20% of such patients do so on a background of active systemic disease, in the majority of cases systemic disease is quiescent or only mildly active. The physician confronted with a patient with SLE and neurological features has to make the important distinction between neurological disease directly due to lupus (primary), opportunistic infection as a secondary cause, and steroid psychosis, since most patients will be on immunosuppressive therapy at the time of presentation. A diverse range of clinical presentations is seen (Table 48.7), reflecting multiple underlying pathogenic mechanisms. At least three

Table 48.7 Neuropsychiatric manifestations of SLE

Organic brain syndrome—cognitive impairment, psychosis[*]	
Seizures	
Cranial neuropathy	
Peripheral neuropathy	Decreasing order
Cerebrovascular accident	of frequency
Movement disorder	
Transverse myelitis	

[*]May be steroid-induced

hypotheses have been proposed to explain the diverse clinical presentations: anti-neuronal antibodies, thrombosis associated with phospholipid antibodies, and cytokine-driven disease.

Regrettably, none of the currently available laboratory markers of SLE is sufficiently specific for the diagnosis of primary neurological lupus. Several studies have shown that abnormalities in anti-DNA and complement (C3, C4) levels in either serum or cerebrospinal fluid (CSF) do not discriminate between neurological and non-neurological disease in SLE. Initial enthusiasm for antibodies directed against neurones (lymphocytotoxic antibodies, which cross-react with brain tissue and antibodies directly targeted against neuronal antigens) as specific markers for neurological lupus were dampened by studies demonstrating their presence in lupus patients without neurological involvement. Equally, recent claims that antibodies directed against ribosomal P proteins are specific markers of lupus psychosis have been refuted by their demonstration in up to 50% of SLE patients without psychosis.

Examination of CSF is mandatory in all patients with neuropsychiatric SLE to enable cases of infection masquerading as NPSLE to be diagnosed. In a recent prospective study of neurological involvement in SLE, infection (cryptococcal, tuberculosis and pyogenic meningitis) was the underlying cause in approximately 50% of cases. The presence of oligoclonal bands exclusively in CSF favours primary NPSLE but may also occur with infection. In the absence of a specific labora-tory marker, the diagnosis of NPSLE remains heavily dependent on traditional clinical acumen.

Assessment of disease activity in SLE

The accurate measurement of disease activity is crucial to the proper management of SLE. Several indices of disease activity have been devised in order to simplify this task and ensure uniformity in clinical studies. Four well-validated systems currently in use are the SLE Disease Activity Index (SLEDAI), Systemic Lupus Activity Measure (SLAM), the British Isles Lupus Activity Group (BILAG) scale and the Lupus Activity Index (LAI). In conjunction with clinical assessment, serological markers of disease activity are a vital aid to the physician in determining the need for immunosuppressive therapy in SLE.

Active disease is accompanied in most patients by a rise in serum anti-DNA levels and a fall in complement (C3, C4) levels. In some patients, however, complement measurements do not mirror disease activity. Since C3 acts as an acute phase reactant, a rise in concentration secondary to inflammation or infection would mask consumption due to active SLE. Serum C3 levels are normal in approximately 50% of patients with active disease, while C4 measurements are of limited value in patients with C4 null alleles. As a result, several studies have assessed the role of complement breakdown products (C3d, C4d, C5b-9) as markers of disease activity.

In general, complement breakdown products are more sensitive markers of active disease (sensitivity 60–80%) than conventional C3 and C4 measurements. Their relative lack of specificity (specificity 45–80%) has, however, prevented its widespread adoption in clinical practice. In the absence of the ideal serological marker of disease activity in SLE, the use of serial anti-DNA antibody levels in conjunction with complement (either C3, or C4, and/or breakdown products) and CRP represents the most useful laboratory profile for assessing disease activity (Table 48.8).

The place of adhesion molecule assays in the routine assessment of disease activity in lupus is currently under investigation. Preliminary studies suggest that serum levels of VCAM-1 (vascular cell adhesion molecule) are markedly raised in lupus nephritis and appear to correlate with disease activity; E-Selectin and ICAM-1 (intercellular adhesion molecule) levels are unhelpful. Whether measurement of VCAM-1 is superior to existing serological markers of activity will depend on the merits of future prospective studies.

Table 48.8 Changes in anti-DNA antibodies, C3, C4 and CRP in relation to disease activity in SLE

	anti-DNA	C3	C4	CRP
Active disease	↑	↓	↓	N or sl ↑
Inactive disease	N or sl ↑	N	N	N
Concomitant bacterial infection	N or sl ↑	N, ↑ or ↓	N, ↑ or ↓	↑

N = normal; sl = slight

Cryoglobulinaemia

Introduction

The term 'cryoglobulinaemia' is used to denote the presence of cryoglobulins in blood. Cryoglobulins are immunoglobulins that precipitate reversibly in the cold (4°C), redissolving at higher temperatures (37°C). Three types of cryoglobulins are recognized on the basis of their immunoglobulin composition and associated diseases (Table 48.9). Type I cryoglobulins are composed entirely of monoclonal immunoglobulin (IgG or IgM) and account for approximately 25% of all cryoglobulins. Type II, which are composed of a mixture of monoclonal IgM with rheumatoid factor activity and polyclonal IgG, account for a further 25%. Type III cryoglobulins are composed entirely of a mixture of polyclonal IgG and IgM and account for the remaining 50%. While the majority of cryoglobulins tend to precipitate at temperatures below 10°C, occasionally a thermolabile cryoglobulin may precipitate in the syringe used for venepuncture if it has not been prewarmed at 37°C. The precise reason(s) for the cryoprecipitation of immunoglobulins is not known.

Aetiology

Cryoglobulinaemia is associated in the majority of cases with an underlying disorder in the form of malignant paraproteinaemia, lymphoma, autoimmune disease or infection. Type I cryoglobulinaemia is associated typically with paraproteinaemia, with only a minority of patients failing to show evidence of underlying lymphoproliferative disease at presentation. In mixed cryoglobulinaemia (types II and III), detailed clinical investigation fails to uncover associated autoimmune disease or infection in up to one-third of patients. These patients were classified originally as having idiopathic or mixed essential cryoglobulinaemia. Since 1992, studies from Italy, USA, France and Switzerland have provided convincing evidence that 60–80% of patients with types II and III

Table 48.9 Classification of cryoglobulins

	Composition	Disease associations
Type I	Monoclonal immunoglobulin, usually IgM or IgG	Waldenström's macroglobulinaemia Myeloma, lymphoproliferative disease
Type II	Monoclonal IgM rheumatoid factor plus polyclonal IgG	Infections • Viral—hepatitis C, hepatitis B, HIV, Epstein–Barr • Bacterial—endocarditis • Spirochaetal—syphilis, Lyme disease • Parasitic—malaria • Fungal—coccidioidomycosis • 'Idiopathic'—mixed essential cryoglobulinaemia
Type III	Polyclonal IgM rheumatoid factor plus polyclonal IgG[*]	Autoimmune • SLE, rheumatoid arthritis, Sjögren's syndrome 'Idiopathic' • Mixed essential cryoglobulinaemia

[*]Trace amount of type III cryoglobulins may be found in some normal individuals

cryoglobulinaemia have underlying hepatitis C infection. Although some patients with mixed cryoglobulinaemia exhibit features of lymphoproliferative disease, such as monoclonal B cell populations in bone marrow and clonal immunoglobulin gene rearrangement in peripheral blood lymphocytes, overt lymphoma is uncommon.

The immunopathogenesis of cryoglobulinaemia is poorly understood. A wide range of primary antigen–antibody complexes has been detected in the cryoprecipitates of types II and III cryoglobulins, in addition to the complex of rheumatoid factor and IgG. This has led to the view that the formation of mixed cryoglobulins is the end result of a sequence of events driven by an antibody response to either infective agents or endogenous antigens, as in SLE.

Clinical features

The clinical manifestations of cryoglobulinaemia are due to a combination of vascular obstruction and immune complex deposition. Type I cryoglobulins may occur in either sex and mainly cause hyperviscosity and vascular obstruction. In contrast, mixed cryoglobulins (types II and III) affect females in particular and present with diverse clinical features, due to deposition of cryoprecipitable immune complexes in blood vessels, causing systemic vasculitis affecting the skin, kidney and joints. Skin biopsies of the characteristic purpuric rash seen in such patients show leukocytoclastic vasculitis with deposition of immunoglobulin and complement. Renal involvement due to membranoproliferative

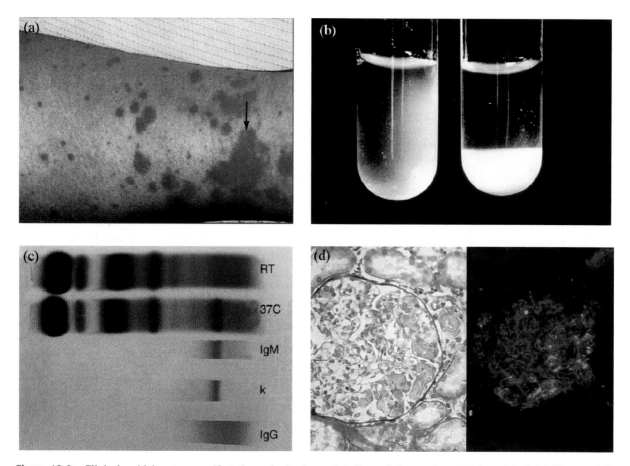

Figure 48.8 Clinical and laboratory manifestations of mixed cryoglobulinaemia in a patient with hepatitis C. (a) Characteristic purpuric rash on lower limbs; arrow indicates an area of palpable purpura. Reproduced from Shakil and Bisceglie (1994), by permission. (b) Stored serum showing cryoprecipitate after 24 hours incubation at 4°C (right), redissolving on heating to 37°C (left). (c) Zone electrophoresis of serum collected at 37°C shows the redissolved cryoprecipitate as a discrete band in the gamma region, which on immunofixation is shown to be composed of monoclonal IgM kappa and polyclonal IgG. Note absence of gamma band on zone electrophoresis of sample collected at room temperature (RT) from the same patient. (d) Renal biopsy showing eosinophilic glomerular deposits of cryoglobulin (pseudothrombi) on routine H&E examination (left) corresponding to coarse deposits (right) of IgG on immunofluorescence. Reproduced from Graham (*Arthrit Rehum* 1992; **35**: 1107), by permission

glomerulonephritis with immunoglobulin and complement deposition occurs in up to 50% of all patients with mixed cryoglobulinaemia. Distinctive histological features of cryoglobulinaemic glomerulonephritis include marked glomerular monocytic infiltration, amorphous Congo red-negative eosinophilic deposits in capillaries and a double-contoured glomerular basement membrane due to an interposition of monocytes. The presence of these features on renal biopsy in a patient with so-called 'idiopathic' glomerulonephritis should prompt a search for cryoglobulins. Impaired liver function with a wide spectrum of histological abnormality, ranging from chronic persistent hepatitis to cirrhosis, occurs in up to 70% of patients and is of interest in view of the strong association of hepatitis C infection and mixed cryoglobulinaemia (Figure 48.8).

Laboratory investigation of suspected cryoglobulinaemia

Processing of samples

The commonest reason for failure to demonstrate circulating cryoglobulins is incorrect sample collection and processing. Meticulous attention in the collection of blood samples is essential. Blood should be collected into a plain tube without anticoagulant and immersed into a flask containing water at 37°C, followed by immediate transfer to the laboratory. Failure to collect samples at 37°C enables cryoglobulins to precipitate with the blood clot, and hence escape detection. Figure 48.9 illustrates the steps in the detection of cryoglobulins in the laboratory.

Other laboratory features suggesting presence of cryoglobulins

Useful pointers to the presence of mixed cryoglobulins are marked depletion of early serum complement components (C4, C1q) due to activation of the classical pathway by immune complexes. The combination of a low serum C4 and IgM rheumatoid factor is a characteristic feature of mixed cryoglobulinaemia, occurring in over 90% of patients. It is a useful rule of thumb that patients with an unexplained low serum C4 and renal or skin disease should be investigated for cryoglobulinaemia.

Cryoglobulins interfere with routine immunochemical measurements of serum immunoglobulins, leading to

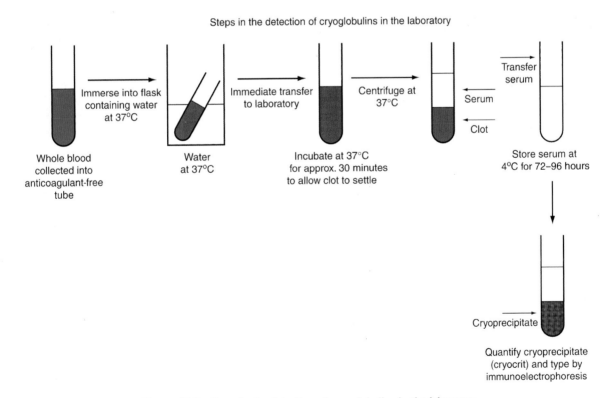

Steps in the detection of cryoglobulins in the laboratory

Figure 48.9 Steps in the detection of cryoglobulins in the laboratory

artefactually low levels; they may also interfere with routine full blood count analysis by automated cell counters leading to spurious leukocytosis and thrombo-cytosis. Collection and analysis of samples at 37°C will prevent these problems.

In addition to characterizing the cryoglobulin, all patients should be investigated for an underlying trigger. In the case of type I cryoglobulinaemia, appropriate investigations for lymphoproliferative disease should be instituted. Patients with mixed cryoglobulinaemia should have hepatitis serology done, including PCR for hepatitis C RNA, in order to select those patients who would benefit from α-interferon therapy. Routine investigation for other infective triggers (endocarditis, syphilis, Lyme disease, malaria, HIV) reportedly associated with mixed cryoglobulinaemia is not warranted in the absence of clues to the contrary.

Further reading

ACR Ad Hoc Committee on Neuropsychiatric Lupus Nomenclature. The American College of Rheumatology nomenclature and case definitions for neuropsychiatric lupus syndromes. *Arthrit Rheum* 1999; **42**: 599–608.

Beddhu S, Bastacky S, Johnson JP. The clinical and morphological spectrum of renal cryoglobulinaemia. *Medicine* 2002; **81**: 398–409.

Bootsma H *et al.* Prevention of relapses in systemic lupus erythematosus. *Lancet* 1995; **345**: 1595–1599.

Bruyn GAW. Controversies in lupus: nervous system involvement. *Ann Rheum Dis* 1995; **54**: 159–167.

Buyon JP *et al.* Assessment of disease activity and impending flare in patients with SLE. Comparison of the use of complement split products and conventional measures of complement. *Arthrit Rheum* 1992; **35**: 1028–1037.

Cervera R *et al.* Systemic lupus erythematosus: clinical and immunologic patterns of disease expression in a cohort of 1000 patients. *Medicine (Baltimore)* 1993; **72**: 113–124.

Chapel H, Haeney M, Misbah S, Snowden N. *Essentials of Clinical Immunology*, 4th Edn. 1999: Blackwell Science, Oxford.

Cross LS, Aslam A, Misbah SA. Antinuclear antibody-negative lupus as a diagnostic entity does it no larger exist? *Q J Med* 2004; **97**: 303–308.

Ferri C, Zignego AL, Pileri SA. Cryoglobulins (review). *J Clin Pathol* 2002; **55**: 4–13.

Gorevic P. Cryopathies: cryoglobulins and cryofibrinogenaemia. In *Samter's Immunologic Diseases*, 5th edn, vol II, Frank MM, Austen KF, Claman HN, Unanue ER (eds). 1994: Little, Brown and Co, Boston, 951–974.

Isenberg D, Smeenk R. Clinical laboratory assays for measuring anti-DNA antibodies. Where are we now? (review). *Lupus* 2002; **11**: 797–800.

Kavanaugh A, Tomar R, Reveille J *et al.* Guidelines for clinical use of the antinuclear antibody test and tests for specific autoantibodies to nuclear antigens. *Arch Pathol Lab Med* 2000; **124**: 71–81.

Levine JS, Branch DW, Rauch J. The antiphospholipid syndrome (review). *New Engl J Med* 2002; **346**: 752–763.

Lock RJ, Unsworth DJ. Measurement of immune complexes is not useful in routine clinical practice. *Ann Clin Biochem* 2000; **37**: 253–261.

Mok CC, Lau CS. Pathogenesis of systemic lupus erythematosus (review). *J Clin Pathol* 2003; **56**: 481–490.

Rose NR, Macario EC, Fahey J, Fredman H, Penn GM. *Manual of Clinical Laboratory Immunology*, 4th edn. 1992: American Society for Microbiology, 731.

Sharp GC *et al.* Mixed connective tissue disease—an apparently distinct rheumatic disease syndrome associated with a specific antibody to an extractable nuclear antigen. *Am J Med* 1972; **52**: 148–159.

Smolen JS *et al.* Reference sera for antinuclear antibodies II. Further definition of antibody specificities in international antinuclear antibody reference sera by immunofluorescence and western blotting. *Arthrit Rheum* 1997; **40**: 413–418.

Trendelenburg M, Schifferli JA. Cryoglobulins in chronic hepatitis C infection (editorial). *Clin Exp Immunol* 2003; **133**: 153–155.

IUIS/WHO. Use and abuse of laboratory tests in clinical immunology: critical considerations of eight widely used diagnostic procedures. Report of an IUIS/WHO working group. *Clin Exp Immunol* 1981; **46**: 662–674.

Wallace DJ, Linker-Israeli M. It's not the same old lupus or Sjögren's any more: one hundred new insights, approaches and options since 1990. *Curr Opin Rheumatol* 1999; **11**: 321–329.

Walport MJ. Complement and systemic lupus erythematosus (review). *Arthrit Res* 2002; **4** (suppl 3): S 279–293.

49

HLA typing

Mark Hathaway

Introduction

Transplantation is now an accepted medical therapy to replace diseased organs. However, the response of the host's immune system to the transplanted organ remains a major obstacle to a successful outcome. Organ transplants are destroyed by an adaptive immune response, principally by T lymphocytes to non-self antigens present on the surface of the grafted tissue. Of the various donor antigens present on allografted tissue that may potentially elicit an immune response, disparate antigens of the major histocompatibility complex (MHC) are the most important.

When donor and recipient are MHC-disparate, an immune response is initiated and directed against a non-self MHC molecule or molecules on the grafted tissue. Although other antigen systems can invoke an allograft-directed immune response, MHC antigens known as human leukocyte antigens, or HLA for short, are the most immunogenic. This is because of their ability to bind directly to the T cell antigen receptor, thus bypassing normal antigen processing which is required to stimulate T cell responses; and the high frequency of circulating T cells in peripheral populations with receptor specificity for non-self MHC.

Since differences in MHC antigens provoke such vigorous rejection of allografts, a considerable amount of work has been directed towards donor:recipient MHC matching. Defining the HLA specificity, in an attempt to minimize rejection, through donor:recipient MHC matching is a process known as HLA typing.

HLA structure and function

The HLA genes of the human MHC consist of multiple class I, class II and class III loci present on the short arm of chromosome 6. They comprise approximately 4×10^6 base pairs, containing at least 50 genes.

HLA class I proteins consist an alpha (α) chain that has three subunits, each resembling an immunoglobulin (Ig) domain. When expressed on the cell surface, HLA class I molecules are non-covalently bound to the peptide β-2-microglobulin (β-2M), which is coded for on a separate chromosome. At present there are three well-defined α-chain genes, designated HLA-A, -B, and -C. HLA-A and HLA-B represent the major class I products and serve as targets for both antibody- and cell-mediated immune responses against transplanted tissue. Their expression is differential, depending on cell type, with cells of the lymphoid lineage having the highest expression and hepatocyes and red blood cells having the lowest. Expression can be altered by inflammatory mediators such as cytokines and this is particularly important in transplantation, since upregulation can promote allograft immunogenicity, or increase the susceptibility of allografts to a pre-existing immune response.

HLA class II proteins differ from those of the class-I region in terms of structure, function and distribution. They consist of two chains, α and β, and are expressed on the cell surface as $\alpha\beta$ heterodimers. HLA class II α and β chain genes are designated HLA-DP, HLA-DQ and HLA-DR, both chains being encoded for in the

The Science of Laboratory Diagnosis, Second Edition Edited by David Burnett and John Crocker
© 2005 John Wiley & Sons, Ltd

class-II region and having two subunits resembling Ig domains. HLA-DR gene clusters contain an extra β chain gene, whose product can pair with any DR α chain. Therefore, three sets of class II genes can give rise to four types of class II molecules. The distribution of class II proteins is largely restricted to B lymphocytes and professional antigen-presenting cells (APCs), although expression on other cells is inducible following activation. The function of class II molecules has been traditionally considered in terms of their ability to stimulate helper T cell responses; however, more recent evidence has shown significant cytotoxic antibody and effector T cell responses directed against class II determinants.

Also encoded for in the MHC are two TAP genes. These are found in the class II region, closely associated with two genes encoding low molecular weight proteins of the proteosome. The genes of the class III region encode, amongst other things, the complement components C4 (C4a and C4b), C2 and factor B, together with those for the cytokine tumour necrosis factor (TNFα and β), the steroid synthesizing enzyme 21-hydroxylase, and two heat shock proteins, Hsp 70 1 and Hsp 70 2.

Genetics of the MHC

The genes coding for HLA class I α chains and class II α and β chains are linked within the MHC. Although the genes coding for each chain are to be found in separate regions, several genes encoding for each chain have been identified within each region. Because the HLA genes are in close proximity to each other, genetic recombination is rare. Therefore, most offspring inherit an intact set of parental alleles, one from each parent. Such sets of linked genes are known as *haplotypes*. Certain alleles in particular haplotypes form in greater or lesser frequencies than would be expected if the alleles were at genetic equilibrium. Such a phenomenon is known as *linkage disequilibrium* and may reflect both the recent origin of some alleles and geographical origins and racial breeding patterns.

The products of HLA class I and class II genes are co-dominantly expressed, therefore heterozygous individuals should express two distinct HLA specificities for each locus (one maternal, one paternal). In addition, because there are three genes for HLA class I and four possible sets for class II, each individual would be expected to express three different MHC class I and four different class II proteins. The number expressed is in fact much higher, due to the extreme *polymorphic nature* of class I and II genes; indeed, more than 70 alleles at the same genetic locus have been identified for some class I proteins. For this reason, the probability of HLA genes in two non-identical individuals encoding the same allele is extremely small. Because HLA proteins are extremely immunogenic, the need in transplantation is to get the closest possible match between allograft and recipient, thus minimizing the risk of graft loss to rejection. The technical process of HLA protein identification in a given individual is known as HLA typing.

The mechanics of HLA typing

Serological typing

Historically, the mixed lymphocyte reaction (MLR) was used to detect HLA variability. In this technique, cells from a potential recipient are co-cultured with 'stimulator' cells of donor origin that have been irradiated so that they cannot respond. T cells from the recipient are stimulated to proliferate and differentiate in response to disparate HLA antigens, usually as a result of CD4$^+$ T cell recognition of HLA class II antigens and recognition of class I antigens by CD8$^+$ T cells. Thus, 'matched' recipients can be readily identified on the basis of their 'non-responsiveness'. Whilst this technique correlates well with rejection, is extremely sensitive and closely reflects the rejection response itself, its application in the clinical setting is of limited or no value, since it takes 5–10 days to obtain results and is cumbersome, expensive and technically difficult to perform.

Until recently, the 'traditional' method used to distinguish HLA non-identical individuals employed antibody. HLA-A and -B locus antigens were the first to be defined in this manner, using allo-antisera obtained from subjects immunized by blood transfusions, pregnancy or renal allograft rejection. Using this technique, called a microcytotoxicity assay, peripheral blood T lymphocytes (HLA class I antigens) and B lymphocytes (HLA-DR, -DQ) from potential allograft recipients of unknown HLA type are incubated with antiserum containing HLA antibody of characterized specificity. These cells are then exposed to complement. If antibody reacts with HLA proteins expressed on the cell surface, complement is activated and the cells are killed—complement-mediated lysis. In the absence of reaction, no lysis occurs. Killing is usually visualized using an ethidium bromide/acridine orange cocktail that colours viable cells green and dead cells red. Killing is determined semi-quantitatively by assessing the percentage of dead cells in each well.

Thus, where lysis occurs, the specificity of the antibody identifies which HLA proteins are expressed.

Several types of error are possible with serological typing. A failure to identify a rare or cross-reactive antigen is a frequent problem. This is principally because the relevant antiserum has not been used or is not available. Linkage disequilibrium, geographical origins and racial breeding patterns are also contributing factors. Moreover, some antigens are expressed at a lower frequency or not at all in certain populations. Such errors are most likely to occur in laboratories using limited numbers of antisera. In addition, a misinterpretation of antiserum reactions can also produce errors. Antiserum may contain more than one antibody, each with differing HLA specificities, and even monospecific HLA antibodies frequently cross-react with other HLA antigens. Furthermore, HLA typing of DR antigens using serology is particularly susceptible to misinterpretation, since B lymphocytes are both more cross-reactive to a wide range of DR antigens and more susceptible to non-specific complement-mediated lysis, giving rise to 'false positive' results. Technical variations also account for a 15–30% inter-laboratory error in serological typing. Variation in complement activity between batches and quality of antiserum are the main contributory factors.

Serology is a rapid method for HLA typing; however, the reagents used are not specific enough to determine the precise structural identity of MHC molecules in genetically non-identical individuals. This can only be achieved by direct analysis of the MHC genes themselves.

Molecular typing

Restriction fragment length polymorphism

In recent years, intensive molecular cloning and mapping of the class II region of the MHC has been achieved. Extensive analysis of the organization of specific gene sequences, using a technique known as Southern blotting, has revealed the existence of polymorphisms in the recognition sites of a group of enzymes called restriction endonucleases. These polymorphisms in restriction sites are, in the majority of cases, allele-specific. Therefore, mapping and elucidation of the restriction fragment length polymorphism (RFLP) patterns associated with HLA alleles should facilitate allelic identification in any given individual. The feasibility of HLA typing by detection of RFLPs using DNA probes was first suggested by Wake *et al.*

(1982), who reported HLA-DR region polymorphisms using a full-length DRβ1 cDNA clone. RFLP typing of HLA-DR and -DQ alleles using full-length cDNA probes for DRβ, DQα and DQβ have since been used extensively in an attempt to accurately define the relationship between RFLPs and serological or cellular defined HLA class II specificities.

RFLP analysis is carried out on genomic DNA samples usually obtained from 'buffy coat' leukocytes. Full-length DNA is extracted via sodium dodecyl sulphate (SDS)/proteinase K digestion of the leukocytes and subjected to restriction digestion using the restriction endonuclease Taq-1 or MSP-1. The digest is then electrophoretically separated on a 2% agarose gel and transferred to a nitrocellulose membrane, using a Southern blotting technique. Restriction fragment patterns are visualized by hybridization of the blot with complimentary radiolabelled cDNA probes, which is then exposed to X-ray film. The hybridization signal patterns generated are then compared with reference tables to enable identification of differing HLA-DR and -DQ specificities.

The merits of this technique are that multiple samples (>30) can be processed simultaneously. Also, DRβ, DQα and DQβ allelic specificities can be identified from a single sample, since restriction digests can be blotted and probed with one HLA gene-specific cDNA (e.g. DRβ) and the blot stripped, washed and re-probed with a cDNA of differing HLA specificity (e.g. DQα or DQβ). Its disadvantages are that RFLP requires extremely careful sample handling and DNA extraction. The DNA must be full-length, not partially degraded, since this can radically alter the restriction pattern, giving rise to incorrect banding. In addition, it cannot be used in the clinical transplant setting to HLA-type cadaveric donors due to inherent time constraints, since it can take up to 3 weeks to obtain results. Moreover, the restriction fragment banding patterns are highly complex and inter-locus cross-hybridization of cDNA probes means that this technique requires considerable expertise in interpretation. However, the latter problem can be circumvented by the use of short region, or exon-specific, cDNA probes. In technical terms, RFLP analysis does not directly identify polymorphic DNA sequences in the region coding for HLA antigens, but restriction sites in strong linkage with them. In addition, it relies on the linkage disequilibrium between HLA-DR and HLA-DQ alleles to discriminate between certain HLA-DR alleles that demonstrate similar RFLP patterns, e.g. DR3 (DQ2) from DR6 (DQ6) and DR7 (DQ2) from DR9 (DQ9). Such an exercise needs great caution when analysing non-Caucasian populations, since particular HLA-DR–DQ associations are not always the same. Indeed, later evidence has since shown that such associations are not always true in Caucasoid populations either.

Polymerase chain reaction

At present, the most convenient method of identifying MHC alleles is by using a technique known as polymerase chain reaction (PCR). This is a rapid method of selectively replicating particular sequences of genomic DNA. In order to amplify specific DNA regions, such as a polymorphic exon of a particular MHC gene, synthetic oligonucleotide primers, complementary to the DNA sequence flanking the region of interest, have to be synthesized. Genomic DNA, extracted in an identical procedure to that for RFLP analysis, is then denatured at high temperature in the presence of excess concentrations of the two synthetic oligonucleotides. Cooling then allows the DNA strands to re-anneal, so that both primers are bound to their complementary sequence on genomic DNA. The thermostable enzyme DNA polymerase (Taq-polymerase), obtained from the bacterium *Thermus aquaticus*, which is added to the reaction, now elongates the primer, using the genomic DNA between the two primers as its template. The replicated DNA is then denatured into single strands by high temperature and the mixture cooled to facilitate new cycles of annealing and replication. The first extension product is random in length, but all subsequent cycles create products of defined length because the template ends at the first primer. Cycles are then repeated until sufficient DNA is available for sequencing.

Once DNA associated with a particular allele has been defined at the sequence level, oligonucleotide probes can be constructed from regions where differences occur. These sequence-specific oligonucleotide (SSO) or allele-specific oligonucleotide (ASO) probes can then be hybridized to Southern-blotted PCR-amplified specific target DNA, using a technique called PCR-SSO/PCR-ASO. Such techniques are rapid, cheap and a sensitive way of defining MHC gene structure. However, PCR-SSO/ASO typing techniques require the preparation of multiple blots and labelled probes, at least one probe for each allele at each locus. RFLP typing, in contrast, requires at most two blots and three probes. Time constraints using PCR-SSO/ASO are similar to DNA-RFLP but the preparation of target DNA is quicker (5–6 hours compared with 24 hours); blotting and probing taking a similar amount of time. Thus, like RFLP, this technique is only of use in non-urgent clinical applica-

tions and therefore cannot be used to HLA-type cadaveric donors.

HLA typing by molecular techniques has been revolutionized by the recent introduction of a PCR-based multiple sequence-specific primer (PCR-SSP) method. Intensive molecular cloning of both HLA class I and class II genes has facilitated the construction of a complete series of SSPs. PCR-SSP maintains the allelic specificity of each primer pair, both by the stringency of the PCR reaction conditions and the design of the oligonucleotide primers, which exploit the ability of Taq polymerase to amplify target DNA sequences that are mismatched to the primer sequence. In reactions where complementarity between DNA and primer is complete, amplification efficiency is 100% and target DNA is replicated. Where there and one or more base pair mismatches between target DNA and the $3'$ end of the primer, amplification efficiency is 0% and no products are synthesized. This system for HLA class I and class II typing uses 192 PCR reactions to define HLA-A, -B, -C, DRβ1, DRβ3, DRβ4, DRβ5 and DQβ1 genes. Reaction products are electrophoretically separated, using a 1% agarose gel containing ethidium bromide, and visualized on a UV transilluminator.

Complete, HLA types can be identified from a single Polaroid photograph, hence this process has been termed 'phototyping'. This technique has sensitivity greater than or equal to serology without cross-reaction problems, and can distinguish most heterozygous allelic combinations. It has the advantage over both DNA-RFLP- and PCR-SSO/ASO-based typing techniques in that it does not require blotting and probing and is therefore cheaper and quicker to perform. Moreover, full HLA typing, from blood to results, can be obtained in 3 hours, making this technique comparable to serology and thus suitable for HLA typing of cadaveric donors. Indeed, PCR-SSP has now superseded serological techniques in many histocompatibility-testing laboratories. Another advantage over DNA-RFLP is that PCR-SSP does not rely on full-length DNA to produce results, therefore partially degraded samples can be utilized.

DNA-based typing via PCR amplification is now a common laboratory procedure. HLA typing requires a second assay to identify the amplified alleles. As outlined above, several types of assay can be used to effect this, but recently, new SSO typing kits have been developed that use a homogeneous multiplex system, such that all SSOs are analysed simultaneously and therefore the entire assay is carried out in a single tube with addition of a single reagent. PCR-SSP uses equimolar concentrations of forward and reverse primers, thus double-stranded products result. However, if one primer is in excess, single-stranded (as well as double-stranded) products arise on exhaustion of the limiting primer. Once denatured, both can hybridize to SSO probes. The most recent development is to attach biotinylated SSO probes to microspheres that can then be analysed using a fluoroanalyser. Each microsphere has a unique signature that can be distinguished by the analyser, and each carries a different biotinylated SSO, therefore a probe mixture can be distinguished by virtue of its association with a particular microsphere. Binding of the probe is visualized using streptavidin-PE. The relative signal from each probe is used to assign positivity and negativity with the amplified DNA. This provides the information required to assign an HLA phenotype and had the distinct advantage of not requiring hazardous chemicals. However, this and other PCR-based techniques are not devoid of problems. Deviation from defined PCR protocols, poor quality DNA (in terms of purity) and unsuitable PCR machines can produce individual PCR failures that result in incorrect or missed antigen assignment. In addition, these high-level molecular techniques are no less demanding than serology and require considerable training and expertise if they are to be performed correctly.

Sequencing-based typing

DNA sequencing techniques were originally developed in the 1970s, but have now advanced sufficiently to be considered rapid, cheap and simple methods for HLA typing. Two basic techniques have emerged, viz. the chemical degradation technique developed by Maxim and Gilbert (1977), and the enzymatic method developed by Sanger et al. (1977). Several reports detailing both HLA class 1 and class 2 sequence data were published in the mid-1980s. However, at that time, the extent of HLA polymorphism, together with the laborious techniques required to amplify DNA regions, meant that sequencing could not be considered realistic for tissue typing. This consideration was rapidly reversed following the introduction of PCR-based methods of DNA amplification. Initial approaches used RNA successfully to sequence both class 1 and class 2 alleles, which is both simple and rapid to isolate, and simplified the amplification of the short exon regions needed. Its principle disadvantage was the requirement for viable material for RNA isolation. In addition, RNA is unstable, making extraction, particularly from archive material, notoriously difficult. At the same time, DNA-based sequence typing techniques were also being developed and it is these that are currently used in most tissue-typing laboratories.

The most popular method for DNA sequencing is the dideoxy-mediated chain termination technique, which itself evolved from an original technique developed in 1975. In short, this technique involves the amplification of the region to be sequenced, which is then denatured to produce single-stranded DNA (ssDNA). A sequencing primer is then annealed to the ssDNA and the DNA chain extended in the 5′ to 3′ direction. Extension will terminate should a 2′3′ dideoxynucleotide be incorporated rather than a conventional deoxynucleotide. Four reactions are set up, each containing one of four dideoxy nucleotides as well as all four deoxynucleotides. Thus, four separate sets of chain-terminated fragments are produced. These fragments remain annealed to the ssDNA that has acted as the template and, by heating or using a denaturing agent, the chain terminated fragments can be released from the template and separated using high-resolution denaturing gel electrophoresis. The sequence of the original DNA is then deduced by comparing the relative position of the products in the four lanes of the gel.

Although the basic method remains unchanged, a number of improvements have been made that improve the speed, simplicity and reliability of DNA sequencing. These include the use of PCR fragments as templates, which provides a rapid method for obtaining large amounts of template material, and the use of biotinylated primer, which means that the biotin-labelled PCR product can be rapidly extracted using streptavidin-labelled magnetic beads. Improvements in enzymes used for sequencing have also contributed. T7 DNA polymerase is now preferred to Klenow polymerase, because it incorporates DNA bases into the extending chain at a more even rate. DNA polymerases derived from *Thermus aquaticus* have been engineered to be more thermostable, which in turn yields more products. Radio–labelled nucleotides are being increasingly replaced with fluorescent labelling methods as a means of detecting sequencing products. In addition, the use of four-colour dyes means that products can be run on a single gel lane. Linking of each dye to separate ddNTPS also means that reactions can be carried out in a single tube. A wide range of automated sequencers are also available that detect fluorescent-labelled products following slab gel or vertical capillary electrophoresis. Moreover, all of these machines transfer data directly to a computer, bypassing the need for manual analysis of raw data, since data is automatically converted into sequence information.

As with most techniques, sequencing is not without problems. Ambiguous allele combinations are the biggest problem. This happens in all loci and occurs when two alleles produce a heterozygous sequence that is identical to the sequence of a different pair of alleles. There may also be problems with PCR and sequencing primer design. Sequencing was thought to hold an advantage over other DNA typing, in as much that it would detect previously unidentified alleles. This is true unless the new allele contains polymorphisms in positions corresponding to the $3'$ end of the PCR or sequencing primers. In addition, the sequence-based typing must sequence the entire gene under study, since the shorter the sequence, the greater the chances of novel polymorphisms being missed. The use of multiple primers for PCR and sequencing can result in preferential amplification or sequencing of a particular allele. This leads to an incorrect assignation of homozygosity. Sequence-based typing techniques are still labour-intensive and require expensive equipment and reagents. This alone is probably the greatest obstacle to its adoption as a front-line technique for HLA laboratories. Moreover, although sequence-based typing provides very high-resolution typing, there is as yet no evidence to suggest that such high-resolution HLA matching is important in solid organ transplantation. For bone-marrow transplantation, however, the picture is different, with clear evidence that matching affects outcome.

Summary

The cell surface glycoproteins of the MHC play a central role in transplant immunology. The MHC was originally determined as the major barrier to transplantation because of the strong rejection response of T lymphocytes to non-self MHC antigens present on the grafted tissue. The HLA proteins of the human MHC are amongst the most polymorphic known, therefore the likelihood of two unrelated individuals expressing the same HLA alleles is very small. Since T cell antigen recognition is profoundly influenced by MHC polymorphism, the HLA proteins of transplant donors and potential recipients must be identified and the closest possible match sought, in order to minimize the risk of graft loss to rejection. The technique of HLA identification, termed 'tissue typing', is indeed used in clinical medicine to match donor to recipient in cadaveric transplant programmes, but can also be used to study the role of the MHC in determining susceptibility to allergic and autoimmune conditions.

MHC genotyping in humans was originally carried out by mixed lymphocyte reaction and then serology. Because of inherent methodological constraints, these methods were superseded by techniques analysing at the genetic expression level. The -DR and -DQ genes of the MHC class II region were the first to be HLA-typed by DNA-RFLP. This technique has largely been replaced by quicker and faster PCR-based methods. Molecular cloning and mapping of the MHC has led to the recent development of a new PCR-based technique that types antigens of both class I and class II regions. Using this technique, HLA genotyping can be carried out on a single sample using multiple PCR and a single gel, with results obtainable from a single Polaroid photograph. This system has either replaced, or is replacing, all previous serological/molecular-based HLA typing procedures in the majority of histocompatibility testing laboratories. Sequence-based DNA techniques provide a high-resolution typing method that is commonly used in the bone marrow transplantation setting.

SECTION 9

MOLECULAR PATHOLOGY

50

Laser capture microdissection

Orla Sheils, Paul Smyth, Esther O'Regan, Stephen Finn,

Richard Flavin and **John O'Leary**

Recent advances in molecular technologies have revolutionized the study of genomics, transcriptomics and proteomics. However, a serious potential drawback in the application of these technologies is the inherent heterogeneity of surgically resected tissues. Erroneous results can be generated, causing distortion of subsequent analysis unless the input material is free of cell populations that are surplus to requirements. Laser microdissection of tissue sections and cytological preparations is a valuable upstream resource to facilitate the procurement of pure cell populations and overcome the hurdle of tissue complexity. It can be coupled with a variety of downstream molecular technologies to generate valid and meaningful results.

Laser capture microdissection (LCM) is a technique originally developed at the National Cancer Institute. Since its inception there have been a number of modifications and a range of instruments are currently available, which essentially fall into two categories, depending on the type of laser [infra-red (IR) or ultraviolet (UV)] employed.

LCM can be applied to an assortment of tissue preparations, from frozen to fixed paraffin embedded sections or cytological preparations. Routine staining using haematoxylin and eosin or toluidine blue is generally used to assist morphological identification of the cellular type of interest and to facilitate navigation around a tissue section. However, histochemical staining, immunohistochemistry or immunofluorescence may also be used to permit selection of cells according to

phenotypic and functional characteristics. Depending on the starting material and the requirements of the selected downstream protocols, DNA, mRNA or protein may be extracted and successfully analysed. In this way the identification of cell specific biomarkers of disease or potential therapeutic targets can be accurately achieved.

One area where this technology has been especially useful is that of cancer research. A major hurdle for cancer researchers lies in the difficulty of characterizing molecular changes that result during cancer progression, where premalignant cells progress to form a malignant tumour. Identification of proteins up- or downregulated during tumour progression that may aid in early cancer detection is hampered by the small cell subpopulation in which these proteins exist. Laser capture microdissection (LCM) allows researchers to compare normal with diseased cells by isolating distinct subpopulations from stained tissue sections.

Arcturus LCM—PixCell™ and AutoPix™

LCM facilitates increased sensitivity and accuracy of molecular assays by starting with samples of homogeneous cell types and multicellular structures isolated from whole tissue or cytology samples. This unique approach to microdissection, developed in 1996 at the National Institutes of Health (USA) and available exclusively from Arcturus, ensures that biological molecules, such as RNA and DNA, remain undamaged during the

The Science of Laboratory Diagnosis, Second Edition   Edited by David Burnett and John Crocker
© 2005 John Wiley & Sons, Ltd

microdissection process. Downstream molecular analysis of these molecules produces accurate and assured results that have led to over 300 peer-reviewed publications by independent researchers.

LCM has enormous flexibility with respect to tissue and cell fixation preparations. LCM effectively extracts cells from both paraffin-embedded and frozen tissue sections, prepared using a wide variety of different dyes, slide surfaces and protocols.

Based on the adherence of selected cells to a thermoplastic membrane, LCM utilizes a low-power infrared laser to melt the membrane above the cells of interest. The microscope stage of the PixCell II LCM instrument uses a joystick to control its movement. Special 'caps' (Figure 50.1) are loaded into the assembly, through which

a microcentrifuge tube containing the buffer solutions required for the isolation of the molecules of interest. The minimum diameter of the laser beam of the LCM microscope is currently 7.5 μm, the maximum diameter 30 μm. Following this procedure, biomolecules may be extracted from the cells using the proprietary or generic nucleic acid or protein extraction kits.

The process of cell capture is direct and easy to perform and there is a range of products optimized for specific downstream applications. The PixCell II LCM System (Figure 50.2) does not use pulsed UV radiation

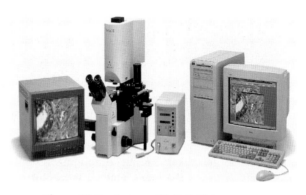

Figure 50.2 Arcturus PixCell 11 instrument

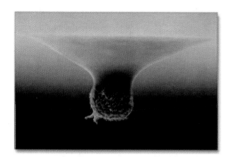

Figure 50.1 Scanning electron micrograph of a CapSure LCM Cap with a single cell laser-captured onto the thermoplastic film. Courtesy of Arcturus

the laser is focused over the cells of interest. These caps, which are coated with a thermoplastic film, are placed over the tissue section or cytology sample. The cap is suspended on a mechanical transport arm and placed on the desired area of the dehydrated tissue section under standard pressure. After visual selection of the desired cells, guided by a positioning beam, laser activation leads to focal melting of the ethylene vinyl acetate (EVA) membrane. The formation of a thin protrusion of melted plastic, which bridges the gap between the cap and tissue and adheres to the target cell, means that when the cap is lifted, the selected cells remain attached and are captured for further analysis. The polymer re-solidifies within milliseconds and forms a composite with the tissue. Laser impulses, usually 0.5–5.0 ms in duration, can be repeated multiple times across the whole cap surface, which allows the rapid isolation of large numbers of cells. The selected tissue fragments are harvested by simple lifting of the cap, which is then transferred to

or other indirect capture techniques, a feature which, the manufacturers assert, reduces potential sample loss or the introduction of electrostatic charges that make the sample difficult to handle. The low energy of the IR laser also avoids potentially damaging photochemical effects.

There is an optional Image Archiving Workstation available with the PixCell II LCM System. This facility provides a user-friendly interface for recording and storing both pre- and post-microdissection images with optional user annotations.

A recent advance to the Arcturus' repertoire in LCM technology is the automated AutoPix™ LCM system. The major advantage of this instrument (Figure 50.3) over the PixCell 11 is that all stage and optical movement, cameras, filters and objectives are completely computer-controlled. This allows areas within numerous fields of view to be visualized, selected, and captured simultaneously. In addition, inbuilt cell and feature recognition algorithms enable the user to teach the software to locate and target specific cells or regions of interest on various samples. The system (Figures 50.4, 50.5, 50.6) also has the ability to pool microdissected cells or regions from multiple samples in one session, facilitating collection of microdissected material.

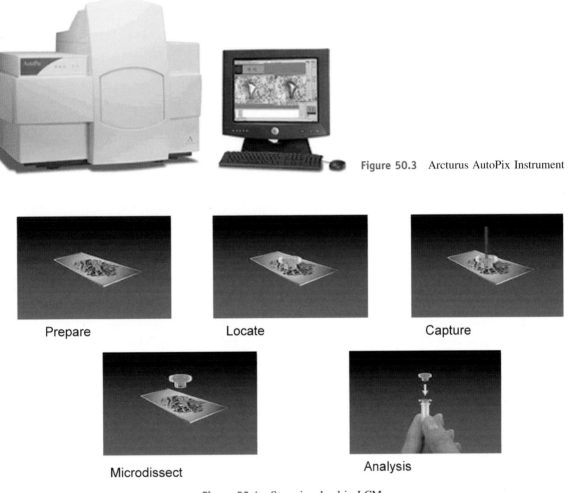

Figure 50.3 Arcturus AutoPix Instrument

Prepare

Locate

Capture

Microdissect

Analysis

Figure 50.4 Steps involved in LCM

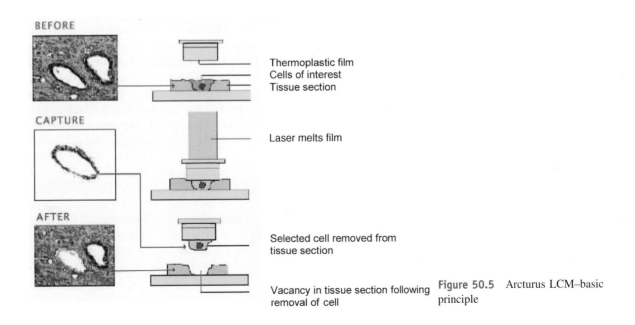

BEFORE

Thermoplastic film
Cells of interest
Tissue section

CAPTURE

Laser melts film

AFTER

Selected cell removed from
tissue section

Vacancy in tissue section following
removal of cell

Figure 50.5 Arcturus LCM–basic
principle

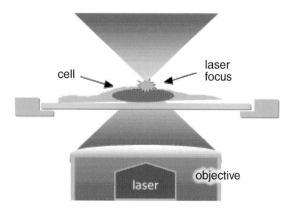

Figure 50.6 Cartoon depicting how a laser beam is focused through a shade to dissect individual cells

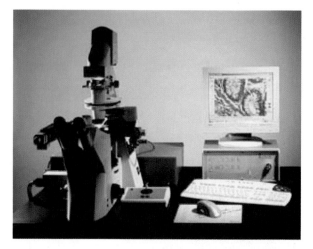

Figure 50.7   PALM microbeam microdissection instrument

Laser microbeam microdissection

Another commercially available advanced laser microdissection technology is available in the form of laser microbeam microdissection (LMM; PALM—Mikrolaser Technologie, Bernried, Germany). The main differentiating principle between LCM and LMM is the choice of laser. The PALM system uses a highly focused UV laser to cut or ablate selected cells from surrounding structures.

The PALM Microbeam (Figure 50.7) is a state-of-the-art microscope designed for the isolation and collection of non-contaminated biological tissue, cells or organelles cut directly from histological sections or cell cultures for downstream analysis, typically for RNA or protein content (Figure 50.8). A pulsed nitrogen UV-A laser at 337 nm is coupled to the epifluorescence or bright-field path of the microscope and programmed to trace any desired cutting pattern before catapulting specimens, either as fragments from normal histological slides, intact cells from special membrane-coated slides, or living cells from membrane-coated culture dishes, directly into an Eppendorf tube for further analysis.

Several additional applications are available with the PALM® system. It uses a pulsed UV laser of high beam quality, which is interfaced into the microscope and focused through an objective to a beam spot size of < 1 μm in diameter. The extremely high photon density in the narrow laser focus can be used to sever or ablate biological structures, making it possible to perform microsurgery on cells and molecules or to microprepare single cells and subcellular particles. The MicroBeam is capable of dissecting cytoplasmatic filaments, flagella or sperm tails. In addition, laser-induced microinjection can be performed, e.g. into the nuclear area of living cells, causing material transport into the cell without mechanical tools or viral vectors.

The lasers of the PALM® MicroLaser systems are interfaced into a research microscope via the epifluorescence path. An objective of high numerical aperture focuses the lasers onto the object plane, yielding spot sizes of < 1 μm in diameter. The system comes equipped with a motorized, computer-controlled microscope stage and/or a micromanipulator (PALM® RoboStage and PALM® CapMover). The systems are air-cooled, foot switch-operated and controlled by the computer mouse.

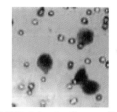
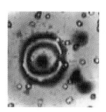
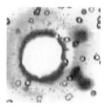

H&E stained cells on a filter   Membrane is cut   and catapulted by LPC   and collected in a microfuge lid.

Figure 50.8   Photographs showing how LPC is achieved from cells as a filter and how cells are collected

All systems can be equipped with fluorescence and with the advanced pattern recognition Metafer P software.

Leica AS LMD

The Leica AS LMD (Figure 50.9) is yet another system offering accurate laser microdissection of cells or cell

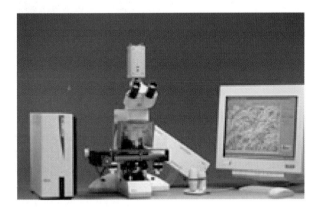

Figure 50.9 Leica AS Laser Microdissection Instrument

groups in preparation for PCR, RT-PCR and proteomics. This system is a 'third-generation' microdissection platform. It was developed combining automated upright microscope architecture, three-dimensional optical control of the dissecting laser beam and the dissected area, non-contact tissue sampling and motorized post-dissection handling.

LCM continues to develop and expand as a technique with advances in instrumentation and computer control of basic function. More precise single-cell techniques are emerging and are being coupled with protocols or extraction kits by suppliers of downstream applications. In a relatively short space of time, LCM has entrenched itself as an invaluable tool for the procurement of pure cell populations from biological material and is an invaluable component of tissue-based protocols in the areas of functional genomics, proteomics and genomics.

Further reading

Banks RE, Dunn MJ, Forbes MA *et al*. The potential use of laser capture microdissection to selectively obtain distinct populations of cells for proteomic analysis—preliminary findings. *Electrophoresis* 1999; **20**: 689–700.

Bohm M, Wieland I, Schutze K, Rubben H. Microbeam moment: non-contact laser microdissection of membrane-mounted native tissue. *Am J Pathol* 1997; **151**: 63–67.

Bonner RF, Emmert-Buck M, Cole K *et al*. Laser capture microdissection: molecular analysis of tissue. *Science* 1997; **278**: 1481–1483.

Craven RA, Totty N, Harnden P *et al*. Laser capture microdissection and two-dimensional polyacrylamide gel electrophoresis: evaluation of tissue preparation and sample limitations. *Am J Pathol*, 2002; **160**: 815–822.

Curran S, McKay JA, McLeod HL, Murray GI. Laser capture microscopy. *J Clin Pathol Mol Pathol* 2000; **53**: 64–68.

DiFrancesco LM, Murthy SK, Luider J, Demetrick DJ. Laser capture microdissection-guided copy number analysis by fluorescence *in situ* hybridization from paraffin sections. *Modern Pathol* 2000; **13**: 105–111.

Eltoum IA, Siegal GP, Frost AR. Microdissection of histologic sections: past, present, and future. *Adv Anat Pathol* 2002; **9**(5): 316–322.

Emmert-Buck MR, Bonner RF, Smith PD *et al*. Laser capture microdissection. *Science* 1996; **274**: 921–922.

Fend F, Raffield M. Laser capture microdissection in pathology. *J Clin Pathol* 2000; **53**: 666–672.

Fend F, Emmert-Buck M, Chuaqui R. Immuno-LCM: laser capture microdissection of immunostained frozen sections for mRNA analysis. *Am J Pathol* 1999; **154**(1): 61–66.

Goldsworthy SM, Stockton PS, Trempus CS, Foley JF, Maronpot RR. Effects of fixation on RNA extraction and amplification from laser capture microdissected tissue. *Mol Carcinogen* 1999; **25**: 86–91.

Liotta L, Petricoin E. Molecular profiling of human cancer. *Nature Rev Genet* 2000; **1**: 48–56.

Mayer A, Stich M, Brocksch D, Schutze K, Lahr G. Going *in vivo* with laser microdissection. *Methods Enzymol* 2002; **356**: 25–33.

Schermelleh L, Thalhammer S, Heckl W, Posl H *et al*. Laser microdissection and laser pressure catapulting for the generation of chromosome-specific paint probes. *Biotechniques* 1999; **27**: 362–367.

Schutze K, Lahr G. Identification of expressed genes by laser mediated manipulation of single cells. *Nature Biotechnol* 1998; **16**: 737–742.

51

Real-Time PCR gene analysis

Cara M Martin, Orla Sheils and **John O'Leary**

Introduction

Real-time quantitative polymerase chain reaction analysis (PCR) is a modification of the original PCR technique, which involves the reliable detection and measurement of products generated during each cycle of the polymerase chain reaction. The technique relies on detection of specific PCR products, based on the use of a fluorescently labelled probe designed to hybridize within the target sequence of the PCR product. During PCR cycling, detection of the increasing fluorescent signal is proportional to the accumulation of amplification products. Therefore, the measurement of fluorescence in a particular sample provides a signal, which is specifically associated with the amplified target and quantitatively related to the amount of PCR product.

Real-time PCR can be performed using a variety of technologies, including the 5′ nuclease assay, hair-pin primers, scorpion probes, intercalating dyes, e.g. SYBR green and FRET (free-resonance energy transfer technology), and using dual-probe hybridization systems (molecular beacons). In this chapter, we will discuss the 5′ nuclease assay known as TaqMan® PCR, and its applications for use in pathology laboratories.

Real-time PCR chemistries

DNA-binding dyes—SyBR green

The basis of non-specific sequence detection methods is the use of intercalating dyes, such as SYBR green or ethidium bromide (Figure 51.1a). The unbound dye exhibits little fluorescence in solution, but during the extension step of the PCR increasing amounts of the intercalating dye bind to the nascent double-stranded DNA. The incorporation of SYBR green into a PCR reaction allows the detection of product accumulation by monitoring the increase in fluoresence emission in real time. This provides greater flexibility by eliminating the need for target-specific fluorescent probes; however, it is important to note that the primers used determine the overall specificity of the reaction. In addition, because the presence of any double-stranded DNA is capable of generating fluorescence, the assay specificity is similar to conventional PCR, and problems can be encountered with binding of the dye to non-specific amplification and primer dimers. The specificity can be improved by generating a dissociation curve to detect non-specific amplification (Ririe *et al.*, 1997). Dissociation curve analysis is performed after a completed PCR. This is achieved by slowly raising the temperature of the PCR reaction from 65°C to 95°C (above the melting temperature of the amplicon) while continuously collecting the fluorescence data. As the temperature increases the PCR product denatures, creating a characteristic melting peak at the melting temperature of the amplicon, which is distinguishable from amplification artifacts that melt at lower temperatures (Figure 51.1b).

Molecular beacons and hybridization probes

In this system, two hybridization probes are employed. One probe carries a fluorescein donor molecule at its 3′ end, whose emission spectrum overlaps with an acceptor probe on the 5′ end of a second probe. In solution, the

The Science of Laboratory Diagnosis, Second Edition   Edited by David Burnett and John Crocker

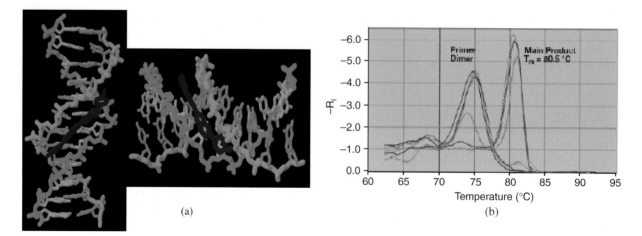

Figure 51.1   (a) SYBR green intercalating dye binds to double-stranded DNA. (b) Dissociation (melting curve), demonstrating primer dimers and the PCR amplicon in a SyBr green assay

two dyes are separate. However, after the denaturation step they hybridize with the target sequence during annealing, and adopt a head-to-tail configuration. This brings the two fluorescent molecules into close proximity, and the fluorescein moiety can transfer its energy to the second. The light energy emitted by the second molecule can then be monitored, and increased levels of fluorescence correspond with the amount of DNA synthesized during the PCR reaction. An additional advantage of this system is the fact that the probes are not hydrolysed, allowing the possibility of the generation of melting curves. These can be used to monitor amplification efficiency.

Hydrolysis probes

The TaqMan® assay uses the 5′–3′ exonuclease activity of Taq or rTth DNA polymerase to hydrolyse a hybridisation probe bound to the target amplicon (Lyamichev et al., 1993; Holland et al., 1991; Lawyer et al., 1989). In this system, three oligonucleotides are required to bind to the target. Two template-specific primers define the endpoints of the amplicon and serve as a first level of specificity. A further level of specificity is achieved by the inclusion of a specific probe, which binds internally to the points defined by the primers. The characteristics of the TaqMan® probe include a fluorescent reporter molecule at the 5′ end, whose emission is quenched by a second molecule at the 3′ end. The spatial proximity of the reporter to the quencher in an intact probe ensures that no net fluorescence is detected. The release of the fluorescence only occurs if target specific amplification

occurs, obviating the need to confirm the amplicon following amplification.

TaqMan PCR chemistry—the 5′ nuclease assay

TaqMan technology is a quantitative real-time PCR technique, based on the 5′ nuclease assay first described by Holland et al. (1991). The technique uses fluorescent probes designed to hybridize within the target sequence and, on the annealing/extension phase of PCR, to generate a signal that accumulates during PCR cycling in proportion to the amount of template prior to the initiation of PCR (Orlando et al., 1998; Gibson et al., 1996).

The basis for this system is to continuously measure PCR products as they accumulate, using a dual-labelled specific fluorogenic oligonucleotide probe called the TaqMan probe (Livak et al., 1995; Lee et al., 1993). The TaqMan probe is composed of a short ($\sim$ 20–25 bases) oligonucleotide labelled with two different dyes, a 3′ quencher dye and a 5′ reporter dye, and a 3′ blocking phosphate to prevent probe extension during PCR (Livak et al., 1995). The fluorescence reporter dye, e.g. FAM (6-carboxy-fluoroscein), VIC® or JOE (2,7-dimethyl-4,5,-dichloro-6-carboxyfluorescein) is covalently linked to the 5′ end of the oligonucleotide probe. TET (tetra-chloro-6-carboxy-fluoroscein) and HEX (hexachloro-6-carboxy-fluoroscein) can also be used as fluorescent reporter dyes in this system. Each of these reporters is quenched by TAMRA (6-carboxy-tetramethyl-rhodamine) (the quencher dye), a non-fluorescent quencher, which is attached by a LAN (linker-arm-modified nucleotide) to the 3' end of the probe. The probe is chemically phosphorylated at its 3' end, which prevents probe extension during PCR applications. The oligonucleotide probe sequence is homologous to an internal region present in the PCR product. When the probe is intact (linearized), energy transfer of the Förster type occurs between the two fluorophores and results in the suppression of the reporter fluorescence (Gibson *et al.*, 1996; Livak *et al.*, 1995).

The TaqMan assay utilizes either Taq or Tth polymerase, isolated from *Thermus aquaticus* and *Thermus thermophilus*, respectively, but any enzyme with 5' nuclease activity can be used. During amplification, the non-extendible probe is cleaved by the 5' exonuclease activity of Taq or Tth DNA polymerase, thereby releasing the reporter from the oligonucleotide quencher and producing an increase in the reporter emission fluorescent intensity. This is monitored in real time during the exponential phase of PCR amplification, using the 7700 Sequence Detector System (Applied Biosystems, Lincoln Centre Drive, Foster City, CA 94404, USA). Cleavage removes the probe from the target strand, allowing primer extension to continue to the end of the template strand. An overview of the process is illustrated in Figure 51.2. Additional reporter dye molecules are cleaved from their respective probes with each cycle, leading to an increase in fluorescence intensity proportional to the amount of amplicon produced. The exonuclease activity of the Taq polymerase acts only if the fluorogenic probe is annealed to the target, since the activity is double-strand-specific, therefore the enzyme cannot hydrolyse the probe when it is free in solution and no reporter fluorescence is detected.

Since the polymerase only cleaves probe while it remains hybridized to its complimentary strand, the temperature conditions of the extension of the PCR must be adjusted to ensure probe binding. The TaqMan system uses a combined annealing and polymerization step at 60–62°C to ensure the probe remains hybridized

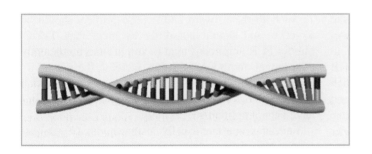

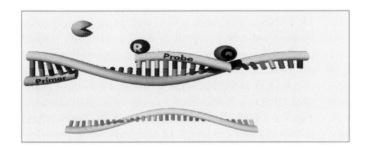

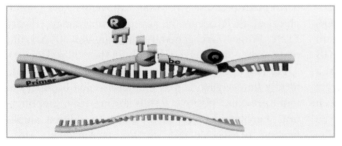

Figure 51.2 Schematic of TaqMan PCR using an internal probe labelled with a reporter and a quencher sequence. TaqMan primers and probe anneal to denatured DNA. During polymerization the probe is cleaved, releasing the reporter dye from the quencher dye, resulting in an increase in fluorescent signal that is proportional to the amount of PCR product that has accumulated

during amplification. Most probes have a melting temperature (T_M) of around 10°C, or at least 5°C higher than the PCR primers (Livak et al., 1995), since binding of the TaqMan probe prior to the primers is crucial to the success of the process. Without it, PCR products will be formed without generation of fluorescence and thus without detection. This ensures that the probe remains bound to its target during the primer extension step and also ensures maximum 5′–3′ exonuclease activity of the Taq and Tth DNA polymerases.

Minor groove binder TaqMan probes

More recently, minor groove binder (MGB) TaqMan fluorogenic probes have been developed that improve the sensitivity of a TaqMan assay. MGBs (naturally occurring antibiotics and synthetic molecules) are able to fit into the minor groove of the helix formed by double-stranded DNA and stabilize DNA duplexes, increasing mismatch discrimination when bound to an oligonucleotide probe. TaqMan MGB fluorogenic probes have a number of characteristics that make them superior to traditional fluorogenic probes. An MGB can be attached to the 3′-end, the 5′-end, or to an internal nucleotide of the oligonucleotide. MGB probes bind more tightly to their complement, which raises the melting temperature (T_m) of the probes and allows for more flexible assay design. Studies have shown that the introduction of an MGB onto a 12-mer probe with a T_m of 20°C increases its T_m to 65°C. This T_m is equivalent to the T_m of a 27-mer probe without an MGB (Kutyavin et al., 2000). It is recommended that probe T_m be >10°C higher than primer T_m, so the introduction of an MGB contributes significantly to assay design, allowing the use of a wider range of primers The use of an MGB allows shorter probes to be used and better mismatch discrimination. MGB-oligonucleotides demonstrate an increased difference between the T_m of match and single-base mismatch oligonucleotides, therefore increasing the discriminatory power of hybridization assays.

Another feature of MGB probes is the low background fluorescence and, as a consequence, a greater signal:-noise ratio. The background fluorescence of intact MGB probes increase slightly with probe length, but is still several times lower than probes without an MGB. MGB probes stabilize A–T bonds more than G–C bonds in a DNA duplex. This reduces the influence of target sequence on T_m (Kutyavin et al., 2000). It has been found also that mismatch discrimination is improved when the mismatch is placed under the MGB. Typically,

an oligonucleotide–MGB conjugate is designed such that the MGB resides at the 3′-end of an oligonucleotide containing an A–T-rich region of about 6–7 bases. It was observed that mismatches positioned within the MGB-binding region were better discriminated, showing an increased free energy difference between match and mismatches for the different mismatch pairs under the MGB (Kutyavin et al., 2000; Orlando et al., 1998; Gibson et al., 1996).

TaqMan primer and probe design

The specificity and sensitivity of a TaqMan PCR assay is determined by the choice of primer and probe sequences. Applied Biosystems have developed a specific software program known as Primer Express, which can be used to design optimal TaqMan PCR assays. The optimal length for TaqMan PCR primers is 15–20 bases with a G/C content of 30–80%, where the last five nucleotides at the 3′ end contain no more than two G and C residues. The T_m of both the forward and reverse primers should be 58–60°C and should not differ by more than 1–2°C. Shorter PCR amplicons tend to amplify more efficiently than longer amplicons and thus increase the sensitivity of the assay. In general, the optimal length for TaqMan PCR amplicons is 50–150 bp, although larger amplicons have been amplified successfully.

TaqMan probes are usually designed with a T_m at least 10°C higher than the PCR primers. This ensures that the probe hybridizes before the primers and remain hybridized during the annealing step. TaqMan probes can be 13–30 bases long, with a G/C content of 50%. TaqMan probes should be designed as close as possible, without overlapping or having complementarity with either of the primers. In addition, TaqMan probes should not contain a G at the 5′ end, as a G adjacent to the reporter dye will quench the fluorescence even after cleavage. The use of MGB TaqMan probes as discussed above greatly reduces the length of the probe while maintaining the required T_m.

Ideally, primer and probe optimization should be performed to assess where the exponential and plateau phase of PCR occurs in any particular assay (Figure 51.3). Primers are generally used in the 50–200 nM range, while the probe is usually in the 100 nM range.

For RNA gene targets, TaqMan RT PCR assays should ideally be designed across the intron–exon boundary to minimize false positive results arising from amplification of contaminating genomic DNA. In addition, amplification of RNA/cDNA in the presence of Mn^{2+}

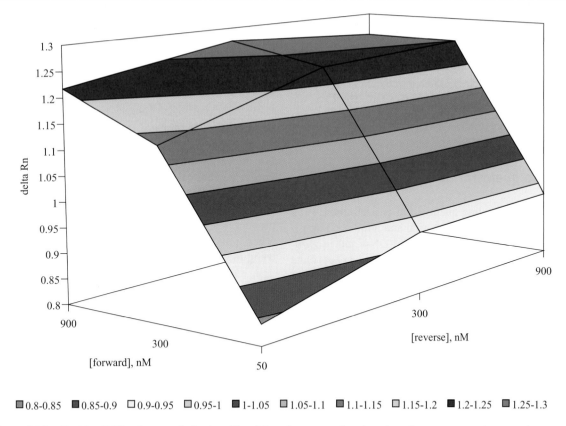

Figure 51.3 TaqMan PCR primer optimization. The ΔR_n values are reduced as the primer concentrations are decreased

minimizes problems that may be caused by amplification of re-annealed DNA fragments (Bauer *et al.*, 1997).

Amplicon detection

The TaqMan procedure is applicable to both end point measurement and to detection of PCR amplification in real time. The increase in fluorescence can be detected using a luminescence spectrophotometer, such as the Applied Biosystems 7900 and 7000 thermal cyclers, which utilize a tungsten halogen lamp and CCD camera system, or the 7700, which utilizes a laser scanning format to detect increases in fluorescence at defined time points in the thermocycling protocol. These DNA sequence detectors can also be used for SYBR green, scorpion probes and molecular beacon technologies with few modifications.

TaqMan end-point detection

End point detection is performed after the TaqMan PCR has been completed and the data is collected (i.e. at cycle

35, 40, etc.). For end-point detection, the increase in fluorescence is compared to the fluorescence of a 'no template control' and interfering fluorescence fluctuations are normalized. This is achieved by dividing the emission intensity of the reporter dye by the emission intensity of the quencher dye to define a ratio known as the RQ (reporter:quencher) for each reaction. The difference between the sample RQ (RQ^+) and the no template control RQ (RQ^-) is defined as the ΔRQ and reliably indicates the magnitude of the signal generated during the PCR.

TaqMan real-time detection

During real-time TaqMan PCR, the fluorescence value measured during each cycle of the PCR represents the amount of product amplified at that cycle. The ABI 7700 sequence detection system collects fluorescent emission at 500–600 nm in each of the 96 wells of the thermal cycler, once every few seconds. A laser directed through fibre-optic cables excites the fluorescent dyes in the tube. These cables then carry the fluorescent emissions back to a CCD camera, where they are detected according to their individual wavelengths. A value called the ΔR_n is then calculated for each sample by subtracting the reporter signal before PCR from the normalized reporter signal. The software also calculates a threshold cycle (C_t), which is the cycle at which a statistically significant increase in PCR product is first detected. The C_t is the basis of all real-time quantitative assays (Higuchi et al., 1993).

Absolute quantitation

TaqMan PCR absolute quantitation is performed using standards of known concentration and similar composition to the target amplicon. Plasmid DNA and in vitro-transcribed RNA are commonly used as absolute standards for TaqMan assays. For measurement of mRNA expression levels, a DNA standard is not the optimal choice; cRNA (copy RNA) or RNA of known concentration is preferable, as it accounts for the efficiency of the reverse transcription reaction. Copy RNA standards can be generated by amplifying a sequence slightly larger than the TaqMan® PCR amplicon, using a set of outer primers. The amplicon can then be cloned into a suitable vector and transcribed into cRNA. Standard curves are generated by amplifying serial dilutions of the standard in the TaqMan PCR assay. Test samples are then plotted along the standard curve to determine the quantity of target in the sample.

Relative quantitation

Relative quantitation is commonly used to quantitatively assess differences in the target sequences among different samples. The objective of a relative quantitative TaqMan experiment is to determine the ratio of a target mRNA or DNA molecule to a different target molecule or to itself under different conditions. The result can then be reported as a fold difference, relative to a calibrator sample. There are two methods for calculating relative quantitation of target gene expression: the standard curve method, and the comparative C_t method (Applied Biosystems, 1997).

Standard curve method

For the standard curve method, standard curves are generated for both the target and the endogenous control assays. For each test sample the amount of target and control quantity is determined from the appropriate standard curve. Then the target amount is divided by the endogenous control quantity to obtain a normalized target value. To calculate the relative expression levels, the normalized target values are divided by the calibrator-normalized target values.

Comparative C_t method

For the comparative C_t method, the relative quantification values are calculated from the threshold cycle (C_t) values generated during the PCR. The C_t value is the cycle at which a statistically significant increase in PCR product is first detected. The comparative C_t method for relative quantitation calculates relative gene expression using the following equation:

$$\text{Relative quantity} = 2^{-\Delta\Delta C_t}$$

The ΔC_t is calculated by normalizing the C_t of the target sample with the C_t of the endogenous control (C_t target $- C_t$ endogenous control). The $\Delta\Delta C_t$ is then calculated by subtracting the average ΔC_t for the calibrator sample from the corresponding average ΔC_t for the target sample. The relative levels of the target gene expression are then expressed as a fold change relative to the calibrator sample (Livak et al., 2001). Relative quantitation using the comparative C_t method is dependent upon similar PCR amplification efficiencies for both the target and the endogenous control genes (Livak et al., 2001; Giulietti et al., 2001).

Housekeeping genes

An important aspect of quantitative PCR experimental design is the choice of an appropriate reference or housekeeping gene. Endogenous control genes can be assayed separately or together with the unknown target and their final ratio calculated. Simultaneous amplification of the target and endogenous control gene minimizes errors that arise due to inaccurate estimation of total nucleic acid concentration and quality in individual samples.

An ideal endogenous control or reference gene should be expressed at a constant level among different tissue types and individuals and should be unaffected by experimental treatment. In addition, expression of the housekeeping gene may be very high compared with that of the unknown target, and in such a situation, the efficiency of amplification between the two targets can differ considerably. For accurate quantitation in reactions that amplify more than one target in the same tube, it is important that the two reactions do not compete. This can be avoided by limiting the concentration of primers used in the PCR, which is dependent on the relative abundance of the different targets.

Three genes are commonly used as endogenous controls for mRNA expression studies. These include mRNAs specific for the housekeeping genes β-actin, glyceraldehyde 3-phosphate dehydrogenase (GAPDH), and ribosomal RNA (rRNA). β-actin mRNA is expressed abundantly in most cell types and encodes a ubiquitous cytoskeleton protein. However, it is important to note that the presence of pseudogenes can interfere with quantitative results (Mutimer et al., 1998).

Ribosomal RNA (rRNA) constitutes 85–90% of the total cellular RNA and is ubiquitously expressed in all tissues. The 18S rRNA housekeeping gene has been shown to be relatively stable in human tissues under varying experimental conditions (Schmittgen et al., 2000). However, rRNA cannot be used as a reference gene when quantitating targets that have been enriched for mRNA, as rRNA is lost during mRNA purification.

GAPDH (glyceraldehyde 3-phosphate dehydrogenase) mRNA is also ubiquitously expressed in all tissues and is commonly used as an endogenous control for quantitative PCR assays. However, there is some evidence that GAPDH expression levels vary during cell culture in vitro (Hamalainen et al., 2001) and between individuals (Bustin et al., 1999), emphasizing the importance of careful validation of endogenous control genes for comparative quantitation.

TaqMan PCR applications in pathology

The potential applications for TaqMan technology in medical diagnostics are enormous. The TaqMan assay has been successfully used to detect and quantify various pathogens and for transcriptional analysis of various mRNA targets. We have previously detected and quantified measles virus RNA in fresh frozen and paraffin-embedded intestinal tissue biopsies from children with a new variant of inflammatory bowel disease, using TaqMan RT PCR technology (Uhlmann et al., 2002; Martin et al., 2002). Our group have also successfully used TaqMan technology to detect and type *Human papilloma virus* (HPV) subtypes in cervical tissue biopsies and ThinPrep liquid-based cytological preparations (Murphy et al., 2003). Similarly, we have used this technology to study fetal cells in the maternal circulation in normal and complicated pregnancies (Turner et al., 2003; Byrne et al., 2003).

Allelic discrimination and SNP genotyping TaqMan assays

Aside from detection and quantification of specific DNA and RNA targets, TaqMan PCR technology using MGB probes and the 5′ nuclease assay can be used for SNP (single-nucleotide polymorphism) genotyping and allelic discrimination assays. In a two-allele system, the technology uses a dual-probe approach with two different fluorescent reporter dyes, namely FAM and VIC (Livak, 1999; Lee et al., 1993), whereby two probes are designed, one specific for each allele or polymorphism. Allelic discrimination assays are performed under competitive conditions, with competition between the wild and mutant specific probes occurring at each PCR cycle, but particularly so in the first rounds of PCR. Fluorescent signals from the FAM and VIC probes are only generated in the presence of complementary target sequence (Figure 51.4). End point fluorescence is measured on the ABI Sequence Detectors (7900 HT, 7000, and the 7700). The data is then analysed using the integrated software package supplied by Applied Biosystems, which allows discrimination between homozygous and heterozygous genotypes (Figure 51.5).

Assays on demand™

Applied Biosystems have recently introduced a new service, which allows TaqMan PCR users access to the recently published public and Celera Corporation genome databases. The assays on demand are available for DNA and RNA assays and consists of designed TaqMan primer and probe sets for all known sequenced genes. Over 19 000 human and 9500 mouse gene-specific assays are available for customers to choose from; these can be obtained from the Applied Biosystems website.

TaqMan microfluidics cards

Recent advances in TaqMan chemistry include the launch of a 384-well version of the platform for high-throughput gene expression analysis. The 384-well microfluidics card (Figure 51.6) is designed for custom array configuration, using the validated Assays on Demand™ gene expression products and the 7900 HT sequence detector system. These cards are capable of evaluating gene expression of 12–384 gene targets in up to eight cDNA samples in a single PCR run, depending on the configuration of the card.

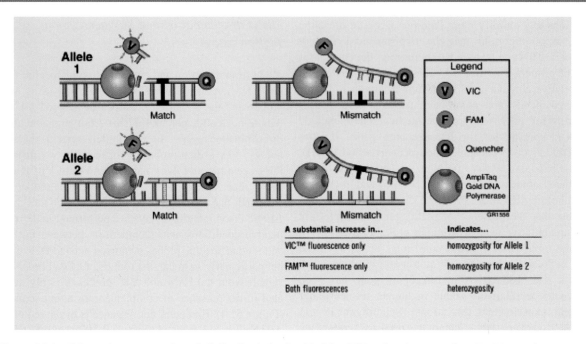

Figure 51.4   Schematic representation of allelic discrimination TaqMan PCR using the two-colour TaqMan probes system

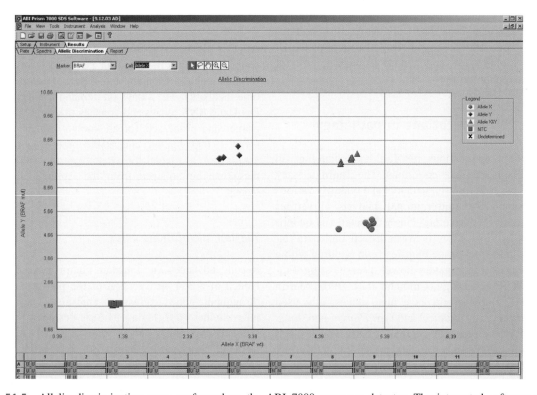

Figure 51.5   Allelic discrimination assay performed on the ABI 7000 sequence detector. The integrated software permits discrimination of different alleles and based on the level of fluorescence detected

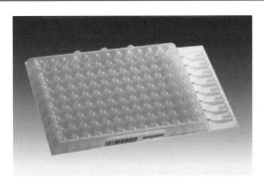

Figure 51.6 High-throughput 384-well microfluidics TaqMan card. These card can be custom-loaded with the validated Assays on Demand™ gene expression products

Another application of this technology is the TaqMan human cytokine microfluidics card for profiling human cytokine gene expression, using the comparative C_t method of relative quantitation. The TaqMan human cytokine card (Applied Biosystems, Foster City, CA, USA) consists of a 96-well consumable divided into 24 sets of replicates, one set for each cytokine assay. The card evaluates a single cDNA sample generated from human total RNA in a two-step RT-PCR experiment.

This assay measures the following 24 cytokines: TNF-α, TNF-β, IFN-γ, TGF-β, LT-β, IL-1α, IL-1β, IL-2, IL-3, IL-4, IL-5, IL-6, IL-7, IL-8 IL-10, IL-12p35, IL-12p40, IL-13, IL-15, IL-17, IL-18, G-CSF, GM-CSF, and M-CSF. Each well contains lyophilized FAM-labelled TaqMan MGB probes and primers for one human cytokine mRNA. A VIC-labelled TaqMan MGB primer and probe set for 18S ribosomal RNA endogenous control was used for multiplex assays.

Relative RNA quantification assays on the cytokine card are performed in a two-step reverse transcription polymerase chain reaction (RT-PCR). In the first step, cDNA is reverse-transcribed from total RNA, using random hexamers and MultiScribe™ reverse transcriptase. The second step includes amplification of the cDNA product, using TaqMan Universal Mastermix and AmpliTaq Gold DNA polymerase. All 96 wells of the card are filled simultaneously with a mixture of cDNA and TaqMan Universal mastermix, through a single port via a channel system. The reaction volume of each well is 1 μl and the total volume required to fill the card is 250 μl. The relative quantity of the specific cytokines in an individual sample is then compared to an appropriate calibrator sample and calculated using the comparative C_t method for relative quantitation (Figure 51.7)

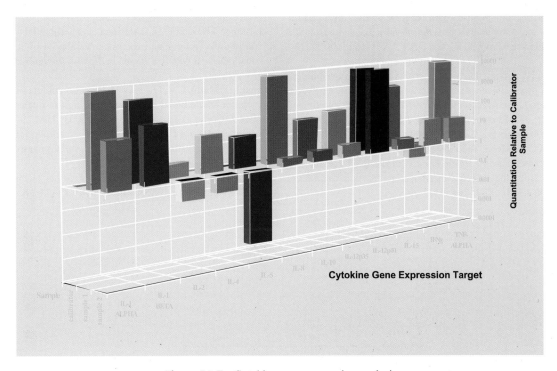

Figure 51.7 Cytokine gene expression analysis

References

Bauer P, Rolfs A, Regits-Zagrosek V, Hildebrandt A, Fleck E. Use of manganese in RT-PCR eliminates PCR artefacts resulting from DNase I digestion. *Biotechniques* 1997; **22**: 1128–1132.

Bustin SA, Gyselman VG, William NS, Dorudi S. Detection of cytokeratins 19/20 and guanylyl cyclase C in peripheral blood of colorectal cancer patients. *Br J Cancer* 1999; **79**: 1813–1820.

Byrne BM, Crowley A, Taulo F, Anthony J, O'Leary JJ, O'Herlihy C. Fetal DNA quantitation in peripheral blood is not-useful as a maker of disease severely in women with preeclampsia. *Hyperkens Pregnancy* 2003; **22**(2): 157–164.

Forster VTH. Zwischenmolekulare Energie-Wanderung und Fluoreszenz. *Ann Physics* 1948; **2**: 55–75.

Gibson UEM, Heid CA, Williams MP. A novel method for real time quantitative RT-PCR. *Genome Res* 1996; **6**: 995–1001.

Giulietti A, Overbergh L, Valckx D *et al*. An overview of real-time quantitative PCR: applications to quantify cytokine gene expression. *Methods* 2001; **25**: 386–401.

Hamalainen HK, Tubman JC, Vikman S *et al*. Identification and validation of endogenous reference genes for expression profiling of T helper cell differentiation by quantitative real time RT-PCR. *Anal Biochem* 2001; **299**: 63–70.

Higuchi R, Fockler C, Dollinger G, Watson R. Kinetic PCR analysis: real-time monitoring of DNA amplification reactions. *Biotechnology* 1993; **11**: 1026–1039.

Holland PM, Abramson RD, Watson R, Gelfand DH. Detection of specific polymerase chain reaction product by utilizing the 5′ to 3′ exonuclease activity of *Thermus aquaticus* DNA polymerase. *Proc Natl. Acad Sci USA* 1991; **88**: 7276–7280.

Kutyavin IV, Afonina IA, Mills A *et al*. 3′-Minor groove binder-DNA probes increase sequence specificity at PCR extension temperatures. *Nucleic Acids Res* 2000; **28**(2): 655–661.

Lakowicz JR. Energy transfer. In *Principles of Fluorescent Spectroscopy*. 1983: Plenum, New York, 303–339.

Lawyer FC, Stoffel S, Saiki RK *et al*. Isolation, characterization, and expression in *Escherichia coli* of the DNA polymerase gene from the extreme thermophile, *Thermus aquaticus*. *J Biol. Chem* 1989; **264**: 6427–6437.

Lee LG, Connell CR, Bloch W. Allelic discrimination by nick-translation PCR with fluorogenic probes. *Nucleic Acids Res* 1993; **21**: 3761–3766.

Livak KJ, Flood SJA, Marmaroj *et al*. Oligonucleotides with fluorescent dyes at opposite ends provide a quenched probe system useful for detecting PCR product and nucleic acid hybridisation. *PCR Methods Appl*, 1995; **4**: 357–362.

Livak KJ, Allelic destination using of fluorogenic probes and the 5′ anclease assay. *Genet Anal* 1999; **14**(5–6): 143-149.

Livak KJ, Schmittgen TD. Analysis of relative gene expression data using real-time quantitative PCR and the 2[ΔΔ C(T)] method. *Methods* 2001; **25**: 402–408.

Lyamichev V, Brow MAD, Dahlberg JE. Structure-specific endonucleolytic cleavage of nucleic acids by eubacterial DNA polymerases. *Science* 1993; **260**: 778–783.

Martin CM, Uhlmann V, Killalea A *et al*. Detection of measles virus in children with ileo-colonic lymphoid nodular hyper-plasia, enterocolitis and developmental disorder. *Mol Psy-chiat* 2002; **7**: 47–48.

Murphy N, Ring M, Killalea AG *et al*. p16INK4A as a marker for cervical dyskaryosis: CIN and cGIN in cervical biopsies and ThinPrep smears. *J Clin Pathol* 2000; **56**: 56–63.

Mutimer H. Deacon N, Crowe S. Sonza S. Pitfalls of processed pseudogenes in RT-PCR. *Biotechniques* 1998; **24**: 585–588.

Orlando C, Pinzani P, Pazzagli M. Developments in quantitative PCR. *Clin Chem Lab Med* 1998; **36**(5): 255–269.

Rhoads RE. Optimization of the annealing temperature for DNA amplification *in vitro*. *Nucleic Acids Res* 1990; **18**: 6409–6412.

Ririe KM, Rasmussen RP, Witter CT. Product differentiation by analysis of DNA melting curves during the polymerase chain reaction. *Anal Biochem* 1997; **245**: 154–160.

Schmittgen TD, Zakrajsek BA. Effect of experimental treatment on housekeeping gene expression: validation by real-time, quantitative RT-PCR. *J Biochem Biophys Methods* 2000; **46**: 69–81.

Turner MJ, Martin CM, O'Leary JJ. Detection of fetal Rhesus D gene in whole blood of women booking for antenatal care. *Eur J. Obstet Gynecol Reprod Biol* 2003; **108**: 29–32.

Uhlmann V, Martin CM, Sheils O *et al*. Potential viral patho-genic mechanism for new variant inflammatory bowel disease. *Mol Pathol* 2002; **55**: 84–90.

Applied Biosystems. *User Bulletin 2. Relative Quantitation*. 1997: Applied Biosystems, Foster City, CA, USA.

52

In-cell PCR

John O'Leary, Cara M Martin and **Orla Sheils**

Introduction

In recent years a number of studies have described 'hybrid' techniques coupling PCR with *in situ* hybridization (Herrington *et al.*, 1992; Haase *et al.*, 1990; Bagasra *et al.*, 1992, 1993, 1994; Boshoff *et al.*, 1995; O'Leary *et al.*, 1994a, 1994b, 1995, 1996, 1998). The techniques initially were not accepted owing to technological problems encountered during amplification of the desired nucleic acid sequence.

In situ amplification technologies have been extended to include a number of modifications of the initially described technique of *in situ* PCR, to include PRINS (primed *in situ* labelling), cycling PRINS, *in situ* PNA PCR (peptide nucleic acid PCR), *in situ* PNA PCR, *in situ* immuno-PCR, *in situ*-TaqMan PCR and allele-specific amplification. Other in-cell amplification technologies, such as nucleic acid base amplification (NASBA), can also be used. These employ T3 and T7 RNA technology and are isothermal replication methodologies for the amplification of RNA in cells and tissue sections.

Overview of methodology

All in-cell PCR techniques attempt to create double-stranded or single-stranded DNA/cDNA amplicons within the cell, which can either be detected directly or following an *in situ* (IS) hybridization step. A fine balance between adequate digestion of cells (allowing access of amplification reagents) and maintaining localization of amplified product within the cellular compartment and preserving tissue/cell morphology must be achieved.

Specific cyclic thermal changes must occur at the individual cell level, akin to what occurs in solution-phase PCR. The first step involves denaturation of double-stranded DNA (dsDNA) to single-stranded form (ssDNA), if one is amplifying a DNA target. For RNA target specific amplification, the RNA template is already single-stranded and reverse transcription is carried out to create a cDNA template.

Second, primers are then annealed to the respective ends of the desired target sequence and a thermostable enzyme (Taq DNA polymerase or Klenow fragment) is then used to extend or ligate, using DNA ligase, an *in situ* ligase chain reaction (IS-LCR), the correctly positioned primers. Specific Taq polymerases have now been designed for use in in-cell PCR analyses, including IS-Taq polymerase, which has a higher concentration and greater unity polymerase activity. Subsequent rounds of thermocycling increase the copy number of the desired target sequence, in a nucleic acid amplification reaction. An exponential increase in the amount of amplified product is never achieved in in-cell amplification reactions, with linear amplification occurring in most situations. This is due to the relative inefficiency of the techniques, owing to problems of accessibility of amplification reagents to the desired nucleic acid sequence, because of the compactness of the nuclear compartment of the cell (containing dsDNA ssDNA pre-mRNA and histone proteins).

Once the amplicon is created, detection must be carried out. If a labelled primer or nucleotide is used, then the amplicon is labelled and can be demonstrated

The Science of Laboratory Diagnosis, Second Edition   Edited by David Burnett and John Crocker
© 2005 John Wiley & Sons, Ltd

directly by immunocytochemical techniques. In general, however, direct labelled nucleotide and labelled primer approaches have largely been abandoned, due to non-specific signal generation and non-specific label incorporation into the PCR amplicon.

Alternatively, and more acceptably, an IS hybridization step (using a single-stranded oligo probe or a double-stranded genomic probe) is carried out post-amplification, adhering to the general rules of standard IS hybridization kinetics and applying stringent post-hybridization washing conditions.

In-cell PCR technologies: definitions

Several techniques (Figures 52.1, 52.2) have been described in the literature, including the following:

- *DNA* in situ *PCR (IS-PCR):* PCR amplification of cellular DNA sequences in tissue specimens using a labelled nucleotide (e.g. dUTP) within the PCR reaction mix. The labelled product is then detected, using standard detection techniques as for conventional in situ hybridization or immunocytochemistry. This technology is not recommended for use.

- *Labelled primer driven* in situ *amplification (LPDISA):* amplification of DNA sequences using a labelled primer within the PCR reaction mix. The labelled product is then detected as for DNA IS-PCR. This technology is not recommended for use.

- *PCR* in situ *hybridization (PCR-ISH):* PCR amplification of cellular DNA sequences in tissue specimens, followed by in situ hybridization detection of the

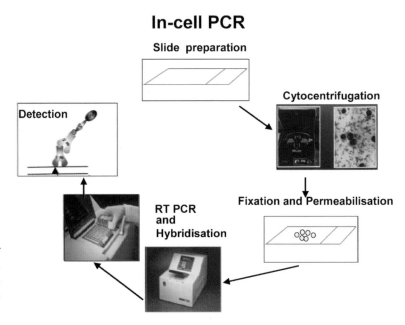

In-cell PCR

Slide preparation

Cytocentrifugation

Detection

Fixation and Permeabilisation

RT PCR and Hybridisation

Figure 52.1 Schematic representation of in-cell PCR, indicating the critical steps involved in the process from cell/tissue adhesion to fixation permeabilization to PCR amplification to detection of amplicon

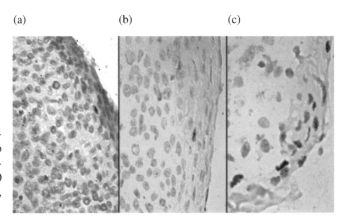

(a)   (b)   (c)

Figure 52.2 *In situ* hybridization and PCR-ISH detection of HPV in a cervical biopsy. (a) ISH, one-step immunocytochemical detection, sensitivity 20–30 genomes/cell. (b) ISH, three-step detection, sensitivity 10–20 genomes/cell. (c) PCR-ISH with three-step detection, sensitivity 1 genome/cell

amplified product, using a labelled internal or genomic probe. The labels used can either be isotopic (e.g. 32P, 35S) or non-isotopic (e.g. biotin, digoxigenin, fluorescein).

- *Reverse transcriptase* in situ *PCR (RT* in situ *PCR):* amplification of mRNA sequences in cells and tissue specimens, by first creating a copy DNA template (cDNA) using reverse transcriptase (RT) and then amplifying the newly created DNA template as for DNA IS-PCR. This technique again has the inherent problems with non-specific label incorporation, and should not be used for the analysis of RNA templates in cells and tissue sections.

- *Reverse transcriptase PCR* in situ *hybridisation (RT-PCR–ISH):* amplification of RNA sequences in cells and tissues specimens by creating a cDNA template using reverse transcriptase (RT). The newly created cDNA is then amplified, and the amplicon probed with an internal oligonucleotide, as in PCR-ISH (see Figure 52.3).

- *PRINS (primed* in situ *amplification) and cycling PRINS:* amplification of specific genetic sequences in metaphase chromosome spreads or interphase nuclei, using one primer to generate single-stranded PCR product. If many rounds of amplification are utilized, then the technique is called cycling PRINS (Gosden *et al.*, 1991).

- In situ *PNA PCR (IS-PNA-PCR) and PCR-PNA-ISH:* IS-PNA-PCR refers to amplification of DNA targets using a DNA mimic molecule, peptide nucleic acid (PNA). PNA is a simple molecule, made up of repeating N-(2-aminoethyl)-glycine units linked by amide bonds. Purine (A and G) and pyrimidine bases (C and T) are attached to the backbone by methylene carbonyl linkages. PNA when used as a primer is not elongated by Taq DNA polymerase and therefore can be used in primer exclusion assays, which allows the discrimination of point mutations and direct individual cell haplotyping. The second reaction, which employs PNA, is PCR-PNA-ISH; here, a 15–20 mer PNA probe is used for the *in situ* hybridization step following amplification. PNAs have higher T_ms (melting temperatures) than DNA oligo probes and single point mutations in a PNA–DNA duplex lower the T_m by approximately 15°C as compared to the corresponding DNA–DNA mismatch duplex (De-Mesmaeker *et al.*, 1995).

- *IS-TaqMan PCR:* amplification of DNA sequences using a conventional primer pair as in standard PCR. However, an internal TaqMan probe is added to the amplification mix. A fluorescent reporter molecule (FAM, HEX, etc.) is placed at the 5′ end of the probe. At the 3′ end, a quencher molecule (again fluorescent, usually TAMRA) is positioned. Once the probe is linearized and intact, the proximity of the quencher to the reporter molecule does not allow any fluorescence from the reporter molecule. Taq DNA polymerases possess two properties important for the reaction: (a) Y-strand fork displacement, which allows Taq DNA polymerase to lift off a single strand in Y configuration; and (b) 5′–3′ endonucleotic activity, which causes cleavage of the linker arm that attaches the reporter molecule to the 5′ end of the TaqMan probe. (see Figure 52.4), thereby giving rise to fluorescence if, and only if, specific amplification has occurred (Figure 52.5) (Lawyer *et al.*, 1989; Holland *et al.*, 1991).

- In situ *allele-specific amplification (IS-ASA):* this technique utilizes amplification refractory mutation system (ARMS) PCR, which has the ability to detect point polymorphisms in human DNA sequences, using artificially created base pair mismatches at the 3′ end of PCR primers. If the polymorphism matching that of the primer sequence is present, amplification of that sequence will preferentially occur.

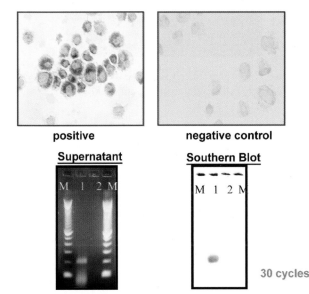

Figure 52.3 RT PCR-ISH detection of dopamine receptor 2 (DRD 2) in hamster ovarian epithelial cells (transfectants) and slab gel and Southern blot analysis of the created amplicon

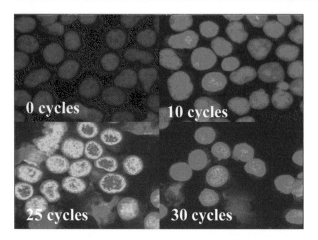

Figure 52.4 Quasi-real time TaqMan PCR analysis of HHV 8 in an effusion lymphoma cell line BC-3. Note diminution of fluorescence after 25 cycles, due to release of the quencher and reporter into the volume limited space of the nucleus in the BC-3 cell line

In-cell amplification of DNA

Equipment

Several instruments are available to perform in-cell PCR, ranging from a standard thermal cycler (using modifications), thermocycling ovens and specifically dedicated thermocyclers (Applied Biosystems Gene Amp *in situ* PCR system 1000; Hybaid Omnigene/Omnislide and MJB slide thermocycler) can be used for in-cell DNA and RNA amplification.

If one uses a standard thermal cycler, then an amplification chamber must be created for the slide. This can be made from aluminium (aluminium foil boat). This boat containing the slide is placed on the thermal cycler, covered with mineral oil and then wrapped completely. However, optimization of thermal conduction is never completely achieved. 'Thermal lag', i.e. differences in

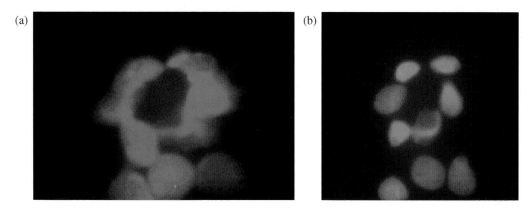

Figure 52.5 RT in-cell PCR analysis of RET/PTC-1 in an immortalized human thyroid cell line. The RET/PTC-1 chimaeric transcript is seen maximally on the luminal border of the cell. (a) FITC channel showing transcripts; (b) DAPI counterstain

- In situ *immuno-PCR: in situ* immunoassays do not allow the detection of the minute numbers of target molecules accessible with *in situ* PCR. *In situ* immuno-PCR is a reaction in which the DNA marker is linked to target molecules through an antibody–biotin–avidin bridge and amplified by *in situ* PCR. Amplified DNA sequences are then detected *in situ* by hybridization. The originators of this technique claim that the technique may be the only one available to detect minute quantities of biological macromolecules such as proteins, carbohydrates and lipids in intact cells or tissue sections (Cao *et al.*, 2000).

temperature between the block face, the glass slide and the PCR reaction mix at each temperature step of the reaction cycle is commonly encountered (O'Leary *et al.*, 1994b). This problem is overcome by use of the specifically designed *in situ* amplification machines, which offer inbuilt slide temperature calibration curves with greater thermodynamic control.

Starting material

In 1990, Haase *et al.* initially described in situ PCR in intact fixed single cells, suspended in PCR reaction buffer. After amplification, cells were cytocentrifuged onto glass slides and the amplified product detected using in situ hybridization (Haase *et al.*, 1990). Initially, some investigators used pieces of glass slides (with cells from cytocentrifuge preparations) in standard Eppendorf tubes, incubated directly in PCR reaction buffer (Spann *et al.*, 1991). More recently, techniques using tissues and cells attached to microscope slides have been used (Bobroski *et al.*, 1995; Cheng and Nuovo, 1994).

For IS-PCR, PCR-ISH, IS-LCR, IS-PNA PCR and IS-TaqMan PCR, fixed cells and tissues, including archival paraffin-embedded material, can be used for amplification. Best results are obtained with freshly fixed cells and tissues, although successful amplification with old archival material (up to 40 years) has been achieved.

Fixed metaphase chromosome spreads and interphase nuclei can be used for the detection of specific subchromosomal regions, using PRINS and cycling PRINS (Gosden *et al.*, 1991). A rigid cellular cytoskeleton must be created, providing a suitable microenvironment, which allows access of amplification reagents with minimal leakage of amplified product. Satisfactory results are obtained with tissues fixed in 1–4% paraformaldehyde, neutral buffered formaldehyde (NBF) and 10% formalin (12–24 hours for biopsy/solid tissue; 10–30 minutes for cytological preparations) (Nuovo *et al.*, 1993; O'Leary *et al.*, 1994b). Less consistent results are obtained with ethanol and acetic acid fixed tissues (Nuovo *et al.*, 1993).

Fixation of cells with formaldehyde fixatives provides a number of drawbacks. Aldehyde groups react with DNA and histone proteins to form DNA–DNA and DNA–histone protein cross-links. Formaldehyde fixation also 'nicks' DNA template (random breaks in dsDNA), which may be non-blunt-ended (i.e. non-overlapping ends). These nicks may subsequently act as potential priming sites for Taq DNA polymerase, leading to incorporation and elongation of labelled and unlabelled nucleotides (i.e. dATP etc) analogous to *in situ* end-labelling for apoptosis. This process occurs at room temperature, leading to spurious results with DNA IS-PCR. This is the predominant reason why in-cell DNA and RNA PCR (i.e. without a hybridization step) have been largely abandoned.

Because repeated cycles of heating and cooling are used during *in situ* amplification, cells and tissues must be adequately attached to a solid support (usually glass), so that detachment does not occur. Glass slides are pretreated with coating agents to ensure maximal section adhesion, the most commonly used being aminopropyltriethoxysilane (APES), Denhardt's solution and Elmer's glue.

Cell and tissue permeabilization

Cells must be adequately digested and permeabilized to facilitate access of reagents. This is can be achieved by protease treatment (e.g. proteinase K, pepsin or trypsin) and/or mild acid hydrolysis (0.01–0.1 N HCl). Maximal digestion times and protease concentrations have to optimized for each tissue/cytological preparation used.

Long digestion times inevitably compromise cellular morphology. Short digestion times result in incomplete dissociation of histone protein–DNA cross-links, which ultimately can hinder the progression of Taq DNA polymerase along native DNA templates. Acid hydrolysis probably acts by driving such cross-links to complete dissociation. Alternatively, microwave irradiation of cells and tissue sections can be used to expose nucleic acid templates. Short pulses of microwave irradiation (with or without proteolysis) using a citrate buffer, analogous to antigen retrieval for immunocytochemistry, allow access of amplification reagents to the desired target sequence and, in addition, facilitate post-amplification immunocytochemistry.

Following this (if a non-isotopic labelling method is used), a blocking step must be employed, depending on the method used for post-amplification detection of product, e.g. peroxidase or alkaline phosphatase detection systems. In the former, endogenous peroxidase is quenched by incubation in a 3% H_2O_2 solution with sodium azide, while 20% ice-cold acetic acid blocks intestinal alkaline phosphatase.

DNA amplification protocols

Successful amplification is governed by: (a) careful optimization of cycling parameters; (b) appropriate design of primer pairs (taking into account their T_m, i.e. specific melting temperature, their ability to form primer dimers and uniqueness); and (c) optimization of Mg^{2+} concentrations, needed to drive the amplification reaction.

Due to reagent sequestration (see below), higher concentrations of amplification reagents are required during *in situ* amplification than for conventional solution-phase techniques, including primers, dNTPs and Mg^{2+}. Mg concentrations in particular have to be carefully optimized, with satisfactory amplification occurring for most applications at 2.5–5.5 mM. Amplification reagent volumes usually vary, depending on the surface area of the cell preparation/tissue section used. This is important, as patchy amplification may occur over the surface of the slide due to volume variations consequent to localized amplification failure. When using the Gene

Amp *in situ* PCR 1000 system, 25–50 µl are typically used.

Initial denaturation of DNA can be achieved before amplification, either during permeabilization or following the fixation process. Alternatively, it may be performed at the beginning of the amplification protocol itself. Denaturation can be achieved using heat, heat/formamide or alkali (Bagasra *et al.*, 1994). In addition, most investigators advocate the use of 'hot start' PCR to reduce mispriming and primer oligomerization and Nuovo (1994) has suggested the addition of single-strand binding protein (SSB) derived from *E. coli*. The precise mode of action of this protein is unknown but it functions in DNA replication and repair by preventing primer mispriming and oligomerization.

Optimization of cycling parameters must be performed for each particular assay. Most protocols employ 25–30 rounds of amplification, exceptionally 50 cycles. Some investigators have performed two successive 30 cycle rounds with the addition of new reagents, including primers and DNA polymerase between each round; a modification of this is 'nested' PCR, where internal primers, 'nested' within the amplicon produced during the first round, are added. However, this is not recommended for routine use.

Primer selection has evolved around two basic strategies: single primer pairs or multiple primer pairs, with or without complementary tails. Multiple primer pairs have been designed to generate longer/overlapping product, with the obvious advantage of localization of amplicons and minimal product diffusion. However, if 'hot-start' PCR is employed, single primer pairs are usually sufficient to ensure successful amplification.

Post-amplification stringency washing and amplicon fixation

Post-fixation with 4% paraformaldehyde and/or ethanol may be employed to maintain localization of amplified product. If one is performing PCR-ISH, an oligonucleotide or genomic probe is applied at this stage. Maximum specificity is achieved using probes hybridizing to sequences internal to the amplified product only. Genomic probes are not restricted to these sequences and appear to provide comparable results.

Following *in situ* amplification, most protocols include a post-amplification washing step, using sodium chloride, sodium citrate (SSC), formamide and varying washing temperatures, to remove diffused extracellular product, which may result in non-specific staining and

generation of false positive results. The 'stringency' of the wash is defined by the set of conditions employed (i.e. SSC concentration, percentage formamide used and the washing temperature). The investigator attempts to achieve a washing 'window' where the signal: background noise ratio is maximal; however, post-hybridization washing stringencies are derived empirically.

Detection of amplicons

Non-isotopic labels (e.g. biotin, digoxigenin, fluorescein) are more widely used and, when used in conjunction with a 'sandwich' immunohistochemical detection technique, appear to provide similar degrees of detection sensitivity to isotopic labels. These may vary from one-step to five-step detection systems, as for conventional immunocytochemistry. The product is finally visualized by either a colour reaction (e.g. NBT/BCIP or AEC chromagens) or fluorescence.

Nuovo has described the performance of post-amplification conventional immunocytochemistry, the obvious advantage being co-localization of product with the cell of interest, e.g. endothelial cell or macrophage. However, attempts to reproduce this by various groups, including our own, have been disappointing and it is likely that most epitopes do not withstand repetitive thermal cycling.

Reaction, tissue and detection controls for use with in-cell DNA PCR assays

Parallel solution-phase PCR, omission of primers and/or Taq DNA polymerase, irrelevant primers and/or probes, known negative controls and reference control genes should be performed with each assay. The number of controls performed depends on the amount of tissue/cells available for the reaction.

The following controls are required in PCR-ISH: (a) reference control gene PCR-ISH, e.g. β-globin, β-actin, etc; (b) DNase digestion of target tissues/cells; (c) RNase digestion of target tissues/cells; (d) target primers with irrelevant probe; (e) irrelevant primers with target probe; (f) irrelevant primers with irrelevant probe; (g) reference control gene primers with the target probe; (h) target primer one only, (asymmetric in-cell PCR); (i) target primer two only; (j) no Taq polymerase; (k) no primers; (l) omit the reverse transcriptase step in RT IS-PCR or RT PCR-ISH; (m) *in situ* hybridization controls for PCR-ISH and RT PCR-ISH; and (n) detection controls for immunocytochemical detection systems.

Reference control genes, including the use of a single-copy mammalian gene such as PDH, are important to assess the degree of amplification in the tissues section/cell preparation. When amplifying DNA targets, the addition of DNAses should abolish the signal. If this does not occur, the signal may have resulted from spurious amplification, or alternatively may represent either RNA/cDNA. RNAse pre-treatment is mandatory in the assessment of RNA targets [*in situ* reverse transcriptase (RT) PCR] and should be included in the amplification of DNA templates to minimize false positive signals originating from cellular RNA. Our group has found that the combination of RNAase A and T1 to provide superior results.

The use of a reference control gene primer pair in conjunction with target specific probe assesses the degree of 'stickiness' of the target probe sequence and the creation of a false positive result. The addition of only one primer in the amplification mix generates an 'asymmetric PCR', with a quantitative reduction in the amount of product synthesized. Irrelevant primers with irrelevant probe should not generate a signal. The specificity of the *in situ* hybridization component of PCR-ISH is assessed by employing an irrelevant probe with target-specific primers.

The role of primer–primer dimerization and primer oligomerization in the generation of false positive signals is assessed by excluding Taq DNA polymerase, whereas the contribution of non-specific elongation of nicked DNA in tissue sections is examined by the exclusion of primers. The latter is an extremely important control for ISH-PCR.

In the assessment of RT-IS PCR, omission of the reverse transcriptase step is important. As in routine *in situ* hybridization, hybridization controls and detection controls are essential to exclude false positive/negative results due to failure of the ISH step or aberrant staining of tissues by the detection system.

In-cell RNA amplification

Cell and tissue preparation

The techniques specifically designed for amplification of RNA targets are RT IS-PCR and RT PCR-ISH. In general, RNA targets are easier to amplify than DNA targets, because of the increased number of starting copies of target. Once cells or tissues are removed from the body, RNA degradation begins almost instantaneously. RNases are ubiquitous in the environment, fingers, gloves and bench-tops being among some of many sources. Fixative solutions contain specific RNases that degrade RNA, and tissue processing again contaminated by RNases minimizes the amount of target RNA that can be amplified.

Initially, an RNase-free working environment should be created. For optimal preservation of RNA in tissue sections, immediate fixation in RNase-free solutions should be carried out. Alcohol, acetic acid:alcohol and neutral-buffered formaldehyde fixatives made up in autoclaved DEPC (diethylpyrocarbonate)-treated water should be used. All protocols for unmasking of nucleic acid again should employ, where possible, RNase-free conditions.

Amplification methodology and chemistries

A cDNA template is created initially using a reverse transcriptase enzyme, usually Moloney mouse leukaemia virus (MMLV) RT, followed by amplification of the newly synthesized cDNA template. A post-amplification *in situ* hybridization step may be employed (RT PCR-ISH), as for DNA PCR-ISH. These techniques employ a two-step approach, i.e. reverse transcription and then amplification. Our group has described a single-step methodology using the rTth DNA polymerase enzyme that obviates the need for splitting the reaction. rTth polymerase possesses both reverse transcriptase and DNA polymerase activity.

Controls for RNA in situ amplification

The same controls are used as in DNA *in situ* amplification. Omission of the reverse transcriptase step will obviously yield a faint or negative result. Parallel DNAse digestion should be carried out in all in-cell RNA assays particularly at the optimization stage.

Problems encountered with in-cell PCR amplification

Many groups have encountered problems with *in situ* PCR (O'Leary *et al.*, 1995, 1996a, 1996b; Teo and Shannak, 1995). Important factors include: the nature of the starting material, fixation conditions and conformational nature of the target that is to be amplified. DNA *in situ* PCR is particularly fraught with difficulties, especially with paraffin-embedded material, where non-specific incorporation of nucleotide sequences may occur in the presence of Taq DNA polymerase, and it is our opinion that this technology should not be used.

PCR-ISH appears to be more specific, especially if a 'hot-start' modification is employed or, alternatively, if multiple primer pairs are used. PCR-ISH protocols, in general, are more sensitive but, in contrast to solution-phase PCR, are less efficient, with apparent linear amplification only. The degree of amplification is difficult to assess. Nuovo *et al.* (1991, 1992, 1993, 1994, 1995) have reported a 200–300 fold increase in product, in contrast to Embretson and colleagues (1993), who estimate an increase of 10–30-fold only. Our experience would tend to support the latter figure.

The major limitation with DNA IS-PCR, as previously mentioned, is the non-specific incorporation of nucleotides into damaged DNA by Taq DNA polymerase. This is cycle- and DNA polymerase-dependent and may occur in the absence of primers and/or with a 'hot-start' modification. Therefore, the routine use of DNA *in situ* PCR is as yet not feasible, due to the risk of generating false signals. Gosden *et al.* (1991) have previously reported the use of strand break joining in chromosomal work, to eliminate spurious incorporation during DNA *in situ* PCR. Pre-treatment with di-deoxy blockage has also been documented to eliminate non-specific incorporation, but this is not always successful. Our group has utilized strand 'super-denaturation,' i.e. where dsDNA is denatured at high temperatures. The DNA is then maintained in a denatured state for an extended period of time (5–10 minutes) but again, this has produced inconsistent results.

Reagent sequestration

Increased concentrations of reagents are required if successful *in situ* amplification is to be achieved (usually of the order of 2–5 times). This results from reagent sequestration, because reagents adhere to slides or to the coating materials used. In addition, reagents may also intercalate with fixative residues left in tissues. Pre-treating slides with 0.1–1% bovine serum albumin (BSA) allows a reduction in reagent concentration, which may function by blocking this sequestration (O'Leary *et al.*, 1995).

Amplicon diffusion and back-diffusion

Product diffusion from the site of synthesis, which may occur as a result of permeabilization and/or cell truncation, is commonly encountered in in-cell PCR analyses. One approach is to reduce the number of cycles. Another frequently employed strategy is to post-fix the slides in ethanol or paraformaldehyde, which helps to maintain localization of product. Alternative approaches include overlaying the tissue section with agarose and/or incorporation of biotin-substituted nucleotides (analogous to *in situ* PCR). This latter modification promotes the generation of bulkier products, which are less likely to diffuse.

Patchy amplification/incomplete amplification

Patchy amplification is commonly encountered, with 30–80% of cells containing the target sequence of interest staining at any one time. There are many reasons for this, including non-uniform digestion with variations in cell permeability, failure to completely disassociate DNA–histone protein cross-linkages and cell truncation. This latter factor is an inevitable consequence of microtome sectioning where cell 'semi-spheres' are created. As a result, the nuclear contents are truncated, giving rise to two possibilities: (a) the desired target sequence may not be present; (b) the target sequence may be present but the product may have diffused out.

Future work with in-cell PCR-based assays

The recent developments of in-cell TaqMan PCR allow investigators to directly quantitate transcripts within cells and tissues specimens. The ability to use two-colour

Table 52.1 Uses of in-cell PCR technologies in cellular pathology

DNA and RNA viruses
HIV 1, 2
HPV 6, 11, 16, 18, 31, 33, etc.
HBV, HCV
CMV
Measles
HHV 6, 7 and 8
HSV DNA
LGV (lymphogranuloma venereum)
Oncogenes, tumour suppressor genes and markers of malignancy
p53 Mutations
ras Mutations (H-Ki, N-ras)
Gene Rearrangements (t11; 22, t11; 14)
Chromosome mapping (PRINS and cyclin PRINS)
T cell receptor rearrangements
Metalloproteinases and their inhibitors
EGF receptor expression
Nitric oxide synthase

detection systems allows simultaneous detection of a housekeeping gene and a target gene.

In-cell TaqMan PCR demonstrates classical TaqMan probe kinetics, with fluorescent quenching visible after a certain number of cycles. This is due to the volume limited space of the cytoplasm/nucleus and is brought about by proximity of quencher and reporter sequences in molar excess in the 'free-state' following hydrolysis of the probe.

The discovery of in-cell TaqMan PCR theoretically should make it possible to introduce TaqMan arrays for direct quantitative analysis. This would offer a major advantage over conventional cDNA and SNP hybridization array platforms, and would for the first time allow gene quantitation of multiple genetic loci simultaneously. Table 52.1 lists the current use of in-cell PCR analyses in cellular pathology.

References

Bagasra O, Hauptman SP, Lischner HW *et al.* Detection of human immunodeficiency virus type 1 provirus in mononuclear cells by *in situ* polymerase chain reaction. *N Engl J Med* 1992; **326**: 1385–1391.

Bagasra O, Seshamma T, Pomerantz RJ. Polymerase chain reaction *in situ*: intracellular amplification and detection of HIV-1 proviral DNA and other gene sequences. *J Immunol Methods* 1993; **158**: 131–145.

Bagasra O, Seshamma T, Hanson J *et al.* Applications of *in situ* PCR methods in molecular biology: I. Details of methodology for general use. *Cell Vision* 1994; **1**: 324–335.

Boshoff C, Schultz TF, Kennedy MM *et al.* Kaposi's sarcoma associated herpes virus (KSHV) infects endothelial and spindle cells. *Nature Med* 1995; **1**: 1274–1278.

Cao Y, Kopplow K, Liu GY. *In situ* immuno-PCR to detect antigens. *Lancet* 2000; **356**(9234): 1002–1003.

Cheng JD, Nuovo GJ. Utility of reverse transcriptase (RT) *in situ* polymerase chain reaction in the diagnosis of viral infections. *J Histotechnol* 1994; **17**: 247–251.

De-Mesmaeker A, Altmann KH, Waldner A, Wendeborn S. Backbone modifications in oligonucleotides and peptide nucleic acid systems. *Curr Opin Struct Biol* 1995; **5**(3): 343–355.

Embretson J, Zupancic M, Beneke J, *et al.* Analysis of human immunodeficiency virus-infected tissues by amplification and *in situ* hybridization reveals latent and permissive infection at single cell resolution. *Proc Natl Acad Sci USA* 1993; **90**: 357–361.

Gosden J, Hanratty D, Starling J *et al.* Oligonucleotide primed *in situ* DNA synthesis (PRINS): a method for chromosome mapping, banding and investigation of sequence organization. *Cytogenet Cell Genet* 1991; **57**: 100–104.

Haase AT, Retzel EF, Staskus KA. Amplification and detection of lentiviral DNA inside cells. *Proc Natl Acad Sci USA* 1990; **87**: 4971–4975.

Herrington CS, de Angelis M, Evans MF *et al.* Detection of high risk human papillomavirus in routine cervical smears: strategy for screening. *J Clin Pathol* 1992; **45**: 385–390.

Holland PM, Abramson RD, Watson R, Gelfand DH. Detection of specific polymerase chain reaction product by utilizing the 5′ to 3′ exonuclease activity of Thermus aquaticus DNA polymerase. *Proc Natl Acad Sci USA* 1991; **88**: 7276–7280.

Lawyer FC, Stoffel S, Saiki RK *et al.* Isolation, characterization, and expression in *Escherichia coli* of the DNA polymerase gene from the extreme thermophile, *Thermus aquaticus. J Biol Chem* 1989; **264**: 6427–6437.

Nuovo GJ, Gallery F, MacConnell P *et al.* An improved technique for the detection of DNA by *in situ* hybridization after PCR amplification, *Am J Pathol* 1991; **139**: 1239–1244.

Nuovo GJ, MacConnell P, Forde A, Delvenne P. Detection of human papillomavirus DNA in formalin fixed tissues by *in situ* hybridization after amplification by PCR. *Am J Pathol* 1991; **139**: 847–850.

Nuovo GJ. *PCR In Situ Hybridization. Protocols and Applications.* 1992: Raven, New York.

Nuovo GJ, Gallery F, Horn R *et al.* Importance of different variables for enhancing *in situ* detection of PCR amplified DNA. *PCR Methods Appl* 1993; **2**: 305–312.

Nuovo GJ. *In situ* detection of PCR-amplified DNA and cDNA: a review. *J Histotechnol* 1994; **17**: 235–246.

Nuovo GJ, MacConnell PB, Simsir A *et al.* Correlation of the *in situ* detection of polymerase chain reaction-amplified metalloproteinase complementary DNAs and their inhibitors with prognosis in cervical carcinoma. *Cancer Res* 1995; **55**: 267–275.

O'Leary JJ, Browne G, Johnson MI *et al.* PCR *in situ* hybridization detection of HPV 16 in fixed CaSki and fixed SiHa cells—an experimental model system. *J Clin Pathol* 1994a; **47**: 933–938.

O'Leary JJ, Browne G, Landers RJ *et al.* The importance of fixation procedures on DNA template and its suitability for solution phase polymerase chain reaction and PCR *in situ* hybridization, *Histochem J* 1994b; **26**: 337–346.

O'Leary JJ, Browne G, Bashir M S, *et al.* Non-isotopic detection of DNA in tissues. In *Non-isotopic Methods in Molecular Biology—A Practical Approach*, Levy E R, Aerrington C S (eds). 1995: IRL Press, Oxford.

O'Leary JJ, Herrington C S (eds). *PCR In Situ Amplification—A Practical Approach.* 1996: IRL Press, Oxford.

O'Leary JJ, Chetty R, Graham AK, McGee J O'D. *In situ* PCR: pathologists' dream or nightmare? *J Pathol* 1996; **178**: 11–20.

O'Leary JJ, Silva I, Uhlmann V, Landers RJ. *In situ* amplification. In *The Science of Laboratory Diagnosis*, Crocker J, Burnett D (eds). 1998: ISIS Medical Media, Oxford, pp 551–563.

Spann W, Pachmann K, Zabnienska H *et al. In situ* amplification of single copy gene segments in individual cells by the polymerase chain reaction. *Infection* 1991: **19**: 242–244.

Teo I A, Shaunak S. Polymerase chain reaction *in situ*: an appraisal of an emerging technique. *Histochem J* 1995; **27**: 647–659.

53

High-density SNP and cDNA array analysis

Orla Sheils, Cara M Martin, Paul Smyth, Jon Sherlock, Stephen Finn, Esther O'Regan, Steve Picton and John O'Leary

Introduction

Fifty years after the discovery of the DNA double helix, the reference sequence for *Homo sapiens* was explicated (Venter *et al.*, 2001; Lander *et al.*, 2001; Consortium IHGS, 2001). The international effort to sequence the 3 billion DNA letters in the human genome has ushered in an exciting new genomic era. DNA microarrays provide an important adjunct in the exploitation of uncharted genomic territory, particularly in the area of gene expression.

It is widely believed that thousands of genes and their products (i.e. RNA and proteins) in a given living organism function in a complicated and orchestrated way, insight into which houses potential for a variety of diagnostic and therapeutic modalities. Traditional methods in molecular biology generally work on a 'one gene in one experiment' basis, which means that the throughput is very limited and the 'whole picture' of gene function is hard to obtain.

In the past several years, a new technology, called DNA microarray, has attracted increasing interest among biologists. This technology comprises assays that simultaneously generate data pertaining to the expression levels of many thousands of genes. This facility represents a dramatic increase in throughput (Elkins & Chu, 1999; Lockhart & Winzeler, 2000; Schena *et al.*, 1995).

An array is an orderly arrangement of samples. It provides a medium for matching known and unknown DNA samples, based on base-pairing rules and automating the process of identifying the unknowns. DNA microarray, or DNA chips, are fabricated by high-speed robotics, on a solid matrix/substrate, for which probes with known identity are used to determine complementary binding, thus allowing massively parallel gene expression and gene discovery studies. The sample spot sizes in microarrays are typically less than 200 μm in diameter and these arrays usually contain thousands of spots.

The microarray market has grown with alarming rapidity over the last number of years. As the price of this technology has fallen, there has been a tendency to shift from home-made DIY options towards the expanding range of commercial devices currently available.

Affymetrix GeneChip technology

The Affymetrix oligonuceotide arrays are synthesized using a process combining photolithography and combinatorial chemistry (Pease *et al.*, 1994). The arrays are composed of a quartz wafer, which is naturally hydroxylated. A set of photolithographic masks is manufactured that allow the sequential addition of specific nucleotides to particular locations on the chip. When ultraviolet light is shone over the mask in the first step of synthesis, the exposed linkers become deprotected and are available for nucleotide coupling. The single type nucleotide solution is then washed over the wafer's surface and attaches to the activated linkers. In the next step, another mask is placed over the wafer for the next round of deprotection and coupling. The process

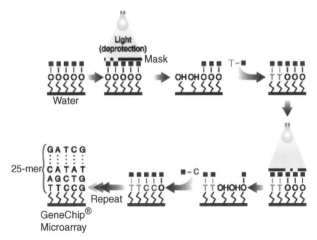

Figure 53.1 Affymetrix uses a combination of photolithography and combinatorial chemistry to manufacture GeneChip Arrays. Image supplied courtesy of Affymetrix©

is sequentially repeated until the probes reach their full length, as illustrated in Figure 53.1.

Individual genes are represented on the GeneChip using a series (typically 11–20) of different 25-mer 'perfect match' oligonucleotides. The HG-U133 set contains 11 probe pairs per probe set. The probe sets are generally located within 600 bp upstream from the poly-A site, as this portion of mRNA is most efficiently converted into labelled target. Probes are selected based on their complementarity to the selected gene or expressed sequence tag (EST), uniqueness relative to other related genes and their predicted hybridization characteristics. For every set of perfect match (PM)

oligonucleotide probes, a paired set of mismatch (MM) probes are also present on the array. The oligonucleotide sequence used for the MM probes are identical to the PM probe but with a single nucleotide substitution in the central position. The specific hybridization signal is determined by subtracting the fluorescence signal from the MM probes from the PM fluorescence signal, and averaged over all the probe pairs representing a particular gene. This average fluorescence signal is a measure of the transcript abundance.

The Affymetrix software detection algorithm uses probe pair intensities to generate a detection p value and assign a present/absent call for each individual gene. Each probe pair in a probe set has a discrimination score, which is calculated for each probe pair and compared to a predefined threshold, *Tau*. The discrimination score is a basic property of a probe pair that describes its ability to detect its intended target. It measures the target specific intensity difference of the probe pair (PM– MM) relative to its overall hybridization intensity. Probe pairs with scores higher than *Tau* vote for the presence of transcript. Probe pairs with scores lower than *Tau* vote for the absence of transcript. A p value is also generated that reflects the confidence of the detection call. This strategy permits high sensitivity at low target concentrations and preserves the ability to discriminate between closely related sequences.

In contrast to cDNA microarrays, which use a two-colour hybridization approach in which labelled target and control are hybridized to the same array, each Affymetrix GeneChip is designed to analyse a single RNA sample (Figure 53.2). mRNA is converted to double-stranded cDNA by reverse transcription, using an oligo

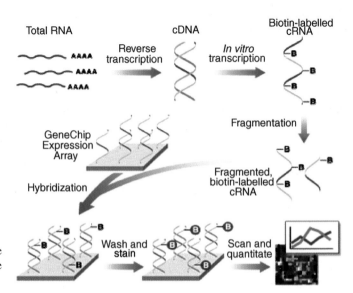

Figure 53.2 Schematic of the procedure for gene expression analysis using affymetrix GeneChips. Image supplied courtesy of Affymetrix©

d(T) primer engineered to contain a T7 RNA promotor site. Biotin-labelled nucleotides are directly incorporated into the cRNA target by *in vitro* transcription with a T7 polymerase. Labelled cRNA is fragmented into < 200 bp fragments and hybridized to the GeneChip. The fluorescent signal is obtained after staining the Gene-Chip with streptavidin phycoerythrin.

SNP profiling and DNA arrays

Complex genetic diseases require many thousands of markers and hundreds of samples to provide sufficient power to identify regions of the genome and genes responsible for a measurable phenotype. Single nucleotide polymorphisms (SNPs) have been estimated to occur on average every 1000 bases in the human genome. These polymorphisms have great potential to be used as genetic markers for many applications, including linkage, association and loss of heterozygosity in cancer.

Current SNP genotyping involves the use of locus-specific primers, a practice which potentially increases cost and limits the number of SNP markers that can be assayed in a single experiment. However, Affymetrix have launched a GeneChip® Mapping 10 K Array. This system can assay more than 10 000 SNPs in a single scalable experiment that does not rely on locus-specific PCR (Mei *et al.*, 2000; Sellick *et al.*, 2003). The company proposes to launch a two-array set (Centurion) in the near future to analyse more than 100 000 SNPs per sample, enabling whole genome association studies.

The GeneChip® Mapping 10 K Array, and subsequent Centurion arrays, rely on the whole genome sampling assay (WGSA). This scheme is a generic approach for complexity reduction of the whole genome to allow efficient hybridization to a microarray containing over 10 000 SNPs (Cutler *et al.*, 2001). The assay runs in four simple steps: restriction digestion of genomic DNA; ligation of a specific adaptor; amplification with a PCR primer; and fragmentation of the DNA; followed by labelling and hybridization to the array (Kennedy *et al.*, 2003).

For the Centurion arrays, the PCR amplification step uses the Pfx enzyme to preferentially amplify fragments of 500–2000 bp, reducing the complexity of the genome to approximately 300 MB total. This complexity reduction allows accurate genotyping by allele-specific hybridization for over 50 000 SNPs on each array, with input requirements of assay requiring only 250 ng human DNA per array, or 500 ng for the set.

Applied biosystems expression array system

The Applied Biosystems Expression Array System is based on a microarray design that represents the whole human genome, utilizes current transcript data and relies entirely upon gene annotations that have been validated by experts in human curation. Each probe is part of a relational database that includes both Celera Genomics annotations and those in the public domain. Combined with specially developed chemiluminescent chemistries, this complete system delivers greater probe and detection sensitivity than previous generations of microarray systems. In addition, annotation information for all of the 31 097 human genes that are represented on the microarray is included in an Oracle® database that is provided with the 1700 system. The manufacturers suggest that the result is a complete system that is capable of rapid and accurate analysis of microarray data for gene expression research. 'Follow-on' experiments from microarrays can be achieved by linking to quantitative real-time PCR TaqMan® probe-based assays, which enable microarray data validation, absolute quantitation of transcript production and investigation of alternative splicing events.

The Applied Biosystems Expression Array System (Figures 53.3–53.6) consists of an analyser (Applied Biosystems 1700 Chemiluminescent Analyzer) that can image arrays in chemiluminescence, to survey and measure the gene expression at very low levels and in fluorescence, to locate and auto-grid features. Designed to incorporate a state-of-the-art CCD camera, the 1700 system precisely images the chemiluminescent signal that results when labelled transcripts are hybridized to a microarray. In addition, the 1700 system images the microarray in a fluorescent mode to grid, normalize and identify features with pinpoint accuracy, even in the absence of gene expression products binding to microarray probes.

The new Applied Biosystems Expression Array System uses the latest genomic data, combined with sensitive detection chemistries to deliver comprehensive gene expression analysis. A variety of complimentary kits are available, including:

- Chemiluminescent RT Labelling Kit, which converts mRNA from cells into digoxigenin-labelled cDNA.

- Chemiluminescent RT-IVT Labelling Kit, which converts mRNA from cells into digoxigenin-labelled cRNA, while simultaneously and linearly amplifying input RNA. The resultant digoxigenin-labelled cDNA

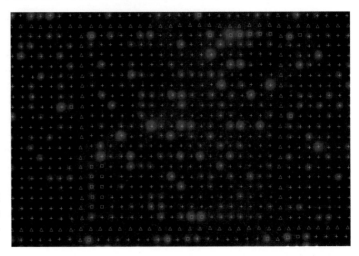

Figure 53.3 Colour representation of Applied Biosystems 1700 grid formation and layout. ▲ = fluorescent signals (used for gridding and quantitation); □ = control; + = probe/target

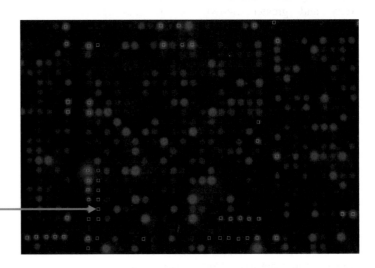

Figure 53.4 Magnified area of a 1700 array, demonstrating chemiluminescent quantitative ladder (arrow)

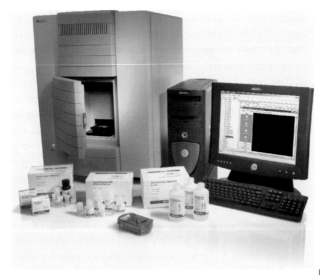

Figure 53.5 Applied Biosystems 1700 array system

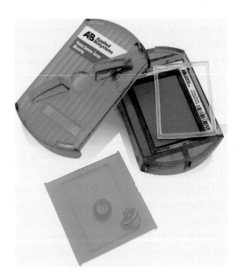

Figure 53.6 Applied Biosystems microarrays are sealed in a plastic disposable container

or cRNA is specifically hybridized to the Applied Biosystems microarray.

- Chemiluminescence Detection Kit, which is used to visualize features that have digoxigenin-labelled cDNA or cRNA bound to the oligonucleotide probes. Visualization is achieved by incubating the microarray with an anti-digoxigenin alkaline phosphatase conjugate. Alkaline phosphatase hydrolyses a chemiluminescent substrate and emits light at a wavelength of ~ 458 nm. The signal intensity is proportional to the mRNA level expressed in the cells.

The manufacturers assert that the resultant chemiluminescent signals on the microarray provide higher sensitivity and greater dynamic range than previous conventional fluorescent microarrays, and further they suggest that high quality data can be obtained with the Applied Biosystems Expression Array System from as little as 100 ng of total RNA starting material.

Applied Biosystems Human Genome Survey Microarrays are designed using public and Celera data for all known genes (31 097). These microarrays contain oligonucleotides with a feature diameter of < 180 µm and a space of > 45 µm (edge-to-edge) between each feature. The oligonucleotides target transcripts for each gene of the human genome. Oligonucleotide probes are synthesized at Applied Biosystems and designed to ensure maximal specificity. Prior to microarray manufacture, all probes undergo analysis by mass spectrometry for quality control. The Applied Biosystems microarrays are sealed in a pre-assembled cartridge, which contains a loading port that can be easily resealed after the labelled cDNA or cRNA samples have been added. When hybridization is complete, the cartridge is disassembled and discarded. The microarrays are then processed in batches and the unbound material is washed away.

Oracle Database for target (gene expression) annotation, which is part of the Applied Biosystems Expression Array System, contains the latest gene annotation data that is essential for all laboratories engaged in today's gene expression studies and provides full storage and query access for all experimental data. The database includes, for example, gene acronyms, gene names, cross-references for gene identification, public (GO) and Celera (Panther™) gene ontologies, and other relevant information. In addition, the manufacturers pledge to continually update the annotations with the most current information about the transcripts targeted by the microarray.

Illumina 'Array of Arrays'™

The expression arrays offered by the company Illumina constitute a fundamentally different way of building arrays: the random self-assembly of beads into patterned microwell substrates. They have utilized technological advances in both the fibre-optics and micro-electromechanical system (MEMS) industries to build substrates that contain multiple thousands of wells across their surfaces (Figure 53.7).

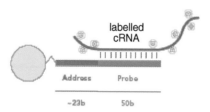

Figure 53.7 Illumina probe design and bead immobilization. Image courtesy of illumina.com

Quantitatively pooled libraries of beads are then self-assembled into the etched microwell substrates, to yield a high-density array platform. Two different Array of Arrays™ formats, the Sentrix™ Array Matrix, and the Sentrix™ BeadChip, are currently available.

The Array Matrix uses fibre-optic bundles containing nearly 50 000 individual light-conducting fibre strands that are chemically etched to create a 3 µm well at the end of each strand. Array bundles are grouped together into a 96-array configuration that matches the well spacing of standard microtitre plates. This unique format allows users to conduct experiments simply and quickly on 96 arrays simultaneously. Moreover, the platform can be readily incorporated into automation routines using standard robotic equipment, leading to reduced error, labour and resource requirements.

The BeadChip format is a slide-sized platform allowing the processing of eight samples at a time and can be scanned on a standard laser scanner.

Independent of the array format, each bead in every array contains hundred of thousands of covalently attached oligonucleotide probes. Up to 1500 unique bead types containing different probe sequences are represented in each array, with an average 30-fold redundancy of each bead type. After bead assembly, a hybridization-based procedure is used to decode the array, determining which bead type resides in each well. This final process validates the performance of each bead type.

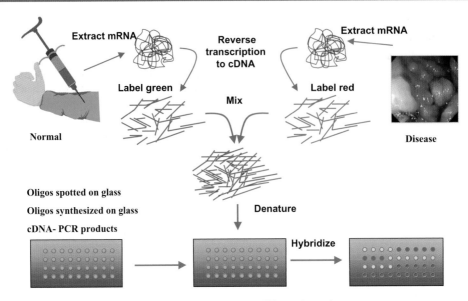

Figure 53.8   Gene expression profiling using microarrays

Dual-colour DNA microarrays (Figure 53.8)

With this technology small quantities of probe are spotted onto a glass slide using a robotic printer. The probes can consist of cDNA, oligonucleotides or PCR products, each probe being complementary to a specific gene. The protocol for target labelling and hybridization to microarrays is different to that used with the Affymetrix GeneChip technology. To compare the relative abundance of each gene in two different RNA samples, a two-colour hybridization experiment is performed. Total RNA is extracted from the two samples, labelled using two different fluorophores. Fluorescent reporters are selected with non-overlapping spectra, Cy3 (green emission at 540 nm) and Cy5 (red emission at 650 nm). These fluorescent labels can be incorporated directly by reverse transcription with an oligo dT primer in the presence of fluorescent nucleotides Cy3-dUTP, or Cy5-dUTP, or indirectly in a T7 RNA amplification step. Labelled cDNA or cRNA from the test and reference sample are mixed together, unincorporated dyes are removed and mixture is hybridized to the microarray. The ratio Cy3:Cy5 is determined and in turn the relative abundance of that specific sequence in the two samples.

MWG microarrays (Figure 53.9)

MWG microarrays are spotted with oligonucleotide sets designed from the CodeSeq® database. The CodeSeq® database is a non-redundant protein-related MWG data-

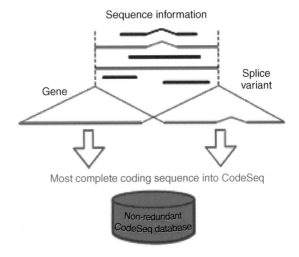

Figure 53.9   MWG probe design

base derived from public sequences for each gene; redundant and partial sequences are removed for each transcript. Specific genes and transcripts on the arrays are represented by specific 50-mer oligonucleotides which are matched in GC content and TM and are free from secondary structures.

Data handling and secondary analysis

The vast quantities of data emanating from array surveys of the human genome may be impressive, but without interpretation that is all it remains—a mass of data. Gene function is one of the key elements researchers want to extract from microarray experiments, and a variety of secondary analytical tools are available to this end.

Perhaps due the relative novelty of microarray technology, or the accelerated pace at which the technology is expanding, presentation of secondary analysis from microarray data has suffered from lack of standardization. Microarray expression studies are capable of producing immense quantities of transcriptomic data. Such data can generate insights into gene function and interaction in various metabolic pathways (Young, 2000; Lockhart & Winzeler, 2000) but only if a standardized approach to data presentation is pursued (Simon *et al.*, 2002; Barrett & Kawasaki, 2003).

Gene expression data is complicated by its nature. It should be analysed in the context of a series of parameters, such as the type of array used, the nature of the biological material examined, the protocols employed with RNA sample and the nature of the calibrator chosen. This final factor is particularly important, given that current microarrays do not measure or quantify expression *per se*; rather, relative or fold changes compared with a calibrator sample are calculated. Lack of standardization among the calibrators used is one of the most important confounding issues when trying to compare data generated by different sources. Different array platforms and experimental design also contribute to non-standardized data, rendering direct comparisons difficult if not impossible.

Recently, Brazma *et al.* (2001, 2002) proposed a system with a view to standardizing microarray data. These authors aspired to define the minimum information that must be reported to ensure the interpretability of the generated results, as well as their potential independent validation. Their system bears the acronym MIAME (the Minimum Information About a Microarray Experiment). With the MIAME system, data and annotations from a microarray experiment needs to comply with the following restrictions: 'the recorded information about each experiment should be sufficient to interpret the experiment and be detailed enough to enable comparisons to similar experiments and permit replication' and 'the information should be structured in a way that enables useful querying and automated data analysis and mining'. A further principle underpinning MIAME is the concession that the area is rapidly developing. It suggests that standards should merely require the description of data in sufficient detail and annotation to facilitate interested parties in understanding how conclusions were reached. The programme details the essential variable components of a microarray experiment and indicates points that need to be included in any manuscript pertaining to this area. Finally, the system acknowledges the use of microarray technology for purposes other than expression analysis (e.g. SNP profiling) and further versions of the systems are planned to accommodate this aspect.

References

Barrett JC, Kawasaki ES. Microarrays: the use of oligonucleotides and cDNA for the analysis of gene expression. *Ding Discov Today* 2003; **8**(3): 134–141.

Brazma A, Hingamp P, Quackenbush J *et al*. Minimum information about a microarray experiment (MIAME)—toward standards for microarray data. *Nature Genet* 2001; **29**(4): 365–371.

Brazma A *et al*. Microarray data representation, annotation and storage. *Adv Biochem Eng Biotechnol* 2002; **77**: 113–139.

Elkins R, Chu FW. Microarrays their origins and applications. *Trends Biotechnol* 1999; **17**: 217–218.

Cutler DJ, Zwick ME, Carrasquillo MM *et al*. High-throughput variation detection and genotyping using microarrays. *Genome Res* 2001; **11**: 1913–1925.

Consortium IHGS (International Human Genome Mapping Consortium). A physical map of the human genome. *Nature* 2001; **409** (6822): 934–941.

Kennedy GC, Matsuzaki H, Dong, S, Liu W *et al*. Large-scale genotyping of complex DNA. *Nature Biotechnol* 2003; **21**: 1233–1237.

Lander ES *et al*. Initial sequencing and analysis of the human genome. *Nature* 2001; **409**: 860–921.

Lockhart D, Winzeler E. Genomics, gene expression and DNA arrays. *Nature* 2000; **405**: 827–836.

Mei R, Galipeau PC, Prass C *et al*. Genome-wide detection of allelic imbalance using human SNPs and high-density DNA arrays. *Genome Res* 2000; **10**: 1126–1137.

Pease AC, Solas D, Sullivan EJ *et al*. Light-generated oligonucleotide arrays for rapid DNA sequence analysis. *Proc Natl Acad Sci USA* 1994; **91**: 5022–5026.

Sellick G, Garrett C, Houlston RS. A novel gene for neonatal diabetes maps to chromosome 10p12.1–p13. *Diabetes* 2003; **52**: 2636–2638.

Schena M, Shalon D, Davis RW, Brown PO. Quantitative monitoring of gene expression patterns with complementary DNA microarray. *Science* 1995; **270**: 467–470.

Simon R, Radmacher MD, Dobbin K. Design of studies using DNA microarrays. *Genet Epidemiol* 2002; **23**: 21–36.

Venter JC *et al*. The sequence of the human genome. *Science* 2001; **291**: 1303–1351.

Young R. Biomedical discovery with DNA arrays. *Cell* 2000; **102**: 9–16.

54

CGH array analysis of human tissues

Esther O'Regan, Paul Smyth, Stephen Finn, Cara M Martin,

Orla Sheils and John O'Leary

Background to CGH and array CGH

Historically, cytogenetic analysis of solid tumours has proved difficult and, although there are many techniques used for detection of genetic changes involved in solid tumours, all have their limitations. Image cytometry, which is used to detect aneuploid clones, is not sensitive enough to detect small genetic changes, while karyotyping presents its own difficulties in the fact that it is highly specialized, time consuming and requires tissue culture of solid tumours, which can be unreliable. Loss of heterozygosity studies and fluorescence *in situ* hybridization (FISH) studies do indeed provide us with very detailed information on one or a small number of specific genes or chromosome regions at a time; however, they cannot give us an overview of the whole genome.

In 1992, Kallioniemi *et al.* developed a molecular cytogenetic method, comparative genomic hybridization (CGH) capable of detecting and mapping relative DNA sequence copy number variation across the whole genome in one single experiment. This revolutionary technique uses a relatively small amount of DNA and allows us to survey the whole genome and detect losses and gains in all chromosomes at once, without the need for cell culture (Hermsen *et al.*, 1996).

Kallioniemi's group at the University of California, San Francisco, initially used CGH to detect novel chromosomal aberrations in 11 cancer cell lines, and since then the body of literature on the use of this technique to detect genetic alterations has been growing and evolving rapidly (Forozan *et al.*, 2000). The advantage of this technique is its genome-wide screening ability, which is less time- and labour-consuming than conventional FISH. The applications of CGH in cancer research include screening of tumours for genetic aberrations, and analysing genetic alteration profiles within tumours in order to increase our understanding of tumour progression and prognosis. While being a powerful diagnostic and research tool, CGH does have a limitation, in that it utilizes condensed states of metaphase chromosomes for visualization, making it difficult to distinguish overlapping signals from genes in close proximity to each other, thus preventing the precise localization of a sequence of interest. The resolution for detecting copy number loss is greater than or equal to 10 MB, and for copy number gains, is no less than 2 MB. Another difficulty presented by CGH is the need for experienced technical staff with training in cytogenetics, with the ability to identify and determine the loci of copy number changes.

In 1995, Schena *et al.* developed the microarray, in which cDNA clones of gene specific hybridization targets from plants were used to quantitatively measure expression of the corresponding plant genes. The success of this novel scientific tool led to the use of microarrays for human genome analysis, thus permitting us to place a representation of the entire human genome on a single slide. Microarrays or 'chips', as they are commonly known, are orderly arrangements of individual nucleic acid samples, which are immobilized in the form of a grid on a solid surface such as glass, chromium, silicon,

The Science of Laboratory Diagnosis, Second Edition   Edited by David Burnett and John Crocker

etc. (Maughan *et al.*, 2001). Microarray analysis is now a foundational technology, allowing the analysis of DNA sequence variation, gene expression, protein levels, tissues and cells in an extensive parallel format (Stears *et al.*, 2003). Since the development of microarrays, recognized limitations of conventional CGH have been overcome by coupling it to microarray technology. Instead of using metaphase chromosomes, CGH is applied to genomic sequences of DNA bound to slides. This system significantly increases resolution for detecting regions of imbalance, and also avoids the need for experienced cytogeneticists.

Overview of comparative genomic hybridization

CGH involves using disease- or tumour-specific DNA labelled with a green fluorochrome, mixed (1:1) with normal (diploid) DNA labelled with a red fluorochrome. This mixture is hybridized to normal metaphase human preparations on a glass slide. The labelled DNA fragments compete for hybridization to their locus of origin on the metaphase spread of chromosomes, and hybridization of tumour DNA is represented by green fluorescence, while hybridization of normal DNA is represented by red fluorescence. The relative amounts of tumour and reference DNA bound at any given locus are dependent on the relative abundance of those sequences in the two DNA samples. The resulting green:red fluorescence ratio is the quantitative representation of loss or gain of genetic material. In short, gene copy number gain (amplification) produces an elevated green:red ratio, and copy number loss (deletion) at a specific locus result in a reduced green:red ratio.

Normal metaphase slides are prepared from phytohaemagglutinin-stimulated peripheral blood lymphocyte cultures from a human with a normal karyotype. The cells are arrested in mitosis, treated with hypotonic KCL, fixed in methanol or acetic acid and mounted on slides, with special attention paid to minimizing the number of overlapping chromosomes. For high-quality preparations there should be little cytoplasm, thus keeping the background levels to a minimum; the chromosomes should be dark when viewed on a phase-contrast microscope; and also they should be of adequate length (approximately 400–500 bands) (Kahru *et al.*, 1997). Of course, as an alternative to this time-consuming work, fully prepared metaphase slides are commercially available.

Advantages

CGH makes it possible to detect and map DNA sequence copy-number increases and decreases anywhere in the genome, providing information on the overall frequency of gains and losses, any clustering of these changes to chromosomal sub-regions, and the size and number of regions affected in any given tumour sample. The ability to survey the whole genome in a single experiment is a distinct advantage over allelic loss studies, which target only one locus at a time. CGH does not require preparation of metaphase spreads from the cells to be analysed, which may prove very difficult in banding analysis of solid tumours, thus CGH is ideal for use in solid tumour analysis, especially since improved DNA extraction technique and universal PCR amplification permit acquisition of higher yields of DNA from almost any kind of clinical specimen, even formalin-fixed, paraffin-embedded tissue.

As no specific probes or previous knowledge of genomic alterations is required, CGH is very suitable for identification and mapping of previously unknown aberrations, which have led to the locations of very significant genes (Mertens *et al.*, 1997).

Limitations

CGH has proved to be a critical tool; however, it does have a number of limitations. First, it can only detect copy gain and loss. It cannot detect any structural chromosomal changes that do not involve copy gain or loss, e.g. balanced translocations or inversions. It is therefore most suitable in the analysis of epithelial tumours, in which the major type of genetic instability is chromosomal imbalance, while it is not as useful in haematological or mesenchymal tumour analysis. Second, because the target DNA within the chromosome is supercoiled, the minimum size of the DNA aberration that can be detected, presents a problem, i.e. the resolution is 10 Mb for loss, and because this level of detectability is a function of both the size of the aberration and the number of excess copies, the resolution for gain is 2 Mb. This limitation prevents precise localization of sequences of interest. It must also be noted that in solid tumour analysis it is difficult to detect small copy number changes because of contamination of the tumour cells with normal cells. Isolation of pure cell populations by microdissection is recommended to reduce the contamination, and thus increase the detection sensitivity.

Also, due to a high number of repetitive sequences in chromosomal regions 1p32, 16p and 19p, the analysis of these regions may be unreliable (Weiss *et al.*, 1999). Finally, non-homogeneous or granular staining patterns can result from sample DNA preparations contaminated with high amounts of protein or from labelled fragments that are either too short or too long.

Clinical applications

The applications of CGH range from cancer genetics to prenatal diagnosis. In cancer, deletions and amplifications contribute to alterations in the expression of tumour suppressor genes and oncogenes. Widespread DNA copy number alteration has a direct effect on global gene expression patterns, supporting the theory that there is a high degree of copy number-dependent expression in solid tumours. Studies on breast cancer and renal cancer, among others, have shown that the number of aberrations may be associated with overall survival rates and patient outcomes, hence the level of genetic instability can be a useful indicator of prognosis (Isola *et al.*, 1995; Moch *et al.*, 1996). CGH is a sensitive screening method for detection and mapping of these critical genes associated with cancer, and has also been used to identify persistent patterns of common clonal genetic abnormalities that are found in many tumours, e.g. loss on chromosome 13 and gain of 8q (Mertens *et al.*, 1997).

Developmental abnormalities, e.g. Down's, Prader-Willi and cri-du-chat syndromes, result from gain or loss of one copy of a chromosome or chromosomal region and, although conventional cytogenetics is used to identify chromosomal aberrations in these disorders, CGH has the added value of allowing the detection of unknown extragenetic material or unbalanced aberrations that could lead to identification of novel regions and genes that are responsible for the patients' phenotype.

Microarrays

The development of the microarray in 1992 by Schena *et al.* has revolutionized the approach to biological research and, since 1992, it has rapidly become a standard tool in many genomic research laboratories, with broad applications in areas including genetic screening, proteomics, safety assessment and diagnostics (Stears *et al.*, 2003; Solinas-Toldo *et al.*, 1997).

Recently the principal of microarray-based CGH has been introduced (Pinkel *et al.*, 1998) and refined (Mantripragada *et al.*, 2003). In this technique, metaphase

chromosomes of the classical CGH technique are replaced by a high-density array of genomic clones in the form of bacterial artificial chromosomes (BACs), yeast artificial chromosomes (YACs) or cosmids on a solid surface. This novel combination of CGH on a chip has avoided some of the limitations of conventional CGH.

First, due to lack of spatial resolution of conventional CGH, the resolution remains at the level of chromosomal banding. However, in combining CGH and microarray technology, this limitation is overcome, thus improving resolution and allowing for identification of genomic imbalances that have not been observed using conventional CGH (Mantripragada *et al.*, 2003). Of note, however, is that the resolution is determined by the size of the cloned DNA insert, therefore this may vary from 100 KB to 40 MB.

The capacity for simultaneous analysis of hundreds of genomic loci vastly improves the precision of the data and reduces the cost as compared to that of serial methods. CGH microarrays provide us with a platform for aberration detection that has improved sensitivity, improved resolution, better reproducibility and higher throughput.

An array is an orderly arrangement of samples and a microarray has spot sizes that are generally less than 200 μm in diameter. They can be either custom-made (Phimister, 1999) or commercially available types can be used. The microarray is fabricated by high-speed robotics on a surface that must allow for stable attachment of array elements and minimal background signals. Arraying and imaging instrumentation can be assembled in-house or purchased directly from a variety of different vendors.

The Vysis Genosensor™ Array 300 platform Figure 54.1 utilizes unique attachment chemistry that allows for 287 large insert clones such as bacterial artificial chromosomes (BACs) and P1artificial chromosomes (PACs) to be spotted onto a chromium-plated surface. Three spots represent each clone and comprise known oncogenes, tumour suppressor genes, known areas of loss of heterozygosity, common microdeletions, subtelomeres and marker clones. The resolution is dependent on the size of the clone and can vary between 100 Kb and 40 Mb.

The Spectral Genomics SpectralChip™ is based on a unique proprietary chemical coupling of DNA fragments to untreated glass surfaces, thus eliminating non-specific binding of the probes to positively charged surfaces. This reduces background noise and fluorescence. The SpectralChip Microarray kit includes two arrays with 1003 non-overlapping BAC clones that span the

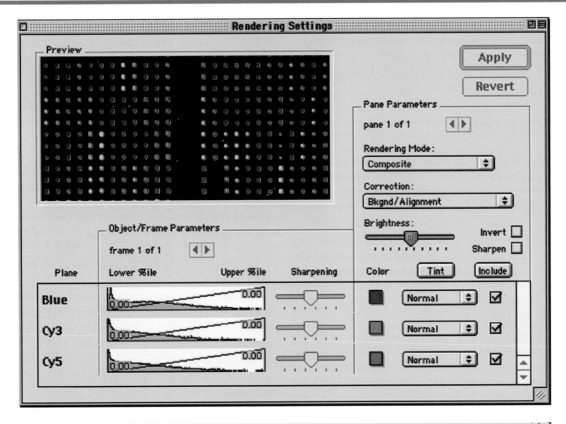

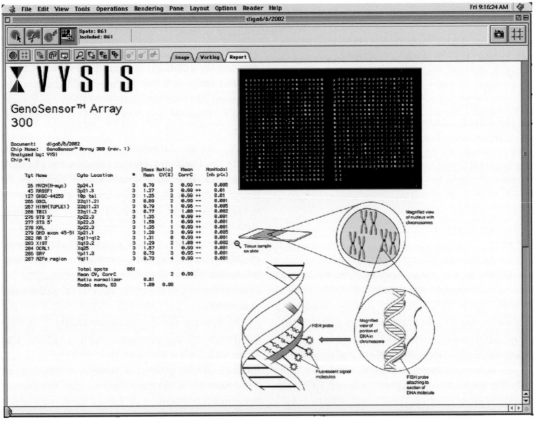

Figure 54.1   Final report output from Genosensor™ array 300 system

genome at intervals of approximately 3 Mb and are spotted in duplicate. This gives a resolution of greater than 3 Mb.

It is important to note some nomenclature disparity in the literature regarding the terms 'probe' and 'target'. We follow the recommendations of Phimister *et al.*, in that 'probe' refers to the bound nucleic acid with the known sequence, while 'target' implies the free nucleic acid sample that one is trying to identify (Emmert-Buck *et al.* 1996).

Starting material

When isolating DNA for CGH analysis, it is imperative that the DNA is of high quality. DNA from solid tumours should be obtained from fresh or frozen tissue, thus avoiding extensive degradation; however, acquisition of tissue in these states is not always feasible.

DNA extracted from formalin-fixed paraffin-embedded tissue will be cross-linked and will consist of highly fragmented DNA, and is thus suboptimal for labelling. To minimize the degradation, a formalin fixation period of less than 24 hours is recommended, and preferably the use of buffered formalin with a neutral pH. Dilution of tumour DNA by DNA from surrounding 'normal/contaminating' stroma can lead to shifts in the ratio of tumour DNA to normal DNA, resulting in failure to detect chromosomal aberrations.

To ameliorate the problem of tissue heterogeneity in solid tumours, it is advantageous to obtain a pure cell population prior to DNA extraction. This can be achieved by microdissection of the sample, either by manual dissection or using a laser capture microdissection (LCM) system.

With the Arcturus PixCell® 2 system, a non-damaging infrared laser melts a low-melting temperature polymer onto the cells of choice, allowing the cells to adhere, thus isolating the morphologically identified cell populations of interest (Telenius *et al.*, 1992).

The use of this valuable tool in obtaining pure tumour DNA has some limitations, however. The technique is time-consuming, requiring laser capture of cells from multiple sections in order to collect sufficient numbers of cells to allow for adequate DNA isolation.

Most CGH studies involve the use of commercially available DNA extraction kits, DNA isolation kits based on affinity columns, and phenol/chloroform extractions. When using formalin-fixed paraffin-embedded samples as the starting material, modifications will have to be made to generic extraction protocols. Because of extensive cross-linking, a prolonged incubation period of up to 3 days in cell lysis solution and repeated addition of proteinase K during this period is advised (Weiss *et al.*, 1999).

For one CGH microarray experiment, 0.1–0.5 µg DNA is required. This may be difficult to obtain, especially from small samples of formalin-fixed paraffin-embedded tissue. To improve the yield, non-specific whole genome amplification of DNA can be performed. Degenerate oligonucleotide primed polymerase chain reaction (DOP-PCR; Speicher *et al.*, 1993; Kuukasjarvi *et al.*, 1997) is an efficient and reliable whole-genome amplification technique.

This type of PCR employs a primer containing degenerate oligonucleotides. The amplification procedure is divided into two steps. The first part involves five PCR cycles performed at low annealing temperatures (32°C), allowing frequent binding of the DOP primer. This generates a pool of DNA sequences from evenly dispersed sites within a given genome. The second step has a more stringent annealing temperature of 62°C for 35 cycles, resulting in more specific priming. The outcome of this two-step procedure is exponential amplification of all the sequences that have been synthesized in the first step, resulting in a large amount of DNA. Several published groups have altered in some way the original DOP-PCR protocol, in an effort to improve both the DNA yield and the reliability of the method (Huang *et al.* 2000).

To test the performance of the method, a mixture of DNAs extracted from tumour cell lines can be used as a positive control. Vysis use CoSH, which is a mixture of the following cell lines: COLO 320 HSR (colonic adenocarcinoma), 35%; SJSA-1 (osteosarcoma), 40%; and BT-474 (breast carcinoma), 25%, with known copy number gains and losses at specific loci.

DNA labelling and hybridization

To obtain uniform, intense hybridization to microarrays, DNA probe fragment size should be 200–400 base pairs, and this is achieved by random labelling the DNA and digesting it to this optimal fragment length. In the direct labelling method recommended by Vysis and Spectral Genomics, fluorophores Cy3 and Cy5 are directly bound to the sample DNA and the whole genomic reference DNA, respectively.

The DNAs are mixed together and co-hybridized to a microarray in the presence of unlabelled human Cot-1 DNA. Cot-1 DNA is placental DNA of 50–100 base pairs in length, which is enriched for repetitive DNA sequences, and its function is to block binding of the labelled DNA to the centromeric and heterochromatic regions, which contain highly polymorphic repeat sequences. Blocking of these regions prevents their inclusion in the analysis, thus allowing for optimal amplitude of the red:green ratio.

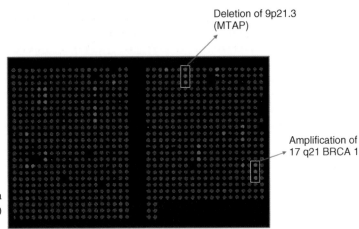

Deletion of 9p21.3 (MTAP)

Amplification of 17 q21 BRCA 1

Figure 54.2 Microarray visualization showing a 9p21.3 (MTAP) deletion (red) and 17q21 (BRCA1) amplification (green)

After hybridization for 2–4 days at 37°C in a humid incubator, the chips are washed to remove any unhybridized probe. 4,6-diamidino-2-penylindole (array DAPI) is applied as a counterstain.

The image capture and storage time for each slide is approximately 1 hour. A fluorescent imaging system captures an image of the hybridized chip in three colour planes: Cy3, Cy5 and DAPI blue. The Vysis Genosensor™ Array 300 uses a CCD camera and a 175 W xenon illumination source to capture three images of each microarray, specific for the DAPI counterstain (blue), the test DNA (green) and the reference DNA (red), respectively. The blue image is used to identify and localize the target spots on the grid. Once identified, the spots can then be quantitatively analysed using specialized software, which integrates the green and red fluorescence intensities, subtracts the local background, and calculates the ratio of test intensity to reference intensity (T:R) for each spot (three replicate spots for each target gene). Figure 54.2 of course, the averaged T:R ratios have to be normalized with respect to a control spot or group of spots. The Vysis system does this by detecting spots that appear to be normal and dividing all T:R ratios by the T:R ratio of the 'normal' targets.

As representation on the microarrays, in particular expression arrays, increases in density, data storage and bioinformatics will become more challenging, and impeccable collection, analysis and interpretation methods are of paramount importance if we are to prevent flawed data that might lead to incorrect conclusions. In an effort to prevent this happening, statistics and bioinformatics are fast becoming more prominent components in the training of molecular biologists.

Conclusion

We have seen a reshaping of molecular biology since the development of microarray technology, and the coupling of this technology with comparative genomic hybridization has emerged as a powerful tool, enabling multi-target assessment in a single test with the ability to detect single-copy changes. This invaluable technique has accelerated the detection of novel genes that may play a role in both the pathogenesis of tumours and the development of genomic profile disease management.

References

Emmert-Buck MR, Bonner RF, Smith PD *et al.* Laser Capture Microdissection. *Science* 1996; **274**(5289): 998–1001.

Forozan F, Mahlamaki EH, Monni O *et al.* Comparative genomic hybridization analysis of 38 breast cancer cell lines: a basis for interpreting complementary DNA microarray data. *Cancer Res* 2000; **60**(16): 4519–4525.

Hermsen MA, Meijer GA, Baak JP *et al.* CGH—a new tool in cancer pathology. *Human Pathol* 1996; **27**(4): 342–349.

Huang Q *et al.* Improving DOP-PCR-CGH for analysis of DNA copy number changes in tumours. *Genes Chromosomes Cancer* 2000; **28**: 395–403.

Isola JJ, Kallioniemi O-P, Chu LW *et al.* Genetic aberrations detected by CGH predict outcome in node-negative breast cancer. *Am J Pathol* 1995; **147**(4): 905–911.

Kahru R, Kahkonen M, Kuukasjarvi T *et al.* QC of CGH: impact of metaphase chromosomes and the dynamic range of hybridization. *Cytometry* 1997; **28**(3): 198–205.

Kallioniemi A, Kallioniemi OP, Sudar D *et al.* Comparative genomic hybridization for molecular cytogenetic analysis of solid tumors. *Science* 1992; **258**(5083): 818–821.

Kuukasjarvi T, Tanner M, Pennanen S *et al*. Optimizing DOP-PCR for universal amplification of small DNA samples in CGH. *Genes Chromosomes Cancer* 1997; **18**(2): 94–101.

Mantripragada KK, Buckley MG, Benetkiewicz M *et al*. High resolution profiling of a 11 Mb segment of human chromosome 22 in sporadic schwannoma using array-CGH. *Int J Oncol* 2003; **22**(3): 615–622.

Maughan NJ, Lewis F, Smith AV. An introduction to arrays. *J Pathol* 2001; **195**(1): 3–6.

Mertens F, Johansson B, Hoglund M, Mitelman F. Chromosomal imbalance maps of malignant solid tumours: a cytogenetic survey of 3185 neoplasms. *Cancer Res* 1997; **57**(13): 2765–2780.

Moch H, Presti JC, Sauter G *et al*. Genetic aberrations detected by comparative genomic hybridization are associated with clinical outcome in renal cell carcinoma. *Cancer Res* 1996; **56**(1): 27–30.

Phimister B. Going global. *Nature Genet* 1999; **21**(suppl 1): 1–6.

Pinkel D, Segraves R, Sudar D *et al*. High resolution analysis of DNA copy number variation using CGH to microarrays. *Nature Genet* 1998; **20**(2): 207–211.

Schena M, Shalon D, Davis RW, Brown PO. Quantitative monitoring of gene expression patterns with a complimentary DNA microarray. *Science* 1995; **270**: 467–470.

Solinas-Toldo L, Stilgenbauer S, Nickolenko J *et al*. Matrix-based CGH: biochips to screen for genomic imbalances. *Genes Chromosomes Cancer* 1997; **20**(4) 399–407.

Speicher MR, du Manoir S, Schrock E, Holtgreve-Grez H *et al*. Molecular cytogenetic analysis of formalin fixed, paraffin embedded solid tumours by CGH after universal DNA amplification. *Hum Mol Genet* 1993; **2**(11): 1907–1914.

Stears RL, Martinsky T, Schena M. Trends in microarray analysis. *Nature Med* 2003; **9**(1): 140–145.

Telenius H, Carter NP, Bebb CE *et al*. Degenerate oligonucleotide-primed PCR: general amplification of target DNA by a single degenerate primer. *Genomics* 1992; **13**(3): 718–725.

Weiss MM, Hermsen MAJA, Meijer GA *et al*. Comparative genomic hybridization. *J Clin Pathol Mol Pathol* 1999; **52**(5): 243–251.

55

DNA sequencing

Cara M Martin, Steven J Picton, Orla Sheils and **John O'Leary**

Introduction

The identification of the chemical deoxyribonucleic acid, DNA, in the mid-1940s by Avery, MacLeod and McCarty showed for the first time that DNA is the material of inheritance, the so-called substance of life. This single discovery laid the foundation for the science that has enabled the establishment of molecular genetics, gene therapy, genetic counselling and the manipulation of gene expression *in vitro*. It has provided the basis for the techniques that now lead to the tabloid outrages inspired by the publication of latest applications of recombinant DNA techniques, such as the cloning of 'Dolly' the sheep at the Roslin Institute, Edinburgh, in Scotland, and facilitated the international effort to sequence the 3 billion DNA letters in the human genome, earlier this decade.

In 1953 the three-dimensional structure of this double-stranded DNA molecule was unravelled and published by James Watson and Francis Crick. The rest, as they say, is history. Since the identity and structure of the molecule responsible for inherited change was discovered, the language of the genetic code, based on the four bases adenine (A), cytosine (C), guanine (G) and thymine (T) has been established. The flow of this information from DNA base sequence to proteins has now been elucidated and clarified beyond any scientific doubt.

Of key events critical to the successful birth and maturation of applied molecular biology, the discovery of methods for determining the individual base sequence of nucleic acids must rank amongst the most important. Sequencing technology is currently used across a diverse number of disciplines, ranging from medical science and forensics to population genetics, phylogenetics and conservation genetics. As we move into an era of comparative genomics, drug discovery and genetic screening, the demand for high-throughput sequencing technologies is greater than ever before. The ability to rapidly determine DNA sequences has revolutionized the science of molecular genetics. DNA sequences from diverse sources have been obtained and vast repositories, such as the EMBL database, DDBJ and GenBank, exist as international stocks of nucleic acid sequences. These databanks serve as a nucleic acid library to which scientists have electronic access in order to study evolution, mutations, phylogeny, and ultimately to apply the sequence information to the characterization of complete biological systems. The purpose of this chapter is to review this sequencing technology and its applications, in particular in the Human Genome Project.

The history of DNA sequencing

Initial attempts at sequencing techniques were performed on short tRNA templates by Robert Holley's group in the mid-1960s. This method involved digesting the RNA with sequence-specific RNases and separating the resulting ribonucleotides by ion exchange chromatography. At the beginning of the 1970s routine DNA sequencing became a reality with the discovery and isolation of DNA restriction enzymes, essentially molecular scissors to cut up the complex genome templates, and DNA polymerases that enabled the template fragments to be copied *in vitro*. These enzymes enabled small DNA fragments to be isolated from much larger sequences

The Science of Laboratory Diagnosis, Second Edition Edited by David Burnett and John Crocker
© 2005 John Wiley & Sons, Ltd

and then used as templates for *in vitro* synthesis of new labelled or tagged DNA.

In 1980 three scientists were awarded the Nobel prize in chemistry for the independent development of two methods of DNA sequencing. These were Maxam & Gilbert, who developed a chemical method of DNA sequencing, and Fred Sanger, who described an enzymatic method for DNA sequencing. Both of these techniques, and modifications to them, are the backbone of most present-day sequencing technologies, with the dideoxy-chain termination method (Sanger) predominating.

Chemical sequencing of DNA

One of the earliest methods of determining the nucleotide sequence of a section of isolated DNA was the chemical sequencing of the DNA strand, more usually referred to as the Maxam–Gilbert technique and published in 1977 (Maxam and Gilbert, 1977). In this method, an isolated DNA fragment is radiolabelled at one end and then partially degraded by subjecting the labelled template to a series of base-specific cleavage reactions. These cleavage reactions generate five populations of radiolabelled molecules that extend from a common point (the radiolabelled terminus) to the site of chemical cleavage. The conditions are designed such that, on average, only one target base in each molecule is modified within a given DNA strand, and these reactions are carried out in two stages: (a) specific bases or types of bases undergo chemical modification; and (b) the modified base is removed from its sugar and the phosphodiester bonds 5′ and 3′ to the modified base are cleaved. Five different chemical modifications occur in separate reaction tubes, which cleave the DNA at specific bases. Following each of the specific chemical reactions, the template in the tube is treated with piperidine, which then cleaves phosphodiester bonds adjacent to the damaged DNA.

The resulting set of end-labelled molecules, whose lengths can range from one to several hundred nucleotides, can be used to identify the position of individual bases by yielding a 'ladder' of fragments that vary in size from one another by a single base. These fragments are separated by gel electrophoresis through a polyacrylamide gel and the sequence read from an autoradiograph of the sequencing gel. The range of this Maxam–Gilbert method is less than that of the Sanger method, with at most 600 bp of sequence being generated from a single set of reactions. The use of this method has dramatically reduced in recent years, largely due to the enormous improvements in enzymatic sequencing

approaches, including automation and tailor-made DNA polymerases. Nonetheless, this approach continues to play a crucial role in many laboratories and is used to establish sequences of oligonucleotide sequences, and in the functional dissection of transcriptional control signals (Carey & Small, 2000).

The dideoxy method of DNA sequencing

The Sanger (Sanger *et al.* 1977) or chain termination method of sequencing DNA is the approach used by the major genome initiatives. The principle of this method is simple; an isolated fragment of DNA or entire plasmid, cosmid or PCR product is denatured to its single-stranded form by heat or alkali treatment. A short synthetic oligonucleotide primer is annealed to its complimentary sequence, encoded on one of the single-stranded templates. The 3′ end of the primer/template duplex is then used as the initiation site for polymerase action and a complimentary DNA strand is synthesized using dNTPs as precursors. Chain termination chemistry has been used in conjunction with labelled oligonucleotide primers (Figure 55.1) or by incorporation of labelled nucleotides during the extension reaction (Figure 55.2). In

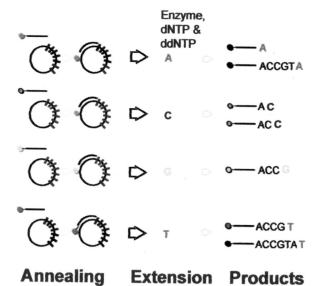

Annealing   Extension   Products

Figure 55.1 Sanger or chain-termination sequencing chemistry employing fluorescent dye-labelled primers. Four different dye-labelled primers (A, C, G and T termination) are used in four separate extension and termination reactions. At completion of the reactions, the contents of the four tubes are pooled and loaded onto a single lane of a polyacrylamide gel. The ladder of dye-labelled products are separated by electrophoresis and detected in real time

**DNA polymerase,
dNTPs and Dideoxy
terminators**

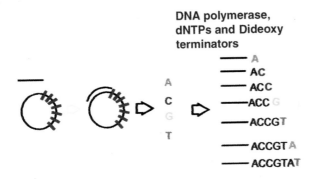

Annealing   Extension   Products

Figure 55.2 Sanger or chain-termination sequencing chemistry employing dye-labelled dideoxy terminators. Dideoxy terminators, with each of the four possible ddNTPs being labelled with a different fluorescent dye, are incorporated by a polymerase during the extension phase of the sequencing reaction. The ladder of dye-labelled products are separated by electrophoresis and detected in real time

sequencing with dye primers, four separate sequencing reactions are carried out for each sample, each reaction containing a different dye-labelled primer. This method is well suited for sequencing projects that use universal primers; however, those that use custom made primers become more cumbersome and expensive, as each primer must be modified in four separate dye-labelling reactions.

In the standard chain termination sequencing approach, four separate synthesis reactions are required. Each of the individual reactions contains a small amount of one of the four 2′,3′ dideoxynucleotide triphosphates (ddNTPs), which differ from deoxynucleotides by having a hydrogen atom attached rather than an OH group (Figure 55.3). When the growing strand of DNA being synthesized incorporates a specific ddNTP, the elongation reaction is terminated, since the ddNTP lacks the 3′-hydroxyl group required by the polymerase to form a phosphodiester bond with the succeeding dNTP. By

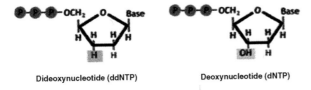

Dideoxynucleotide (ddNTP)   Deoxynucleotide (dNTP)

Figure 55.3 Chemical structures of dideoxynucleotides and deoxynucleotides. The replacement of the hydroxyl group by a hydrogen prevents dideoxynucleotides from undergoing further chain extension during DNA synthesis

careful control of the ratio of ddNTP to dNTP in each of the four reactions, one achieves a random but low-level incorporation of each of the ddNTPs into the growing strands of DNA and creates an array of fragments with a common 5′ end, defined by the primer, but terminating at each possible position where the specific ddNTP could have been incorporated. The average length of such chains can be manipulated by altering the ddNTP:dNTP ratios to ensure that all of the products can be easily resolved by polyacrylamide gel or capillary electrophoresis.

By carrying out four reactions, each with one of the four ddNTPs present, and then resolving the four reactions, A-, C-, G- and T-terminated, side-by-side on a resolving gel or by capillary electrophoresis, we again produce the characteristic ladder of fragments that enables the sequence to be read. Common labelling strategies include incorporation of fluorescently or radiolabelled dNTPs, followed by capillary electrophoresis, autoradiography or chemiluminescent detection of the terminated products. Major advances have been made in this technique, largely due to the improvements in fluorophore chemistry. It is now possible to label each of the ddNTPs, with different dyes, which enables the sequencing reaction to be carried out with one primer in a single tube, sparing considerable time and expense. At present there are two types of dye terminators available, one incorporating dichlororhodamine dyes (dRhodamine Terminator, Applied Biosystems) and the other incorporating BigDyes (BigDye terminator, Applied Biosystems).

Early sequencing chemistries employed polymerases such as the Klenow fragment of DNA polymerase I, or used the bacteriophage-derived T7 DNA polymerase or its variants. In more recent times thermostable polymerases, such as AmpliTaq DNA polymerase and its variants, have been exploited to carry out the chain termination chemistry by the marriage of chain termination and the PCR process. Such an approach is termed cycle sequencing (Figure 55.4). The harnessing of PCR to the dideoxy method in cycle sequencing (Carothers *et al.*, 1989) greatly improved the sensitivity of sequencing. Cycle sequencing is in many ways similar to the standard DNA sequencing reaction. It begins with a standard sequencing reaction mixture of buffer, template, primer, dNTPs and ddNTPs. A thermostable DNA polymerase replaces the standard polymerase. This mixture is subjected to the usual rounds of denaturation, annealing and extension steps of an amplification reaction. Unlike a normal DNA amplification, which uses two primers to exponentially amplify the template, cycle sequencing uses one primer only to

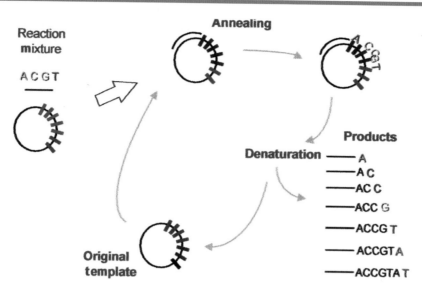

Figure 55.4   Chain termination cycle sequencing. In a combination of the Sanger chain-termination method and the PCR process, the original DNA serves as a template for a linear PCR reaction. In each of 25 rounds of PCR cycling, a ladder of dye-labelled terminated fragments are produced from the templates. Following the extension step, the subsequent denaturation then allows the same DNA molecules to serve again as a template for production of more dye-labelled products

linearly amplify the extension products. Because of the repeated cycling of the reaction, less template is required for cycle sequencing than for the older dideoxy methods. Additionally, by denaturing the double-stranded template before each primer annealing step during the temperature cycling round, the need to prepare single-stranded templates for DNA sequencing is eliminated. Furthermore, the double-stranded templates have the benefit of permitting the sequencing of both strands of DNA. This sequencing approach is also much more amenable to automation than were traditional sequencing approaches.

Automated sequencing

The throughput of sequencing technology was the major rate-limiting step in large-scale sequencing projects, such as the human genome project. The most significant advance in DNA sequencing technologies has been the automation of the technique. This has occurred largely in three main areas, as mentioned above—the improvements in fluorophore chemistries, the discovery of more and more thermostable polymerases and the development of the PCR technique. At the outset of the sequencing of nucleic acids, radioisotopic markers were the only method for the detection of the fragments and such labelled fragments were separated by acrylamide gels and the isotopic bands visualized following auto-

radiography. Four reactions, A, C, G and T, were required for each template and the reactions were then loaded into adjacent lanes on the gel. Following separation and autoradiography, the sequence was determined by 'reading' the band pattern from the bottom to the top of the autoradiograph, representing fragments of ever-increasing length until the resolving power of the gel became limiting. The requirement to use four lanes for each template reaction was a major limitation on the number of samples that could be processed simultaneously on one gel, and further required high levels of template. The manual reading of the autoradiographs, as those from the pre-automation days will bear witness to, was a lengthy and tedious job. Manual reading is also highly prone to human error, in both interpretation of the data on the X-ray film and errors in transcription from the sequence on the autoradiograph to the sequence on a piece of paper or typed directly onto a computer. In many cases the resulting X-ray films were read by two people for verification and DNA sequence was required and compared from reactions carried out on both of the DNA strands, giving both the forward and reverse sequence for comparison.

Current automated methods are capable of generating up to 2 million bases a day, compared with a maximum of 300–500 bases/day by manual polyacrylamide gel electrophoresis (PAGE). As sequencing chemistry, particularly the Sanger chain-termination methodology, has become more robust, the DNA template requirements for the reactions are less demanding. The vital development for the automation of the sequencing process arose from the use of fluorescent reporter dyes as the molecule for the detection of the sequencing ladder. In conjunction with laser excitation of the dyes as they migrate through the gel, and direct optical detection of the fluorescent fragments in real time, full automation of the data acquisition became possible.

There have been two main automation strategies for the separation of DNA fragments; thin slab gel and capillary gel electrophoresis. The first generation of automated sequencers consisted of long vertical polyacrylamide gels, which were run in an electrophoresis tank with integrated fluorescent detection systems. Fluorescently labelled fragments are excited by a laser beam, which passes through a narrow window at the bottom of the sequencing gel. The fluorescent data are then collected and a virtual gel image constructed (Figure 55.5). The separation times in gel electrophoresis can be reduced significantly if higher voltages are used and ultra-thin gels are used as a separation medium.

The second and currently most widely used strategy, which has replaced gel-based sequencing, uses thin liquid polymer-filled capillary tubes. Thin-walled capillaries of varying diameters and lengths allow for the rapid separation of labelled DNA fragments, thus reducing the separation times by up to a factor of 25 when compared with standard gel electrophoretic techniques. Automated capillary sequencers work in the following manner: an automated syringe driver slowly fills the capillary with polymer, the automated sample tray containing sequencing reactions moves such that the capillary is immersed into a specific sample on the tray, and a small aliquot of the sequencing reaction is drawn into the capillary. A current is then applied until all the DNA fragments have resolved and passed the optical window towards the end of the capillary. A laser excites the fluorescently labelled fragments and a CCD camera collects the fluorescence data for their subsequent analysis (Figure 55.6). Between samples, the capillary is refilled with fresh polymer before continuing the process for the next sequencing reaction.

Capillary sequencers have a greater throughput than slab gel sequencers and eliminate the tedious gel preparation and loading steps. The first commercial capillary sequencers became available in early 2000. One current sequencer has 96 capillaries, which operate in parallel for high-throughput sequence analysis. This system is capable of analysing up to 2 million bp DNA in 24 hours.

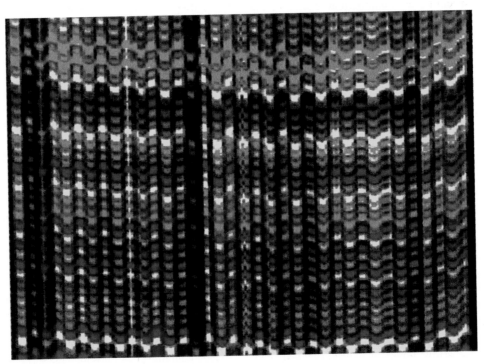

Figure 55.5   Virtual image of a sequencing gel. This electronic image represents the fluorescent sequencing ladders from multiple templates that were loaded and separated simultaneously on a four-dye single-lane instrument

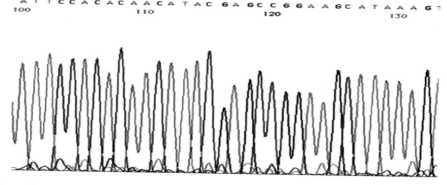

Figure 55.6 Electropherogram generated on an automated DNA capillary sequencer. The four DNA bases are colour-coded, with peaks representing each base. C, blue; A, green; G, black; and T, red

The human genome project

The major advances in sequencing technology in the last decade have resulted in the successful completion of the Human Genome Project (HGP) in 2003, 2 years ahead of schedule. This project represents one of the major achievements in the history of science. The international effort formally commenced in 1990 as a $3 billion, 15 year effort, to sequence the 3 billion base pairs in the human genome. It has been considered by many to be one of the most ambitious scientific undertakings of all time, even paralleled with landing on the moon. In 2001, ahead of schedule, the first working draft sequence of the human genome was published in special editions of *Science* (Venter *et al.*, 2001) and *Nature* (Lander *et al.*, 2001). Since then, researchers have worked to convert this draft sequence into finished sequence, or sequence with fewer than 1 error per 10 000 bases and highly contiguous.

The sequencing approach taken by the HGP Consortium was to adopt a 'map-based' or 'hierarchial shotgun' sequencing method (Figure 55.7). In this approach, genomic DNA was fragmented into large overlapping pieces of approximately 150 Mb and inserted into a special type of vector, called a bacterial artificial chromosome (BAC). This was achieved by partial digestion with restriction enzymes with common recognition sites. The resulting BAC vectors were then transformed into *E. coli* to create a BAC library. Individual BAC clones were fully digested, using additional restriction enzymes, to produce a unique pattern or fingerprint. The BAC inserts were subsequently isolated and mapped to determine the order of each cloned fragment. Once mapped, the individual BAC clones were fragmented randomly into smaller pieces (∼ 2000 bp long), which were in turn

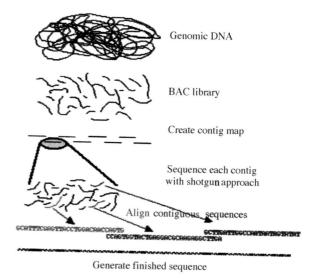

Genomic DNA

BAC library

Create contig map

Sequence each contig
with shotgun approach

Align contiguous sequences

Generate finished sequence

Figure 55.7 Hierarchical shotgun sequencing approach adopted by the HGP consortium

cloned into a plasmid vector (shotgun clone) and sequenced on both strands. Using advanced computer programs, these sequences were aligned such that identical sequences overlapped and the contiguous pieces assembled into finished sequence after each strand had been sequenced at least four times.

The strategy developed by Celera Genomics, who started their quest much later than the HGP consortium, is known as whole genome shotgun sequencing (Figure 55.8). Shotgun sequencing involved randomly shearing genomic DNA into small pieces (2000–10 000 bp long), which were cloned directly into plasmids and sequenced at random on both strands, thus eliminating

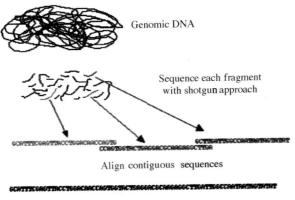

Genomic DNA

Sequence each fragment
with shotgun approach

Align contiguous sequences

Generate finished sequence

Figure 55.8 Whole genome shotgun sequencing approach adopted by Celera Genomics

the BAC step used by the HGP approach. The challenge with this approach was in the assembly of the sequences. Celera commissioned supercomputers, which were capable of handling over 80 terabytes of data and performing the five hundred million trillion sequence comparisons required for the initial assembly. The advantages for Celera were that they already had access to the HGP sequence data, which provided them with reference sequence to work with.

The information we have gained from the human genome sequence is enormous and some of the highlights are mentioned below. The genome is far more heterogeneous than was first expected, and the total number of human genes is less than was expected, with a current consensus of around 30 000 genes.

Advancing areas in nucleic acid sequencing

The importance of the human genome sequence cannot be overstated; however, the human genome represents only one source of information that is required for elucidating complex biological mechanisms. Understanding the genomes of other organisms will play a huge role in our understanding genes that cause diseases, their regulatory mechanisms and the pathophysiology of diseases. The recent sequencing of the mouse genome, the most important animal model of human disease, also represents a significant achievement in the area of genomics. For the foreseeable future, large-scale sequencing will continue to play an enormous role in facilitating progress in scientists' understanding of disease processes. Efforts are also being made to re-sequence

genomes. In this regard, higher levels of automation are required, which will allow researchers to perform sample preparation, sequencing and data analysis on the same platform. Aside from the requirement of highly automated systems, other sequencing approaches that are currently being pursued as alternative separation and detection methods include matrix-assisted laser desorption/ionization time-of-flight mass spectrometry (MALDI–TOF–MS) and sequencing by hybridization or chip-based sequencing. Advances in these areas will serve to reduce the cost of sequencing and allow researchers to focus their sequencing efforts on the more important functional regions of the genome.

Sequencing by MALDI–TOF–MS is a method for separating DNA fragments generated using the Sanger technique. The DNA fragments are mixed with a carrier matrix, such as 3-hydroxypicolinic acid (Wu *et al.*, 1993), and painted on the desorption target surface (a stainless steel plate). After the small organic material crystallizes, the plate is placed in a mass spectrometer for analysis. A laser then desorbs and ionizes the DNA fragments, while acceleration in a mass spectrometer allows determination of fragment length by time-of-flight detection. The advantages to using this type of technique include higher sequencing speed and enables shorter DNA fragments to be sequenced. It is also a label-free technique, so the cost is considerably lower than existing sequencing technologies. With the rapid discovery of new genes and disease-associated mutations, mass spectrometry might be a valuable and economical tool for re-sequencing applications to complement the existing sequencing technologies.

The other emerging strategy is sequencing by hybridization or chip–based sequencing. This can be carried out by immobilizing several thousands short pieces of DNA of known sequences (oligonucleotides) to a glass or silicone surface at defined locations. The target DNA whose sequence is to be determined is fluorescently labelled and then hybridized to the chip. The target sequence is deduced from the subset of oligonucleotide probes that have bound to the target DNA. One of the major constraints with this approach for generating a universal sequencing chip is that the total number of combinatorial variants for an oligonucleotide of 15 bp in length required to represent the whole genome is too large to fit on a single DNA chip, which is currently capable of holding about 400 000 oligonucleotides (Fedrigo *et al.*, 2004). Nonetheless, this approach may be useful for re-sequencing experiments or for sequencing individual genes with mutation hot spots.

To conclude, advances in DNA sequencing and analysis technologies, through automation and integration with other related technologies, will continue to revolutionize biological research.

References

Sanger F, Nicklen S, Coulson AR. DNA sequencing with chain-terminator inhibitors. *Proc Natl Acad Sci USA* 1977; **74**: 5463–5467.

Maxam AM, Gilbert W. A new method for sequencing DNA. *Proc Natl Acad Sci USA* 1977; **74**: 560–564.

Carey M, Small ST. *Transcriptional regulation in eukaryotes: concepts, strategies, and techniques.* 2000: Cold Spring Harbor Laboratory Press, New York.

Carothers AM, Urlaub G, Mucha J *et al*. Point mutation analysis in a mammalian gene: rapid generation of total RNA, PCR amplification of cDNA and Taq sequencing by a novel method. *BioTechniques* 1989; **7**: 494–499.

Venter JC *et al*. The sequence of the human genome. *Science* 2001; **291**: 1303–1351.

Lander ES *et al*. Initial sequencing and analysis of the human genome. *Nature* 2001; **409**: 860–921.

Wu KJ, Steding A, Becker CH. Matrix-assisted laser desorption time-of-flight mass spectrometry of oligonucleotides using 3-hydroxypicolinic acid as an ultraviolet-sensitive matrix. *Rapid Commun Mass Spectrom* 1993; **7**(2): 142–146.

Fedrigo O, Naylor G. A gene-specific DNA sequencing chip for exploring molecular evolutionary change. *Nucleic Acids Res* 2004 **32**(3): 1208–1213.

Further reading

Sambrook J, Russell DW. *Molecular Cloning: A Laboratory Manual.* 3rd edn. 2001: Cold Spring Harbor Laboratory Press: New York.

Tabor S, Richardson CC. DNA sequence analysis with a modified bacteriophage T7 DNA polymerase. *Proc Natl Acad Sci USA* 1987; **84**: 4767–4771.

Smith LM, Sanders JZ, Kaiser RJ *et al*. Fluorescence detection in automated DNA sequence analysis. *Nature (Lond)* 1986; **321**: 674–679.

Prober JM, Trainor GI, Dam RJ *et al*. A system for rapid DNA sequencing with fluorescent chain-terminating dideoxynucleotides. *Science* 1987; **238**: 336–341.

Ansorge W, Sproat B, Stegemann J *et al*. Automated DNA sequencing: ultrasensitive detection of fluorescent bands during electrophoresis. *Nucleic Acids Res* 1987; **15**: 4593–4602.

Innis MA, Myambo KB, Gelfand DH, Brow MA. DNA sequencing with *Thermus aquaticus* DNA polymerase and direct sequencing of polymerase chain reaction–amplified DNA. *Proc Natl Acad Sci USA* 1988; **85**: 9436–9440.

Hunkapillar T, Kaiser RJ, Koop BF, Hood L. Large-scale and automated DNA sequencing determination. *Science* 1991; **254**: 59–67.

Adams MD, Fields C, Venter JC (eds). *Automated DNA Sequencing and Analysis.* 1994: Academic Press, London.

Howe CJ, Ward ES (eds). *Nucleic Acids Sequencing* 1992: IRL Press, Oxford.

Index

Index compiled by Christine Boylan